BETA-LACTAM ANTIBIOTICS FOR CLINICAL USE

CLINICAL PHARMACOLOGY

Series Editor

MURRAY WEINER

Division of Clinical Pharmacology and Toxicology
University of Cincinnati
College of Medicine
Cincinnati, Ohio

Volume 1 Nicotinic Acid: Nutrient-Cofactor-Drug, *by Murray Weiner and Jan van Eys*

Volume 2 Drugs in Central Nervous System Disorders, *edited by David C. Horwell*

Volume 3 Clinical Application of Interferons and Their Inducers, Second Edition, *edited by Dale A. Stringfellow*

Volume 4 Beta-Lactam Antibiotics for Clinical Use, *edited by Sherry F. Queener, J. Alan Webber, and Stephen W. Queener*

Volume 5 Receptor Binding in Drug Research, *edited by Robert A. O'Brien*

Volume 6 Drug Therapy in Hypertension, *edited by Jan I. M. Drayer, David T. Lowenthal, and Michael A. Weber*

BETA-LACTAM ANTIBIOTICS FOR CLINICAL USE

edited by

Sherry F. Queener
Indiana University School of Medicine
Indianapolis, Indiana

J. Alan Webber
Lilly Research Laboratories
Indianapolis, Indiana

Stephen W. Queener
Eli Lilly and Co.
Indianapolis, Indiana

Marcel Dekker, Inc. • New York and Basel

Library of Congress Cataloging in Publication Data

Beta-lactam antibiotics for clinical use.

(Clinical pharmacology ; v. 4)
Includes index.
1. Beta lactam antibiotics. I. Queener, Sherry F.
II. Webber, J. Alan, [date]. III. Queener, Stephen W.
IV. Series.
RM666.B46B48 1986 615'.329 86-8984
ISBN 0-8247-7386-1

MARCEL DEKKER, INC.
270 Madison Avenue, New York, New York 10016

Current printing (last digit):
10 9 8 7 6 5 4 3 2 1

PRINTED IN THE UNITED STATES OF AMERICA

Series Introduction

There is perhaps no better example of the accomplishments of human intelligence in the control of man's natural enemies than that of the development of antibacterial agents in general and the beta-lactams in particular. The initial observation that a product secreted by one organism (a fungus) attacked another (a bacterium) represents such a common phenomenon in nature that it is perhaps more surprising that it was not ignored altogether than that its potential utility was not immediately recognized. Fortunately a long line of the right questions were asked by the right people and a collection of immensely important and interrelated facts was generated. As a result there now exists a battery of highly effective, well-understood beta-lactams that is preventing or controlling thousands of miserable infections on a daily basis. Some of the major steps were accomplished by knowledgeable, freely associating specialists in less time than it now takes to prepare a National Institutes of Health research grant request and wait for it to be reviewed, evaluated, and funded.

In this volume, Sherry F. Queener, J. Alan Webber, and Stephen W. Queener have collected a remarkable spectrum of major contributions ranging from fundamental laboratory observations through brilliant solutions of production problems, and finally an understanding of mechanisms of action that makes possible rational effective clinical utility and the ongoing development of newer agents designed to address specific clinical problems.

I have no doubt that this volume will be very much appreciated. I consider it an important member of our evolving series of clinical pharmacology books.

Murray Weiner
Series Editor

Preface

Beta-Lactam Antibiotics for Clinical Use represents the effort of experts in widely divergent fields who have focused their talents upon the beta-lactam antibiotics in order to produce a full view of these fascinating compounds. Part 1 presents the current state of knowledge on such basic topics as mode of action of beta-lactam antibiotics, potential mechanisms of resistance, and clinically observed resistance to these agents. The biosynthesis of penicillin and cephalosporin is described by Dr. E. P. Abraham, a man whose continuous involvement in beta-lactam antibiotics began with the pioneering work of the Oxford Group. The history of beta-lactam antibiotics is briefly related in Chapter 1.

The second part of the book features the penam group of beta-lactams, the drugs commonly called penicillins. The manufacture of these drugs, their pharmacological properties, and applications to clinical medicine are described in three detailed and well-referenced chapters.

The third section of the book features cephalosporins, compounds sharing the ceph-3-em nucleus but differing widely in the substituents attached to that nucleus. The chapters in this section cover in detail the manufacture, pharmacology, and clinical applications of cephalosporins so that treatment parallels that in the section dealing with penicillins. The parallel organization should enable the reader to make comparisons more readily.

The last five chapters of the book describe special beta-lactam antibiotics that are not members of the penicillin or cephalosporin classes. Within each chapter in this part the authors have briefly summarized the history of the compounds, their origins, resistance patterns, manufacture, pharmacology, and clinical uses of the particular agents. The organizational motif in the multichapter treatment of penicillins and cephalosporins thus appears again within each chapter that deals with a new nonclassical beta-lactam.

Chemists, microbiologists, pharmacologists, and clinicians have all contributed to this volume, as an inspection of the list of contributors readily illustrates. We have drawn upon such a varied group because we wished to present as complete a picture as possible, rather than to present excessively specialized information. We have also avoided excessive specialization by restricting our coverage to beta-lactam compounds that are now used clinically or are shortly expected to be so used. In creating this sort of book, we have tried to be of service to teachers, managers in pharmaceutical houses, researchers, clinicians in infectious disease, and others who need a reference in this area. We hope that the volume would be useful as the first book such a person would seek out. For more detailed studies, each chapter is fully referenced from the current literature.

Sherry F. Queener
J. Alan Webber
Stephen W. Queener

Contributors

Sir Edward P. Abraham, D.Phil. Sir William Dunn School of Pathology, University of Oxford, Oxford, England

Richard F. Bergstrom, Ph.D. Lilly Laboratory for Clinical Research, Lilly Research Laboratories, Eli Lilly and Company, Indianapolis, Indiana

Jerome Birnbaum, Ph.D. Department of Microbiology and Agricultural Research, Merck Sharp & Dohme Research Laboratories, Rahway, New Jersey

Charles A. Bunnell, Ph.D. Technical Services, Tippecanoe Laboratories, Eli Lilly and Company, Lafayette, Indiana

Christopher M. Cimarusti, Ph.D.* Department of Organic Chemistry, The Squibb Institute for Medical Research, Princeton, New Jersey

George M. Eliopoulos, M.D. Infectious Diseases Section, New England Deaconess Hospital, Boston, Massachusetts

Sharon A. Henry, M.D. Medical Development, The Squibb Institute for Medical Research, Princeton, New Jersey

---

**Current affiliation*: Department of Chemical Development, Squibb Chemical Division, Princeton, New Jersey

Edward S. Inamine, Ph.D. Department of Fermentation Microbiology, Merck Sharp & Dohme Research Laboratories, Rahway, New Jersey

Bill G. Jackson, Ph.D. Process Research Division, Eli Lilly and Company, Indianapolis, Indiana

George A. Jacoby, M.D. Infectious Disease Unit, Massachusetts General Hospital, Boston, Massachusetts

Frederick M. Kahan Department of Exploratory Biological Research, Merck Institute for Therapeutic Research, Rahway, New Jersey

Robert B. Kammer, M.D. Clinical Investigation and Regulatory Affairs Division, Eli Lilly and Company, Indianapolis, Indiana

Richard B. Kohler, M.D. Division of Infectious Diseases, Department of Medicine, Indiana University School of Medicine, Indianapolis, Indiana

Helmut Kropp Department of Exploratory Biological Research, Merck Sharp & Dohme Research Laboratories, Rahway, New Jersey

David A. Lowe, Ph.D. Fermentation Development Laboratories, Bristol-Myers Company, Syracuse, New York

Wayne D. Luke, Ph.D. Antibiotic Technical Services, Tippecanoe Laboratories, Eli Lilly and Company, Lafayette, Indiana

James S. MacDonald, Ph.D. Department of Safety Assessment, Merck Sharp & Dohme Research Laboratories, West Point, Pennsylvania

Christopher M. Martin, M.D. Infectious Diseases, Merck Sharp & Dohme Research Laboratories, West Point, Pennsylvania

Antone A. Medeiros, M.D. Departments of Medicine and Laboratory Medicine, The Miriam Hospital and Brown University, Providence, Rhode Island

Charles H. Nightingale, Ph.D. Department of Pharmacy Services, Hartford Hospital, Hartford, Connecticut

Fred M. Perry, Jr., Ph.D. Technical Services, Eli Lilly and Company, Tippecanoe Laboratories, Lafayette, Indiana

Karen I. Plaisance, Pharm. D.* Department of Pharmacy Services, Hartford Hospital and School of Pharmacy, University of Connecticut, Hartford, Connecticut

John F. Quay, Ph.D. Department of Drug Disposition, Lilly Research Laboratories, Eli Lilly and Company, Indianapolis, Indiana

Sherry F. Queener, Ph.D. Department of Pharmacology and Toxicology, Indiana University School of Medicine, Indianapolis, Indiana

Richard Quintiliani, M.D. Division of Infectious Diseases, Department of Medicine, Hartford Hospital, Hartford, Connecticut

Christopher Reading, Ph.D. Biochemical Services Unit, Beecham Pharmaceuticals Research Division, Chemotherapeutic Research Centre, Betchworth, Surrey, England

José Ignacio Santos, M.D.† Departments of Pediatrics and Pathology, Boston University School of Medicine and Boston City Hospital, Boston, Massachusetts

Brian Slocombe, Ph.D. Bacteriological Services Unit, Beecham Pharmaceuticals Research Division, Chemotherapeutic Research Centre, Betchworth, Surrey, England

Edward O. Stapley, Ph.D. Department of Basic Microbiology, Merck Institute for Therapeutic Research, Rahway, New Jersey

Edward A. Swabb, M.D., Ph.D.‡ Department of Clinical Research, Anti-infectives/Anti-inflammatory, The Squibb Institute for Medical Research, Princeton, New Jersey

Richard B. Sykes, Ph.D. Infection and Inflammation Research Division, The Squibb Institute for Medical Research, Princeton, New Jersey

Donald J. Tipper, Ph.D. Department of Molecular Genetics and Microbiology, University of Massachusetts Medical School, Worcester, Massachusetts

---

**Current affiliation*: Clinical Pharmacy Department, School of Pharmacy, University of Maryland, Baltimore, Maryland

†*Current affiliation*: Departamento de Enfermedades Infecciosas y Parasitarias, Hospital Infantil de Mexico, Mexico City, Mexico

‡*Current affiliation*: Gastrointestinal Research, G. D. Searle, Chicago, Illinois

Lawrence Joseph Wheat, M.D. Infectious Diseases Division, Department of Medicine, Indiana University School of Medicine, Indianapolis, Indiana

Arthur C. White, M.D. Infectious Diseases Division, Department of Medicine, Indiana University School of Medicine, Indianapolis, Indiana

Hideo Yamada, M.D. Pharmacokinetics and Biopharmaceutics Division, Shionogi Research Laboratories, Shionogi and Company, Osaka, Japan

Mitsuru Yoshioka, Ph.D. Organic Chemistry Division, Shionogi Research Laboratories, Shionogi and Company, Osaka, Japan

Contents

Part 3 Cephalosporins

BETA-LACTAM ANTIBIOTICS FOR CLINICAL USE

PART 1

BETA-LACTAM ANTIBIOTICS: GENERAL CONSIDERATIONS

1

History and Origins of Beta-Lactam Antibiotics

SHERRY F. QUEENER
Indiana University School of Medicine, Indianapolis, Indiana

I. ORIGINS IN NATURE

Fleming discovered penicillin in a mold-contaminated bacterial Petri plate in the summer of 1928. Because of the subsequent importance of penicillin, the discovery of the drug stands sharply illuminated to our view, isolated from the events that preceded and surrounded it in real time. In fact the conceptual framework that made the discovery of penicillin possible developed gradually over the 50 years or so preceding Fleming's actual isolation of the penicillin-producing organism.

The possibility of one organism interfering with the growth of another was the subject of active investigation in the early days of microbiology. Pasteur and Joubert are often cited as examples of this early work, perhaps because in their 1877 paper they mention the therapeutic possibilities of such antagonism (1). Other workers contributed more to understanding the mechanisms that produced microbial antagonism. In 1885 Cornil and Babes reported experiments on microbial antagonism in vitro that suggested the phenomena could be traced to a chemical from one organism acting as an inhibitor to the other (2). The work of Cornil and Babes was firmly supported in 1887 by Garre, who demonstrated that a substance from *Bacillus fluorescens* diffused through solid media and inhibited *Staphylococcus pyrogenes* (3). In 1889 Vuillemin gave this phenomenon a name when he coined the term *antibiosis*, defining it much as we would today: life against life (4).

In this early literature we also find studies that foreshadowed the work that would yield beta-lactam antibiotics some 50 years later. A series of English workers reported on the ability of *Penicillium* to inhibit bacterial growth under various conditions (5). In 1871 Sanderson reported that bacteria failed to grow in a simple culture broth when the broth contained *Penicillium* (6). Joseph Lister reported the same phenomenon using urine as a culture broth (7). William Roberts (8) and John Tyndall (9) added their observations of similar phenomena by 1881.

Among this group of early workers on *Penicillium*, only two seem to have had the idea that an antibacterial substance might be involved: Lister and Roberts. Lister is reported anecdotally to have used *Penicillium* in 1884 as an adjunct in treating infected wounds (5).

By the end of the nineteenth century the concept was clear: Microbial antagonism could be caused by a specific substance released by one of the interacting organisms. The idea became reality when *Penicillium* was used as the source of the first antibiotic isolated from fermentation broths. In 1896 Gosio succeeded in crystallizing a phenolic substance (later named mycophenolic acid) from culture broth supporting growth of the mold (10,11). A solution of this substance had a powerful antiseptic action against *Bacillus anthracis.*

Some of the work on antagonism between molds and bacteria was outside the mainstream of microbiology and would never have become well known had penicillin not become so important. In 1897 a young French medical student, E. A. C. Duchesne, acting on the scientific advice of Gabriel Roux, described antagonism between *Escherichia coli* and *Penicillium glaucum.* Duchesne discovered that *E. coli* did not survive when transferred onto an actively growing culture of *Penicillium.* Duchesne extended his observation to include testing for antagonism in animals. He injected guinea pigs with *E. coli* and typhoid bacteria, withholding treatment from half the animals but injecting the others with the nutrient broth that had supported the growth of *Penicillium.* The control animals died but the treated animals survived (12,13). These remarkable studies bore no fruit; Duchesne left the laboratory for good after receiving his M.D. in 1897 and no one took up the study. The thesis in which Duchesne's results were published was not widely circulated and was only rediscovered after some 40 years later, when *Penicillium* had been independently developed as a source of clinically useful antibiotics. The identity of the active compound in Duchesne's cultures may never be known for certain.

In the years immediately preceding the actual discovery of penicillin, developments in physiology and medicine also established important principles that contributed to the discovery of penicillin. The early work of Alexander Fleming himself illustrates the development of research along two important lines: the role of host defenses (primarily leukocytes) in infections and bacterial cell lysis.

Working with infected wounds in World War I, Fleming and others were intrigued by the interplay between antiseptics and the leukocytes mobilized by the body to fight infection. Except for the treatment of syphilis, Paul Ehrlich's concept of selective toxicity had not been successfully applied to therapy at this time. Antiseptics that were powerful antibacterials were known but were so damaging to human tissues that they could not be given systemically. Fleming, whose work in this area continued for many years, devised a simple system to test the effect of antiseptics and other chemicals on isolated leukocytes. Fleming observed that all of the antiseptics then known were at some concentrations more damaging to leukocytes than to bacteria. He and others were well aware that an ideal antiseptic should destroy bacteria but not harm leukocytes or other human tissues (14).

Fleming was also the discoverer of lysozyme, an enzyme that dissolves bacterial cell walls, causing lysis of the bacteria (15). This new enzyme activity was discovered after Fleming placed nasal mucus on a plate containing growing bacteria and observed lysis where bacteria contacted the mucus. Further testing showed the lytic activity was present in saliva and other natural fluids. This discovery was of fundamental importance for several reasons, but in terms of advancing chemotherapy it suggested one mechanism by which organisms might attack and defeat bacterial pathogens.

II. DEVELOPMENT OF CLINICAL POTENTIAL

The uninterrupted history of beta-lactam antibiotics leading to modern uses of these compounds begins with that most famous of all laboratory contaminations in which Fleming observed that *Penicillium* lysed *Staphylococcus aureus* growing on an agar plate (16). The *Penicillium*, originally described as *Penicillium rubrum* by Fleming himself, was later classified as *Penicillium notatum* (17) and probably was accidentally carried into Fleming's laboratory from a mycologist's laboratory in the same building (18). To the man who discovered lysozyme, it was the bacterial lysis produced by growth of this organism that was intriguing. Fleming carefully subcultured and preserved the *Penicillium*, but he was less successful at isolating the lytic agent released by the organism into the culture broth. At Fleming's suggestion, S. Craddock and F. Ridley, who were studying with Fleming at this time, attempted to extract the active agent from aqueous media into ether, as well as other solvents. Although Craddock's notebooks suggest that the antibacterial activity was successfully extracted into ether, acetone, and alcohol, the procedure was tedious and conducted on a very small scale (18). In reporting the results, Fleming mentioned briefly that the compound was soluble in alcohol and insoluble in ether or chloroform (16). In the latter two statements he seems to be misreporting the data of Craddock and Ridley, although we must remember that the surviving records in the scientific notebooks covering that period are incomplete (18). Moreover, as we now know, the solubilities of the free acid and salt forms of penicillin are different.

Outside his area of expertise with these chemical studies, Fleming quickly became discouraged with the chemical purification and concentration of the antibacterial activity he named penicillin. He returned to using the crude culture broth in his work. He showed that *Staphylococci*, *Streptococcus pyrogenes*, and pneumococcus cultures were inhibited by penicillin broth even up to dilutions of 1:800. More strikingly, Fleming noted that penicillin was the first compound he had tested that was more harmful to bacteria than to leukocytes. Fleming also tested the toxicity of the broth on animal tissues, applying it directly to wounds and even into human eyes. The material was confirmed to be nonirritating and nontoxic (16). Although Fleming injected the broth into mice and rabbits to test for toxicity, he did not extend his experiment by testing the broth in infected animals. Fleming did suggest that penicillin might be useful as a dressing on infected wounds, but he published nothing further on this use of penicillin. Fleming continued to use penicillin as a laboratory tool in his bacteriological researches (16,19).

Recognizing that penicillin might be of interest if it could be isolated in quantity, Clutterbuck and colleagues began work using the *Penicillium* strain from Fleming (17). They showed that penicillin could be produced when the mold was grown on synthetic media rather than the nutrient broth used by Fleming. They also reported the extraction of penicillin from acidified culture broth into ether and the adsorption of the compound to charcoal. To their frustration, they also discovered that oxidants and many other factors, including bacterial contaminants, were capable of rapidly destroying the tiny amount of penicillin found in crude broths. These workers did not continue research on penicillin.

Although apparently discouraged from work on penicillin by the chemical problems he and others had encountered, Fleming continued to maintain the original *Penicillium* culture and sent it to several interested researchers in other laboratories, including some in the United States. R. D. Reid of the Pennsylvania State College, using the culture modification reported by Clutterbuck et al., attempted to modify production of penicillin and extract it from the penicillium broth. He found that the compound was destroyed by distillation, lost on dialysis, and either not formed or destroyed when the culture was exposed to ultraviolet light or oxygen gas (20). Another American investigator, S. Bornstein of Beth Israel Hospital in New York City, using Fleming's strain and his culture conditions to study the effects of penicillin on enterococci and other streptococci (21). Like Fleming before him, Bornstein employed penicillin as a laboratory tool, using susceptibility to penicillin as one criterion for differentiating the various streptococci. Bornstein's studies were submitted for publication August 1, 1939. About that same time in Oxford, England, H. W. Florey received the first $5000 of a proposed 5-year, $25,000 grant from the Rockefeller Foundation (22). The subject was penicillin.

The Oxford group has become legendary for the prodigious progress it made on penicillin in a very short time. When they began their work in 1939 the compound could not be produced in quantity and could not be assayed in any systematic way. By August of 1940 they reported successful use of penicillin to cure infections in animals (23); in 1941 they reported the first clinical use in humans (24). Along the way they solved many of the problems that had resisted the best efforts of everyone else who had ever worked on penicillin.

The Oxford group was successful because each of the extremely talented individuals in it brought special expertise that was dedicated to a common goal (22,25). H. W. Florey, Head of the Sir William Dunn School of Pathology, was a physiologist by training and had a strong interest in lytic compounds such as lysozyme, pyocyanase, and penicillin. He recruited Dr. Ernst Chain to develop biochemical research at the school. Chain suggested a systematic survey of antimicrobial substances produced by microorganisms as a subject for study. Later it was Chain who introduced freeze-drying, a major advance in processing penicillin. N. G. Heatley specialized in problems relating to the production of penicillin. He was responsible for devising the step of re-extracting penicillin into a neutral aqueous solution from an organic solvent and for devising the cylinder-plate method used for the microbiological assay of the material (22). A. D. Gardner and J. Orr-Ewing contributed bacteriological expertise. M. A. Jennings along with H. W. Florey contributed to the biological and pharmacological studies. A. G. Sanders was ultimately responsible for one of the large-scale production plants required to produce sufficient penicillin for the studies of the group. E. P. Abraham, a gifted biochemist, introduced the use of chromatography for the preparation of penicillin suitable for clinical use. The clinical trials were guided by H. W. Florey, C. M. Fletcher, and M. E. Florey (25).

The first trials were in patients suffering from infections caused by staphylococci or streptococci, organisms shown by Fleming and others to be susceptible to penicillin in vitro. Case 1 was an Oxford policeman severely ill with abcesses and osteomyelitis arising from a staphylococcal infection. Treatment was begun on February 12, 1941, and improvement was rapid. Therapy continued until all the available drug was used up—4.4 g in 5 days. Thereafter the patient relapsed and ultimately died. The next patient, a boy with osteomyelitis caused by hemolytic streptococcus, received newly isolated penicillin as well as some material recovered from the urine of the first case. The boy improved on receiving the drug but relapsed 3 weeks later, following surgery. These patients were treated in February 1941. Experience with these two cases caused H. W. Florey to realize for the first time the amount of penicillin that would be required for successful therapy of serious infections. The Oxford group suspended trials for 2 months while they accumulated more drug. The next patient, treated in early May, recovered uneventfully from a serious, necrotizing carbuncle. Case 4, a moribund 4-year-old with a staphylococcal infection spreading from the sinuses, responded dramatically to the drug but died suddenly of a stroke. Despite the tragic outcome, the researchers considered this case as a hopeful sign, for autopsy revealed the child had been largely cleared of the infection at the time of his death. From this point on the tide seemed to turn. A 14-year-old boy with staphylococcal septicemia and osteomyelitis required 17.2 g of a crude penicillin preparation but was cured. A 6-month-old infant was cured of a severe *Staph. aureus* urinary tract infection. Four patients were cured of severe eye infections by topical application of penicillin.

These early clinical trials were carried out with extremely crude penicillin preparations. The researchers had been deceived by the unparalleled potency of penicillin into believing that the material was much purer than it turned out to be. The Oxford group later reported that the first treatment in humans was done with penicillin ranging from 0.3 to 7% pure (see Ref. 25, p. 647). The contaminants were not altogether innocuous. The first two human beings ever to receive intravenous penicillin suffered fever and chills. The pyrogen was largely eliminated from the penicillin preparations used in the clinical trials, but occasional batches were still contaminated. Chills and pyrexia were reported in three of the five patients who received parenteral penicillin in these first trials.

III. EXPANDING THE AVAILABILITY OF PENICILLIN

Although the first clinical trials were promising, they were not unqualified successes. More patients with serious diseases needed to be treated before the drug would be established in medical practice; therefore much more penicillin would be required. Florey realized that the Oxford group had reached its reasonable limit in producing penicillin. If more was needed for clinical trials, it had to come from elsewhere. He turned again to the Rockefeller Foundation. With the encouragement of Dr. Weaver of that institution, Florey and Heatley arranged to go to America to seek aid in producing penicillin for further clinical trials (see Ref. 25, p. 649).

Arriving in the United States in late June, Florey and Heatley consulted acquaintances on the East Coast who referred them ultimately to Dr. C. Thom of the Bureau of Plant Industry at Beltsville, Maryland. Dr. Thom was the recognized world's authority on *Penicillium* taxonomy. He introduced Heatley and Florey to Dr. Wells at the U.S. Department of Agriculture in Washington, D.C., who sent the British workers to meet the one group of scientists most able to help them: the fermentation experts of the Northern Regional Research Laboratory (NRRL) of the U.S. Department of Agriculture in Peoria, Illinois. Created during the Great Depression, this laboratory was charged with the development of commercial uses for agricultural products or by-products.

On July 14, 1941, Dr. May, who was the director of the NRRL, and Dr. R. Coghill, director of the fermentation division, met with Florey and Heatley on the penicillin problem. By the end of the year A. J. Moyer of the NRRL, working with Heatley, had improved penicillin production over 10-fold by adding corn-steep liquor to the fermentation (26). This contribution was the first of three critical advances made during the next 4 years by NRRL scientists. The second involved developing techniques for the cultivation of *Penicillium* suspended in an aerated medium rather than the tedious and limiting surface culture used in 1941. The third contribution was the isolation of new strains of *Penicillium* that would produce high amounts of penicillin in submerged culture. This work was begun in 1942. Dr. Kenneth Raper of the NRRL examined several hundred strains of *Penicillium* isolated from various sources, including soil samples sent to Peoria from all over the world by Army Transport Command (27). The best strain obtained in this screen was isolated in July of 1943 from a moldy canteloupe bought in a Peoria market (26). This strain, identified as *Penicillium crysogenum* (NRRL 1951) was immediately used to select an improved variant (NRRL 1951.B25) that could give yields of 250 units/ml in the small tanks used for stirred fermentations in those days. In the spring of 1944 this culture was shared with industry, as well as with other laboratories working on penicillin. The strains used today in penicillin manufacture worldwide trace their lineage to this culture (26,28).

The early American effort on penicillin was not limited to the activities of the NRRL. After leaving Heatley in Peoria in 1941, Florey visited American scientists interested in penicillin, later making mention of the groups at the Mayo Clinic led by Dr. Herrell, Dr. Heilman, and Dr. Heilman (29) and at Columbia University (Dr. Dawson, Dr. Hobby, Dr. Meyer, and Dr. Chaffee) (30,31) as contributing much to the early acceptance in America of the clinical promise of penicillin (see Ref. 25, p. 650). Florey also stimulated interest in penicillin production at several pharmaceutical firms. Penicillin projects were begun about this time at E. R. Squibb & Sons, Charles Pfizer & Co., Lederle, and Merck & Co.

At America's entry into the war in December 1941, penicillin fell under the authority of the Committee on Medical Research of the Office of Scientific Research and Development. Dr. A. N. Richards, who headed this committee and was well acquainted with H. W. Florey, devoted large amounts of government money and extraordinary effort into getting penicillin produced in sufficient quantity for clinical trial and subsequent military use (32). The program was remarkably successful. At the time when Heatley and Florey had first come to America in 1941, British production of penicillin was in surface culture in small, flat porcelain containers. The broth contained 1-2 units/ml of penicillin. Treatment of a few seriously ill patients was sufficient to deplete the world's supply of the drug. By the end of 1942 about 122 million units of penicillin (roughly equivalent to 73 g of pure material) had been produced in the United States (see Ref. 25, p. 651). Since the doses used in those early trials were very low by modern standards (10,000-15,000 units every 3 hr), over 100 patients were able to receive therapy (see Ref. 25, p. 656).

The results of these trials and independently initiated trials in England and in the United States began to appear in late 1942 and continued into 1943 (33-40), a year in which penicillin production rose exponentially. By 1944 improved fermentation techniques and strains producing up to 250 units/ml combined to bring penicillin production in the United States alone to over 3000 lb. By 1946 British industry was producing enough penicillin to allow 370 million units a month to be exported; U.S. production was even higher (see Ref. 25, p. 671). Penicillin was at last available on the open market.

IV. CHEMICAL EXPANSION OF THE CLASS

Penicillium produces different penicillins, depending upon the strain, available nutrients, and culture conditions. This fact was brought to light when extensive strain development and media improvement work was carried out by the American scientists at the NRRL. Florey and co-workers in England grew the Oxford strain of *Penicillium*, which traced its lineage to Fleming's original isolate, on modified Czapek-Dox medium with glucose and yeast extract supplements (24). The American workers modified this minimal medium by adding corn-steep liquor to stimulate penicillin production; lactose was generally substituted for glucose (26). At the same time new *Penicillium* strains were being isolated and tested, with the ultimate goal of growing *Penicillium* commercially in submerged culture. This goal was achieved with the discovery that NRRL 832, a *P. notatum* strain originally from the laboratory of Biourge in Belgium, produced 40-50 units/ml of penicillin in submerged culture.

At this stage in early 1943 studies on the structure of penicillin, which had lagged far behind the biological studies, finally caught up. Crystalline penicillin was prepared at Squibb and the elemental analysis was firmly established (see Ref. 25, p. 770). The Oxford group quickly thereafter crystallized their penicillin and established that the elemental analysis of English penicillin differed from the American analysis. It was also clear at this time that hydrolysis of pure American penicillin yielded phenylacetic acid, a product never obtained by hydrolysis of English penicillin. The inevitable conclusion was that two different penicillins were being studied. The American penicillin (called penicillin G by the Americans and penicillin II by the British) was predominantly benzylpenicillin. The early clinical trials in England were done primarily with 2-pentenylpenicillin (penicillin F or I). Both forms of penicillin contained the unprecedented beta-lactam ring system, a structure that was not conclusively proven until 1945 (see Ref. 25, p. 669).

By 1949 six natural penicillins were known, differing from one another exclusively in the side chain. The natural side chains were 2-pentenyl, 3-pentenyl, p-hydroxybenzyl, benzyl, n-amyl, and n-heptyl groups (see Ref. 25, p. 786). Of these compounds, benzylpenicillin was the most potent and the only one exploited for medical use.

Chemists were eager to go beyond what nature had supplied, but they needed a controlled way to alter the side chain of the penicillin molecule. Guidance came from the fermentation work that had gone before. It was known by this time that one reason why the American fermentations yielded penicillin G rather than penicillin F was that corn-steep liquor provided a rich source of precursors for the side chain of penicillin G. Phenylacetic acid could be incorporated in high yield into penicillin G under appropriate culture conditions. This precursor could also redirect synthesis. For example, Wis. Q-176 produced 900 units/ml penicillin K (a mixture of n-amyl- and n-heptylpenicillin) on standard media but produced primarily penicillin G when phenylacetic acid was added to the medium (26).

This experience with natural penicillins suggested to the chemists that new penicillins might be formed if unusual compounds that could serve as precursors for the penicillin side chain were added to the fermentations. The early use of this technique, called precursing, is illustrated in a series of papers by Behrens and co-workers (41-44). By using phenoxyacetic acid for its derivatives as precursors, Behrens and his colleagues formed phenoxymethylpenicillin (penicillin V) in 1948 (43). However, since the compound was less potent than penicillin G, its potential usefulness was overlooked until Brandl and Margreiter showed that penicillin V was more stable in acid than penicillin G and therefore more likely to survive oral administration (45).

Precursing was ultimately not useful for making other penicillins for two reasons: First, many of the desirable side chain precursors were toxic to the *Penicillium* culture; second, many of the compounds were incorporated in very low yields into the penicillin molecule (43). The chemists needed to escape the limitations of the biological system altogether and devise a way to chemically control the addition of the side chain to the penicillin molecule.

The key to chemical modifications of penicillins was 6-aminopenicillanic acid (6-APA), the penicillin nucleus (41). Although apparently observed in the early 1950s in Japan, the substance was not immediately exploited (46). In 1956 Dr. J. C. Sheehan synthesized 6-APA and converted it to the naturally occurring penicillin V by an acylation reaction in which the side chain was added to the preformed nucleus (47). Among other things, this impressive work opened the possibility of forming novel penicillins by adding unusual side chains. When scientists at Beecham Laboratories in England learned how to obtain large amounts of inexpensive 6-APA from fermentations, this material became the logical precursor for a whole group of new compounds (48). The semisynthetic penicillins were the result.

The first semisynthetic penicillin to be introduced was phenethicillin (phenoxyethylpenicillin), which appeared in 1959 from Beecham Laboratories. This drug was not significantly different from penicillin V. The first semisynthetic penicillin with unique properties was methicillin, approved for clinical use in the United States in 1960. This drug was designed to resist hydrolysis by penicillinases, thereby adding an extremely valuable property to the penicillin family.

Semisynthetic penicillins have been developed continuously since 1959 (49); as of 1985, 18 of them are used in medical practice in the United States. The properties of these drugs are discussed in the penicillin section of this book (Part 2).

V. RETURN TO NATURE

In 1961 Abraham and Newton described a new beta-lactam, cephalosporin C, produced by a strain of *Cephalosporium acremonium* isolated in Sardinia from sewage (50). This compound quickly generated an entirely new family of beta-lactam antibiotics as chemists learned to form the nucleus 7-aminocephalosporanic acid (7-ACA) and subsequently reacylate it to form new semisynthetic cephalosporin antibiotics. The complex and elegant chemistry of these compounds is reviewed in Chapters 5 and 11.

The discovery of the cephalosporins showed that the beta-lactam family might be larger than originally expected. Returning to natural fermentation sources, scientists discovered several related compounds with important antibiotic activity. Carbapenems were obtained from *Streptomyces* (Chap. 14), cephamycins from actinomycetes (Chap. 13), and monobactams from *Pseudomonas*, *Gluconobacter*, and *Chromobacterium* (Chap. 16). Development of these exciting new classes of beta-lactams is just beginning, as is well documented in the last third of this volume.

Dr. J. C. Sheehan, who spent most of his scientific career working with the penicillin nucleus, called the beta-lactam structure an enchanted ring (51). That fascinating ring still enchants basic scientists today, and the practical benefits of that enchantment enrich all our lives.

REFERENCES

1. L. Pasteur and J. Joubert. Charbon et septicémie. *C. R. Acad. Sci. Paris*, *85*: 101–115 (1877).
2. C. V. Cornil and V. Babes. Concurrence vitale des bactéries; atténuation de

leurs propriétés dans de milieux nutritifs modifiés par d'autres bactéries: Tentative de thérapeutique bactériologique. *J. Conaiss. Med. Prat. Pharmacol.* 7:321–323 (1885).

3. C. Garre. Uber Antagonisten unter den Bacterien. *Corresp. Bl. Schweiz. Aerzte, 17*:384–392 (1887).
4. P. Vuillemin. Antibiose et symbiose. *C.R. Assoc. Fr. Av. Sci., 2*:525–543 (1889).
5. S. Selwyn. Pioneer work on the "penicillin phenomenon," 1870–1876. *J. Antimicrob. Chemother., 5*:249–255 (1979).
6. J. B. Sanderson. Appendix No. 5. Further report of researches concerning the intimate pathology of contagion. The origin and distribution of microzymes (bacteria) in water, and the circumstances which determine their existence in the tissue and liquids of the living body. 13th Report of the Medical Officer of the Privy Council [John Simon], with Appendix 1870. Her Majesty's Stationery Office, London, 1871, pp. 56–66.
7. J. A. Lister. A contribution to the germ theory of putrefaction and other fermentative changes, and to the natural history of torulae and bacteria. *Trans. R. Soc. Edinburgh, 27*:313 (1875).
8. W. Roberts. Studies of biogenesis. *Philos. Trans. R. Soc. London, 164*:457–477 (1874).
9. J. Tyndall. *Essays on the Floating Matter of the Air in Relation to Putrefaction and Infection,* Appleton, New York, 1881.
10. B. Gosio. Ricerche batteriologiche e chimiche sulle alterazioni del mais; contributo all'etiologia della pellagra. *Riv. Ig. Sanit. Pubbl. Roma, 7*:825, 869, 961 (1896).
11. C. L. Alsberg and O. F. Black. U.S. Dept. of Agriculture Bureau of Plant Industry, Bulletin No. 270, 1913.
12. E. A. C. Duchesne. Contribution à l'étude de la concurrence vitale chez les micro-organisms. Antagonisme entre les moisissures et les microbes. Thesis, University of Lyons. Quoted in H. W. Florey, Historical introduction, in *Antibiotics,* Vol. 1 (H. W. Florey, E. Chain, N. G. Heatley, M. A. Jennings, A. G. Sanders, E. P. Abraham, and M. E. Florey, eds.), Oxford University Press, London, 1949, p. 58.
13. R. A. Kyle and M. A. Shampo. Ernest August Clement Duchesne. *J. Am. Med. Assoc., 240*:847 (1978).
14. A. Fleming. History and development of penicillin, in *Penicillin. Its Practical Application.* Blakiston, Philadelphia, 1946, pp. 1–23.
15. A. Fleming. Lysozyme; president's address. *Proc. R. Soc. Med., 26*:71–84 (1932).
16. A. Fleming. On the antibacterial action of cultures of a penicillium, with special reference to their use in the isolation of *B. influenzae. Br. J. Exp. Pathol., 10*:226–236 (1929).
17. P. W. Clutterbuck, R. Lovell, and H. Raistrick. Studies in the biochemistry of micro-organisms. XXVI. The formation from glucose by members of the *Penicillium chrysogenum* species of a pigment, an alkali soluble protein and penicillin—The antibacterial substance of Fleming. *Biochem. J., 26*:1907–1918 (1932).

18. R. Hare. New light on the history of penicillin. *Med. Hist., 26*:1–24 (1982).
19. A. Fleming. On specific antibacterial properties of penicillin and potassium tellwrite; incorporating method of demonstrating some bacterial antagonisms. *J. Pathol. Bacteriol., 35*:831–842 (1932).
20. R. D. Reid. Some properties of a bacterial-inhibitory substance produced by a mold. *J. Bacteriol., 29*:215–221 (1935).
21. S. Bornstein. Action of penicillin on enterococci and other streptococci. *J. Bacteriol., 39*:383–387 (1940).
22. E. Chain. The early years of the penicillin discovery. *Trends Pharmacol. Sci., 1*:6–11 (1979).
23. E. Chain, H. W. Florey, A. D. Gardner, N. G. Heatley, M. A. Jennings, J Orr-Ewing, and A. G. Sanders. Penicillin as a chemotherapeutic agent. *Lancet, 2*:226–228 (1940).
24. E. P. Abraham, C. M. Fletcher, H. W. Florey, A. D. Gardner, N. G. Heatley, and M. A. Jennings. Further observations on penicillin. *Lancet, 2*:177 (1941).
25. E. P. Abraham, E. Chain, H. W. Florey, M. E. Florey, N. G. Heatley, M. A. Jennings, and A. G. Sanders. Historical introduction, in *Antibiotics,* Vol. 2 (H. W. Florey, E. Chain, N. G. Heatley, M. A. Jennings, A. G. Sanders, E. P. Abraham, and M. E. Florey, eds.), Oxford University Press, London, 1949, p. 639.
26. K. B. Raper. The penicillin saga remembered. *ASM News, 44*:645–653 (1978).
27. K. B. Raper, D. F. Alexander, and R. D. Coghill. Penicillin II. Natural variation and penicillin production in *Penicillium notatum* and allied species. *J. Bacteriol., 48*:639–659 (1944).
28. S. Queener and R. Swartz. Penicillins: Biosynthetic and semisynthetic, in *Economic Microbiology,* Vol. 3. (A. H. Rose, ed.), Academic, New York, 1979, pp. 35–122.
29. D. H. Heilman and W. E. Herrell. Comparative bacteriostatic activity of penicillin and gramicidin. *J. Bacteriol., 43*:12 (1942).
30. M. H. Dawson, G. L. Hobby, R. Meyer, and E. Chaffee. Penicillin as a chemotherapeutic agent. *J. Clin. Invest., 20*:434 (1941).
31. G. L. Hobby, K. Meyer,M. H. Dawson, and E. Chaffee. The antibacterial action of penicillin. *J. Bacteriol., 43*:11 (1942).
32. A. N. Richards. Penicillin. Statement released by the Committee on Medical Research. *J. Am. Med. Assoc., 122*:235–236 (1943).
33. G. L. Hobby, K. Meyer, and E. Chaffee. Chemotherapeutic activity of penicillin. *Proc. Soc. Exp. Biol. Med., 50*:285–288 (1942).
34. W. E. Herrell, D. H. Heilman, and H. L. Williams. The clinical use of penicillin. *Proc. Staff Meet. Mayo Clin., 17*:609–616 (1942).
35. W. E. Herrell. Further observations on the clinical use of penicillin. *Proc. Staff Meet. Mayo Clin., 18*:65–76 (1943).
36. H. W. Florey and M. E. Florey. General and local administration of penicillin. *Lancet, 1*:387–397 (1943).

37. C. H. Rammelkamp and C. S. Keefer. The absorption, excretion, and distribution of penicillin. *J. Clin. Invest., 22*:425–437 (1943).
38. C. H. Rammelkamp and C. S. Keefer. Penicillin: Its antibacterial effect in whole blood and serum for the hemolytic *Streptococcus* and *Staphylococcus aureus. J. Clin. Invest., 22*:649–657 (1943).
39. C. S. Keefer, F. G. Blake, E. R. Marshall, Jr., J. S. Lockwood, and W. B. Wood, Jr. Penicillin in the treatment of infections. A report of 500 cases. Statement by the Committee on Chemotherapeutic and Other Agents, Division of Medical Sciences, National Research Council. *J. Am. Med. Assoc., 122*:1217–1224 (1943).
40. A. Fleming. Streptococcal meningitis treated with penicillin; measurement of bacteriostatic power of blood and cerebrospinal fluid. *Lancet, 2*:434–438 (1943).
41. O. K. Behrens, J. Corse, R. G. Jones, M. J. Mann, Q. F. Soper, F. R. Van Abeele, and M. C. Chiang. Biosynthesis of penicillins. 1. Biological precursors for benzylpenicillin (penicillin G). *J. Biol. Chem., 175*:751–764 (1948).
42. O. K. Behrens, J. Corse, R. G. Jones, E. C. Kleiderer, Q. F. Soper, F. R. Van Abeele, L. M. Larson, J. C. Sylvester, W. J. Haines, and H. E. Carter. Biosynthesis of penicillins. II. Utilization of deuterophenylacetyl-N^{15}-DL-valine in penicillin biosynthesis. *J. Biol. Chem., 175*:765–769 (1948).
43. O. K. Behrens, J. Corse, D. E. Huff, R. G. Jones, Q. F. Soper, and C. W. Whitehead. Biosynthesis of penicillins. III. Preparation and evaluation of precursors for new penicillins. *J. Biol. Chem., 175*:771–792 (1948).
44. O. K. Behrens, J. Corse, J. P. Edwards, L. Garrison, R. G. Jones, Q. F. Soper, F. R. Van Abeele, and C. W. Whitehead. Biosynthesis of penicillin. IV. New crystalline biosynthetic penicillin. *J. Biol. Chem., 175*:793–809 (1948).
45. E. Brandl and H. Margreiter. Ein saurestabiles biosynthetisches Penicillin. *Oesterr. Chem. Ztg., 55*:11 (1954).
46. E. P. Abraham. Introduction, in *Chemistry and Biology of Beta-Lactam Antibiotics,* Vol. 1 (R. B. Morin and M. Gorman, eds.), Academic, New York, 1982, pp. xxi–xxxviii.
47. J. C. Sheehan and K. R. Henery-Logan. A general synthesis of the penicillins. *J. Am. Chem. Soc., 81*:5838–5839 (1959).
48. F. R. Batchelor, F. P. Doyle, J. H. C. Nayler, and G. N. Rolinson. Synthesis of penicillin: 6-Amino penicillinac acid in penicillin fermentations. *Nature, 183*:257–258 (1959).
49. G. N. Rolinson. 6-APA and the development of the beta-lactam antibiotics. *J. Antimicrob. Chemother., 5*:7–14 (1979).
50. E. P. Abraham and G. G. F. Newton. The structure of cephalosporin C. *Biochem. J., 79*:377–393 (1961).
51. J. C. Sheehan. *The Enchanted Ring,* MIT Press, Cambridge, Mass., 1982.

2

Mode of Action of Beta-Lactam Antibiotics

DONALD J. TIPPER
University of Massachusetts Medical School, Worcester, Massachusetts

I. INTRODUCTION

It is, by now, well established that beta-lactam antibiotics affect sensitive bacteria by inhibiting late stages in the biosynthesis of their cell wall peptidoglycan. Because this polymer is responsible for maintaining the shape and integrity of the cell walls of which it forms a part, interference in its synthesis is potentially lethal. Although considerable variation in peptidoglycan structure is found among pathogenic bacteria, sequence analysis of their peptides (see Refs. 1 and 2 and below) demonstrates that the basic mechanism of crosslink formation by transpeptidation, the specific target of beta-lactam antibiotics, is ubiquitous. Thus almost all pathogenic bacteria are potentially susceptible, and since peptidoglycan and its crosslinking mechanism are found only in bacteria, the selective toxicity of these antibiotics can be exceedingly high. Their use in a given patient is usually limited only by allergic reactions. The efficacy of a given beta-lactam antibiotic against a bacterial infection is primarily dependent on the intrinsic susceptibilities of transpeptidase targets located in the cytoplasmic membrane of the particular bacterial strain. Growth rate and local osmolarity may modify the lethal consequences of interaction of the drug with the target. Access to this target by permeation of the bacterial cell wall, access to the site of infection, and various pharmacological factors related to uptake, secretion, sequestration, and stability of the drug also influence efficacy. In most instances the most significant determinants of efficacy are the ability to permeate the bacterial cell wall and susceptibility to bacterial beta-lactamases, primary determinants of the effective drug concentration at the site of action.

In spite of these generalizations, the bewildering variety of beta-lactam antibiotics currently in clinical use or under evaluation attests to the fact that the design of these selective inhibitors has still not been perfected. This continuing effort is necessary because of the intrinsic variation in bacterial susceptibility and because of the humbling capacity of bacteria to render the latest modified beta-lactam antibiotics ineffective by acquiring resistance by mutation or (more commonly) by acquisition of beta-lactamase-producing R-factor plasmids. Knowledge of the enemy is always half the battle, but in the case of beta-lactam antibiotics, knowledge has always lagged behind use. The consequence has been a series of setbacks, starting with the very early selection of penicillin-resistant beta-lactamase-producing *Staphylococcus aureus* strains. The fairly recent selection of beta-lactamase-producing *Hemophilus influenzae* and gonococcus strains, the realization of the potential of certain bacterial species (principally gram positive) for intrinsic or acquired tolerance to killing by penicillins (3), and documentation of the role of beta-lactamases in nonhydrolytic mechanisms of resistance of opportunistic gram-negative bacterial pathogens to the newest beta-lactam antibiotics (4) are only the latest chapters in the history of this struggle.

The desire to understand the primary mode of action of beta-lactam antibiotics has been the major impetus behind investigation of the complexities of bacterial cell wall peptidoglycan structure and synthesis. Over the past 10 years it has become clear that multiple transpeptidases and related enzymes are involved in this process; that their roles in the normal cycle of cell growth, morphogenesis, and division are complex and carefully orchestrated; and that the physiological consequences of interfering with different components of this process are equally complex and not completely understood. These targets are identified biochemically as penicillin-binding proteins (PBPs) (5,6), the cytoplasmic membrane components which form stable, acylated derivatives with labeled benzylpenicillin ("penicillin") or other beta-lactam antibiotics.

The objective of this review is to summarize current understanding of peptidoglycan biosynthesis, with emphasis on the roles of specific PBPs, and to describe what is known about the mechanism and physiological consequences of their inhibition. This information should clarify the effects of different beta-lactam antibiotics on specific pathogens and the potential use of such information in predicting the consequences of the use of mixtures of beta-lactam antibiotics. The design of new beta-lactam variants remains an empirical exercise in medicinal chemistry. Incisive analysis of the interactions of beta-lactam antibiotics with crucial PBP targets, beta-lactamases and gram-negative porin cell wall permeation components (7), should gradually convert this art into an exact science.

II. STRUCTURE OF BACTERIAL CELL WALL PEPTIDOGLYCAN

The glycan component of peptidoglycan is an alternating polymer of N-acetylglucosamine (GlcNAc) and N-acetylmuramic acid (MurNAc) with chitinlike properties (2). MurNAc, the 3-O-D-lactyl derivative of GlcNAc, is the hallmark of eubacterial (9) cell wall peptidoglycan (Fig. 1). MurNAc provides the carboxyl group to which the peptide components of peptidoglycan are attached. The peptide, in turn, contains the dibasic amino acids that act as the branch points for crosslink formation between different peptides and their associated glycan strands. The peptidoglycan therefore forms a two- or three-dimensional array (Fig. 2), the "murein sacculus" (8), which surrounds the entire bacterial cell and whose integrity is responsible for the mechanical strength and shape-maintaining abilities of the cell wall.

The evolution of peptidoglycan with this general pattern as the major protective component of bacterial cell walls is an extremely ancient event, occurring several billion years ago following the divergence of the precursors of contemporary archaebacteria, eubacteria, and eukaryotic cells (9). The eubacteria, consisting of prokaryotes containing this type of MurNAc-based peptidoglycan, comprise all known human bacterial pathogens and normal flora, with the exception of the mycoplasmas. These wall-less prokaryotes are apparently also derived from eubacteria by a more recent loss of the capacity to produce cell wall peptidoglycan (9). They alone among known human bacterial pathogens clearly lack intrinsic susceptibility to beta-lactam antibiotics. The obligate intracellular pathogens are protected by their location.

Bacterial cell wall peptidoglycan has therefore successfully met and adapted to the challenges of our terrestrial environment for countless generations. The most extreme structural variants are found in gram-positive bacteria, especially in the type B peptidoglycans (see below) of certain corynebacteria and other ancient genera. The single pattern found in all gram-negative bacteria examined suggests that this group represents a relatively late and highly successful step in bacterial evolution (1). The peptidoglycan of these bacteria has an A1γ structure (see below) of minimal complexity and quantity, sufficient for survival when accompanied by the unique external permeability barrier provided by the gram-negative outer membrane. Peptidoglycan may effectively be a monolayer in these organisms, as schematically represented in Figure 2. It is a thicker, multilayered structure in gram-positive cell walls. The gram-negative outer membrane, by controlling the environment of the periplasm (which lies between the outer and cytoplasmic membranes, and in which the peptidoglycan layer lies) provides the gram-negative bacterium with unique control over the immediate environment of its cytoplasmic membrane. In particular, the periplasm provides a compartment for secreted enzymes and proteins which modify or trap ligands passing through the porin-defined diffusion channels of the outer membrane (7), giving control over import, export, and modification of such ligands, including, of course, hydrolysis and binding of beta-lactam antibiotics.

Peptidoglycans are classified according to their peptide structure (1,2), major examples of which are shown in Figure 3. The general form is (A)-D-Glu-(B)-D-

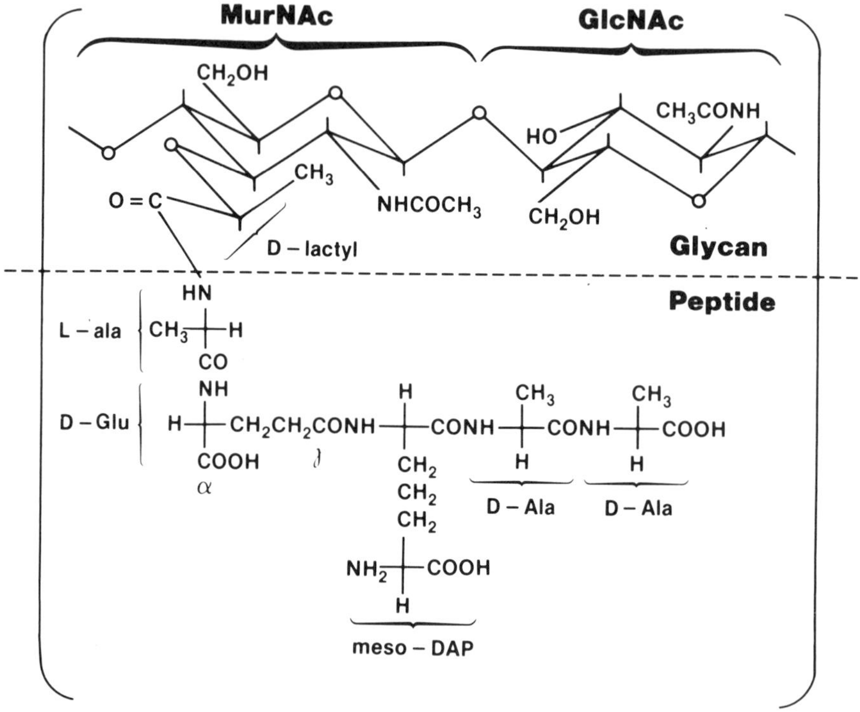

Figure 1 Structure of peptidoglycan: the repeating subunit of the nascent, crosslinked peptidoglycan of the type A1γ peptidoglycan of *Escherichia coli.* The repeating disaccharide of the β-1,4-linked glycan is shown in the flat-ribbon conformation of chitin, in which it is probably fixed by hydrogen bonds (not shown; see Fig. 6) (2). N-Acetylmuramic acid (MurNAc) is the 3-O-D-lactyl derivative of GlcNAc. The alternation of MurNAc and GlcNAc is assured by biosynthesis of this disaccharide-peptide subunit prior to polymerization (see Fig. 4). The pentapeptide L-Ala-γD-Glu-mDAP-D-Ala-D-Ala is attached to each MurNAc residue of the repeating subunit. mDAP is meso-diaminopimelic acid. It is linked at its L center to the γ-COOH of D-glutamate and to D-alanyl-D-alanine. In the convention used, an α-peptide linkage is shown as a horizontal line. Linkages from or to non-α-COOH or NH_2 groups are represented by vertical lines. Subsequent transpeptidation will link the penultimate D-alanine residue to the amino group at the D center of mDAP (see Fig. 4).

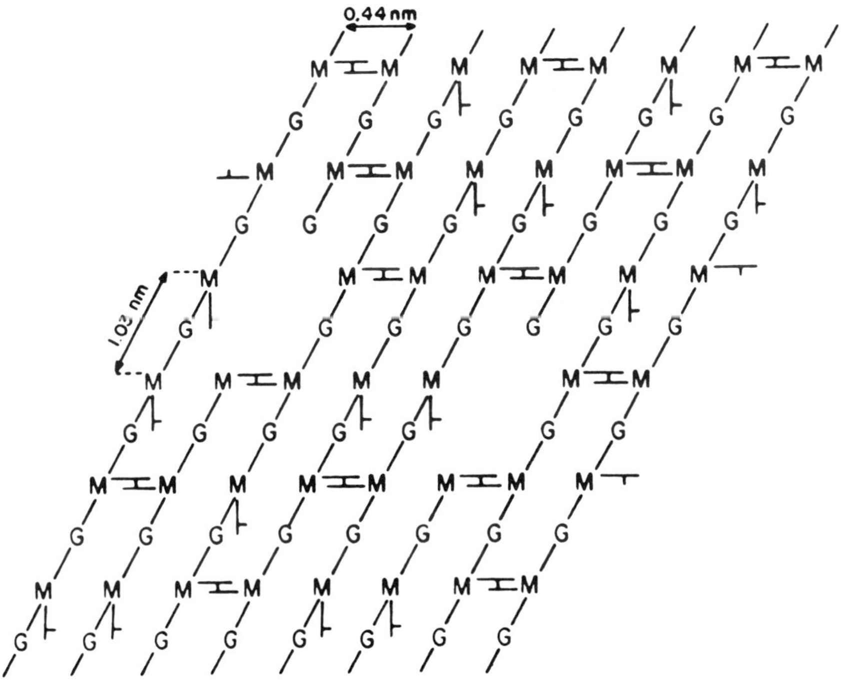

Figure 2 Schematic presentation of a portion of a two-dimensional array of peptidoglycan subunits in the cell wall of *E. coli.* In these walls, the glycan chains average 50 disaccharide units in length and the peptides consist almost entirely of uncrosslinked monomers (vertical lines) or crosslinked dimers (horizontal "H girders"). Dimers comprise about two-thirds of the peptide units, giving an average degree of crosslinking of 33%. [Redrawn from D. J. Tipper and A. Wright, in *The Bacteria*, Vol. 7 (J. R. Sokatch and L. N. Ornston, eds.), New York, 1979, p. 313, with permission of Academic Press.]

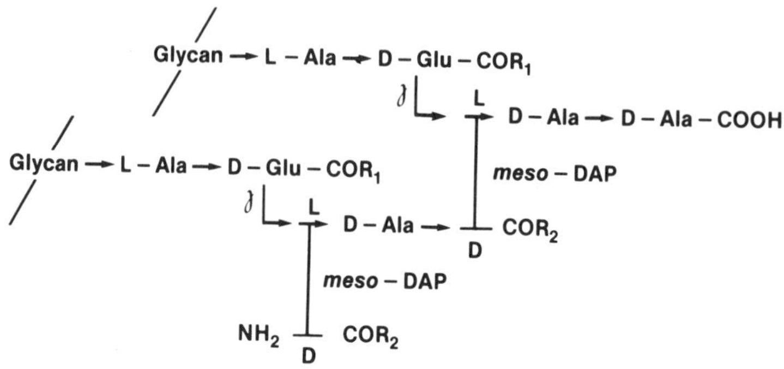

E. coli

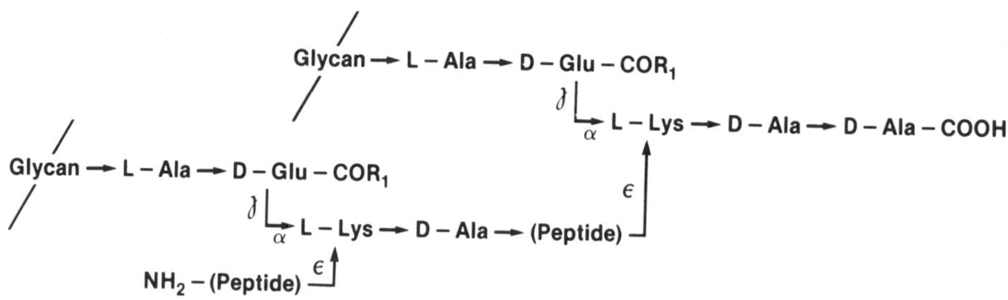

S. aureus

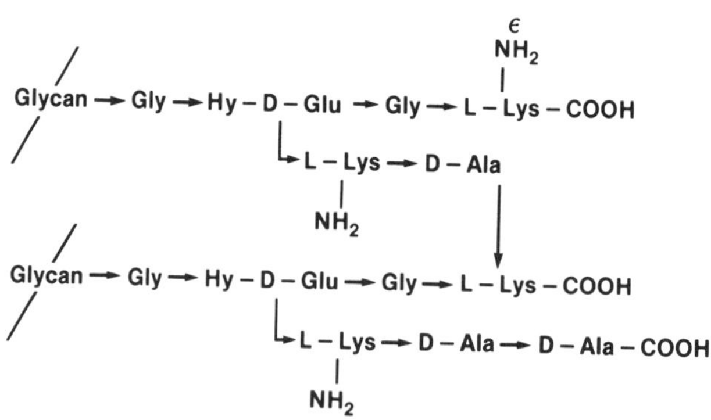

M. lacticum

Ala-D-Ala, where A is linked to MurNAc and is usually L-alanine and B is usually a dibasic amino acid. Type A1 structures lack additional crosslink peptide residues. Crosslinks are formed directly between the ω-amino group of B and the penultimate D-alanine residue, as shown for the type A1γ structure (Fig. 3, top) found in all gram-negative bacteria and some gram-positive bacteria. The A1γ subunit is shown in nascent, uncrosslinked form in Figure 1. In this structure B is meso-diaminopimelic acid (m-DAP). In bacteria L-lysine is derived from m-DAP by decarboxylation at its D center. Amidation of free COOH groups in peptidoglycan is species specific; examples include the type A1γ structures of *Escherichia coli* and *Bacillus subtilis* (Fig. 3, top). In both species C-terminal peptide subunits do not retain both of the D-alanine residues found in the nascent subunit (Figs. 1 and 3): One or both are removed by sequential D,D- and L,D-carboxypeptidase action.

In type A2, A3, and A4 structures additional amino acid residues form crosslinks between B (dibasic) and the penultimate D-alanine residue (Fig. 3, center).

Figure 3 Representatives of peptidoglycan types (1). All types are derived from a basal pentapeptide with the sequence (A)-D-Glu-(B)-D-Ala-D-Ala, where A is usually L-alanine, B is usually a dibasic amino acid, and D-Glu is linked to B via its γ-COOH group.

In type A1γ (*E. coli*), the third amino acid is mDAP, which is directly crosslinked to the D-alanine in position 4 (see Fig. 1). Peptide C termini have one or both D-alanine residues removed by sequential D,D-, and L,D-carboxypeptidase action (not shown). In *E. coli*, R_1=R_2=OH. In *B. subtilis* (gram positive) R_1=OH and R_2=NH_2 in the vegetative cell wall, while R_1=R_2=OH in the spore cortical peptidoglycan. Other variations in amidation occur in other bacterial species.

In type A2 (e.g., *S. aureus*), the third amino acid is dibasic and is most commonly L-lysine, as shown, and is crosslinked to D-alanine in position 4 via an intervening peptide. In *S. aureus* this peptide is predominantly pentaglycine, though some L-serine residues also are found.

In type B peptidoglycans the third amino acid is not involved in crosslinkage and it not always dibasic, though it is in the example shown (*M. lacticum*). Instead, a cross-bridge peptide incorporating a dibasic amino acid (here also L-lysine) is attached to the α-COOH of D-glutamate at position 2, and this cross-bridge dibasic amino acid acts as the acceptor for crosslink formation to the D-alanine in position 4. D-Glu is oxidized to β-hydroxy-D-glutamate in this particular peptidoglycan, an unusual modification. [Redrawn from D. J. Tipper and A. Wright, in *The Bacteria*, Vol. 7 (J. R. Sokatch and L. N. Ornston, eds.), 1979, pp. 324–326, with permission of Academic Press.]

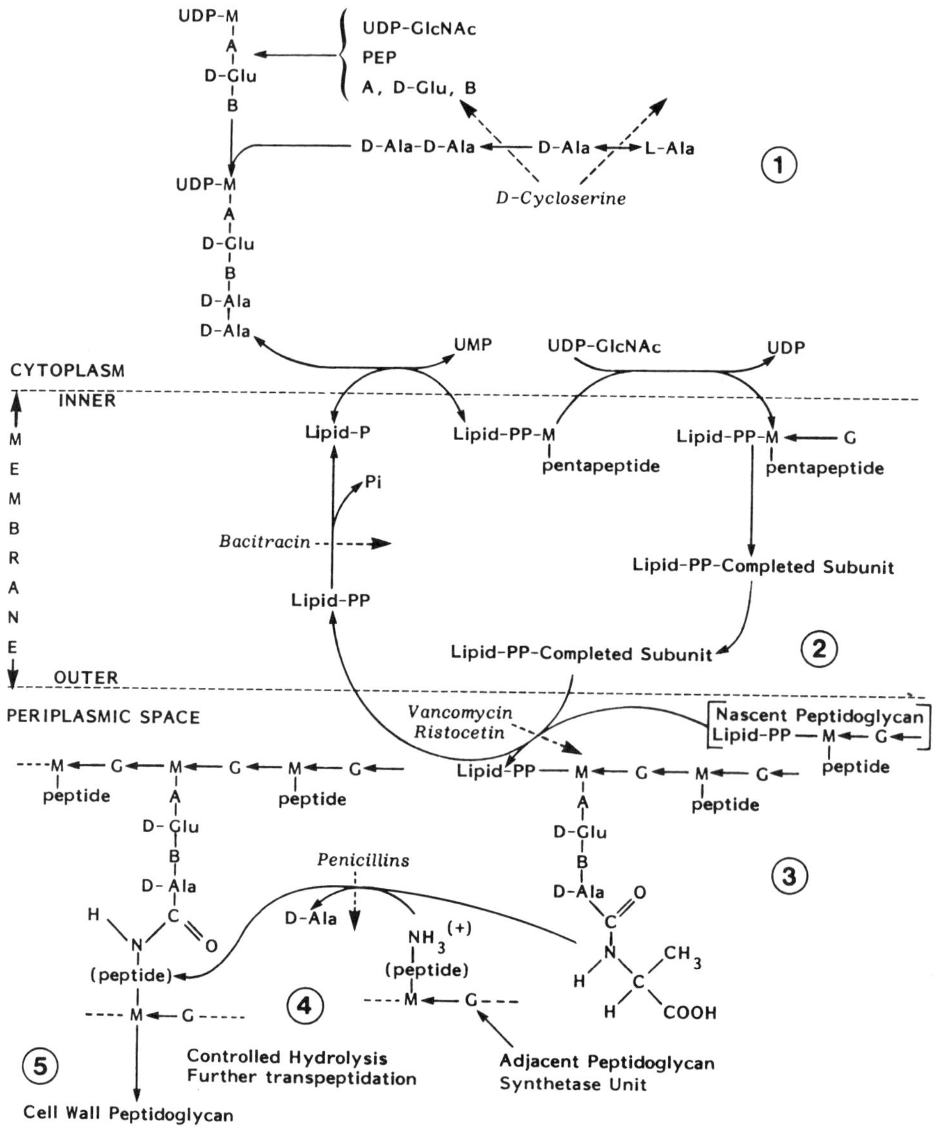

Figure 4 Biosynthesis of peptidoglycan. Peptidoglycans of all of the types found in eubacteria, including the three types shown in Figure 3, are synthesized according to this general scheme.

The first stage (top) involves cytoplasmic enzymes, substrates, and products, and results in synthesis of UDP-MurNAc-pentapeptide [(A)-D-Glu-(B)-D-Ala-D-

In *S. aureus*, this peptide is usually pentaglycine. Many variants are known among gram-positive bacteria (10). In type B peptidoglycans the cross-bridge peptide extends from the α-COOH of D-glutamate to the penultimate D-alanine residue and must contain a dibasic amino acid. In the example shown (Fig. 3, bottom), *Microbacterium lacticum*, this bridge is glycyl-L-lysine. D-Glutamate residues and D-alanyl-D-alanine COOH termini are universally present at least in the nascent subunits of all eubacterial peptidoglycans. The γ linkage of D-glutamate presumably defines an essential conformational component of the peptide. The D-Ala-D-Ala terminus provides the substrate for beta-lactam antibiotic-sensitive enzymes which produce and control crosslinkage of the peptidoglycan.

III. BIOSYNTHESIS OF PEPTIDOGLYCAN

Before bacterial cell wall structures had been analyzed in any detail, it was observed that the action of penicillin on sensitive bacteria leads to cell wall rupture and lysis, unless cells are protected by a medium of high osmolarity, in which case osmotically sensitive spheroplasts are formed (11). Park's observation (12) that *S. aureus* cells exposed to penicillin accumulate a nucleotide-peptide, later

---

Ala]. The fourth and fifth amino acids are invariably added as the presynthesized dipeptide D-alanyl-D-alanine.

The second stage (center) involves both cytoplasmic and membrane-bound substrates. The enzymes and products are bound to the inner surface of the cytoplasmic membrane. The first step in this "lipid cycle" is transfer of phospho-MurNAc-pentapeptide to lipid-P. Lipid-P is undecaprenyl phosphate, the carrier lipid for bacterial exocellular polysaccharide biosynthesis. Addition of GlcNAc completes the disaccharide. The peptide subunit is completed by species-specific modifications: addition of cross-bridge amino acids, amidation of D-Glu or mDAP, oxidation of D-Glu to Hy-D-Glu (Fig. 3), and others not shown. The completed subunit then translocates to the exterior surface of the membrane for polymerization, releasing lipid-pyrophosphate (lipid-PP). This is converted back to lipid-P acceptor by the bacitracin-sensitive membrane-bound pyrophosphatase, completing the cycle.

The third and fourth stages, initiated by polymerization, include crosslink formation by transpeptidation and D,D-carboxypeptidase action, both resulting in loss of the terminal D-alanine residue. The enzymes are located on the outer surface of the cytoplasmic membrane. Other cell wall polymers are covalently attached to nascent peptidoglycan at this stage (not shown). In stage 5 controlled hydrolysis and delayed transpeptidation of peptidoglycan modify the maturing structure to allow cell expansion, morphogenesis, and separation.

shown to be a precursor of the peptidoglycan, was a major breakthrough in both structural and biosynthetic studies of bacterial cell wall peptidoglycan, to which Strominger and his colleagues have made major contributions (13). Further details can be found in a recent review (10).

The biosynthetic process has three major stages (Fig. 4). In the first stage soluble cytoplasmic enzymes synthesize UDP-MurNAc-pentapeptide, the Park nucleotide (12) which accumulates in *S. aureus* treated with penicillin. UDP-MurNAc is synthesized from UDP-GlcNAc by addition of phosphoenolpyruvate (PEP) and reduction. UDP-MurNAc acts as the acceptor for sequential addition of (A), D-Glu, and (B) (Fig. 4). This UDP-MurNAc-tripeptide is then the substrate for addition of presynthesized D-alanyl-D-alanine, forming the pentapeptide. Incorporation of this dipeptide provides the common donor substrate for transpeptidation. D-Cycloserine and a variety of related alanine analog antibiotics inhibit alanine racemase, D-Ala-D-Ala synthetase, or the dipeptide ligase (14).

The second stage of synthesis is initiated by transfer of phospho-MurNAc-pentapeptide to undecaprenyl phosphate (Fig. 4). The membrane-bound MurNAc-pentapeptide, anchored by pyrophosphate linkage to this carrier lipid, is then modified on the inner surface of the cytoplasmic membrane to form a complete nascent peptidoglycan subunit (e.g., Fig. 1). This modification includes addition of GlcNAc from UDP-GlcNAc, addition of cross-bridge amino acids (if any), amidation of free carboxyl groups on D-Glu or mDAP, and other minor modifications (10). This stage terminates with translocation of the completed subunit, activated for polymerization by the pyrophosphate linkage, to the exterior of the cytoplasmic membrane.

The third stage of synthesis is initiated by polymerization of peptidoglycan by transglycosylation (Fig. 4). Newly inserted subunits retain their lipid-PP and act as acceptors. The donor is probably a nascent polymeric glycan retaining lipid-PP, though characterization of this polymerization intermediate is incomplete. Lipid-PP released from the acceptor recycles through the membrane and is hydrolyzed to the lipid-P acceptor for phospho-MurNAc-pentapeptide by the bacitracin-sensitive pyrophosphatase (15). Vancomycin and related antibiotics inhibit the transglycosylase by binding to the D-alanyl-D-alanine peptide termini of its substrates (16).

The third stage of synthesis continues with transpeptidation, illustrated in general form in Figure 4 (reaction 4). This reaction binds soluble uncrosslinked, nascent peptidoglycan to the pre-existing, crosslinked, insoluble cell wall peptidoglycan matrix (Fig. 2). Modification by D,D-carboxypeptidase action may be an alternative at this stage, resulting in removal of the terminal D-alanine residue without transpeptidation.

The reactions of D,D-carboxypeptidases and transpeptidases are functionally analogous, as illustrated in Figure 5. Both activities, in various ratios, are found

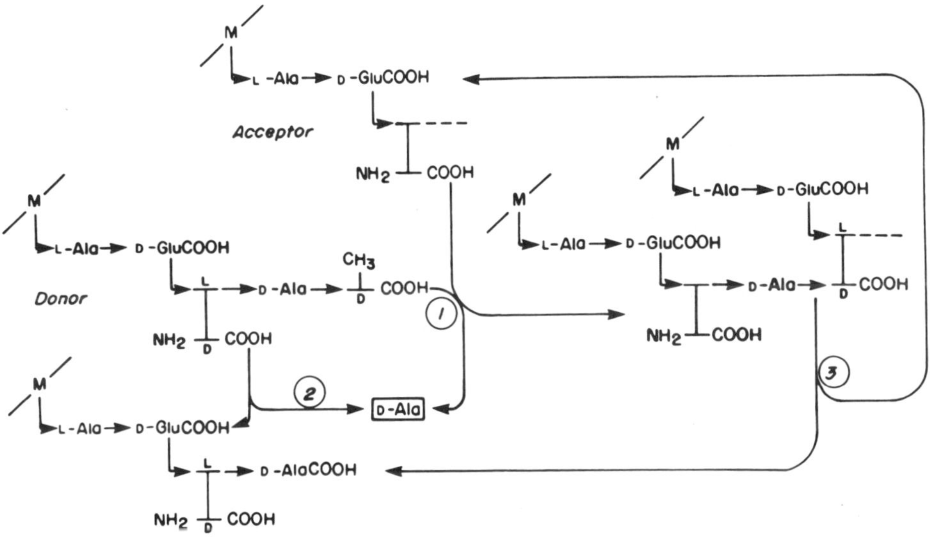

Figure 5 Relationship between transpeptidase, D,D-carboxypeptidase, and D,D-endopeptidase functions of PBPs. The substrate shown is the Alγ peptidoglycan of *E. coli* cell walls. A PBP that is primarily a transpeptidase (e.g., PBP 1A or 1B), binds a nascent peptidoglycan subunit to its donor site, producing acyl-D-Ala-ENZ (Fig. 7), with release of the terminal D-alanine residue. Binding of a suitable peptidoglycan subunit in the acceptor site leads to transpeptidation (reaction 1). Binding of water to the acceptor site (e.g., of PBP 5 or 6) leads to D,D-carboxypeptidase action (reaction 2). Binding of previously crosslinked peptidoglycan (e.g., to PBP4; reaction 3) leads, by a reversal of reaction 1, to release of an amino terminal peptide fragment and acyl-D-Ala-ENZ formation. Hydrolysis of the latter by water (reaction 2) completes the D,D-endopeptidase hydrolysis of the crosslink. It could also act as a transpeptidation donor (Fig. 7), potentially resulting in a reorientation of crosslinks. [Redrawn from D. J. Tipper and A. Wright, in *The Bacteria*, Vol. 7 (J. R. Sokatch and L. N. Ornston, eds.), 1979, p. 365, with permission of Academic Press.]

in the purified and semipurified PBPs of several bacteria (5,6,17,18). In *E. coli* and similar organisms a balance between carboxypeptidase and transpeptidase action may control the extent of crosslinkage. However, data from *E. coli* mutants lacking specific carboxypeptidase components suggest that such effects, if real, may be subtle (see below). In *Gaffkya homari* an unusual pattern of transpeptidation exists in which only the tetrapeptide products of D,D-carboxypeptidase action on nascent subunits can act as acceptors for transpeptidation, while the donor pentapeptides derive from the pre-existing cell wall peptidoglycan matrix (19). Clearly in this organism, and probably in others, the activities of D,D-

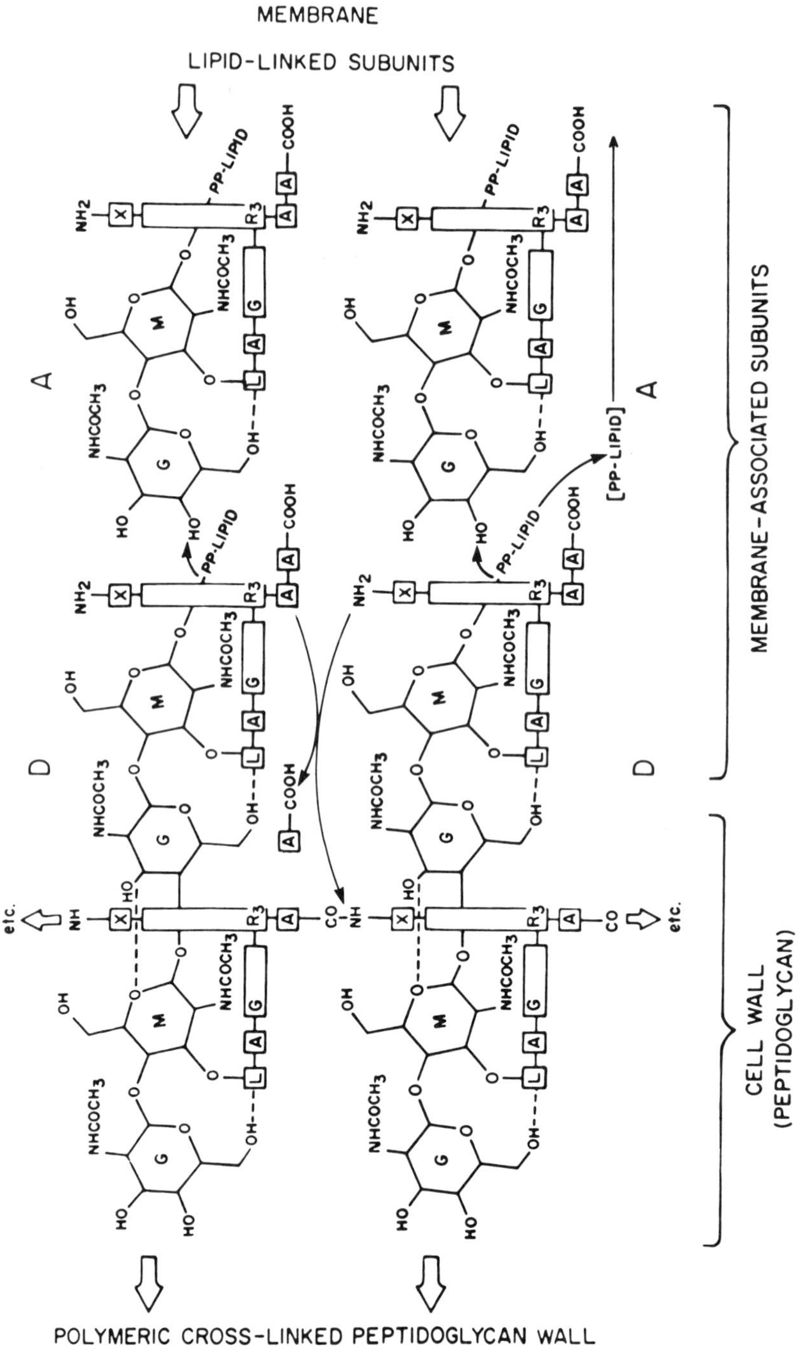
MEMBRANE
LIPID-LINKED SUBUNITS
MEMBRANE-ASSOCIATED SUBUNITS
CELL WALL (PEPTIDOGLYCAN)
POLYMERIC CROSS-LINKED PEPTIDOGLYCAN WALL
PP-LIPID
[PP-LIPID]
NHCOCH3
COOH
NH2
etc.

carboxypeptidases and transpeptidases are integrated and require careful control if peptidoglycan with a normal crosslinkage pattern is to be produced. Clusters of PBPs with the appropriate activities may act in concert at or near sites of peptidoglycan polymerization.

Recent analyses of in vitro function of the essential PBPs of *E. coli* (PBPs 1A, 1B, 2, and 3) have indicated that they have both transglycosylase and transpeptidase activity (20–24). It was previously hypothesized (10) that these two activities would need to be temporally and physically integrated to ensure an efficient and functional pattern of transpeptidation, as illustrated in Figure 6. A synthetic site is schematically shown as an "assembly line," possibly all within the active site of a single membrane-associated PBP, whose transpeptidase activity depends on the availability of acceptor due to association with other assembly sites in a close functional array. In vivo evidence apparently at variance with this model indicates the existence of a short, transient, soluble peptidoglycan intermediate (25) and of a slow increase in crosslinkage of presynthesized peptidoglycan with time (26,27). The evidence for the nascent, uncrosslinked polymer is not strong and is disputed (28). The slow postpolymerization increase in transpeptidation is better documented and is probably due to secondary transpeptidases (see below). The situation in any single bacterial cell may be too complex for simple generalization. Concomitant polymerization and crosslinkage, delayed

---

Figure 6 Polymerization and crosslinking by transpeptidation of a nascent type A2 Peptidoglycan. Two parallel peptidoglycan-polymerizing sites are shown. Each consists of an acceptor (A) and a donor (D) site. A nascent subunit in the A site consists of GlcNAc (G), MurNAc (M) with its 3-O-D-lactyl moiety (L), linked to a pentapeptide A-G-R_3-AA-COOH (A = alanine) substituted on the dibasic amino acid R_3 by a cross-bridge peptide X-NH_2. This is the acceptor for transglycosylation from nascent glycan in the D site. Both substrates are bound to membrane by lipid-PP. Transglycosylation releases one molecule of lipid-PP and results in translocation of the newly added subunit to the D site. Hydrogen bonds defining the chitinlike conformation of the glycan are shown as dotted lines.

Transpeptidation (or other PBP activity, such as D,D-carboxypeptidase action) is shown as a concomitant event, involving a PBP in close proximity to or as part of the transglycosylase, resulting in crosslink formation between the amino acceptor X–NH_2 and the penultimate D-alanine residue of the donor subunit, with release of a terminal D-alanine (A-COOH) residue. Both donor and acceptor substrates shown here are nascent peptidoglycan, possibly as occurs during cross-wall formation (see text). [Redrawn from D. J. Tipper and A. Wright, in *The Bacteria*, Vol. 7 (J. R. Sokatch and L. N. Ornston, eds.), 1979, p. 316, with permission of Academic Press.]

incorporation by transpeptidation of nascent, soluble polymer, and modification of "older" peptidoglycan by further transpeptidation, all catalyzed by different PBPs, may occur at different sites in the cell wall, with different functions and various rates dependent on the cycle of cell growth and division.

Modification of "mature," crosslinked, insoluble peptidoglycan involves hydrolysis (Fig. 4, reaction 5). Uncontrolled peptidoglycan hydrolysis leads to weakening and solubilization of the wall. The activities causing these effects are called autolysins. Walls of many gram-positive bacterial species undergo turnover through the agency of controlled autolysins. Others, such as some *E. coli* strains, undergo little or no turnover. All bacteria are presumed to require controlled peptidoglycan hydrolysis to allow cell expansion, morphogenesis, and separation. Some species, such as *E. coli*, contain PBPs which have in vitro D,D-endopeptidase activity (PBP4; see below) that are formally analogous in function to D,D-carboxypeptidases (Fig. 5) and which may, in vivo, be involved either in hydrolysis or in rearrangement of crosslinks by transpeptidation.

Some bacterial species have very little autolytic capacity, as determined by response to lethal concentrations of beta-lactam antibiotics or cell disruption. Others which do autolyse under these conditions can undergo marked reduction in autolytic capacity by mutation without loss of viability in the laboratory. The persistence of potentially suicidal levels of autolytic activity in the wild-type cells is therefore difficult to explain. It must be supposed that species survival in their natural habitat is enhanced by their presence.

IV. INHIBITION OF TRANSPEPTIDATION BY BETA-LACTAM ANTIBIOTICS

High-affinity binding sites for penicillin (now called PBPs) were identified early as membrane-bound components of unknown function (29) well before analysis of peptidoglycan structure led to the hypothesis that its integrity depended on crosslinks derived from transpeptidation. Analysis of the relationship between PBPs and transpeptidation is still continuing. The first direct evidence for the mode of action of beta-lactam antibiotics derived from an analysis of the effects of penicillin on *S. aureus* peptidoglycan structure. Biosynthetic studies in *S. aureus* subcellular preparations had failed to demonstrate penicillin sensitivity in any of the stages up to polymerization of soluble peptidoglycan by transglycosylation (Fig. 4), and since structural analyses indicated that the crosslinks in *S. aureus* involved the penultimate D-alanine residue, it was hypothesized that the terminal residue was lost in a transpeptidation reaction (30,31). Labeling (30) and chemical analytical (31) studies showed that penicillin caused a decrease in cell wall crosslinkage and an increase in peptidoglycan subunits retaining the acyl-D-Ala-D-Ala-COOH termini of their nucleotide pentapeptide precursor.

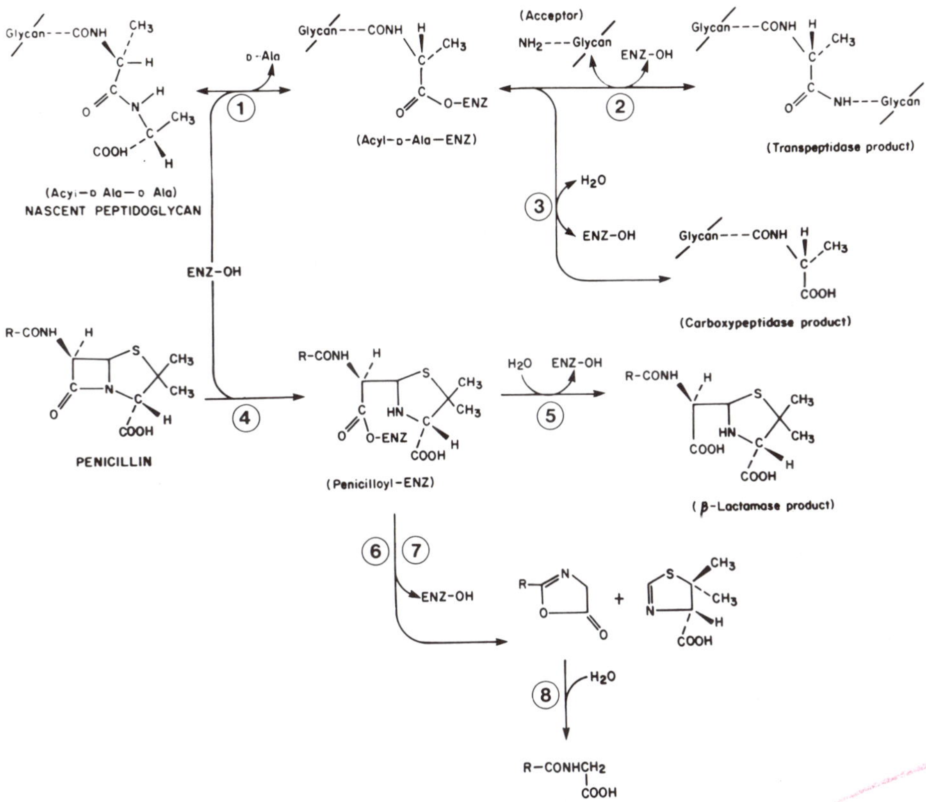

Figure 7 Transpeptidation and its inhibition by beta-lactam antibiotics. A nascent polymerized peptidoglycan subunit (Fig. 1) binds to the transpeptidase PBP (ENZ-OH), leading to acylation of the active site serine residue (acyl-D-Ala-ENZ) and release of the terminal D-Ala residue (reaction 1). Binding of the N-terminal acceptor group of an adjacent peptidoglycan subunit (NH_2---glycan) results in peptide crosslink formation and release of PBP (ENZ-OH; reaction 2). If the PBP is a D,D-carboxypeptidase, water acts as the acceptor (reaction 3).

Beta-lactam antibiotics, such as the penicillin shown, act as donor substrate analogs, binding to and acylating the L-serine residue in the donor site of the PBP, producing penicilloyl-ENZ (reaction 4). This may be a very stable product, causing inhibition of PBP function. Rapid hydrolysis by water (reaction 5) will produce beta-lactamase action, regenerating active PBP (ENZ-OH). Other breakdown pathways may occur less efficiently, such as the fragmentation shown (reactions 6, 7, and 8), that also slowly regenerate active PBP. Other pathways for fragmentation of unstable acylated PBP derivatives may produce stable, permanently inactivated enzyme derivatives (not shown). [Redrawn from D. J. Tipper and A. Wright, in *The Bacteria*, Vol. 7 (J. R. Sokatch and L. N. Ornston, eds.), 1979, p. 361, with permission of Academic Press.]

It was further suggested (31) that the acyl-D-Ala-D-Ala substrate of the (then hypothetical) transpeptidase reacted with an acceptor in the active site to form an acyl-D-Ala-ENZ intermediate (Fig. 7), with release of D-alanine. Penicillin was believed to acylate this transpeptidase as a structural analog of its acyl-D-Ala-D-Ala substrate, forming a stable product (penicilloyl-ENZ; Fig. 7) and inhibiting transpeptidation. It was anticipated that this product corresponded to the previously described penicillin-binding sites. These predictions have been borne out by investigations of several penicillin-sensitive proteins. It was further hypothesized that beta-lactamases are "modified transpeptidases" (31), derived from a common ancestral gene, in which the same mechanism is employed, but in which hydrolysis of the penicilloyl-ENZ intermediate is very rapid. This hypothesis seems to hold true for the major classes of beta-lactamases.

Transpeptidation and its inhibition by penicillin was soon demonstrated in *E. coli* membrane preparations (32), studies that also led to the first observations of D,D-carboxypeptidase activity. This activity, clearly analogous to transpeptidation in mechanism (Fig. 5), was found to be exquisitely sensitive to penicillin, also consistent with the role of penicillin as an analog of the acyl-D-Ala-D-Ala carboxypeptidase substrate (31). The D,D-carboxypeptidase activity was later shown to reside in several low molecular weight *E. coli* PBPs. These and similar D,D-carboxypeptidases from gram-positive organisms have, because of their abundance, solubility, and ease of purification, been the principal models for in vitro analysis of PBP function and inhibition by beta-lactam antibiotics (18, 33).

V. DEFINITION AND COMPLEXITY OF PENICILLIN-BINDING PROTEINS

Early studies of the binding of $[^{35}S]$ penicillin to sensitive bacteria, summarized by Cooper (29), demonstrated the presence of a small number of high-affinity sites, whose saturation required penicillin concentrations correlating well with minimal inhibitory concentrations (MICs). Bound labeled antibiotic was stable to boiling 2% SDS or phenol, and was not removed by exposure to beta-lactamase or a large excess of unlabeled penicillin. Covalent attachment by penicilloyl ester formation was suggested. Proof of this covalent bond was found more than 20 years later.

Following the development of the acyl-enzyme intermediate hypothesis for the mode of action of transpeptidases, early attention focused on the penicilloyl derivatives of the readily solubilizable D,D-carboxypeptidases of *B. subtilis, Bacillus stearothermophilus, Streptomyces,* and *E. coli* (18,33). A penicilloyl derivative is formed which has the stability of an ester following denaturation by SDS, but which can be readily transferred to a suitable acceptor, such as hydroxylamine, if the enzyme remains in active conformation. Hydroxylamine may therefore be used to elute PBPs in active form from ampicillin affinity columns (33).

These studies demonstrated the presence of multiple PBPs in these organisms and identified two classes: abundant, relatively low molecular weight PBPs with D,D-carboxypeptidase activity, not absolutely required for growth, and larger species of unknown function corresponding to the probable lethal targets of penicillin action and presumed to be transpeptidases. Spratt and Pardee (34) developed a simple and rapid technique for the visualization of PBPs: isolation of cytoplasmic membrane preparations, incubation with [^{14}C] penicillin, denaturation with SDS, fractionation by SDS-PAGE, and autoradiography. To be identified in this manner, PBPs must form stable, covalent adducts with penicillin which remain intact in boiling 2% SDS. All evidence suggests that this class of PBPs includes all of the significant targets, and that no cytoplasmic, markedly unstable, or noncovalent PBPs need be implicated in the mode of action of beta-lactam antibiotics.

Affinity of PBPs for other beta-lactam antibiotics has usually been inferred from data on competition with labeled penicillin. Use of other labeled beta-lactam antibiotics, for example, ampicillin, mecillinam (an amidinopenicillin), cefoxitin (a cephamycin), moxalactam (an oxacephem), and furazlocillin, has detected no additional binding proteins which fail to bind penicillin. Penicillin seems to be least selective in its ability to interact with PBPs, but many beta-lactam antibiotics bind preferentially to only one or two PBPs. Thus the naming of these beta-lactam antibiotic targets as "penicillin"-binding proteins remains valid. Use of a ^{125}I-labeled Bolton-Hunter derivative of ampicillin allowed detection of a minor *E. coli* PBP (PBP1C) not seen with agents of lower specific radioactivity (35). This component is of unknown significance and is not discussed in this review.

The use of high specific activity [^{3}H] penicillin (e.g., see Ref. 36) allows in vivo study of the competition of different beta-lactam antibiotics for individual PBPs, providing the most meaningful data on sites of action. Correlations between binding inhibition caused by an unlabeled beta-lactam antibiotic and the concentration dependence of its physiological effects allow identification of the PBPs which are "lethal targets" for this antibiotic, that is, those whose inactivation is responsible for lethality. The best studied PBPs are those of *E. coli*, whose structures and functions are summarized below.

VI. *ESCHERICHIA COLI* PBPs

Escherichia coli contains seven PBPs, not including PBP1C (see Ref. 5 and Table 1). The role each plays in peptidoglycan synthesis and cell morphogenesis is gradually becoming clarified through three types of investigations: studies of the physiological effects of beta-lactam antibiotics that bind preferentially to single

Table 1 Properties of *E. coli* PBPs[a]

PBP	Molecular weight	Molecules per cell	Gene name(s)	Map position	Selective inhibitors	Consequences of inactivation	Functions
1A	92,000	200	*pon A mrc A*	73.5		Rapid cell lysis if both inactivated	Transglycosylases and "primary" transpeptidases; essential for cylindrical cell wall synthesis
1Bs	∿90,000	250	*pon B mrc B*	3.3	Cephaloridine, cefsulodin		
2	66,000	20	*pbp A mrd A*	14.4	Mecillinam, clavulanic acid	Spherical, nongrowing cells	Transpeptidase required
					N-Formimidoyl thienamycin		Initiation of cylindrical wall growth at sites of septation
3	60,000	50	*pbpB ftsI*	1.8	Cephalexin, cefuroxime, aztreonam, furazlocillin	Filamentous, nonseptate cells	A transglycosylase/transpeptidase required for septum cross-wall synthesis
4	49,000	110	*dacB*	68		Delayed transpeptidation absent	A secondary transpeptidase, D,D-carboxypeptidase, or D,D-endopeptidase acting maturing peptidoglycan
5	42,000	1,800	*dacA*	13.7		None obvious	A D,D-carboxypeptidase
6	40,000	600	*dacC*			None obvious	A D,D-carboxypeptidase

[a]The molecular weights given are for the mature forms of the enzymes. As demonstrated for PBPs 1B, 3, and 5, each probably has a leader peptide in its gene which is removed during secretion to the exterior of the cytoplasmic membrane. PBPlc, detected only with an iodinated derivative of ampicillin (35), is not listed, since little is known about its properties. Beta-lactam antibiotics which interact with strong preference with individual "essential" PBPs (PBPs 1B, 2, and 3) are listed. Most react strongly with PBP1A, but since this is not lethal if active PBP1Bs remain, this is not usually significant. The *dacC* mutant (46) has not been mapped.

species (Table 1), studies of mutants in the genes for these PBPs that confer resistance to these selective antibiotics and/or which mimic the physiological effects of their interaction (Table 1), and studies of the in vivo effects of overproduction of these PBPs or in vitro activities of the purified PBPs themselves (Table 1). Although some redundancy in function is apparent, these investigations indicate that, in *E. coli* and related rod-shaped gram-negative bacteria, different transpeptidases are involved in cylindrical cell wall extension, in septum cross-wall formation, and in the initiation of cylindrical wall growth at sites of septation. This dispersion of function probably exists to various degrees in all eubacteria, since all eubacteria investigated have multiple PBPs, ranging in number from 3 to 8 (as distinct bands on SDS gels) (6). This specialization presumably provides a mechanism for control of wall architecture during the cell division cycle. Since PBP components may have markedly different relative affinities for different beta-lactam antibiotics, such antibiotics at their minimal inhibitory concentrations (MICs) may primarily affect different cell-cycle-dependent aspects of peptidoglycan synthesis, with different morphological and physiological consequences. Thus cephaloridine at its MIC causes lysis of *E. coli* without cell elongation, but cephalexin and ampicillin cause primarily filament formation owing to inhibition of septation. Ampicillin, at higher concentrations, causes lysis. Mecillinam, on the other hand, leads to the formation of lysis-resistant spherical cells at its MIC, or even at several-fold higher concentrations.

These effects are correlated with PBP affinities (Table 1): cephaloridine at its MIC and ampicillin at high concentrations saturate PBPs 1A and 1Bs. Cephalexin and ampicillin at their MICs saturate PBP3. Mecillinam reacts primarily with PBP2 at all concentrations. Other beta-lactam antibiotics with similar differential PBP affinities cause similar physiological effects, though mixed effects are common owing to low levels of discrimination between different PBPs. Since all of the antibiotics listed in Table 1 are bactericidal, inhibition of either PBP1A plus 1Bs, PBP2, or PBP3 is lethal, even if the other PBPs remain active. Thus *E. coli* has at least three "lethal targets" for beta-lactam antibiotics. Simultaneous attack on these targets by nonselective antibiotics or by mixtures of PBP-selective antibiotics might be expected to enhance lethality.

In *E. coli*, as in most other bacteria studied (6), the high and low molecular weight PBPs form two distinct groups. The high molecular weight group (PBPs 1A, 1Bs, 2, and 3) comprises the lethal targets and has relatively high affinities for both penicillins and cephalosporins; PBPs 1A, 1Bs, and 3 appear to be "primary" transpeptidases involved in concerted peptidoglycan polymerization and crosslinking reactions (see below). The low molecular weight group has low affinity for cephalosporins and includes enzymes acting primarily as D,D-carboxypeptidases, endopeptidases, or secondary transpeptidases (Fig. 5), all acting to modify presynthesized peptidoglycans. Their functions appear to be dispensable for growth in the laboratory.

A. PBPs 1A and 1Bs

The highest molecular weight *E. coli* PBPs were originally identified as a single species called PBP1; however, the use of SDS gels with higher resolving power showed this to comprise two distinct species: a minor PBP1A component and a major PBP1B component that itself gives rise to at least three bands on such gels (PBP1Bs). However, PBP1Bs arises from a single gene, since mutations in this gene (*ponB* or *mrcB*; see Table 1) cause concomitant loss of all PBP1B species, and all return on reversion (37,38). Mutation in a separate gene, *ponA* or *mrcA* (Table 1) causes loss of PBP1A (38). Mutation in a locus *iap*, involved in the proteolytic processing of alkaline phosphatase, results in formation of a single PBP1B component (quoted in Ref. 6). Thus PBP1Bs are probably derived by the processing of a single protein, the *ponB* gene product.

PBP1A and PBP1Bs appear to function interchangeably in cylindrical cell wall synthesis. Both *ponA*⁻ and *ponB*⁻ mutants are viable, but a cell carrying a temperature-sensitive (ts) *ponA* mutations and a *ponB*⁻ mutation lyses at 42°C (38). PBP1A has a much higher affinity for beta-lactam antibiotics than PBP1Bs, being saturated well below the MIC of most cephalosporins. Apparently inhibition of PBP1A function is not lethal and, as might be expected, *ponA*⁻ mutants have little alteration in phenotype. In contrast, *ponB*⁻ mutants are hypersensitive to many beta-lactam antibiotics (38). Thus in wild-type cells cephalothin saturates PBP1A well below its MIC, PBP3 at its MIC, but PBP1Bs (and also causing rapid lysis) only at higher concentrations. In a *ponB*⁻ mutant cephalothin has a reduced MIC and causes lysis at this concentration, owing to inhibition of PBP1A activity. Apparently inhibition of the bulk of both PBPs 1A and 1Bs function is necessary to cause lysis of growing *E. coli* cells. The combined enzyme activity of these PBPs appears to be present in excess in normal cells. Inactivation apparently leads to suicidal levels of autolysin activation (see below).

Both PBPs 1A and 1Bs catalyze a partially coupled transglycosylation and transpeptidation reaction using undecaprenyl-PP-disaccharide-pentapeptide (Fig. 3) as substrate (20–22). The peptidoglycan synthesized by PBP1A was hypercrosslinked (39), suggesting that PBP1A is not identical to PBP1Bs in activity and may serve an unknown specialized function in normal cells, a function apparently not essential for growth in the laboratory in the presence of functional PBP1Bs.

B. PBP3

Many penicillins and cephalosporins, such as ampicillin and cephalothin, have a higher affinity for PBP3 than for PBP1Bs and their MIC is correlated with the concentrations necessary for PBP3 saturation. When PBP3 is inactivated by these antibiotics, the consequence, as for growth of a ts PBP3 mutant at nonpermissive temperature (40), is the formation of filamentous, nonseptate cells with bulges at the normal sites of cell division. Heat-resistant revertants of the ts PBP3 mutant regain normal PBP3, confirming that this gene product is responsible for the ts growth phenotype (5,40). Apparently PBP3 is essential for septum cross-wall synthesis (Table 1). It has been suggested (41) that, while the acceptor for cylindrical wall synthesis is pre-existing peptidoglycan, the one for cross-wall synthesis is a second chain of nascent peptidoglycan, as shown in Figure 5. Whatever the mechanisms of transpeptidation involved in elongation and septation, their transpeptidases are apparently not interchangeable.

C. PBP2

Only amidinopenicillins and derivatives of thienamycin and clavulanic acid bind preferentially to PBP2 (Table 1), causing the formation of osmotically stable, nonviable spherical cells that lyse only after several hours (42). Mutants in *pbpA* (*mrd A*), the gene for PBP2, cause related morphological effects: mecillinam-resistant round cells with no detectable PBP2 activity (38) or cells exhibiting this phenotype only at high temperature (43). This is the least abundant PBP in normal cells (Table 1) and has been the most difficult *E. coli* PBP to study. It probably has transpeptidase activity, since cells carrying multiple copies of cloned *pbpA* and overproducing PBP2 have mecillinam-sensitive in vitro transpeptidation activity (24). Transglycosylation by PBP2 has yet to be assessed. As suggested (44), PBP2 activity apparently controls the production of new zones of cylindrical cell wall growth at sites of septal cross-wall synthesis.

D. PBPs 4, 5, and 6

Escherichia coli mutants lacking all detectable PBP 4, 5, or 6 activity (38,45, 46) (*dacB*$^-$, *dacA*$^-$, or dacC$^-$, respectively; see Table 1) are viable, as is the *dacA*$^-$, *dacC*$^-$ double mutant lacking both PBP4 and PBP5 activity (38). It is possible that these PBPs can function interchangeably, that the residual activity of each of these PBPs in these mutants is sufficient for viability, or that these activities are truly dispensable. PBP4 has D,D-endopeptidase activity in vitro (Table 1) and may function as a secondary transpeptidase in vivo, responsible for the slow increase in crosslinkage of newly synthesized *E. coli* peptidoglycan (47). This activity is absent in *E. coli dacB*$^-$ mutants. Such a role has been clearly demonstrated for the nonessential *S. aureus* PBP4, where mutational loss or selective inactivation by cefoxitin causes a marked decrease in average cell wall crosslinking (48).

PBPs 5 and 6 appear to act as D,D-carboxypeptidases in vivo as well as in vitro. Overproduction of PBP5 causes spherical cell production (49) and PBP5 activity is increased on initiation of septation (50), suggesting that D,D-carboxypeptidase action may play an important role in septal cross-wall synthesis. The transpeptides formed in nascent peptidoglycan by the activity of PBP5 or PBP6 may be preferentially utilized as acceptors for transpeptidation in cross-wall synthesis (50).

In conclusion, in *E. coli*, PBP3 and at least part of the PBP5 and PBP6 activities are involved in septum formation. PBP2 controls the initiation of cylindrical wall synthesis, a process catalyzed by PBPs 1A and 1Bs, and PBP4 is involved in modification of the crosslinkage of recently polymerized peptidoglycan. Because the high molecular weight species play indispensible roles in the cell-cycle-coupled process of cell wall biosynthesis, inactivation of any one of them is potentially lethal. Death is only accompanied by rapid lysis following inhibition of PBPs 1A and 1Bs, apparently because the activities of PBPs 2 and 3 are not coupled to autolysin action.

VII. PBPs OF GRAM-POSITIVE BACTERIA

Relatively little information is available concerning the functions of the high molecular weight PBPs of gram-positive bacteria. Mutants of *B. subtilis* (51) selected for resistance to cloxacillin had a parallel decrease in the affinity of PBP2a for cloxacillin, but not for penicillin. The mutants retained the penicillin sensitivity of their parent. Other changes, including modification in the rod diameter in the mutants (51), suggest functional specialization of PBPs as in *E. coli*. It is likely that cephalosporins have a different PBP (2b) as their primary target in *B. subtilis* (6).

Penicillin inhibits the transpeptidase activity of membrane-wall preparations of *Bacillus megaterium*. Activity is recovered in parallel with the release of bound penicillin from PBP1 (52). The most intriguing data on *B. megaterium* PBPs concerns PBP4, which was purified as a peptidoglycan transglycosylase prior to detection of its penicillin-binding capacity (53). The possible relationship to bifunctional *E. coli* PBPs is obvious. Detection of transglycosylase and low-level transpeptidase activity in high molecular weight *Bacillus* sp. PBPs has recently been reported (6).

The most significant data relating gram-positive PBPs to lethal targets probably derives from analysis of beta-lactam antibiotic-resistant clinical isolates. Marked decreases in PBP2 and PBP3 affinity have been reported in methicillin-resistant staphylococci (54,55) and in the PBPs 1a,1b,2a, and 2b of penicillin-resistant pneumococci (56). The intrinsic penicillin resistance of group D streptococci has been correlated with the relatively low affinities of their PBPs. Comparison of in vivo and in vitro affinities failed to detect the previously postulated permeability barrier (36).

In conclusion, it is probable that in most gram-positive bacteria, as in *E. coli*, PBP transpeptidases are functionally differentiated, playing critical roles in different aspects of cell wall growth and division. This diversity provides multiple lethal targets for beta-lactam antibiotics, possibly with preferential affinities for specific drugs. This variety of PBP functions indicates that generalizations concerning efficacy of beta-lactam antibiotics against gram-positive bacterial pathogens must be interpreted with caution, and we must be on the alert for the appearance of additional resistant mutants with modified PBPs.

VIII. ACYLATION OF PBPs BY BETA-LACTAM ANTIBIOTICS AND BY NASCENT PEPTIDOGLYCAN: RELATIONSHIP TO BETA-LACTAMASES

Demonstration that penicillin and model acyl-D-alanyl-D-alanine substrates acylate the same serine residue in several penicillin-sensitive low molecular weight PBPs (D,D-carboxypeptidases) has effectively proven the substrate analog theory (31) of beta-lactam antibiotic action for these enzymes. This process has also been demonstrated for the soluble D,D-carboxypeptidases of *Streptomyces* R61 and *Actinomadura* R39, so effectively studied by Ghuysen and his co-workers as model penicillin-sensitive enzymes (17,18). These workers were the first to interpret the interaction of such enzymes with their normal substrates and with beta-lactam antibiotics according to simple kinetic schemes of the form

$$E + S \underset{k_{-1}}{\overset{k_1}{\rightleftharpoons}} E{\cdot}S \xrightarrow[\text{D-Ala}]{k_2} E\text{–}P \xrightarrow[H_2O]{k_3} E{\cdot}POH \underset{k_{-4}}{\overset{k_4}{\rightleftharpoons}} E + P\text{–}OH$$

where E·S and E·POH are noncovalent complexes with substrate and product, respectively, whose concentrations depend on their dissociation constants. For an efficient D,D-carboxypeptidase, E·S formation is rapid, k_2 and k_3 are both efficient reactions and E·POH dissociates rapidly. The ability to trap the acyl-enzyme intermediate E–P depends on the ratio of k_2 to k_3. Ghuysen et al. (17) pioneered the use of diacetyl-L-Lys-D-Ala-D-Ala as a model substrate for D,D-carboxypeptidases. For *S. aureus* PBP4, $k_2 > k_3$ with this substrate, and an acyl enzyme was trapped by rapid denaturation (57). The use of the depsipeptide analog, diacetyl-L-Lys-D-Ala-D-lactate, for which k_2 is markedly accelerated, has allowed isolation of similar derivatives of several other D,D-carboxypeptidases (58,59), confirming the existence of the acyl-enzyme catalytic intermediates. Similar studies of high molecular weight PBPs have been difficult, since they apparently have much more specific substrate requirements (e.g., for nascent peptidoglycan).

Isolation of stoichiometric penicilloyl derivatives of PBPs is, by contrast, relatively facile, since, for penicillins to be effective, k_3 (or other mechanisms of deacylation; e.g., see Fig. 7) must be very slow. Analysis of the sequences acylated by both depsipeptide substrates and penicillin has demonstrated that both react with the same serine residue, presumably part of the active site, in the D,D-carboxypeptidases of *B. subtilis* (PBP5), *B. stearothermophilus* (PBP5), *E. coli* (PBP5), and the *Streptomyces* R61 exocellular enzyme (data summarized in Refs. 5 and 6), firmly establishing the validity of the substrate analog hypothesis. Apparently neither the Zn^{2+}-containing beta-lactamase of *Bacillus cereus* nor the unusual, penicillin-insensitive low molecular weight Zn^{2+}-containing D,D-carboxypeptidase of *Streptomyces albus* G (60) employ an acyl-enzyme mechanism. However, for the far more prevalent class A and C beta-lactamases, acyl intermediates have been identified by a variety of techniques.

Because of the interest in establishing the mechanisms of action of beta-lactamases and investigating their relatedness to PBPs, various beta-lactam derivatives that inactivate these enzymes by forming stable acyl derivatives have been used to investigate their active sites (e.g., see Ref. 61). For class A enzymes, such as the *S. aureus* and R-TEM enzymes, distinct sequence homology to the PBP5 carboxypeptidases is apparent around the active serine acylation sites (62), supporting the original hypothesis (31) of a common evolutionary origin. The class C chromosomal beta-lactamases of *E. coli* (*ampC*) and *Pseudomonas aeruginosa* show much less distinct but still probably significant homology (data summarized in Refs. 5 and 6).

The N-terminal sequences of the *PBP5s* of *B. subtilis, B. stearothermophilus,* and *E. coli* can be aligned without gaps (5). Variable short N-terminal extensions result in location of the active site serine residues at positions 36, 36, and 44, respectively. The corresponding residue in the *E. coli* R-TEM enzyme is at position 45 (5,61). Maximum similarity in sequence and predicted secondary structure is found in these N-terminal regions of the PBP5s and the class A beta-lactamases. The C-terminal regions are quite different, presumably reflecting evolution for different functions (5).

The complete sequence of *E. coli* PBP3 is now known (5). It shows similarity to the sequence of PBP5 in only one short region, the same region in PBP5 that shows homology to beta-lactamases. This region may be the active site in PBP3. In contrast to PBP5, this site is located far away from the N terminus, near the middle of PBP3. The large N-terminal domain of PBP3 may have the transglycosylase function of PBP3, and the C-terminal region the transpeptidase function (5). This point may be clarified by sequence comparisons with other transpeptidase/transglycosylase PBPs.

The binding of model peptide substrates and beta-lactam antibiotics to the R61 D,D-carboxypeptidase has recently been visualized by x-ray crystallography at high resolution (63), allowing comparison of the intimate details of how each type of ligand interacts with the active site. Extension of such analyses to PBPs more closely related to "lethal targets" should be a giant step toward the rational design of inhibitors.

IX. STRUCTURE-ACTIVITY RELATIONSHIPS AMONG BETA-LACTAM ANTIBIOTICS

To be effective, a beta-lactam antibiotic must have a sufficiently high affinity for essential PBPs of a sufficiently broad range of bacterial genera to give it a useful spectrum of activity. This affinity, defined in the general kinetic model as the dissociation constant for the E·S complex (k_{-1}/k_1), must be accompanied by a high acylating activity (high k_2) and low deacylation rate (low k_3) in order that an inactivated acyl enzyme be produced.

The basic requirement for acylating activity appears to be a beta-lactam ring activated for nucleophilic attack on its carbonyl group by electron-withdrawing groups attached to the adjacent corners (e.g., the ring amide nitrogen and C_6 in penams) (64). The earlier concept (31) of a requirement for suppression of the beta-lactam amide resonance by the distortion about the nitrogen caused by a nonplanar bicyclic ring structure, as in penams and cephems, had to be replaced by this more general model to account for the activity of highly effective monobactams such as aztreonam. The postulated analogy (31) between the amide bond of beta-lactam antibiotics and a monovalent transition state during cleavage of the normal D-Ala-D-Ala substrate received some support from molecular orbital calculations (64). It remains viable in the general sense of bond stability and reactivity, if not in absolute structural mimicry.

Analysis of D,D-carboxypeptidases (18) indicates that the PBPs themselves do not have a particularly high affinity for model substrates such as diacetyl-L-Lys-D-Ala-D-Ala, and that affinity for penicillin is no higher, contrary to one aspect of the original postulate (31). Instead, only an adequate "fit" to the active site (18) accompanied by high acylating activity is required. Studies of the R61 enzyme crystals (63) indicate that, apart from the serine acylation site, the components of the active site involved in binding the model substrates and beta-lactam inhibitors are not coincidental. The only common requirement is probably that of a negative charge strategically located close to the amide nitrogen (64), as for the C_3 carboxylate in penams, equivalent to the carboxylate of a C-terminal D-alanine residue.

Analysis of the role played by other antibiotic substituents in binding to PBP targets is complicated by the bewildering variety of active beta-lactam antibiotics. Design of new inhibitors which are not simple ad hoc variants of known antibiotics will require more specific information on target enzymes than is available in the large volume of existing structure/function data (64). Mecillinam was not designed as a selective inhibitor of PBPs similar to *E. coli* PBP2, and attempts at such specific design may require detailed analysis of the active sites of each class of PBP. While an antibiotic activity spectrum limited, for example, to aerobic gram-negative rods could be extremely valuable against contemporary opportunistic pathogens, current knowledge of the variety and functions of essential PBP targets in such organisms only suggests that this may be possible, without providing design characteristics. Knowledge of the relationship between structure and outer membrane permeability for organisms such as *P. aeruginosa* is just as important and difficult to acquire and rationalize.

Once acylated by a beta-lactam antibiotic, the PBP derivative must be stable. The characteristics involved in a low k_3 (kinetic model), appear to be restraints on approach by H_2O or other potential acceptor molecules to the ester linkage. Fortunately, it has been possible to construct beta-lactams resistant to beta-lactamase hydrolysis which retain all the characteristics necessary for PBP acylation. The complex of essential PBPs seems to have more flexibility in accommodating these substrate analogs than do the beta-lactamases. Since the class A and C beta-lactamases employ the same acyl intermediate mechanism as PBPs, resistance to beta-lactamases can be achieved by reducing affinity, acylation rate, or deacylation (solvolysis) rate. A reduced rate of deacylation would seem to be most compatible with persistence of antibiotic activity. Most of the newer beta-lactam-resistant derivatives seem to acylate class A beta-lactamases poorly, but still react rapidly with class C enzymes, producing stable acyl-beta-lactamase derivatives. Unfortunately, while this confers resistance to hydrolysis, a slow rate of outer membrane permeation, coupled with acylation and effective induction of these periplasmic gram-negative beta-lactamases, results in resistance due to stoichiometric binding of the drug (4). This mechanism is effective because of the aforementioned modest affinity of these antibiotics for their PBP targets. The active monobactams, which seem to have low reactivity with class C beta-lactamases, may provide one route for avoiding this latest road block thrown up by gram-negative pathogenic bacteria to beta-lactam antibiotics. Resistance mechanisms not based on beta-lactamases are discussed below. Clearly, overproduction of a PBP with high affinity for a given beta-lactam antibiotic could protect the producing cell as well as does production of nonhydrolyzing beta-lactamase. It is perhaps fortunate that the abundant, smaller PBPs of gram-negative bacteria have low affinities for many nonpenam antibiotics.

X. NON-BETA-LACTAMASE MECHANISMS OF ACQUIRED RESISTANCE

The widespread use of beta-lactamase-resistant antibiotics, besides uncovering the nonhydrolytic beta-lactamase-dependent resistance mechanism described above, is also leading to increased reports of clinical antibiotic resistance related to mutations in PBPs leading to reduced penicillin binding. These changes presumably require amino acid substitutions in the PBPs causing modifications in the active site compatible with normal function, but not with facile and stable acylation by beta-lactams. This process must be related to the differences in the components of the active site involved in binding of substrate and inhibitors (63).

This process is typically a consequence of several small, incremental steps in resistance, as seen in *Neisseria gonorrhoeae* following indiscriminate use of penicillin and prior to selection of the beta-lactamase-producing strains. Not all of this increase in resistance is due to PBP modification; decrease in outer membrane permeability is also involved. This mechanism is more difficult to document but is potentially available in all gram-negative bacteria. Changes in PBP patterns have been demonstrated for *N. gonorrhoeae* (65) and more recently for pneumococci (56). At least one class of methicillin resistance in *S. aureus* is due to a PBP modification (54,55). This has the atypical characteristic of a single-step mutation to high resistance, as does mutation to mecillinam resistance in *E. coli* (43). Other examples can be anticipated as use of powerful beta-lactamase-resistant beta-lactams such as moxalactam and aztreonam accelerates.

XI. TOLERANCE AND THE MECHANISMS OF LETHALITY OF BETA-LACTAM ANTIBIOTICS

Beta-lactam antibiotics are bactericidal in their action against most pathogens, a characteristic of importance in specific clinical circumstances where phagocytosis and its enhancement by complement and specific immunity are defective. Treatment failures of staphylococcal infections (66) emphasized the potential role of tolerance as a resistance mechanism.

As summarized by Tomasz (3,67), numerous data implicate endogenous autolysins (peptidoglycan hydrolases; see Fig. 4) as mediators of cell death by lysis following exposure to beta-lactams. Pneumococci are prime examples, having a highly active MurNAc–L–alanine amidase autolysin. Viable, autolysin-defective mutants retain the low MIC of penicillin characteristic of their parents, but are killed only slowly. This phenomenon has been called tolerance, since penicillin has become a bacteriostatic antibiotic for these mutants. Oral streptococci, such as *Streptococcus sanguis* and *Streptococcus mutans*, are intrinsically tolerant and have very low autolytic capacity. In *Streptococci* and *Staphylococci*, autolysis activity is controlled by inhibitory interaction with lipoteichoic acids. The pathway of autolysin activation following exposure of growing cells to beta-lactams is not clear but involves release of these inhibitory polymers from the cells, presumably a secondary consequence of inhibition of some specific aspect of peptidoglycan biosynthesis. Release may still occur in tolerant bacteria, but is not coupled to autolysin activation. The negative control of autolysins exhibited by nongrowing cells appears to be paramount in all bacteria, accounting for the dependence of the bactericidal response to beta-lactam antibiotics on an adequate rate of bacterial cell growth.

Autolysins may also be under positive control: For example, choline in the cell wall teichoic acid of pneumococci is required for autolysin activation (3,67). Coupling of autolysin activation to the cycle of cell growth and division probably explains why interaction of beta-lactams is coupled to autolysis only when specific PBPs are involved (e.g., the PBP1 complex of *E. coli*). While inhibition of *E. coli* PBP2 and PBP3 is lethal, this is not due to activation of massive autolysis. Group A streptococci are highly sensitive to penicillin, but exposure does not lead to gross lysis. Both tolerant mutants of group A streptococci and resistant mutants with altered PBPs have been obtained in the laboratory (68), but fortunately only rare tolerant isolates have been reported in the clinic, in spite of the widespread use of very low concentrations of penicillin (supplied in depot form) in long-term prophylaxis of group A streptococcal infections. The ability of osmotic support to protect group A streptococci against killing suggests that limited autolysis may play a role in lethality even in these organisms (68).

In conclusion, autolysin activation appears to be a prevalent mechanism of lethality for beta-lactam antibiotics, but is not the only mechanism. Tolerance can be found when PBP inactivation is reversible and triggering of irreversible autolysis is very slow. The tolerant response implies that PBP interactions with beta-lactams can lead to inhibition of general macromolecular synthesis. Perhaps the nonautolytic mechanisms of lethality are simply a nonreversible inhibition of this type, determined by the rate of deacylation of the inhibited critical PBP. Inhibition of macromolecular synthesis needs to be maintained until some critical cell component becomes irreversibly damaged. Peptidoglycan hydrolysis is only one possibility; proteolytic degradation to protein and RNA synthetic machineries and sufficient damage to membrane lipids are only some of the others.

REFERENCES

1. K. H. Schleifer and O. Kandler. Peptidoglycan types of bacterial cell walls and their taxonomic implications. *Bacteriol. Rev., 36*:407–477 (1972).
2. D. J. Tipper. The structure of bacterial cell wall peptidoglycans. *Int. J. Syst. Bacteriol., 26*:361–377 (1970).
3. A. Tomasz. The mechanism of the irreversible antimicrobial effects of penicillins: How the beta-lactam antibiotics kill and lyse bacteria. *Annu. Rev. Microbiol., 33*:113–137 (1979).
4. C. C. Sander. Inducible β-lactamases and non-hydrolytic resistance mechanisms. *J. Antimicrob. Chemother., 13*:1–2 (1984).
5. G. Spratt. Penicillin-binding proteins and the future of β-lactam antibiotics. *J. Gen. Microb., 129*:1247–1260 (1983).
6. D. J. Waxman and J. L. Strominger. Penicillin-binding proteins and the mechanism of action of β-lactam antibiotics. *Annu. Rev. Biochem., 52*:825–869 (1983).

7. H. Nikaido. Outer membrane permeability of bacteria: Resistance and accessibility of targets, in *β-Lactam Antibiotics* (M. Salton and G. D. Shockman, eds.), Academic, New York, 1981, pp. 249–260.
8. W. Weidel and H. Pelzer. Bag-shaped macromolecules — A new outlook on bacterial cell walls. *Adv. Enzymol., 26*:193–232 (1964).
9. G. E. Fox, E. Stackebrandt, R. B. Hespell, J. Gibson, J. Maniloff, T. A. Dyer, R. S. Wolfe, W. E. Balch, R. S. Tanner, L. J. Magrum, L. B. Zablen, R. Blakemore, R. Gupta, L. Bonen, B. J. Lewis, D. A. Stahl, K. R. Luehrsen, K. N. Chen, and C. R. Woese. The phylogeny of prokaryotes. *Science, 209*: 457–463 (1980).
10. D. J. Tipper and A. Wright. The structure and biosynthesis of bacterial cell walls, in *The Bacteria*, Vol. 7 (J. R. Sokatch and L. N. Ornston, eds.), Academic, New York, 1979, pp. 291–426.
11. J. L. Strominger. How penicillin kills bacteria: A short history, in *Microbiology* (D. Schlessinger, ed.), American Society for Microbiology, Washington, D.C., 1977, pp. 177–181.
12. J. T. Park. Uridine 5'-pyrophosphate derivatives. III. Amino acid-containing derivatives. *J. Biol. Chem., 194*:897–904 (1952).
13. J. L. Strominger. Penicillin-sensitive enzymatic reactions in bacterial cell wall synthesis. *Harvey Lect., 64*:179–213 (1970).
14. F. C. Neuhaus and W. P. Hammes. Inhibition of cell wall biosynthesis by analogues of alanine. *Pharmacol. Ther., 14*:265–320 (1981).
15. W. H. Toscano and D. R. Storm. Bacitracin. *Pharmacol. Ther., 16*:199–210 (1982).
16. H. R. Perkins. Vancomycin and related antibiotics. *Pharmac. Ther., 16*:181–197 (1982).
17. J.-M. Ghuysen, J.-M. Frere, M. Leyh-Bouille, H. R. Perkins, and M. Nieto. The active centres in penicillin-sensitive enzymes. *Philos. Trans. R. Soc. London B, 289*:285–301 (1980).
18. J.-M. Ghuysen, J.-M. Frere, M. Leyh-Bouille, O. Dideberg, J. Lamotte-Brasseur, H. R. Perkins, and J. L. DeCoen. Penicillins and Δ^3-cephalosporins as inhibitors and mechanism-based inactivators of D-alanyl-D-Ala peptidases, in *Topics in Molecular Pharmacology* (A. S. V. Burgen and G. C. K. Roberts, eds.), Elsevier/North-Holland, New York, 1981, pp. 63–97.
19. W. P. Hammes and O. Kandler. Biosynthesis of peptidoglycan in *Gaffkya homari*. The incorporation of peptidoglycan into the cell wall and the direction of transpeptidation. *Eur. J. Biochem., 70*:97–106 (1976).
20. J. Nakagawa, S. Tamaka, and M. Matsuhashi. Purified penicillin binding proteins 1Bs from *Escherichia coli* membrane showing activities of both peptidoglycan polymerase and peptidoglycan cross-linking enzyme. *Agric. Biol. Chem., 43*:1379–1380 (1979).
21. H. Suzuki, Y. van Heijenoort, T. Tamura, J. Mizoguchi, Y. Hirota, and J. van Heijenoort. In vitro peptidoglycan polymerization catalyzed by penicillin binding protein 1B of *Escherichia coli* K12. *FEBS Lett., 110*:245–249 (1980).
22. F. Ishino, S. Mitsui, S. Tamaki, and M. Matsuhashi. Dual enzyme activities

of cell wall peptidoglycan synthesis, peptidoglycan transglycosylase and penicillin-sensitive transpeptidase, in purified preparations of *Escherichia coli* penicillin-binding protein 1A. *Biochem. Biophys. Res. Commun., 97*: 287–293 (1980).
23. F. Ishino and M. Matsuhashi. Peptidoglycan synthetic enzyme activities of highly purified penicillin-binding protein 3 in *Escherichia coli*: A septum-forming reaction sequence. *Biochem. Biophys. Res. Commun., 101*:905–911 (1981).
24. F. Ishino, S. Tamaki, B. G. Spratt, and M. Matsuhashi. A mecillinam-sensitive peptidoglycan cross-linking reaction in *Escherichia coli. Biochem. Biophys. Res. Commun., 109*:689–696 (1982).
25. H. Mett, R. Bracha, and D. Mirelman. Soluble nascent peptidoglycan in growing *Escherichia coli* cells. *J. Biol. Chem., 255*:9584–9890 (1980).
26. W. D. Fordham and C. Gilvarg. Kinetics of cross-linking of peptidoglycan in *Bacillus megaterium. J. Biol. Chem., 249*:2478–2482 (1974).
27. P. Dezelee and G. D. Shockman. Studies on the formation of peptide cross-links in the cell wall peptidoglycan of *Streptococcus faecalis. J. Biol. Chem., 250*:6806–6816 (1975).
28. E. W. Goodell, Z. Markiewicz, and U. Schwarz. Absence of oligomeric murein intermediates in *Escherichia coli. J. Bacteriol., 156*:130–135 (1983).
29. P. D. Cooper. Site of action or radiopenicillin. *Bacteriol. Rev., 70*:28–48 (1956).
30. E. M. Wise and J. T. Park. Penicillin: Its basic site of action as an inhibitor of a peptide cross-linking reaction in cell wall mucopeptide synthesis. *Proc. Nat. Acad. Sci. U.S.A., 54*:75–81 (1965).
31. D. J. Tipper and J. L. Strominger. Mechanism of action of penicillins: A proposal based on their structural similarity to acyl-D-alanyl-D-alanine. *Proc. Nat. Acad. Sci. U.S.A., 54*:1133–1141 (1965).
32. K. Izaki, M. Matsuhashi, and J. L. Strominger. Glycopeptide transpeptidase and D-alanine carboxypeptidase: Penicillin-sensitive enzymatic reactions. *Proc. Nat. Acad. Sci. U.S.A., 55*:656–663 (1966).
33. P. M. Blumberg and J. L. Strominger. Interaction of penicillin with the bacterial cell: Penicillin-binding proteins and penicillin-sensitive enzymes. *Bacteriol. Rev., 38*:291–335 (1974).
34. B. G. Spratt and A. B. Pardee. Penicillin-binding proteins and cell shape in *E. coli. Nature London, 254*:516–517 (1975).
35. U. Schwarz, K. Seeger, F. Wengenmayer, and H. Strecker. Penicillin-binding proteins of *Escherichia coli* identified with a ^{125}I-derivative of ampicillin. *FEMS Microbiol. Lett., 10*:107–109 (1981).
36. R. Williamson, S. B. Calderwood, R. C. Moellering, Jr., and A. Tomasz. Studies on the mechanism of intrinsic resistance to β-lactam antibiotics in group D streptococci. *J. Gen. Microbiol., 129*:813–822 (1983).
37. S. Tamaki, S. Nakajima, and M. Matsuhashi. Thermosensitive mutation in *Escherichia coli* simultaneously causing defects in penicillin-binding protein 1Bs and in enzyme activity for peptidoglycan synthesis in vitro. *Proc. Nat. Acad. Sci. U.S.A., 74*:5472–5476 (1977).

38. H. Suzuki, Y. Nishimura, and Y. Hirota. On the process of cellular division in *Escherichia coli*: A series of mutants of *E. coli* altered in the penicillin-binding proteins. *Proc. Nat. Acad. Sci. U.S.A., 75*:664–668 (1978).
39. S. Tomioka, F. Ishino, S. Tamaki, and M. Matsuhashi. Formation of hyper-cross-linked peptidoglycan with multiple cross-linkages by a penicillin-binding protein, 1A, of *Escherichia coli. Biochem. Biophys. Res. Commun., 106*:1175–1182 (1982).
40. B. G. Spratt. Temperature-sensitive cell division mutants pf *Escherichia coli* with thermolabile penicillin-binding proteins. *J. Bacteriol., 131*:293–305 (1977).
41. D. Mirelman. Biosynthesis and assembly of cell wall peptidoglycan, in *Bacterial Outer Membranes* (M. Inouye, ed.), Wiley, New York, 1979, pp. 115–166.
42. F. Lund and L. Tybring. 6β-Amidinopenicillanic acids — A new group of antibiotics. *Nature New Biol., 236*:135–137 (1972).
43. M. Iwaya, R. Goldman, D. J. Tipper, B. Feingold, and J. L. Strominger. Morphology of an *Escherichia coli* mutant with a temperature-dependent round cell shape. *J. Bacteriol., 136*:1143–1158 (1978).
44. B. G. Spratt. Distinct penicillin binding proteins involved in the division, elongation, and shape of *Escherichia coli. Proc. Nat. Acad. Sci. U.S.A., 72*: 2999–3003 (1975).
45. B. G. Spratt. Deletion of the penicillin-binding protein 5 gene of *Escherichia coli. J. Bacteriol., 14*:1190–1192 (1980).
46. J. K. Broome-Smith and B. G. Spratt. Deletion of the penicillin-binding protein 6 gene of *Escherichia coli. J. Bacteriol., 152*:904–906 (1982).
47. M. DePedro and U. Schwarz. Heterogeneity of newly inserted and preexisting murein in the sacculus of *Escherichia coli. Proc. Nat. Acad. Sci. U.S.A., 78*:5856–5860 (1981).
48. A. W. Wyke, J. B. Ward, M. V. Hayes, and N. A. C. Curtis. A role in vivo for penicillin-binding protein 4 of *Staphylococcus aureus. Eur. J. Biochem., 119*:389–393 (1981).
49. Z. Markiewicz, J. K. Broome-Smith, U. Schwarz, and B. G. Spratt. Spherical *E. coli* due to elevated levels of D-alanine carbosypeptidase. *Nature London, 297*:702–704 (1982).
50. D. Mirelman, Y. Yashouv-Gan, and U. Schwarz. Regulation of murein biosynthesis and septum formation in filamentous cells of *Escherichia coli PAT 84. J. Bacteriol., 129*:1593–1600 (1977).
51. C. E. Buchanan. Altered proteins in penicillin-resistant mutants of *Bacillus subtilis*, in *Microbiology* (D. Schlessinger, ed.), American Society for Microbiology, Washington, D.C., 1977, pp. 191–194.
52. P. E. Reynolds, S. T. Shepherd, and H. A. Chase. Identification of the binding protein which may be the target of penicillin action in *Bacillus megaterium. Nature London, 271*:568–570 (1978).
53. A. Taku, M. Stuckey, and D. P. Fan. Purification of the peptidoglycan transglycosylase of *Bacillus megaterium. J. Biol. Chem., 257*:5018–5022 (1982).
54. B. Hartman and A. Tomasz. Altered penicillin-binding proteins in methicil-

lin-resistant strains of *Staphylococcus aureus. Antimicrob. Agents Chemother., 19*:726–735 (1981).

55. A. W. Wyke, J. B. Ward, and M. V. Hayes. Synthesis of peptidoglycan *in vivo* in methicillin-resistant *Staphylococcus aureus. Eur. J. Biochem., 127*: 553–558 (1982).
56. R. Williamson, S. Zighelboim, and A. Tomasz. Penicillin-binding proteins of penicillin-resistant and penicillin-tolerant *Streptococcus pneumoniae*, (M. Salton and G. D. Shockman, eds.), Academic, New York, 1981, pp. 215–225.
57. J. W. Kozarich and J. L. Strominger. A membrane enzyme from *Staphylococcus aureus* which catalyses transpeptidase, carboxypeptidase and penicillinase activities. *J. Biol. Chem., 253*:1272–1278 (1978).
58. J. R. Rasmussen and J. L. Strominger. Utilization of a depsipeptide substrate for trapping acyl-enzyme intermediates of penicillin-sensitive D-alanine carboxypeptidases. *Proc. Nat. Acad. Sci. U.S.A., 75*:84–88 (1978).
59. R. R. Yocum, D. J. Waxman, J. R. Rasmussen, and J. L. Strominger. Mechanism of penicillin action: Penicillin and substrate bind covalently to the same active site serine in two bacterial D-alanine-carboxypeptidases. *Proc. Nat. Acad. Sci. U.S.A., 76*:2730–2734 (1979).
60. B. Joris, J. Van Beeumen, F. Casagrande, C. Gerday, J.-M. Frere, and J.-M. Ghuysen. The complete amino acid sequence of the Zn^{2+}-containing D-alanyl-D-alanine-cleaving carboxypeptidase of *Streptomyces albus G. Eur. J. Biochem., 130*:53–69 (1983).
61. V. Knott-Hunziker, S. G. Waley, B. S. Orlek, and P. G. Sammes. Penicillinase active sites: Labelling of serine-44 in β-lactamase I by 6β-bromopenicillanic acid. *FEBS Lett., 99*:59–61 (1979).
62. D. J. Waxman and J. L. Strominger. Sequence of active site peptides from the penicillin-sensitive D-alanine carboxypeptidase of *Bacillus subtilis. J. Biol. Chem., 255*:3964–3976 (1980).
63. J. A. Kelly, P. C. Moews, J. R. Knox, J.-M. Frere, and J.-M. Ghuysen. Penicillin target enzymes and the antibiotic binding site. *Science, 218*:479–481 (1982).
64. D. B. Boyd. Theoretical and physicochemical studies on β-lactam antibiotics, in *The Chemistry and Biology of β-Lactam Antibiotics*, Vol. 1 (R. B. Morin and M. Gorman, eds.), Academic, New York, 1982, pp. 437–535.
65. T. J. Dougherty, A. E. Koller, and A. Tomasz. Penicillin-binding proteins of penicillin-susceptible and intrinsically resistant *Neisseria gonorrhoeae. Antimicrob. Agents Chemother., 18*:730–737 (1980).
66. L. D. Sabath, M. Laverdiere, N. Whieler, D. Blazevic, and B. J. Wilkinson. A new type of penicillin resistance of *Staphylococcus aureus. Lancet, 1*:443–447 (1977).
67. A. Tomasz. Penicillin tolerance and the control of murein hydrolases, in *β-Lactam Antibiotics* (M. Salton and G. D. Shockman, eds.), Academic, New York, 1980, pp. 227–247.
68. L. Butmann and A. Tomasz. Penicillin-resistant and penicillin-tolerant mutants of group A streptococci. *Antimicrob. Agents Chemother., 22*:128–136 (1982).

3

Beta-Lactamase-Mediated Resistance

ANTONE A. MEDEIROS
The Miriam Hospital and Brown University, Providence, Rhode Island

GEORGE A. JACOBY
Massachusetts General Hospital, Boston, Massachusetts

I. INTRODUCTION

Beta-lactamases are enzymes that inactivate beta-lactam antibiotics by splitting the amide bond of the beta-lactam ring. The resistance to beta-lactam antibiotics of most bacterial pathogens is due to the production of these enzymes. Numerous beta-lactamases exist, some encoded by chromosomal genes and others by plasmids or transposons. This review will focus on the distribution of plasmid-mediated beta-lactamases and their R factors (1).

Beta-lactamase production by bacteria was discovered as early as 1940. Abraham and Chain (2) crushed a suspension of *Escherichia coli* to produce an extract that inactivated penicillin. Because papain digestion and heat inactivated the extract, the authors postulated that the active component was an enzyme, which they termed "penicillinase." They also found the enzyme in another penicillin-resistant gram-negative rod, but not in a strain of penicillin-susceptible *Staphylococcus*. In 1944 Kirby (3) showed that penicillinase production was strongly correlated with the penicillin resistance of clinical isolates of *Staphylococcus aureus*. The prevalence of these penicillinase-producing staphylococci rose rapidly after the introduction of penicillin G, first in hospitals and then in the community. With the advent of semisynthetic penicillins and cephalosporins which resisted hydrolysis by staphylococcal beta-lactamase, spread of penicillinase-producing staphylococci within institutions decreased. At the same time increased use of the broad-spectrum penicillin ampicillin fostered a rise in the incidence of infections due to ampicillin-resistant gram-negative bacilli. These pathogens produced a large variety of beta-lactamases capable of destroying the newer penicillins and cephalosporins (4). It was then discovered that the more common types of beta-lactamases were encoded by plasmids (5) and transposons (6), which are capable of widespread transfer to other genera. Consequently, attention shifted from staphylococcal beta-lactamase to the beta-lactamases of gram-negative bacilli that had replaced staphylococci as the major threat to the hospitalized patient. Search for new beta-lactam antibiotics resistant to the beta-lactamases of gram-negative bacilli became a major thrust of the pharmaceutical industry. As new classes of beta-lactam antibiotics have come into clinical use (7), pathogens producing new types of beta-lactamases have emerged.

II. CLASSIFICATION OF BETA-LACTAMASES

A. ·Gram-Positive Bacteria

Among the gram-positive bacteria staphylococci are the major pathogens that produce beta-lactamase. Four types (A–D) of closely related staphylococcal beta-lactamases have been distinguished by serological and enzymological criteria (8,9). These enzymes have a molecular weight of 28,000 and preferentially hydrolyze penicillins. With the exception of type D, all types are inducible and are excreted extracellularly (10). Staphylococcal beta-lactamases share extensive sequence homology with beta-lactamases found in *Bacillus* species (10,11). The beta-lactamases of both *Bacillus cereus* and *Staph. aureus* have been found to be thioether lipoproteins (12). The genes determining staphylococcal beta-lactamases are usually carried on small plasmids that can be transferred from cell to cell via transduction with bacteriophage. Larger plasmids carrying a beta-lactamase gene and resistance to other antibiotics have been described recently (13, 14). These genes can transfer by conjugation, not only between strains of *Staph. aureus* but also between *Staph. aureus* and *Staphylococcus epidermidis* (13,14).

In an extensive survey of the beta-lactamases produced by various clinical pathogens, Matthew and Harris (15) found two strains of streptococci, one of *Streptococcus uberis* and one of *Streptococcus faecalis*, which produced beta-lactamase. More recently Murray and Mederski-Samoraj (16) described a strain of *Str. faecalis* that produced a plasmid-determined beta-lactamase. None of the streptococcal beta-lactamases have been well characterized.

B. Gram-Negative Bacteria

Gram-negative bacteria produce a much greater variety of beta-lactamases than do gram-positive bacteria. This diversity has led to several classification schemes. The relative rates at which different beta-lactam antibiotics are hydrolyzed, that is, the substrate profile, provided the basis for the earliest of the classification schemes (17,18). Inhibition of beta-lactamase by various compounds and reaction to antisera provided additional distinction. Richmond and Sykes (19) divided the beta-lactamases into five classes according to these criteria. Their class 1 beta-lactamases, characterized by a high rate of hydrolysis of cephalosporins, included the chromosomally determined beta-lactamases of most of the enterobacteriaceae and *Pseudomonas.* The chromosomal beta-lactamases of *Proteus* and *Klebsiella*, which are more active against penicillins, made up classes 2 and 4, respectively. Class 3 consisted of the plasmid-determined beta-lactamases that were active against both penicillins and cephalosporins but not carbenicillin or isoxazolyl penicillins. This classification includes the TEM-type enzymes discussed in the next section. Class 5 was a heterogeneous grouping that contained oxacillin-hydrolyzing and carbenicillin-hydrolyzing beta-lactamases, also discussed in the next section. Difficulty in determining substrate and inhibitor profiles using crude enzyme preparations and the heterogeneity within some of these classes have often made it difficult to utilize the classification just described, especially when multiple beta-lactamases coexist within a bacterial cell.

A major advance in the classification of beta-lactamases occurred when Matthew et al. (4) showed that specific beta-lactamases could be identified by flatbed isoelectric focusing in polyacrylamide gel. Bands corresponding to specific beta-lactamases were identified by developing the gel with an overlay of nitrocefin, a chromogenic cephalosporin that changes color with hydrolysis. Specific beta-lactamases often showed patterns consisting of a main band and several accessory bands that were reproducible and characteristic of that enzyme. An unknown beta-lactamase could be readily identified in a crude cell extract by comparing its isoelectric point and banding pattern with reference enzymes run on the same gel. Using concentrated cell extracts, Matthew et al. detected discrete beta-lactamase bands in virtually all gram-negative bacteria studied.

The beta-lactamases of staphylococci are exceptional in that they form a nondescript blur when focused on a bed of polyacrylamide gel (A. A. Medeiros, unpublished observations), perhaps because their lipid component masks the net electrical charge of the amino acids in the protein. The plasmid-determined beta-lactamase of *Str. faecalis* JH2-7 (16) produces a similar blur when focused on polyacrylamide gel electrophoresis (A. A. Medeiros, unpublished observations).

Ambler (11) and Bergstrom et al. (20) have defined three evolutionarily distinct classes of beta-lactamases based on amino acid and nucleotide sequence studies. Class A beta-lactamases have molecular weights around 29,000, possess a serine residue at their active site, show significant amino acid homology, and preferentially hydrolyze penicillins. The TEM-1 beta-lactamase widely prevalent in gram-negative bacilli and enzymes from *Staph. aureus* and *Bacillus licheniformis* are included in this group. Class B beta-lactamase is a metalloenzyme with a molecular weight of 23,000 that attacks cephalosporins preferentially and is produced only by *Bacillus cereus*. Class C includes the chromosomally determined beta-lactamase of *E. coli*, which shares extensive sequence homology with chromosomally mediated beta-lactamases of *Shigella* and *Klebsiella* species, and lesser homology with those of *Serratia, Salmonella*, and *Pseudomonas* species.

These enzymes are relatively large proteins, of molecular weight about 39,000, and they also have serine at their active site but share no homology with the class A beta-lactamases (20–22). Undoubtedly, as additional beta-lactamases or their genes are sequenced, additional classes will need to be added.

The sequence around the active site serine of the class A beta-lactamase shares homology with the amino acid sequence around the penicillin-binding sites of the D-alanine carboxypeptidases of *Bacillus* species. This observation supports the hypothesis that these beta-lactamases could be derived from penicillin-binding proteins involved in peptidoglycan synthesis (23–25).

C. Beta-Lactamases Determined by Plasmids and Transposons

Matthew et al. (26,27) described 11 types of plasmid-determined beta-lactamases, all of which are produced constitutively, and grouped them into three broad classes: (a) those that hydrolyze benzylpenicillin and cephaloridine at similar rates (broad-spectrum enzymes); (b) those that hydrolyze oxacillin and related penicillins rapidly (oxacillinases); and (c) those that readily break down carbenicillin (carbenicillinases). All of these enzymes possess a unique isoelectric point and most have a characteristic banding pattern on flat-bed isoelectric focusing. The patterns usually consist of a single major band and several satellite bands that develop late after overlay of nitrocefin onto the polyacrylamide gel. Figure 1 shows the band patterns of 19 plasmid-determined beta-lactamases in polyacrylamide gel approximately 20 min after the overlay of nitrocefin. The satellite bands of several are evident and in some instances bands representing weaker chromosomally determined beta-lactamases of the host strain are also seen. A matrix of highly purified agarose has also been used for isoelectric focusing of beta-lactamases, producing similar banding patterns and permitting shorter focusing times (28).

The properties of the 11 plasmid-determined beta-lactamases characterized by Matthew (26) are summarized in Tables 1 and 2. The broad-spectrum penicillinases (TEM-1, TEM-2, SHV-1, and HMS-1) all have nearly equal activity against benzylpenicillin and cephaloridine. The oxacillinases, on the other hand, hydrolyze oxacillin rapidly, as exemplified by OXA-1, OXA-2, and OXA-3. The PSE enzymes have high activity against carbenicillin. One of them, PSE-2, resembles the oxacillinases in having a high relative activity against oxacillin as well. Table 1 also shows that three of these beta-lactamases (OXA-1, PSE-1, and PSE-2) hydrolyze cefotaxime at a significant rate (30).

Cloxacillin inhibits the broad-spectrum enzymes but does not inhibit the other classes. Sodium chloride inhibits the oxacillinases but does not inhibit the broad-spectrum beta-lactamases. Inhibition by p-chloromercuribenzoate is more variable (Table 2). The OXA-2 and OXA-3 beta-lactamases are known to be dimers with molecular weights of 44,600 and 41,200, respectively (32), whereas

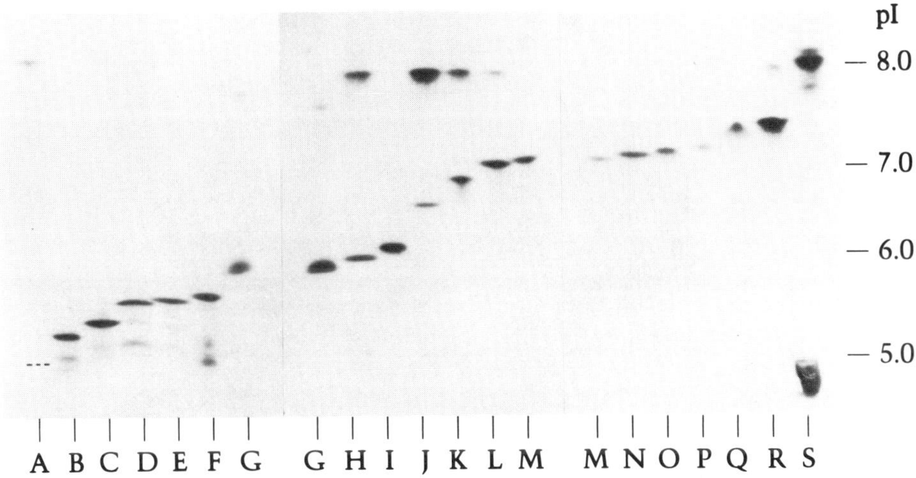

Figure 1 Composite of isoelectric focusing gels showing the band patterns of 19 beta-lactamases determined by plasmids or transposons: (A) HMS-1 (the position of the faint band is indicated by the dotted line), (B) PSE-4, (C) TEM-1, (D) TLE-1, (E) TEM-2, (F) PSE-1, (G) LCR-1, (H) AER-1, (I) PSE-2, (J) PSE-3, (K) OXA-3, (L) OXA-1, (M) OXA-4, (N) SHV-1, (O) OXA-5, (P) OXA-7, (Q) OXA-6, (R) OXA-2, and (S) ROB-1. The producing strain was *E. coli* for all beta-lactamases, except PSE-4 and LCR-1, which were produced by *P. aeruginosa*, and ROB-1, which was produced by *H. influenzae.* An additional band representing the chromosomally determined beta-lactamase of *E. coli* is seen in lanes A, H, J, K, L, and R and that of *P. aeruginosa* in lane G. An irregular accumulation of activity at the anodic loading site, typical of ROB-1, is seen in lane S.

the molecular weights of the other beta-lactamases range between 12,000 and 32,000.

Immunological cross-reaction is observed within but not between these classes of beta-lactamases (Table 2) (33,34). Antisera to TEM-1 cross-react with TEM-2 and also partially inactivate SHV-1. They do not, however, inactivate HMS-1, the OXA- or PSE-type beta-lactamases. Antisera to OXA-1 do not react with the other oxacillin-hydrolyzing enzymes. Antisera to PSE-2 do not react with any of the other plasmid-determined beta-lactamases. However, antiserum prepared against a beta-lactamase termed CARB-3, which may be plasmid-determined, cross-reacts with PSE-1 and PSE-4, indicating their close immunological relationship.

Table 3 shows the terminology used by Matthew along with the nomenclature employed by other authors to describe the same plasmid-determined enzymes.

Table 1 Spectrum of Activity of the Well-Established Plasmid-Determined Beta-Lactamases[a]

Beta-lactamase type	Relative rate of hydrolysis													
	Penicillin G = 100											Cephaloridine = 100		
	Amp	Carb	Oxa	Meth	Clox	Cer	Cet	Lex	Cxm	Mez	Pip	Cez	Cem	Ctx
Broad spectrum														
TEM-1	106	10	5	0	0	76	20	<10	<2	92	77	26	63	<1
TEM-2	107	10	5	0	0	74	20	<10	<2			25	55	0
SHV-1	212	8	0	<2	<2	56	8	14	4	133	147			0
HMS-1	253	14	<2	<2	<2	183	3	<2	<2				<2	
Oxacillinases														
OXA-1	382	30	197	332	190	30	15	0	<2	116	52		26	22
OXA-2	179	15	646	23	200	37	25	<5	<2					0
OXA-3	178	10	336	29	350	44	10	<5	2					0
Carbenicillinases														
PSE-1	90	97	<2	<2	<2	18	<2	0	<2					27
PSE-2	267	121	317	803	371	32	<2	11	4					16
PSE-3	101	253			3	10								<1
PSE-4	88	150	8	16	<2	40	4	8	<2					1

[a]Antibiotic abbreviations and sources of data are as follows: amp = ampicillin (27), carb = carbenicillin (27), cem = cefamandole (29), cer = cephaloridine (27), cet = cephalothin (27), cez = cefazolin (29), clox = cloxacillin (27), ctx = cefotaxime (30), cxm = cefuroxime (27), lex = cephalexin (27), meth = methicillin (27), mez = mezlocillin (31), oxa = oxacillin (27), pip = piperacillin (31).

Table 2 Inhibition Patterns, Cross-Reactivity, and Physical Properties of the Well-Established Plasmid-Determined Beta-Lactamases

Beta-lactamase type	Inhibited by			Molecular weight (x 1000)	pI	Neutralized by antiserum to				
	Clox	pCMB	NaCl			TEM-1	SHV-1	OXA-1	PSE-2	CARB-3
Broad spectrum										
TEM-1	+	–	–	22.0	5.4	+	–	–	–	–
TEM-2	+	–	–	23.5	5.6	+	–	–	–	–
SHV-1	+	+/–	–	17.0	7.6	+/–	+		–	–
HMS-1	+	+	–	21.0	5.2	–				
Oxacillinases										
OXA-1	–	+/–	+	23.3	7.4	–	–	+	–	–
OXA-2	–	–	+	44.6	7.7	–	–	–	–	–
OXA-3	–	–	+	41.2	7.1	–	–	–	–	–
Carbenicillinases										
PSE-1	–	+		28.5	5.7	–	–	–	–	+
PSE-2	–	+	+	12.4	6.1		–		+	
PSE-3		–		12.0	6.9		–			
PSE-4	–	–		32.0	5.3	–	–	–	–	+

Table 3 Nomenclature of Plasmid-Determined Beta-Lactamases

Matthew	Mitsuhashi	Pitton	Labia and Philippon	Richmond and Sykes
TEM-1	Type Ia	Type I		IIIa
("Temoniera," a patient's name)				
TEM-2	Type Ib	Type I		IIIa
SHV-1		Type 2		
(sulfhydryl variable)				IV
HMS-1				
(Hedges, Matthew, and Smith)				
OXA-1	Type II			Va
(oxacillin hydrolyzing)				
OXA-2	Type III			Vb
OXA-3				V
PSE-1	Type IV		CARB-2	V
(*Pseudomonas* specific)				
PSE-2				V
PSE-3				V
PSE-4			CARB-I	V

The original source of the common abbreviations is also shown. Since the carbenicillin-hydrolyzing enzymes were originally found only in *Pseudomonas* species, they were designated as *Pseudomonas*-specific enzymes, or PSE; however, PSE-1 and PSE-2 have since been found in eight genera of Enterobacteriaceae (35–37) and, more recently, PSE-3 was found in strains of *Klebsiella* (38). Hence it is apparent that the PSE designation should be revised and a more logical nomenclature for these beta-lactamases is sorely needed.

D. Newly Discovered Beta-Lactamases

Several novel beta-lactamases determined by plasmids or transposons have been discovered in recent surveys of the types of beta-lactamases produced by clinical isolates (Table 4). Whether these novel beta-lactamases have a more recent origin or are newly detected because the sensitive technique of isoelectric focusing has been applied to isolates from previously unsampled geographical areas is not yet clear. Four new isolates have TEM-like substrate profiles, five are OXA-type beta-lactamases, four are carbenicillinases, and another preferentially hydrolyzes cephalosporins.

A survey of several hundred clinical isolates of ampicillin-resistant *E. coli* revealed the first of the novel TEM-like enzymes (39). *Escherichia coli* 7604 was one of 70 Brazilian strains studied. It produced two beta-lactamases: TEM-1 and another enzyme with a substrate profile and molecular weight similar to those of TEM-1 but with a different isoelectric point. The strain contained two plasmids, each of which determined a different beta-lactamase.

The second novel TEM-like beta-lactamase was found in *Hemophilus influenzae* ROB, a type b strain isolated from a child with meningitis (40). This strain produced a beta-lactamase which resembled TEM-1 but hydrolyzed carbenicillin at a slightly higher rate and cephaloridine at a lower rate relative to benzylpenicillin. *Escherichia coli* C600 was transformed to ampicillin resistance by plasmid DNA from *H. influenzae* ROB and shown by isoelectric focusing to synthesize the ROB beta-lactamase. Extracts of both the wild-type *Hemophilus* isolate and the *E. coli* transformant demonstrated an enzyme band at pI 8.1 and an unusual accumulation of activity remaining at the anodic loading site on the gel. This observation suggested that the enzyme was membrane bound or possibly a lipoprotein similar to the beta-lactamases of *Staph. aureus.* An additional strain of *H. influenzae* producing ROB-1 beta-lactamase was detected in a survey of 50 ampicillin-resistant clinical isolates from the United States (A. A. Medeiros and L. Rubin, unpublished observations).

Simpson et al. (41) identified a third TEM-like beta-lactamase encoded by an incompatibility group P-2 plasmid in a carbenicillin-resistant *Pseudomonas aeruginosa* burn isolate. Isoelectric focusing showed a single band nearly equidistant between those of PSE-1 and PSE-2, clearly distinguishing the LCR-1 beta-lactamase from TEM-1. The LCR-1 enzyme was similar in substrate profile to TEM-1 but had a slightly higher activity against methicillin.

A fourth broad-spectrum beta-lactamase has been identified in an environmental isolate of *Enterobacter cloacae* from a hospital in Cleveland, Ohio (D. Shlaes and A. A. Medeiros, unpublished observations). The OHIO-1 beta-lactamase has an isoelectric point of 7.0 and a substrate profile similar to that of TEM-1. Several clinical isolates of *Ent. cloacae* and *Enterobacter aerogenes* have since been found to produce the same beta-lactamase.

Four novel OXA-like beta-lactamases have been found: two among the *E. coli* isolates from Brazil and two in *P. aeruginosa* (42). An additional oxacillinase has been found in a strain of *Bacillus fragilis* isolated in Japan and shown to be transferable by mating (43). All five of these OXA-like beta-lactamases have distinct isoelectric points ranging from 6.9 to 7.68. The OXA-6 enzyme and the beta-lactamase from *B. fragilis* have molecular weights of 40,000 and 41,500, respectively, whereas the molecular weights of the other OXA-like enzymes range between 23,000 and 25,000.

Four novel beta-lactamases have been detected that preferentially hydrolyze carbenicillin and are determined by plasmids, transposons, or transposon-like elements. Labia et al. (44) studied a strain of *P. aeruginosa* that produced an enzyme termed CARB-3 with a substrate profile similar to those of PSE-1 and PSE-

Table 4 New Beta-Lactamases Determined by Plasmids or Transposons

Name	Original host	Origin	Plasmid	Phenotype[a]	Beta-lactamase substrate profile	Molecular weight (x 10^3)	pI
TLE-1	*Escherichia coli* 7604	Brazil	pMG204b	ApCmKmSmSu	TEM-like	19.8	5.55
ROB-1	*Hemophilus influenzae* Rob	Baltimore	R_{Rob}	Ap	TEM-like		8.1
LCR-1	*Pseudomonas aeruginosa* 2293E	London	pMG76	CbGmSmSuTmHgTer	TEM-like	44.0	6.5 (5.85)[b]
OHIO-1	*Enterobacter cloacae*	Cleveland	p075	ApGmKmTm	TEM-like		7.0
OXA-4	*Escherichia coli* 7259	Brazil	pMG203	ApCmSmSuTp	OXA-like	23.0	7.5
OXA-5	*Pseudomonas aeruginosa* 76072601	London	pMG54	CbGmSmSuTcTmHg	OXA-like	27.0	7.62
OXA-6	*Pseudomonas aeruginosa* Ming	Chicago	pMG39	CbGmKmSmSuTm	OXA-like	40.0	7.68
OXA-7	*Escherichia coli* 7181	Brazil	pMG202	ApCmGmKmSuTmHg	OXA-like	25.3	7.65

—[c]	*Bacillus fragilis* GN11499	Japan	—	ApTc	OXA-like	41.5	6.9
CARB-3	*Pseudomonas aeruginosa* Cilote	Paris	—	CbCmSmSu	PSE-like	31.0	5.75
—[c]	*Proteus mirabilis* N-3	Japan	pCS203	ApCmKmSmSuHg	PSE-like	24.0	6.0
—[c]	*Proteus mirabilis* N-29	Japan	pCS229	ApCmSmSuHg	PSE-like	22.0	6.9
AER-1	*Aeromonas hydrophila* VL 7711	India	—	CbCmSmSu	PSE-like	22.0	5.9
CEP-1	*Proteus mirabilis* 22	Greece	R22K	ApSm	Cephalosporinase	37.5	8.0
CEP-2	*Achromobacter* MULB 912	Quebec	pLQ3	Ap	Cephalosporinase	36.2	8.1

[a]Resistance abbreviations: Ap = ampicillin, Cb = carbenicillin, Gm = gentamicin, Hg = mecuric chloride, Km = kanamycin, Sm = streptomycin, Su = sulfonamide, Tc = tetracycline, Ter = potassium tellurite, Tm = tobramycin, Tp = trimethoprim.
[b]The pI value in parentheses was obtained in our laboratory under experimental conditions different from those of Simpson et al. (41).
[c]Not yet named.

4, but with a higher molecular weight and distinct isoelectric point (5.75). Antisera to CARB-3 inactivated PSE-1 and PSE-4, indicating an immunological relationship as well between these enzymes. The CARB-3 gene is carried on a transposon, and the *Pseudomonas* strain producing the enzyme contains plasmid DNA, but whether the gene for CARB-3 has a plasmid or chromosomal location is not yet known (G. A. Jacoby and A. Philippon, unpublished observations). Takahashi et al. (45) have described two novel carbenicillin-hydrolyzing beta-lactamases in strains of *Proteus mirabilis* that are plasmid mediated. These enzymes, which have not yet been named, have substrate profiles and molecular weights similar to those of PSE-1 and PSE-4, cross-react immunologically with each other and these PSE beta-lactamases, but have distinct isoelectric points at 6.0 and 6.9. Another carbenicillin-hydrolyzing beta-lactamase designated AER-1 has been found in *Aeromonas hydrophila.* The parent strain produced several beta-lactamase bands on isoelectric focusing, but only a single enzyme with an isoelectric point of 5.9 was transferred to *E. coli* by mating when a conjugative plasmid was introduced into the *Aeromonas* host (45a).

There have been two reports of plasmid-determined beta-lactamases with predominant cephalosporin activity. Bobrowski et al. (46) described a plasmid originating in *Prot. mirabilis* that appeared to produce a beta-lactamase identical in enzymological and immunological properties to the chromosomal enzyme of *E. coli* K-12. Levesque et al. (47,48) have described a cephalosporinase determined by a plasmid from *Achromobacter*. This enzyme, which has been termed CEP-2 to indicate a relationship to the *Proteus* cephalosporinase or CEP-1, differed from CEP-1 in its ability to hydrolyze carbenicillin and its resistance to cloxacillin inhibition.

Murray and Mederski-Samoraj (16) described a clinical isolate of enterococcus which produced a beta-lactamase that cotransferred with gentamicin resistance. This is the first report of beta-lactamase transfer among streptococci. By isoelectric focusing in polyacrylamide gel the enterococcal beta-lactamase produces a nondescript blur at the anodic loading site, similar to that seen with staphylococcal beta-lactamase (A. A. Medeiros, unpublished observations).

III. PLASMIDS AND TRANSPOSONS DETERMINING BETA-LACTAMASES

The distribution of beta-lactamases on different plasmid types has been investigated in both enterobacteria and *P. aeruginosa* (26,49,50). In general, those beta-lactamases that are found in a variety of bacterial hosts are also found on many plasmid types, and the properties of the plasmids involved can, in some cases at least, account for the distribution of certain beta-lactamases to particular bacterial species.

The R plasmids are classified into groups by the property of incompatibility. Compatible plasmids can coexist in the same cell while incompatible plasmids cannot (51). Although only a relatively small portion of the plasmid genome determines incompatibility specificity, plasmids of the same incompatibility group usually share a number of other biological properties and considerable overall DNA homology (52). The properties most relevant to explain beta-lactamase gene distribution are plasmid host range and self-transmissibility by conjugation.

Conjugative plasmids are found in both gram-positive and gram-negative bacteria. With very few exceptions, there is an absolute barrier to plasmid transfer between these two bacterial groups. Similarly, little if any plasmid transfer occurs between facultative and strictly anaerobic gram-negative organisms. Hence it is not surprising that distinct beta-lactamases are found in gram-positive and gram-negative organisms and that different beta-lactamases occur in *Bacteroides* than in facultative enteric organisms.

Among the plasmids found in facultative and aerobic gram-negative rods, some have a broad host range while others are restricted to a particular genus (53–55). The broad host range plasmids can be considered as shuttle vectors capable of spreading beta-lactamase and other resistance mechanisms promiscuously, while a beta-lactamase specified by a nonconjugative or narrow host range plasmid may be contained within a particular species unless it can transpose to another plasmid vector.

Matthew has published the distribution of the 11 plasmid-mediated beta-lactamases known in 1979 on 363 plasmids found in gram-negative bacteria (26). A total of 62% specified TEM-1 and 15.4% TEM-2 beta-lactamase. TEM-1 was produced by plasmids belonging to at least 18 incompatibility groups, and TEM-2 was determined by at least 7 incompatibility types. OXA-1 beta-lactamase was the next most common, being determined by 8.8% of the plasmids. OXA-2 followed at 4.7%, SHV-1 at 4.1%, and OXA-3 at 1.9%. Only one plasmid was known to code for HMS-1 and only a few *Pseudomonas* plasmids specified PSE-type enzymes. The plasmids determining PSE beta-lactamases were either of limited host range or non-self-transmissible, perhaps accounting for the distribution of these enzymes to *Pseudomonas* (50).

The properties of the plasmid vectors, however, are only part of the explanation for distribution of resistance genes. Many resistance determinants are specified by segments of DNA that can transpose from one DNA site to another. Hedges and Jacob, who discovered the transposability of the TEM-2 beta-lactamase gene, coined the name *transposon* for such units (6). Transposons determining TEM-2 and TEM-1 have been intensively studied (56,57). They are very similar 5-kilobase (kb) units that contain three sites and two genes essential for transposition (58). Two essential sites are 38 base pair sequences of DNA that occur at the ends of the unit in inverse orientation while a third internal site is involved in the resolution of cointegrate intermediates in the transposition process. The essential genes are *tnpA*, a gene determining the enzyme transposase involved in replicative recombination, and *tnpR,* the gene determining a product that both regulates *tnpA* expression and resolves cointegrate intermediates.

An important feature of transposition is that replication accompanies transposition so that integration at a new site is not accompanied by loss of the transposon from the original site. Another feature is that transposition is independent of the host cell's machinery for homologous or *recA*-dependent recombination. Tn*3* determining TEM-1 shows a regional specificity for adenine- and thymine-rich sites in target DNA but generally finds many suitable insertion sites in a target molecule.

Tn*1* (specifying TEM-2) and Tn*3* are very similar transposons, differing only in a few restriction endonuclease recognition sites and possessing 85% overall DNA homology (59). Presumably, after the beta-lactamase gene was incorporated into a transposon, mutation led to the change in isoelectric point that distinguished the two enzymes. Incorporation into a transposable unit accounts for the distribution of TEM-1 on plasmids of so many different incompatibility groups and also for the spread of TEM-1 to plasmids of *H. influenzae, Neisseria gonorrhoeae*, and *Hemophilus ducreyi.*

In *H. influenzae* TEM-1 production is determined by 30- to 38-megadalton (Md) conjugative plasmids that contain all of Tn*3* in transposable form and by 4- to 5-Md transfer-deficient plasmids that carry only a portion of Tn*3* (60). Penicillin-resistant gonococci from Europe and Africa generally contain a 3.2- to 3.4-Md beta-lactamase plasmid, while resistant strains from the United States and Asia usually contain a 4.7- to 5.8-Md beta-lactamase plasmid (61). Both of these types of plasmids carry only part of Tn*3* and are transfer deficient but can be mobilized for transfer by a coexisting 24-Md conjugative plasmid. *Hemophilus ducreyi* resistant to penicillin contains transfer-deficient plasmids of 5.7 or 7.0–7.4 Md. These plasmids are identical to the two types of beta-lactamase plasmids found in *N. gonorrhoeae*, except that they carry complete Tn*3* sequences (62). A few strains of *H. ducreyi* contain a 3.6-Md beta-lactamase plasmid with only part of Tn*3* (63). Not only are the plasmids of the two *Hemophilus* species related, but beta-lactamase plasmids from *N. gonorrhoeae* and *H. influenzae* have 85% or more base sequence homology; suggesting a common evolutionary origin (64).

TEM-1 is also specified by a larger 24-kb transposon, Tn*4*, which carries resistance to streptomycin (Sm), spectinomycin (Sp), and sulfonamide (Su) as well (Table 5). Tn*4* can transpose as a unit or the TEM-1 gene can transpose independently of the other resistances as Tn*3* (65). Tn*4* thus consists of Tn*3* inserted into an SmSpSu transposon. Tn*21* is such a unit, a 20-kb transposon specifying SmSpSu and mercuric ion (Hg) resistance which is closely related to Tn*4*. In fact, Tn*4* can be thought of as arising from Tn*21* by insertion of Tn*3* into the Hg resistance gene inactivating its expression. The inverted repeats at the ends of

Table 5 Beta-Lactamase Transposons

Transposon	Beta-lactamase	Origin	Phenotype	Size (kb)	Reference
Tn*1*	TEM-2	*Pseudomonas aeruginosa*	Ap	5	6
Tn*3*	TEM-1	*Salmonella paratyphi* B	Ap	5	65
Tn*4*	TEM-1	*Salmonella paratyphi* B	ApSmSpSu	24	65
Tn*A*	TEM-1	*Serratia marcescens*	ApSm	14.3	125
Tn*1699*	TEM-1	*Serratia marcescens*	ApGmKm	9.3	126
Tn*1700*	TEM-1	*Serratia marcescens*	ApGmKmTm	9.3	126
—[a]	SHV-1	*Proteus mirabilis*	Ap	14.3	99
Tn*2603*	OXA-1	*Escherichia coli*	ApSmSpSuHg	20	127
Tn*2410*	OXA-2	*Salmonella typhimurium*	ApSuHg	18.5	69
Tn*1401*	PSE-1	*Salmonella typhimurium*	ApSmSpSuHg	12	35
Tn*1403*	PSE-1	*Pseudomonas aeruginosa*	ApCmSmSp	18	35
Tn*1404*	PSE-2	*Pseudomonas aeruginosa*	ApGmKmSmSp SuTm	9.6	128
Tn*2521*	PSE-4	*Pseudomonas aeruginosa*	ApSmSpSu	6.8	72
Tn*2610*	PSE-like	*Escherichia coli*	ApSmSu	24	70
Tn*798*	AER-1	*Aeromonas hydrophila*	ApCmSmSpSu		45a

[a]Tn number not assigned.

Tn*4* and Tn*21* are identical and are related to the inverted repeats of Tn*3* but differ in about half of the 38 nucleotides (66). Tn*4* and Tn*21* have *tnpA* and *tnpR* genes that are functionally interchangeable with each other but not with those of Tn*3* (67). Thus Tn*4* and Tn*21* are members of the Tn*3* family of transposons in overall organization but have evolved their own specificity.

Table 5 lists other beta-lactamase types that have been shown to be transposable. All the beta-lactamase transposons except Tn*1*, Tn*3*, and the transposon for SHV-1 carry genes for resistance to compounds other than beta-lactams. Furtermore, the linked resistances are strikingly similar, usually involving Sm and Sp (determined by a single adenyltransferase gene) and Su, with resistance to chloramphenicol, gentamicin, kanamycin, tobramycin, and Hg associated less commonly. Tn*2603*, which determines OXA-1 beta-lactamase and resistance to SmSpSuHg, is organized very much like Tn*21* and Tn*4* (68) and has a functionally similar *tnpR* gene (G. A. Jacoby and R. Levesque, unpublished observations). However, in Tn*2603* the OXA-1 beta-lactamase gene is not independently transposable and is found near *tnpR* rather than in the Hg resistance gene. The beta-lactamase gene is similarly located in Tn*2410* specifying OXA-2 (69), in Tn*1401* specifying PSE-1 (G. A. Jacoby and R. Levesque, unpublished observations), and in Tn*2610* determining another PSE-type enzyme (70). How the various beta-lactamase genes become incorporated into multiresistance transposons is not presently known. A site near *tnpR* could be a hot spot for DNA insertion. Alternatively, evolution could have operated on a primitive multiresistance unit so as to alter the properties of the beta-lactamase gene while maintaining its linkage to other resistance determinants that are common to the various transposons.

The transposability of the genes for various beta-lactamases helps explain their distribution on various plasmids. Since the frequency of transposition decreases with transposon size (71), all of the units larger than Tn*1* and Tn*3* may pay a price for their size in terms of diminished transposability. However, a larger size allows resistance to multiple antibiotics to be incorporated into the same package so that beta-lactam and aminoglycoside resistance, for example, can spread as a unit with selection for resistance to either class of antibiotic promoting the spread of resistance to the other.

Typically transposons can integrate into any replicon, whether plasmid, bacteriophage, or chromosomal DNA. Tn*2521*, determining PSE-4, is unusual in that it is found naturally in the chromosome of resistance *P. aeruginosa* isolates at a particular site, although it can transpose to a plasmid location (72). Ω7711, determining AER-1, also has a unique chromosomal site on transfer to *E. coli* and, although it can be mobilized for transfer by a conjugative plasmid, it has not been shown to integrate into plasmid DNA (45a). The resistances carried by Ω7711 are common to other multiresistance beta-lactamase transposons. Ω7711 can thus be considered a defective transposon. Such units may be fairly common. For example, many plasmids determining OXA-2, although they specify the other resistance of Tn*2410*, fail to transpose beta-lactamase production (G. A. Jacoby, unpublished observations). Just as addition and deletion of DNA may be invoked to explain the evolution of multiresistance transposons, if such events involve sites or genes essential for transposition, transposability can be lost. This process has occurred with 4.4-Md *H. influenzae* beta-lactamase plasmids, where only one of the essential terminal inverted repeat segments of Tn*3* has been retained (64).

IV. DISTRIBUTION IN CLINICAL ISOLATES

The existence of beta-lactamase genes on plasmids and transposons ensures that a beta-lactamase originally confined to one group of bacteria may sooner or later appear in other groups. Widespread use of antibiotics fosters selection of the resistant organisms that rise in prevalence locally and then spread worldwide. A prime example of this process occurred with the TEM-1 beta-lactamase common in enterobacteria. In 1974 strains of *H. influenzae* producing TEM-1 were first discovered in the United States. Rare at first, they have since reached a prevalence of 38% in some regions (73). In 1976 strains of *N. gonorrhoeae*- producing the plasmid-determined TEM-1 beta-lactamase appeared in England and 1 year later in the United States (61,74). At first most of the cases were importations from Africa and the Far East, but eventually major outbreaks due to endemic transmission occurred in metropolitan areas. The incidence in the United States rose from 328 cases in 1979 to 3424 cases reported in the first 9 months of 1982, while similar increases in incidence occurred in other countries (75). Recently, a beta-lactamase-producing strain of *Neisseria meningitidis* carrying a 4.5-md plasmid identical to one found in Far Eastern strains of penicillinase-producing *N. gonorrhoeae* was isolated from a mixed culture of a patient in Canada. It is believed that the isolate originated in the genitourinary tract and acquired the plasmid by transfer in vivo from a strain of penicillinase-producing *N. gonorrhoeae* (76).

The distribution of plasmid-determined beta-lactamases, as determined by isoelectric focusing, is summarized in Table 6. The data are a composite of results previously reported by Matthew (26) combined with our own results on several hundred clinical isolates and other reports (39,77–79a). The largest number of different types of beta-lactamases were found in *P. aeruginosa* (12), *E. coli* (11), and *Prot. mirabilis* (9), followed by *Klebsiella* (8), *Salmonella* (5), and *Providencia* (5) species.

In addition to the novel beta-lactamases, new findings include OXA-2 in *P. aeruginosa*, HMS-1 in *Klebsiella* and *Citrobacter*, and the detection of PSE-1, PSE-2, and PSE-3 in Enterobacteriaceae. PSE-1 production has been detected in *E. coli* (35), *Prot. mirabilis* (36), various *Salmonella* species (35), and *Shigella sonnei* (35), while PSE-2 has been found in *E. coli, Ent. cloacae, Klebsiella pneumoniae,* and *Providencia stuartii* (37), and PSE-3 in *Klebsiella* (38). The occurrence of "*Pseudomonas*-specific" enzymes in these enterobacteria emphasize the danger of designating a beta-lactamase type as species specific. Genes for these PSE beta-lactamases are found on transposons (Table 5), which permit

Table 6 Distribution in Gram-Negative Bacilli of Plasmid-Determined Beta-Lactamases (Species Producing Two or More Types of Beta-Lactamase)

	TEM-1	TEM-2	SHV-1	HMS-1	OXA-1	OXA-2	OXA-3	PSE-1	PSE-2	PSE-3	PSE-4	Novel	Total
Pseudomonas aeruginosa	+	+				+	+	+	+	+	+	LCR-1, OXA-4, OXA-5, OXA-6	12
Escherichia coli	+	+	+		+	+	+	+	+			TLE-1, OXA-4, OXA-7	11
Proteus mirabilis	+	+	+	+	+	+		+				Enzymes specified by strains N-3 and N-29	9
Klebsiella sp.	+	+	+	+	+		+		+	+			8
Salmonella sp.	+		+		+	+		+					5
Providencia sp.	+	+			+		+		+				5
Proteus (indole positive)	+	+	+						+				4
Enterobacter sp.	+				+				+				3
Shigella sp.	+	+						+					3
Citrobacter sp.	+	+		+									3
Hemophilus influenzae	+											ROB-1	2
Morganella sp.	+				+								2
Serratia sp.	+					+							2

their spread to various plasmid types in bacterial hosts different from those in which they were originally detected.

The rarest of the well-established beta-lactamases is HMS-1; which has been found in only three isolates, a *Prot. mirabilis* (27), a *Klebsiella*, and a *Citrobacter* (79a). The most common, on the other hand, is TEM-1, which occurred with an overall frequency of 62% among strains studied by Matthew (26). Table 7 shows the beta-lactamases found in surveys of isolates of ampicillin-resistant *E. coli* from different countries. Most were random samplings of clinical isolates, except for those from Indonesia and Thailand (enteropathogenic strains) and England (urinary isolates) (79). Overall, 76% produced TEM-1, whereas 8% produced OXA-1. A total of 11% produced only chromosomal beta-lactamase. The Brazilian collection was extraordinary in that three novel beta-lactamases and PSE-1 were found. It is curious also that no Brazilian strains had resistance due to chromosomal beta-lactamase, which was also true of the strains from Indonesia, Thailand, and Spain. In contrast, a high percentage of isolates from South Africa produced only chromosomal-type beta-lactamase. These data suggest that the distribution of beta-lactamase types within a particular species is not homogeneous worldwide, although certain overall patterns are apparent.

In other species TEM-1 is not the most prevalent beta-lactamase. Marre found that all of 16 ampicillin-resistant strains of *Prot. mirabilis* isolated in Germany produced TEM-2 (R. Marre, personal communication). Philippon et al., on the other hand, found that of 1400 carbenicillin-resistant *Pseudomonas* strains isolated in Paris, 51% produced PSE-1, 30% OXA-2, 7% OXA-1, and 5% TEM-1 (80). In another region of France, Jouvenot et al. (81) found that 70% of carbenicillin-resistant isolates of *P. aeruginosa* produced PSE-1. The extent to which these distributions represent the continued recirculation of a single resistant strain within a particular geographical region is unknown. However, the frequency of PSE-1 in clinical isolates of *P. aeruginosa* is much greater than its frequency on carbenicillin resistance plasmids in this organism (50), which suggests that in many strains the PSE-1 gene has a chromosomal location.

There is evidence, also, that beta-lactamase genes may circulate between animal and human isolates (Table 8). In a study of 113 human and 146 animal isolates of ampicillin-resistant salmonellae from the United States, 81 and 77% of human and animal isolates, respectively, produced TEM-1, similar to results with *E. coli* (78) (A. A. Medeiros and T. F. O'Brien, unpublished observations). However, the second most common beta-lactamase in both human and animal isolates was OXA-2, an uncommon type in *E. coli.* Moreover, most of the isolates producing OXA-2 belonged to a relatively rare serotype, *Salmonella typhimurium* var. *Copenhagen*. This unexpected association in both human and animal isolates suggested that they shared the same resistance determinants. Indeed, endonuclease digests of plasmids from animal and human isolates from different regions of the United States were often identical (82).

Table 7 Types of Beta-Lactamases in Clinical Isolates of Ampicillin-Resistant *E. coli* from Different Regions

Geographical origin	Number tested	Chromosomal only	Beta-lactamase type								
			TEM-1	OXA-1	SHV-1	OXA-2	PSE-1	Novel	TEM-1 + PSE-1	TEM-1 + OXA-1	TEM-1 + novel
Brazil	98	0	71 (72)[a]	10 (10)	6		2	3	2	3	1[b]
Providence	50	6 (12)	41 (82)	2 (4)		1					
Paris	21	3 (14)	16 (76)			2					
Indonesia	11	0	9 (82)	1 (9)			1				
South Africa	47	16 (34)	23 (49)	5 (11)						3	
Boston	34	6 (18)	27 (79)	1 (11)							
Bangkok	29	0	27 (93)						1	1	
England[c]	110	18 (16)	73 (66)	17 (16)	1					1	
Germany[d]	84	13 (16)	62 (74)	8 (10)	1						
Spain[e]	90	0	86 (96)	2 (2)						1	1[f]
Total	574 (100)	64 (11)	435 (76)	46 (8)	8 (1)	3	3	3	3	9 (2)	2

[a]Percent of total in parentheses.
[b]TLE-1.
[c]See Ref. 79.
[d]R. Marre, personal communication.
[e]See Ref. 38.
[f]An uncharacterized beta-lactamase of pI 5.2.

Table 8 Types of Beta-Lactamase in 113 Human and 146 Animal Isolates of Ampicillin-Resistant Salmonellae from the United States

	Beta-lactamase type									
	TEM-1		OXA-2		OXA-1		TEM-1 + PSE-1		TEM-1 + OXA-1	
Serotype	Human	Animal	Human	Animal	Human	Animal	Human	Animal	Human	Animal
S. typhimurium	33	34	4	16	0	2	0	0	0	0
S. typhimurium var. *Copenhagen*	3	6	11	9	0	0	0	0	0	0
Other serotypes	55	72	3	7	1	0	1	0	2	0
Total	91 (81)[a]	112 (77)	18 (16)	32 (22)	1	2	1	0	2	0

[a]Percent total in parentheses.

Table 9 Isolates Producing Multiple Plasmid-Determined Beta-Lactamases

Beta-lactamase type	Species	Origin	Number of isolates
TEM-1 + OXA-1	*E. coli*	Spain	
	E. coli	Thailand	1
	E. coli	Brazil	3
	E. coli	South Africa	3
	Prot. mirabilis		1
	S. St. Paul	United States	1
TEM-1 + OXA-2	*Serratia* sp.	Spain	
	E. coli	Paris	1
	Prov. stuartii	Argentina	1
	S. typhimurium var. *Copenhagen*	United States	1
TEM-1 + OXA-3	*K. pneumoniae*	Boston	1
TEM-1 + PSE-1	*P. aeruginosa*	Boston	1
	Sh. sonnei	Canada	1
	E. coli	Brazil	2
	E. coli	Thailand	1
	S. heidelberg	United States	1
	S. johannesberg	Hong Kong	1
TEM-1 + SHV-1	*Morganella morganii*	England	1
	K. pneumoniae	Boston	1
TEM-1 + TLE-1	*E. coli*	Brazil	1
OXA-2 + PSE-1	*P. aeruginosa*	Boston	4
TEM-1 + OXA-2 + PSE-1	*P. aeruginosa*	Boston	1
TEM-1 + TEM-2	*Klebsiella* sp.	Spain	1
TEM-1 + PSE-3	*Klebsiella* sp.	Spain	1

The prevalence of different beta-lactamases can be expected to vary in time and place when strains become epidemic. Ampicillin-resistant strains of *S. typhimurium, Salmonella typhi,* and *Salmonella wien* which caused large-scale epidemics of salmonellosis in Europe, Africa, and the Middle East were found to produce OXA-1, whereas *Salmonella ordonnez*, which was epidemic in Africa, produced the SHV-1 beta-lactamase (A. A. Medeiros and J. Threlfall, unpublished observations).

Table 9 lists isolates producing two and, in one instance, three plasmid-determined beta-lactamases. In all but one case TEM-1 was one of the beta-lactamases produced. The strain of *P. aeruginosa* that produced OXA-2 plus PSE-1 as well as the single isolate that also produced TEM-1 came from an outbreak of infections in a children's hospital in Boston. Interestingly, a single plasmid (pMG209) found in a Brazilian strain of *E. coli* carried both the TEM-1 and PSE-1 genes (35). The high proportion of strains from South America and the Far East that were found to produce two plasmid-mediated beta-lactamases or which had novel plasmid-mediated beta-lactamases suggests that the bacterial flora of these regions provides fertile ground for cultivating new resistance genes and combinations of resistance.

V. BETA-LACTAMASES DETERMINED BY CHROMOSOMAL GENES

Matthew and Harris (15) found that virtually all gram-negative bacteria produce some chromosomally determined beta-lactamase and that the types of beta-lactamase produced are often specific for species and sometimes for subspecies (83, 84). The amount of beta-lactamase activity is frequently very low, particularly in ampicillin-susceptible isolates, but may increase owing to induction or to alterations in the number of beta-lactamase genes on the chromosome or their regulation (85,86). These genetic alterations are often accompanied by resistance to beta-lactam antibiotics.

Most of the chromosomally determined beta-lactamases preferentially hydrolyze cephalosporins, including many of the compounds that are resistant to hydrolysis by the plasmid-determined beta-lactamases (Table 10). Sawai (87) described two major groups: (1) cephalosporinases with broad substrate specificity that hydrolyze benzylpenicillin, ampicillin, and carbenicillin as well as cephalosporins, and (2) "typical cephalosporinases" that have little or no activity against these penicillins.

A prototypic enzyme of the first group is the inducible beta-lactamase produced by *Proteus vulgaris*. Another important broad-spectrum enzyme is that produced by *K. pneumoniae*, which some classify as a "penicillinase." Indole-positive strains of *Klebsiella* have been described that have activity against cefuroxime and monobactam, that is, *Klebsiella aerogenes* K1 (88) and *Klebsiella oxytoca* (89). Gentamicin-resistant strains of the latter species caused an outbreak in a Liverpool hospital (89). One of the isolates from that outbreak, *K. oxytoca* strain 3859, produces a beta-lactamase active against moxalactam and ceftazidime as well as cefuroxime.

Beta-lactamases of many species comprise the second group. They are the constitutive enzymes produced by *B. fragilis, Citrobacter freundii, Ent. cloacae, E. coli,* and *Morganella morganii.* Inducible enzymes produced by *Acinetobacter calcoaceticus, Ent. aerogenes, Ent. cloacae, Providencia rettgeri, P. aeruginosa,* and *Serratia marcescens* also belong to this latter category. As newer beta-lactam antibiotics have become available, their interaction with beta-lactamases has led to further classification schemes. Thus Mitsuhashi classifies the beta-lactamases

Table 10 Some Beta-Lactamases That Hydrolyze the Newer Beta-Lactam Antibiotics

Antibiotic	Beta-lactamase type: Chromosomal	Plasmid
Cefuroxime or cefotaxime	*Prot. cepacia* GN11164 (93)[a]	OXA-1
	Prot. vulgaris GN7919 (94)	OXA-4
	B. fragilis MULB-1008 (95)	OXA-5
	K. oxytoca R30 (96)	OXA-6
	K. aerogenes K1 (88)	OXA-7
		PSE-1
	Prot. vulgaris 85 (97)	PSE-2
Ceftazidime		OXA-1
		OXA-2
Moxalactam	*K. oxytoca* 3859 (89)	OXA-4
		OXA-5
		PSE-2
		PSE-3
Monobactam	*K. oxytoca* 3859 (89)	
	K. aerogenes K1 (98)	
Imipenem	*P. maltophilia* GN12873 (91)	
	B. fragilis G-237 (92)	

[a]Reference.

of *Pseudomonas cepacia, Prot. vulgaris*, and *B. fragilis* as cefuroximases, while Labia divides the beta-lactamases into groups based on their affinity for moxalactam and the degree to which they are inactivated by it (90). There is a serious need to establish a reference collection of strains producing defined chromosomal beta-lactamases similar to that provided by Matthew for plasmid-determined enzymes.

Saino et al. (91) have found a novel beta-lactamase in *Pseudomonas maltophilia* GN 12873 that destroys imipenem. Also, Yotsuji et al. (92) purified a beta-lactamase from *B. fragilis* G-237 that hydrolyzes most of the cephalosporins, including the cephamycins, penicillins, and imipenem at a high rate. Thus it appears likely that no class of beta-lactam antibiotic escapes attack by some beta-lactamase. Table 10 lists beta-lactamases, both chromosomally and plasmid mediated, which hydrolyze newer beta-lactam antibiotics. Strains producing both plasmid- and chromosomally determined enzymes pose a potentially serious threat.

None of these chromosomally determined beta-lactamases, with one exception, are identical in their biochemical properties to the plasmid-determined enzymes. The exception is a chromosomal beta-lactamase found in many isolates of *K. pneumoniae* that is indistinguishable by kinetic analysis and isoelectric focusing from the SHV-1 beta-lactamase. Nugent and Hedges (99) found that a *K. pneumoniae* strain carried two copies of the SHV-1 structural gene, one on a plasmid and another on a nontransmissible replicon, probably the bacterial chromosome. They suggest that the SHV-1 beta-lactamase gene evolved as a chromosomal gene in *Klebsiella* and was later incorporated into a plasmid. As yet no such ancestral chromosomal gene has been found for the much more common TEM-1 beta-lactamase or for any of the other plasmid-determined beta-lactamases. Thus the origins of most of the plasmid-determined beta-lactamases remain unknown.

There is evidence, also, that the chromosomal beta-lactamases of ampicillin-resistant *E. coli* may have been acquired through interspecies transfer. Olsson et al. (99a) found that five of six ampicillin-resistant clinical isolates of *E. coli* hyperproduced a chromosomal *ampC* beta-lactamase that had a DNA sequence identical to that of the beta-lactamase produced in low levels by a clinical isolate of *Sh. sonnei.* They postulate that transfer of chromosomal DNA from *Shigella* to *E. coli* occurred in vivo and a one-step promoter mutation produced ampicillin resistance in these strains of *E. coli.*

VI. CONTRIBUTION OF BETA-LACTAMASES TO BETA-LACTAM ANTIBIOTIC RESISTANCE

Several parameters contribute to the level of antibiotic resistance mediated by a particular beta-lactamase in a population of bacteria. The efficiency of the beta-lactamase in hydrolyzing an antibiotic depends both on its rate of hydrolysis (V_{max}), conveniently expressed as a ratio relative to benzylpenicillin or cephaloridine, and its affinity for the antibiotic (K_m), a value often difficult to obtain with substrates that are weakly hydrolyzed. Another variable is the amount of beta-lactamase produced by the bacterial cell. Since the amount may vary with phase of cell growth or even conditions of incubation (86), a single value may be misleading. An example is J53(R997), an *E. coli* K12 strain which produces the plasmid-determined HMS-1 beta-lactamase. The strain is highly resistant to ampicillin, yet we could find barely detectable levels of beta-lactamase activity in sonic extracts of cells grown overnight. Extracts of cells in log phase, however, unexpectedly yielded values 100 times greater (100).

Within the bacterial cell, beta-lactamases contribute to antibiotic resistance in several ways. The simplest model is that of penicillinase-producing staphylococci, in which the bacteria, upon exposure to penicillin, begin to produce beta-lactamase which they excrete into the media. Two events then take place concurrently: (1) Penicillin lyses bacteria and (2) beta-lactamase hydrolyzes penicillin. If viable bacterial cells remain after the level of penicillin has fallen below the minimal inhibitory concentration, regrowth of bacteria occurs (101).

The second model shows a similar kinetic effect. It is exemplified by gram-negative bacilli which (1) produce a beta-lactamase that remains trapped in the periplasmic space and (2) have no barrier to antibiotic penetration. An example is *H. influenzae* strains that produce the TEM-1 beta-lactamase (102). In both this model and the first one discussed, a marked inoculum effect occurs, in that the minimal inhibitory concentration for a large inoculum (10^6 organisms/ml) may be 1000-fold greater than with a small inoculum (10^2 organisms/ml). The low level of resistance of single cells has made it possible for ampicillin to cure some infections caused by beta-lactamase-producing strains of *H. influenzae* when the inoculum of infecting bacteria was low (103,104).

The third model is exemplified by resistance to ampicillin of *E. coli* strains that produce the TEM-1 beta-lactamase. These bacteria have a barrier to entry of beta-lactam molecules (the outer membrane) and they produce a beta-lactamase that remains localized to the periplasmic space. In this model the kinetics are more complicated. The enzyme is strategically situated between the barrier to antibiotic penetration (outer membrane) and the antibiotic targets (penicillin-binding proteins on the cytoplasmic membrane). In this position the enzyme can sequentially destroy antibiotic molecules as they make their way through the barrier, analogous to a sharpshooter with abundant ammunition who aims at targets passing through a single entry point. As a consequence, high levels of resistance occur with single bacterial cells, unlike the previous example (101,105, 106).

Variations on this model may occur when the amount of beta-lactamase produced increases with exposure to a beta-lactam (induction) as occurs in *Enterobacter* and *Pseudomonas* species. High levels of beta-lactamase are produced only after a period of exposure to the inducing antibiotic, and hence resistance may be expressed late. This situation sometimes causes a problem for the clinical microbiologist, in that the disk susceptibility test may falsely indicate susceptibility. An example occurs with disk testing of susceptibility to cefamandole for *Enterobacter* strains, which appear falsely susceptible unless preincubated with cefamandole prior to testing. A further problem arises when *Enterobacter* strains are exposed to two beta-lactam antibiotics, one of which is a potent inducer (e.g., cefoxitin) of a beta-lactamase highly active against the other (e.g., cefamandole). Antagonism between the two antibiotics results (107).

One of the more puzzling aspects of this antagonism, however, is that for some antibiotics the induced enzyme hydrolyzes the "antagonized" antibiotic (e.g., carbenicillin) poorly or not at all. It has been postulated that the beta-lactamases protect the cell by binding rather than cleaving the antibiotic, acting in a sense as periplasmic sponges that prevent the antibiotic from reaching its target sites on the inner plasma membrane (108–110). However, not all antibiotics (e.g., imipenem) that bind tightly to the induced *Enterobacter* beta-lactamase are antagonized (111), which suggests that additional mechanisms may be operative.

Documented treatment failures due to emergence of resistance during therapy were rare prior to the use of third-generation cephalosporins (112). Recently such reports have increased, mainly in patients treated with cefamandole, cefoxitin, cefotaxime, moxalactam, ceftazidime, and ceftriaxone for infections due to *Enterbacter, Serratia*, and *Pseudomonas* species (113–116). A disturbing feature of some of these reports is that the strains isolated during therapy with one cephalosporin have decreased susceptibility to other cephalosporins, such as moxalactam, cefamandole, cefotaxime, and cefoperazone (117). Studies of treatment failures due to emergence of resistance in *Enterobacter* during cefamandole therapy have shown that the resistant strains produce increased amounts of beta-lactamase (118), probably owing to mutation in the locus regulating beta-lactamase expression (119). Increase in the production of chromosomal beta-lactamase has been found also in strains of *E. coli* isolated from patients who failed treatment with cephalothin (120) and ampicillin (121).

Acquired resistance to cephalosporins has been found also in a strain of *S. typhimurium* isolated from a patient during treatment with cephalexin, in which the resistant isolate had acquired a permeability barrier to cephalosporins but showed no increase in beta-lactamase production. Production of outer membrane porins, which beta-lactam antibiotics permeate, was almost completely repressed in the resistant mutant, thus providing an example of another type of resistance mechanism acquired during therapy (122,123). Goldstein et al. have described emergence of simultaneous resistance to both beta-lactam and aminoglycoside antibiotics in a strain of *Ser. marcescens*, associated with a change in outer membrane proteins (124). The potential threat of selecting resistant strains during therapy with the newer beta-lactam antibiotics has led some clinicians to recommend combined therapy with aminoglycosides, especially in treating *Enterobacter, Serratia,* and *Pseudomonas* infections.

REFERENCES

1. A. A. Medeiros. Beta-lactamases. *Br. Med. Bull., 40*:18–27 (1984).
2. E. P. Abraham and E. Chain. An enzyme from bacteria able to destroy penicillin. *Nature, 373*:837 (1940).
3. W. M. M. Kirby. Extraction of a highly potent penicillin inactivator from penicillin. *Science, 99*:452–453 (1944).
4. M. Matthew, A. M. Harris, M. J. Marshall, and G. W. Ross. The use of analytical isoelectric focusing for detection and identification of β-lactamases. *J. Gen. Microbiol., 88*:169–178 (1975).

5. N. Datta and P. Kontomichalou. Penicillinase synthesis controlled by infectious R-factors in Enterobacteriaceae. *Nature, 208*:239–241 (1965).
6. R. W. Hedges and A. E. Jacob. Transposition of ampicillin resistance from RP4 to other replicons. *Mol. Gen. Genet., 132*:31–40 (1974).
7. A. G. Brown. β-Lactam nomenclature. *J. Antimicrob. Chemother., 10*:365–372 (1974).
8. M. H. Richmond. Wild-type variants of exopenicillase from *Staphylococcus aureus. Biochem. J., 94*:584–593 (1965).
9. V. T. Rosdahl. Naturally occurring constitutive β-lactamase of novel serotype in staphylococcus aureus. *J. Gen. Microbiol., 77*:229–231 (1973).
10. K. G. H. Dyke. β-Lactamases of *Staphylococcus aureus,* in *Beta-Lactamases* (J. M. T. Hamilton-Miller and J. T. Smith, eds.), Academic, London, 1979, pp. 291–310.
11. R. P. Ambler. The structure of β-lactamases. *Philos. Trans. R. Soc. London, 289*:321–331 (1980).
12. J. B. K. Nielsen and J. O. Lampen. Glyceride-cysteine lipoproteins and secretion by gram-positive bacteria. *J. Bacteriol., 152*:315–322 (1982).
13. R. W. McDonnell, H. M. Sweendy, and S. Cohen. Conjugational transfer of gentamicin resistance plasmids intra- and inter-specifically in *Staphylococcus aureus* and *Staphylococcus epidermidis. Antimicrob. Agents Chemother., 23*:151–160 (1983).
14. R. V. Goering and E. A. Ruff. Comparative analysis of conjugative plasmids mediating gentamicin resistance in *Staphylococcus aureus. Antimicrob. Agents Chemother., 24*:450–452 (1983).
15. M. Matthew and A. M. Harris. Identification of β-lactamases by analytical isoelectric focusing: Correlation with bacterial taxonomy. *J. Gen. Microbiol., 94*:55–67 (1976).
16. B. E. Murray and B. Mederski-Samoraj. Transferrable β-lactamase. A new mechanism for in vitro penicillin resistance in *Streptococcus faecalis. J. Clin. Invest., 72*:1168–1171 (1983).
17. T. Sawai, S. Mitsuhashi, and S. Yamagishi. Comparison of β-lactamases in gram-negative rod bacteria resistant to α-aminobenzylpenicillin. *Jpn. J. Microbiol., 12*:423–434 (1968).
18. G. W. Jack and M. H. Richmond. A comparative study of eight distinct β-lactamases synthesized by gram-negative bacteria. *J. Gen. Microbiol., 61*: 43–61 (1970).
19. M. H. Richmond and R. B. Sykes. The β-lactamases of gram-negative bacteria and their possible physiological role, in *Advances in Microbial Physiology,* Vol. 9 (A. H. Rose and D. W. Tempest, eds.), Academic, London, 1973, pp. 31–88.
20. S. Bergstrom, O. Olsson, and S. Normack. Common evolutionary origin of chromosomal beta-lactamase genes in enterobacteria. *J. Bacteriol., 150*:528–534 (1982).
21. B. Jaurin and T. Grundstrom. *ampc* cephalosporinase of *Escherichia coli* K-12 has a different evolutionary origin from that of β-lactamases of the penicillinase type. *Proc. Nat. Acad. Sci. U.S.A., 78*:4897–4901 (1981).

22. V. Knott-Hunziker, S. Petursson, G. S. Jayatilake, S. G. Waley, B. Jaurin, and T. Grundstrom. Active sites of β-lactamases. The chromosomal β-lactamases of *Pseudomonas aeruginosa* and *Escherichia coli*. *Biochem. J., 201*: 621–627 (1982).
23. R. R. Yocum, D. J. Waxman, J. R. Rasmussen, and J. L. Strominger. Mechanism of penicillin action: Penicillin and substrate bind covalently to the same active site serine in two bacterial D-alanine carboxypeptidases. *Proc. Nat. Acad. Sci. U.S.A., 76*:2730–2734 (1979).
24. D. J. Waxman, H. Amanuma, and J. L. Strominger. Mechanism of penicillin action: Penicillin and substrate bind covalently to the same active site serine in two bacterial D-alanine carboxypeptidases. *Proc. Nat. Acad. Sci. U.S.A., 76*:2730–2734 (1979).
25. D. J. Waxman, H. Amanuma, and J. L. Strominger. Amino acid sequence homologies between *Escherichia coli* penicillin-binding protein 5 and class A β-lactamases. *FEBS Lett., 139*:159–163 (1982).
26. M. Matthew. Plasmid-mediated β-lactamase of gram-negative bacteria: Properties and distribution. *J. Antimicrob. Chemother., 5*:349–358 (1979).
27. M. Matthew, R. W. Hedges, and J. T. Smith. Types of β-lactamase determined by plasmids in gram-negative bacteria. *J. Bacteriol., 138*:657–662 (1979).
28. C. Vecoli, F. E. Prevost, J. J. Ververis, A. A. Medeiros, and G. P. O'Leary, Jr. A comparison of polyacrylamide and agarose gel thin-layer isoelectric focusing for the characterization of β-lactamase. *Antimicrob. Agents Chemother., 24*:186–189 (1983).
29. C. H. O'Callaghan. Effects of partially purified β-lactamases on some cephalosporin compounds, related to the susceptibility of cephaloridine, cited in *Antibiotic and Chemotherapy* (L. P. Garrod, H. P. Lambert, and F. O. O'Grady, eds.), Churchill Livingstone, Edinburgh, 1981, p. 105.
30. I. N. Simpson, S. J. Plested, and P. B. Harper. Investigation of the β-lactamase stability of ceftazidime and eight other new cephalosporin antibiotics. *J. Antimicrob. Chemother., 9*:357–368 (1982).
31. A. Elwell and R. Wise. The β-lactamase stability of acylureidopenicillins. *J. Antimicrob. Chemother., 10*:560–561 (1982).
32. J. W. Dale and J. T. Smith. The dimeric nature of an R-factor mediated β-lactamase. *Biochem. Biophys. Res. Commun., 68*:1000–1005 (1976).
33. R. B. Sykes and M. Matthew. Detection, assay and immunology of β-lactamases, in *Beta-Lactamases* (J. M. T. Hamilton-Miller and J. T. Smith, eds.), Academic. London, 1979, pp. 17–49.
34. G. Paul, A. Philippon, M. Barthelemy, R. Labia, and P. Nevot. Immunological distinction between constitutive β-lactamases of gram-negative rods with antisera TEM-1 and CARB-3, in *Program and Abstracts of the 21st Interscience Conference on Antimicrobial Agents and Chemotherapy,* American Society for Microbiology, Chicago, 1981.
35. A. A. Medeiros, R. W. Hedges, and G. A. Jacoby. Spread of a "*Pseudomonas*-specific" β-lactamase to plasmids of enterobacteria. *J. Bacteriol., 149*:700–707 (1982).

36. K. Katsu, M. Inoue, and S. Mitsuhashi. Plasmid-mediated carbenicillin hydrolyzing β-lactamases of *Proteus mirabilis. J. Antibiot., 43*:1504–1506 (1981).
37. D. Livermore, J. P. Maskell, and J. D. Williams. Detection of PSE (*Pseudomonas*-specific enzyme)-2 β-lactamase in Enterobacteriaceae isolates. *Antimicrob. Agents Chemother., 25*:268–272 (1984).
38. C. Roy, A. Foz, C. Segura, M. Tirado, C. Fuster, and R. Reig. Plasmid-determined β-lactamases identified in a group of 204 ampicillin-resistant Enterobacteriaceae. *J. Antimicrob. Chemother., 12*:507–510 (1983).
39. A. A. Medeiros, J. Ximenez, K. Blickstein-Goldworm, T. F. O'Brien, and J. Acar. Beta-lactamases of ampicillin-resistant *Escherichia coli* from Brazil, France and the United States, in *Current Chemotherapy and Infectious Diseases* (J. D. Nelson and C. Grassi, eds.), American Society for Microbiology, Washington, D.C., 1980, pp. 761–762.
40. L. G. Rubin, A. A. Medeiros, R. H. Yolken, and E. R. Moxon. Ampicillin treatment failure of apparently beta-lactamase-negative *Haemophilus influenzae* type b meningitis due to novel β-lactamase. *Lancet, 2*:1008–1010 (1981).
41. I. N. Simpson, S. J. Plested, M. J. Budin-Jones, J. Lees, R. W. Hedges, and G. A. Jacoby. Characterization of a novel plasmid-mediated β-lactamase and its contribution to β-lactam resistance in *Pseudomonas aeruginosa. FEMS Microbiol. Lett., 19*:23–27 (1983).
42. A. A. Medeiros, M. Cohenford, and G. A. Jacoby. Five novel plasmid-determined β-lactamases. *Antimicrob. Agents Chemother., 27*:715–719 (1985).
43. K. Sato, Y. Matsuura, M. Inoue, and S. Mitsuhashi. Properties of a new penicillinase type produced by *Bacteriodes fragilis. Antimicrob. Agents Chemother., 22*:579–584 (1983).
44. R. Labia, M. Guionie, M. Barthelemy, and A. Philippon. Properties of three carbenicillin-hydrolysing β-lactamases (CARB) from *Pseudomonas aeruginosa*: Identification of a new enzyme. *J. Antimicrob. Chemother., 7*:49–56 (1981).
45. I. Takahashi, K. Tsukamoto, M. Harada, and T. Sawai. Carbenicillin-hydrolyzing penicillinases of *Proteus mirabilis* and the PSE-type penicillinases of *Pseudomonas aeruginosa. Microbiol. Immunol., 27*:995–1004 (1983).

45a. R. W. Hedges, A. A. Medeiros, M. Cohenford, and G. A. Jacoby. Genetic and biochemical properties of AER-1, a novel carbenicillin-hydrolyzing beta-lactamase from *Aeromonas hydrophila. Antimicrob. Agents Chemother., 27*:479–484 (1985).

46. M. M. Bobrowski, M. Matthew, P. T. Barth, N. Datta, N. J. Grinter, A. E. Jacob, P. Kontomichalou, J. W. Dale, and J. T. Smith. Plasmid-determined β-lactamase indistinguishable from the chromosomal β-lactamase of *Escherichia coli. J. Bacteriol., 125*:149–157 (1976).
47. R. Levesque, P. H. Roy, R. Letarte, and J.-C. Pechere. A plasmid-mediated cephalosporinase from *Achromobacter* species. *J. Infect. Dis., 5*:753–761 (1982).

48. R. Levesque and P. H. Roy. Mapping of the plasmid (pLQ3) from *Achromobacter* and cloning of its cephalosporinase gene in *Escherichia coli. Gene, 18*:69–75 (1982).
49. M. Matthew and R. W. Hedges. Analytical isoelectric focusing of R factor-determined β-lactamases: correlation with plasmid compatibility. *J. Bacteriol., 125*:713–718 (1976).
50. G. A. Jacoby and M. Matthew. The distribution of β-lactamase genes on plasmids found in *Pseudomonas. Plasmid, 2*:41–47 (1979).
51. N. Datta. Epidemiology and classification of plasmids, in *Microbiology—1974* (E. Schlessinger, ed.), American Society for Microbiology, Washington, D.C., pp. 9–12.
52. S. Falkow, P. Guerry, R. W. Hedges, and N. Datta. Polynucleotide sequence relationships among plasmids of the I compatibility complex. *J. Gen. Microbiol., 85*:65–76 (1974).
53. N. Datta and R. W. Hedges. Host ranges of R factors. *J. Gen. Microbiol., 70*:453–460 (1972).
54. G. A. Jacoby. Classification of plasmids in *Pseudomonas aeruginosa,* in *Microbiology—1977* (D. Schlessinger, ed.), American Society for Microbiology, Washington, D.C., pp. 119–126.
55. Y. Murooka, N. Takizawa, and T. Harada. Introduction of bacteriophage Mu into bacteria of various genera and intergeneric gene transfer by RP4::Mu. *J. Bacteriol., 145*:358–368 (1981).
56. F. Heffron, R. Kostriken, C. Moirta, and R. Parker. Tn*3* encodes a site-specific recombination system: Identification of essential sequences, genes, and the actual site of recombination. *Cold Spring Harbor Symp. Quant. Biol., 45*:259–268 (1981).
57. M. J. Casadaban, J. Chou, P. Lemaux, C.-P. Tu, and S. N. Cohen. Tn*3*: Transposition and control. *Cold Spring Harbor Symp. Quant. Biol., 45*:269–273 (1981).
58. F. Heffron. Tn*3* and its relatives, in *Mobile Genetic Elements* (J. A. Shapiro, ed.), Academic, New York, 1983, pp. 223–260.
59. C. Rubens, F. Heffron, and S. Falkow. Transposition of a plasmid deoxyribonucleic acid sequence that mediates ampicillin resistance: Independence from host *rec* functions and orientation of insertion. *J. Bacteriol., 128*:425–434 (1976).
60. J. De Graaff, L. P. Elwell, and S. Falkow. Molecular nature of two β-lactamase-specifying plasmids isolated from *Haemophilus influenzae* type b. *J. Bacteriol., 126*:439–446 (1976).
61. P. I. Perine, W. Schalla, M. S. Siegel, C. Thornsberry, J. Biddle, K.-H. Wong, and S. E. Thompson. Evidence for two distinct types of penicillinase-producing *Neisseria gonorrhoeae. Lancet, 2*:993–995 (1977).
62. J. Brunton, M. Meier, N. Ehrman, I. MacLean, L. Slaney, and W. L. Albritton. Molecular epidemiology of β-lactamase-specifying plasmids of *Haemophilus decreyi. Antimicrob. Agents Chemother., 21*:857–863 (1982).
63. P. A. Totten, H. H. Handsfield, D. Peters, K. K. Holmes, and S. Falkow. Characterization of ampicillin resistance plasmids from *Haemophilus*

ducreyi. Antimicrob. Agents Chemother., 21:622–627 (1982).

64. R. Laufs, P.-M. Kaulfers, G. Jahn, and U. Teschner. Molecular characterization of a small *Haemophilus influenzae* plasmid specifying β-lactamase and its relationship to R factors from *Neisseria gonorrhoeae. J. Gen. Microbiol., 111*:223–231 (1979).
65. D. J. Kopecko, J. Brevet, and S. N. Cohen. Involvement of multiple translocating DNA segments and recombinational hotspots in the structural evolution of bacterial plasmids. *J. Mol. Biol., 108*:333–360 (1976).
66. D. R. Hyde and C.-P. D. Tu. Insertion sites and the terminal nucleotide sequences of the Tn4 transposon. *Nucleic Acids Res., 10*:3981–3993 (1982).
67. J. Grinsted, F. De La Cruz, J. Altenbuchner, and R. Schmitt. Complementation of transposition of *tnpA* mutants of Tn3, Tn21, Tn501, and Tn1721. *Plasmid, 8*:276–286 (1982).
68. M. Tanaka, H. Harafuji, and T. Yamamoto. A gene and its product required for transposition of resistance transposon Tn*2603*. *J. Bacteriol., 151*:723–728 (1982).
69. J. Kratz, F. Schmidt, and B. Wiedemann. Transposition of a gene encoding OXA-2 β-lactamase. *J. Gen. Microbiol., 129*:2951–2957 (1983).
70. T. Yamamoto, M. Watanabe, K. Matsumoto, and T. Sawai. Tn*2610*, a transposon involved in the spread of the carbenicillin-hydrolyzing β-lactamase gene. *Mol. Gen. Genet., 189*:282–288 (1983).
71. M. Chandler, M. Clerget, and D. J. Galas. The transposition frequency of IS*1*-flanked transposons in a function of their size. *J. Mol. Biol., 154*:229–243 (1982).
72. M. I. Sinclair and B. W. Holloway. A chromosomally located transposon in *Pseudomonas aeruginosa. J. Bacteriol., 151*:569–579 (1982).
73. C. Thornsberry and L. K. McDougal. Ampicillin-resistant *Haemophilus influenzae*: Incidence, mechanism, and detection. *Postgrad. Med., 71*:135–145 (1982).
74. A. Percival, J. Rowlands, J. E. Corkhill, C. D. Alergant, O. P. Arya, and E. Rees. Penicillinase-producing gonococci in Liverpool. *Lancet, 2*:1379–1382 (1976).
75. Centers for Disease Control. Global distribution of penicillinase-producing *Neisseria gonorrhoeae* (PPNG). *Conn. Med., 42*:223 (1982).
76. J. R. Dillon, M. Pauze, and K. H. Yeung. Spread of penicillinase-producing and transfer plasmids from the gonococcus to *Neisseria meningitis. Lancet, 1*:779–781 (1983).
77. G. A. Jacoby, L. Sutton, and A. A. Medeiros. Plasmid-determined β-lactamase of *Pseudomonas aeruginosa*, in *Current Chemotherapy and Infectious Diseases*, (J. D. Nelson and C. Grassi, eds.), American Society for Microbiology, Washington, D.C., 1980, pp. 769–771.
78. A. A. Medeiros, E. S. Gilleece, and T. F. O'Brien. Distribution of plasmid type β-lactamases in ampicillin-resistant salmonellae from humans and animals in the United States, in *Molecular Biology, Pathogenicity, and Ecology of Bacterial Plasmids* (S. Levy, R. Clowes, and E. Koenig, eds.), Plenum, New York, 1981, p. 634.

79. I. N. Simpson, P. B. Harper, and C. H. O'Callaghan. Principal β-lactamases responsible for resistance to β-lactam antibiotics in urinary tract infections. *Antimicrob. Agents Chemother., 17*:929–936 (1980).
79a. W. Cullmann, W. Opferkuch, M. Steiglitz, and W. Dick. Influence of spontaneous and inducible β-lactamase production on the antimicrobial activity of recently developed β-lactam compounds. *Chemotherapy, 30*:175–181 (1984).
80. A. Philippon, A. Thabaut, and M. Meyran. Beta-lactamases of *Pseudomonas aeruginosa* responsible for resistance to carboxypenicillins in France (1982), in *Abstracts of the 23rd International Conference on Antimicrobial Agents and Chemotherapy,* American Society for Microbiology, Las Vegas, 1983, page 248.
81. M. Jouvenot, P. Bonin, and Y. Michel-Briand. Frequency of β-lactamases that are markedly active against carbenicillin in the *Pseudomonas aeruginosa* strains isolated in a Medical School Hospital. *J. Antimicrob. Chemother., 12*:451–458 (1983).
82. T. F. O'Brien, J. D. Hopkins, E. S. Gilleece, A. A. Medeiros, R. L. Kent, B. O. Blackburn, M. B. Holmes, J. P. Reardon, J. M. Vergeront, W. L. Schell, E. Christenson, M. L. Bissett, and E. V. Morse. Molecular epidemiology of antibiotic resistance in *Salmonella* from animals and human beings in the United States. *N. Engl. J. Med., 307*:1–6 (1982).
83. M. Matthew, G. Cornelis, and G. Wauters. Correlation of serological and biochemical groups of *Yersinia enterocolitica* with the β-lactamases of the strains. *J. Gen. Microbiol., 102*:55–59 (1977).
84. R. Marre, A. A. Medeiros, and A. W. Pascule. Characterization of the β-lactamases of six species of *Legionella. J. Bacteriol., 151*:216–221 (1982).
85. S. Normark, T. Edlund, T. Grundstrom, S. Bergstrom, and H. Wolf-Watz. *Escherichia coli* K-12 hyperproducing chromosomal β-lactamase by gene repititions. *J. Bacteriol., 132*:912–922 (1977).
86. B. Jaurin, T. Grundstrom, T. Edlund, and S. Normark. The *E. coli* β-lactamase attenuator mediates growth rate-dependent regulation. *Nature, 290*: 221–225 (1981).
87. T. Sawai, M. Kanno, and K. Tsukamoto. Characterization of eight β-lactamases of gram-negative bacteria. *J. Bacteriol., 152*:567–571 (1982).
88. M. H. Richmond. The β-lactamase stability of a novel β-lactam antibiotic containing a 7-methoxyoxacephem nucleus. *J. Antimicrob. Chemother., 6*: 445–453 (1980).
89. C. A. Hart and A. Percival. Resistance to cephalosporins among gentamicin-resistant klebsiellae. *J. Antimicrob. Chemother., 9*:275–286 (1982).
90. R. Labia. Moxalactam: An oxa-beta-lactam antibiotic that inactivates β-lactamases. *Rev. Infect. Dis. Suppl., 4*:S529–S535 (1982).
91. Y. Saino, F. Kobayashi, M. Inoue, and S. Mitsuhashi. Purification and properties of inducible penicillin β-lactamase isolated from *Pseudomonas maltophilia. Antimicrob. Agents Chemother., 22*:564–570 (1982).
92. A. Yotsuji, S. Minami, M. Inoue, and S. Mitsuhashi. Properties of novel β-lactamase produced by *Bacteroides fragilis. Antimicrob. Agents Chemother.,*

24:925–929 (1983).

93. K. Hirai, S. Iyobe, M. Inoue, and S. Mitsuhashi. Purification and properties of a new β-lactamase from *Pseudomonas cepacia*. *Antimicrob. Agents Chemother.*, *17*:355–358 (1980).
94. N. Matsubara, A. Yotsumi, K. Kumano, M. Inoue, and S. Mitsuhashi. Purification and some properties of a cephalosporinase from *Proteus vulgaris*. *Antimicrob. Agents Chemother.*, *19*:185–187 (1981).
95. J. C. Pechere, R. Guay, J. Dubois, and R. Letarte. Hydrolysis of cefotaxime by a β-lactamase from *Bacteroides fragilis*. *Antimicrob. Agents Chemother.*, *17*:1001–1003 (1980).
96. R. Labia, A. Kazmierczak, M. Guionie, and J. M. Masson. Some bacterial proteins with affinity for cefotaxime. *J. Antimicrob. Chemother., Suppl. 6A*:19–23 (1980).
97. L. Pagani, M. Perduca, and E. Romero. A β-lactamase from *Proteus vulgaris* that hydrolyzes newly introduced cephalosporins. *Microbiologica, 6*:163–168 (1983).
98. R. B. Sykes, D. P. Bonner, K. Bush, N. H. Georgopapadakou, and J. S. Wells. Monobactams–Monocyclic β-lactam antibiotics produced by bacteria. *J. Antimicrob. Chemother. Suppl. E8*:1–16 (1981).
99. M. E. Nugent and R. W. Hedges. The nature of the genetic determinant for the SHV-1 β-lactamase. *Mol. Gen. Genet.*, *175*:239–243 (1979).

99a. O. Olsson, S. Bergstrom, F. P. Lindberg, and S. Normark. *ampC* β-lactamase hyperproduction in *Escherichia coli*: Natural ampicillin resistance generated by horizontal chromosomal DNA transfer from *Shigella*. *Proc. Nat. Acad. Sci.*, *80*:7556–7560 (1983).

100. J. W. Bisson and A. A. Medeiros. Effect of growth phase on production of plasmid-determined β-lactamase by β-lactam resistant bacteria, in *Abstracts of the Annual Meeting of the American Society of Microbiology*, American Society for Microbiology, Dallas, 1981, p. 11.
101. R. B. Sykes and M. Matthew. The β-lactamases of gram-negative bacteria and their role in resistance to β-lactam antibiotics. *J. Antimicrob. Chemother.*, *2*:115–157 (1976).
102. A. A. Medeiros and T. F. O'Brien. Ampicillin-resistant *Haemophilus influenzae* type B possessing a TEM-type β-lactamase but little permeability barrier to ampicillin. *Lancet*, *1*:716 (1975).
103. E. R. Moxon, A. A. Medeiros, and T. F. O'Brien. Beta-lactamase effect on ampicillin treatment of *Haemophilus influenzae* B bacteremia and meningitis in infant rats. *Antimicrob. Agents Chemother.*, *12*:461–464 (1977).
104. D. Murphy and J. Todd. Treatment of ampicillin-resistant *Haemophilus influenzae* in soft tissue infections with high doses of ampicillin. *J. Pediatr.*, *94*:983–987 (1979).
105. A. Percival, W. Brumfitt, and J. de Louvois. The role of penicillinase in determining natural and acquired resistance of gram-negative bacteria to penicillins. *J. Gen. Microbiol.*, *32*:77–89 (1963).
106. A. A. Medeiros, R. L. Kent, and T. F. O'Brien. Characterization and prevalence of the different mechanisms of resistance to β-lactam antibiotics

in clinical isolates of *Escherichia coli. Antimicrob. Agents Chemother.*, *6*:791–801 (1974).
107. W. E. Graham and A. A. Medeiros. Antagonism of carbenicillin by cephalosporins in gram-negative bacilli, in *Current Chemotherapy and Infectious Diseases* (J. D. Nelson and C. Grassi, eds.), American Society for Microbiology, Washington, D.C., 1980, pp. 489–491.
108. C. Sanders. Novel resistance selected by the new expanded-spectrum cephalosporins: A concern. *J. Infect. Dis.*, *147*:585–589 (1983).
109. R. Labia, R. Bequin-Bellecoq, and M. Guionie. Behavior of ceftazidime towards β-lactamases. *J. Antimicrob. Chemother. Suppl. 8B*:141–146 (1981).
110. T. Yokota and E. Azuma. Biochemical aspects of bacterial resistance to new β-lactam drugs non-hydrolyzable by β-lactamases, in *Antibiotic Resistance Transposition and Other Mechanisms* (A. Mitsuhashi, L. Rosival, and V. Kremery, eds.), Springer-Verlag, Berlin, 1980, pp. 333–337.
111. C. C. Sanders, W. E. Sanders, and R. V. Goering. In vitro antagonism of β-lactam antibiotics by cefoxitin. *Antimicrob. Agents Chemother.*, *21*: 968–975 (1982).
112. D. Sugarman and E. Pesanti. Treatment failures secondary to *in vivo* development of drug resistance by microorganisms. *Rev. Infect. Dis.*, *2*:153–168 (1980).
113. L. C. Preheim, R. G. Penn, C. C. Sanders, R. V. Goering, and D. K. Giger. Emergence of resistance to β-lactam aminoglycoside antibiotics during moxalactam therapy of *Pseudomonas aeruginosa* infections. *Antimicrob. Agents Chemother.*, *22*:1037–1041 (1982).
114. D. G. Beckwith and J. A. Jahre. Role of a cefoxitin-inducible β-lactamase in a case of breakthrough bacteria. *J. Clin. Microbiol.*, *12*:517–520 (1980).
115. C. C. Sanders, R. C. Moellering, Jr., R. R. Martin, R. L. Perkins, D. G. Strike, T. D. Gooty, and W. E. Sanders, Jr. Resistance to cefamandole: A collaborative study of emerging clinical problems. *J. Infect. Dis.*, *145*: 118–125 (1982).
116. R. L. Then and P. Angehrn. Trapping of nonhydrolyzable cephalosporins by cephalosporinases in *Enterobacter cloacae* and *Pseudomonas aeruginosa* as a possible resistance mechanism. *Antimicrob. Agents Chemother.*, *21*: 711–717 (1982).
117. P. R. Murray, G. G. Granich, D. J. Krogstad, and A. C. Niles. *In vivo* selection of resistance to multiple cephalosporins by *Enterobacter cloacae. J. Infect. Dis.*, *147*:590 (1983).
118. B. Olson, R. A. Weinstein, C. Nathan, and S. A. Kabins. Broad spectrum β-lactam resistance in *Enterobacter*: Emergence during treatment and mechanisms of resistance. *J. Antimicrob. Chemother.*, *11*:299–310 (1983).
119. T. D. Gootz, C. C. Sanders, and R. V. Goering. Resistance to cefamandole: Depression of β-lactamases by cefoxitin and mutation in *Enterobacter cloacae. J. Infect. Dis.*, *146*:34–42 (1982).
120. S. A. Kabins, H. M. Sweeney, and S. Cohen. Resistance to cephalothin in vivo associated with increased cephalosporinase production. *Ann. Intern.*

Med., 65:1271–1277 (1966).

121. A. A. Medeiros and M. D. Mandel. In vivo acquired resistance to β-lactam antibiotics due to hyperproduction of β-lactamase, in *Abstracts of the Annual Meeting of the American Society for Microbiology,* American Society for Microbiology, Los Angeles, 1979, p. 6.
122. A. A. Medeiros and T. F. O'Brien. Acquisition of resistance to different β-lactam antibiotics without change in isolate β-lactamase activity, in *Proceedings of the 13th Interscience Conference on Antimicrobial Agents and Chemotherapy,* American Society for Microbiology, 1973, p. 151.
123. H. Nikaido. Outer membrane permeability and β-lactam resistance, in *Microbiology–1984* (D. Schlesinger, ed.), American Society for Microbiology, Washington, D.C., 1984, pp. 381–384.
124. F. W. Goldstein, L. Gutmann, R. Williamson, E. Collatz, and J. F. Acar. *In vivo* and *in vitro* emergence of simultaneous resistance to both β-lactam and aminoglycoside antibiotics in a strain of *Serratia marcescens. Ann. Microbiol., Inst. Pasteur, 134A*:329–337 (1983).
125. R. W. Hedges, M. Matthew, D. I. Smith, J. M. Cresswell, and A. E. Jacob. Properties of a transposon conferring resistance to penicillins and streptomycin. *Gene, 1*:241–253 (1977).
126. C. E. Rubens, W. F. McNeill, and W. E. Farrar, Jr. Evolution of multiple-antibiotic-resistance plasmids mediated by transposable plasmid deoxyribonucleic acid sequences. *J. Bacteriol., 140*:713–719 (1979).
127. T. Yamamoto, M. Tanaka, C. Nohara, Y. Fukunaga, and S. Yamagishi. Transposition of the oxacillin-hydrolyzing penicillinase gene. *J. Bacteriol., 145*:808–813 (1981).
128. A. M. Philippon, G. C. Paul, and G. A. Jacoby. Properties of PSE-2 β-lactamase and genetic basis for its production in *Pseudomonas aeruginosa. Antimicrob. Agents Chemother., 24*:362–369 (1983).

4

Resistance to Beta-Lactam Antibiotics in Hospitals

JOSÉ IGNACIO SANTOS*
Boston University School of Medicine and Boston City Hospital, Boston, Massachusetts

I. INTRODUCTION

Advances in antimicrobial therapy over the past three decades have been accompanied by microbial accommodations to new therapeutic agents. As a result, a progressive erosion of antibiotic effectiveness has been seen in the clinical application of many of these drugs. These general trends have been mirrored in the beta-lactam family of agents. The development of potent beta-lactam antibiotics with prolonged half-lives, broader antimicrobial spectra, and increased resistance to inactivating enzymes has promised control of more and more pathogenic bacteria. However, hospitals have reported ever-increasing declines in the susceptibility of clinically isolated, common bacterial pathogens to many beta-lactam antimicrobials. Although the basis for these changes is not entirely clear, many factors, including the widespread, perhaps even injudicious, use of beta-lactam antibiotics for prophylaxis and treatment of community and hospital-acquired infections, have been implicated. This development of beta-lactam resistance, encountered with greater frequency in hospitals, is a constant and growing threat to the usefulness of these drugs. Careful evaluation of this dilemma is necessary for the formulation of a wise policy of antibiotic therapy and should include review of epidemiological reports of the emergence and spread of resistance, correlation of antibiotic policy with geographical flux in resistance, and examination of changes in the susceptibility of clinically isolated bacteria to beta-lactam antibiotics.

**Current affiliation:* Hospital Infantil de Mexico, Mexico City, Mexico.

II. LABORATORY METHODS USED TO DETECT CHANGES IN ANTIBIOTIC RESISTANCE

Studies on the emergence of beta-lactam resistance in hospitals have been limited by the methods used to detect changes in the susceptibility of clinically isolated bacteria. These methods include antimicrobial susceptibility testing in broth and agar (1, 2), determination of bacterial beta-lactamase production (3), and serum bactericidal tests (4). In general, in vitro methods have been designed and used to investigate antibiotic resistance as a guide for antimicrobial therapy. To a lesser extent, these methods have been used for epidemiological purposes.

Quantitative dilution methods in broth or agar expose a known inoculum of bacteria to various concentrations of the antibiotic being tested and permit the observer to determine the minimal concentration of agent that inhibits growth (MIC). After subculture on an antibiotic-free medium, the minimal bactericidal concentration (MBC) also can be determined. The Steers inoculum-replicating apparatus (5) has permitted more efficient quantitative dilution testing of larger numbers of strains on suitable solid media.

Antimicrobial susceptibility tests are perhaps the most commonly used means to detect antimicrobial resistance. For purposes of in vitro testing, an organism is generally considered susceptible if the concentration of antimicrobial agent necessary to inhibit its growth is lower than that usually attainable in blood and other body fluids. Unfortunately, the results of these tests may vary from laboratory to laboratory because of the influence of several variables: the type, composition, and pH of the medium; the preparation of the antibiotic in question; the inoculum size of the organism; the duration and temperature of incubation; and the definition of inhibitory endpoints (1/4).

Of the currently available susceptibility tests, the only one that attempts to control for these variables is the disk diffusion method. This technique has been standardized by the World Health Organization and approved by the National Committee for Clinical Laboratory Standards and the Food and Drug Administration for in vitro susceptibility testing (6, 7).

The quantitative broth or agar dilution method and the standardized agar diffusion procedures are quite different, yet both methods of susceptibility testing have been widely used for tracking the chronological changes in patterns of bacterial resistance. The key to the reliability of either test in a given laboratory is a combination of quality control procedures and the inclusion of appropriate laboratory control organisms, selected on the basis of repeated and documented performance in the same test system being used (6, 7). Thus maintaining a consistant methodological approach has permitted investigators to report on the emergence of antibiotic resistance by comparing information at any given time to information previously derived from that same laboratory.

In vitro determination of susceptibility of groups of hospital strains collected over a period of time or of strains within the same species collected at other hospitals enable us to document temporal and/or geographical changes in patterns of resistance. If quantitative dilution methods are used, the data usually are presented in tables giving the number or percentage of strains inhibited or killed by increasing concentrations of the antimicrobial agent being tested, expressed as the minimal inhibitory concentration (MIC) or minimal bactericidal concentration (MBC). For the standardized disk susceptibility test, the diameter of the zone of inhibitation measured instead of the MIC. However, it is possible to calculate an MIC correlate for a given zone diameter by using regression analysis (1).

Susceptibility data also are often presented graphically by plotting the number or percentage of strains on the ordinates and the quantitative data (MIC, MBC, or zone diameter) on the abscissa (8). Charting the cumulative percentage of distribution as the ordinate permits one to compare several curves at a time. The graphic presentation of data facilitates the comparison of strains of the same same species collected at different times and tested with the same antibiotic, even if the data derived do not follow a normal distribution.

III. CHANGES IN SUSCEPTIBILITY OF CLINICALLY ISOLATED BACTERIA TO BETA-LACTAM ANTIBIOTICS

The interval between the introduction of beta-lactam antibiotics and the appearance of resistant strains of microbial organisms has varied widely. For example, the group A beta-hemolytic streptococci still have not developed significant resistance to penicillin. In contrast some portion of natural populations of staphylococci probably were resistant to penicillin G before it was even made commercially available (9); moreover, resistance spread rapidly after penicillin G was introduced and became widespread within a decade. Methicillin-resistant *Staphylococcus aureus* did not emerge as a significant pathogen in the United States until a full 20 years after the antibiotic was introduced clinically.

In the last 30 years the so-called "era of chemotherapy for infectious disease" (10), we have witnessed not only a constantly changing pattern of microbial resistance but also an evolution of nosocomial infections. In the 1940s hospital-acquired infections were usually caused by gram-positive cocci, especially beta-hemolytic streptococci and staphylococci. Late in the 1950s *Staphylococcus* strains resistant to many common antibiotics emerged as a major cause of hospital epidemics. The threat of uncontrollable *Staphylococcus* infections in hospitals subsided in the 1960s only to be replaced by threats from increasingly resistant strains of enteric gram-negative bacilli and enterococci (8, 11).

Although many organisms have exhibited changes in their pattern of susceptibility to beta-lactam antibiotics since the introduction of these drugs, we shall focus on the bacterial species isolated most frequently in hospitalized patients for the following discussion.

A. Pneumococcus: *Streptococcus pneumoniae*

All strains of *Streptococcus pneumoniae* isolated in U.S. hospitals before 1969 were inhibitable over a relatively narrow range of penicillin concentrations (11). Subtle changes in susceptibility patterns were noted at the Boston City Hospital in 1972-1973, when pneumococci were tested with a large number of antibiotics, including several analogs of penicillin G and some of the cephalosporins (8). From the late 1960s to the late 1970s numerous hospitals in the United States and other countries reported isolates of pneumococci with increased resistance to penicillin and other antibiotics (12, 13). Of major importance in this regard was the emergence in South Africa in 1977 of a multiply resistant strain of pneumococcus (14-17). In 1978 one-third of 57 strains of pneumococci isolated from patients with severe pneumococcal infections in New Guinea were penicillin-resistant (18). A total of 21 serotypes were identified, of which 10 showed diminished sensitivity to penicillin. Since that time pneumococci with reduced sensitivity or resistance to penicillin have been recovered from patients with pneumonia, meningitis, and bacteremia in the United States (19). Relatively penicillin-insensitive organisms accounted for 14% of strains of *Strep. pneumoniae* isolated from a group of Navajo Indian tribes (20).

The emergence of multiply resistant pneumococcal strains emphasizes the need for routine antibiotic and sensitivity testing of pneumococci isolated from patients with serious infection. Anderson and co-workers recently reported on the usefulness of the oxacillin disk screening for penicillin resistance of pneumococci (21).

Pneumococci may be described as sensitive to penicillin, resistant, or tolerant to the drug. Sensitive strains are lysed by penicillin. Resistant strains grow normally at high concentrations of beta-lactam antibiotics. The growth of tolerant strains is inhibited by beta-lactam antibiotics, but the cells are not killed and do not lyse. Penicillin-binding proteins have been studied in these three types of pneumococcal strains (22). Resistant strains (including a highly resistant clinical isolate from South Africa) contain several altered forms of penicillin-binding proteins with lowered affinity for beta-lactam antibiotics. Tolerant organisms seem to contain normal penicillin-binding proteins and may resist lysis because of deficiencies in the autolytic pathways (22). Studies such as these have suggested that the resistance among pneumococci is independent of beta-lactamase production. Beta-lactamase production was not demonstrated among the resistant pneumococci from South Africa (14).

B. Streptococcus

1. Group A Beta-Hemolytic Streptococcus

Group A streptococci have retained their sensitivity to penicillin G. In contrast, resistance to tetracyclines, chloramphenicol, and erythromycin has varied cyclically and dramatically, as illustrated in studies from Japan (23). In 1971 only 8.5% of group A beta-hemolytic streptococci isolated in Japan were resistant to erythromycin, but by 1974, 72.3% of all isolates were reported to be resistant to the drug. During this period erythromycin and other macrolides were used regularly throughout Japan for treating upper respiratory tract infections. Rheumatic heart disease in children during this same period fell dramatically.

The practice of intensive antibiotic usage in Japan may have contributed to the development of erythromycin-resistant strains of group A beta-hemolytic streptococci (24). Such practice might be expected to increase the risk of emergence of clinically important resistance to penicillin G in group A streptococci, but to date such resistance has not appeared.

2. Group B Beta-Hemolytic Streptococcus

Group B streptococci are a principle cause of bacteremia and meningitis among neonates (25, 26). Infections arising within 5 days of birth are associated with vertical transmission (from the birth canal of the mother); group B streptococci are commonly the causative organisms. Infections arising beyond 1 week of age are associated with horizontal transmission (nosocomial or community acquired) and are more likely to be caused by other organisms (27).

Although the minimum inhibitory concentration (MIC) of penicillin G for group B streptococci is considerably higher than that of group A strains (11, 12, 25, 28), the group B streptococci are usually reported to be susceptible. Despite continued susceptibility to penicillin in in vitro testing, group B streptococci show a poorer clinical response to antibiotic therapy than do group A strains (25).

Group B streptococci may be killed slowly at growth-inhibiting concentrations of penicillin G. In a recent study 100 isolates of group B streptococci from the blood and cerebrospinal fluid of infected neonates were examined; 4% were tolerant to penicillin (25). Tolerant group B streptococci resist not only penicillin-induced killing during logarithmic growth but also the synergistic effect of penicillin plus gentamicin. Tolerant strains appeared to possess lower autolytic activity in their cell walls than did nontolerant strains (25). The clinical importance of tolerance is not known; however, at least one case of relapse of infection has been attributed to a strain tolerant to penicillin (26).

The reports cited above coupled with the observation that the combination of ampicillin and gentamicin exhibits synergistic in vitro killing of nontolerant group B streptococci has prompted some authors to recommend this combination for systemic disease.

3. Enterococci (Group D Streptococci)

Enterococci classified within the group D streptococci exhibit MIC values for penicillin on the order of 100- to 200-fold higher than for group A streptococci and 10- to 100-fold higher than for group B streptococci (12, 28). The susceptibility of enterococci to penicillin for strains isolated at Boston City Hospital during three time periods has been compared (11). Strains isolated during 1949 were differentiated only by resistance to treatment for 30 min at 60°C. Strains isolated in 1953-1954 and 1968-1969 were identified by serology as group D streptococci; further delineation was carried out by means of biochemical reactions. The MIC for penicillin G in the heterogeneous group of strains isolated in 1949 showed a bimodal distribution as a result of a few strains being highly sensitive to the drug. However, with the more discriminating classification of strains carried out with the 1953-1954 and 1968-1969 groups, no highly penicillin-sensitive strains were included. In contrast to tetracyclines, aminoglycosides, and erythromycin, susceptibility to penicillin G varied little for *Streptococcus liquefaciens, Streptococcus zymogenes,* and *Streptococcus faecalis* between 1953-1954 and 1968-1969. These three species constituted the majority of the enterococcus group in this study. Inhibition occurred over a narrow range of concentrations of penicillin G, with the exception of a few strains of *Strep. liquefaciens* from the 1968-1969 group that were highly resistant to penicillin. Strains of *Streptococcus faecium* of this era showed a bimodal distribution toward penicillin G and ampicillin (8). More recent isolates show a clear bimodal distribution indicative of increased incidence of resistance (8).

Highly resistant as well as tolerant strains of *Strep. faecalis* have now been identified (12, 29). Penicillin tolerance in this organism, like others, is apparently related to deficient autolysin activity (30). The intrinsic high resistance of *Strep. faecalis* toward certain beta-lactam antibiotics may result from the relatively poor binding of many of these compounds to the penicillin-binding proteins PBP1 and PBP3 (30). Although susceptibility toward penicillin G and ampicillin may be demonstrated for many strains, cephalosporins, including the newer agents, are generally without effect (12, 28, 31).

C. Staphylococcus

Staphylococci that produce the enzyme penicillinase probably existed in natural populations of the organism long before penicillin became available for therapeutic use (9). Certainly these penicillinase-producing staphylococci soon gained prevalence in every corner of the world after the use of penicillin became widespread.

Penicillinase production is the most common mechanism for resistance among staphylococci (see Chap. 3). Resistance via this mechanism was thwarted by the development of the penicillinase-resistant penicillins, such as methicillin, nafcillin, and the isoxazolyl penicillins (8; see also Part 2). Methicillin was introduced in the United States in 1960, and the isoxazolyl penicillins shortly thereafter. Although initially rare, methicillin resistance was quickly recognized among hospitalized patients. The first report of a methicillin-resistant staphylococcus in England in 1961 was quickly followed by reports in other European countries (8, 12, 32, 39). Although the first case of methicillin-resistant staphylococci in the United States appeared in 1960, these organisms did not gain prevalence until the end of the decade (8, 40, 44). The appearance of methicillin-resistant staphylococcus strains, which have become endemic in hospital-acquired infections, is more closely related to total antibiotic use than to specific usage of the penicillinase-resistant penicillins (12, 39).

The mechanism by which *Staphylococcus* acquires resistance to methicillin is not completely understood. Resistance is not gained by inactivation of the antibiotic. Cell walls may be altered (12, 45). Methicillin resistance is always accompanied by resistance to penicillin G, isoxazolyl penicillins, nafcillin, and cephalosporins (12, 47). The chromosomal event leading to resistance to these beta-lactam antibiotics frequently also causes resistance to unrelated antibiotics, such as streptomycin, tetracycline, chloramphenicol, and erythromycin (12, 45, 46).

D. *Neisseria*

1. *Neisseria gonorrhoeae*

The incidence of strains of *Neisseria gonorrhoeae* resistant to penicillin and the level of resistance in these strains has risen steadily since the widespread use of penicillin to treat gonorrhea (11, 12, 48, 49). The incidence of resistant organisms is high in many areas worldwide, including the Far East, West Africa, and the Philippines. Resistance is less common in other areas but has recently become severe enough in the United States to warrant concern (12, 49).

Resistance to penicillins in *N. gonorrhoeae* is of two types: relative and absolute. Relative resistance to penicillin first appeared about 20 years ago and has increased steadily since (12). A single gene mutation seems to confer resistance to the beta-lactam antibiotics, as well as to an array of unrelated antibiotics (12). Cell wall changes are noted in these relatively penicillin-resistant strains; penicillin binding is more than an order of magnitude lower than that observed with normal cell walls from *N. gonorrhoeae* (50). Enzymatic degradation of penicillin does not contribute to this type of resistance (51).

Absolute resistance to penicillin in *N. gonorrhoeae* occurs by production of beta-lactamase (12). At least two types of penicillinase-producing strains have been well documented. Far Eastern strains contain a plasmid reported to be 5.8×10^6 daltons; these strains are tetracycline resistant and may also carry additional plasmids which can transfer R plasmids. West African strains contain a smaller plasmid coding for a penicillinase molecule; these strains are sensitive to tetracycline and do not bear additional plasmids like those in the Far Eastern strains (12).

2. *Branhamella catarrhalis*

Branhamella catarrhalis is a pathogen associated with otitis and sinusitis in children and lower respiratory tract infections in patients with generalized immunosuppression or chronic chest disease. Smokers or former smokers also are highly represented in bronchopulmonary infections due to this pathogen.

A recent report from the Princess Margaret Hospital of New Zealand (52) showed beta-lactamase production in 38 of 99 isolates of *B. catarrhalis* and increased resistance to amoxicillin and ampicillin, which had been given before the results of the antibiotic susceptibility testing were known. Erythromycin, tetracycline, or trimethoprim/sulfamethoxazole were appropriate choices for chemotherapy. Amoxicillin-sensitive *Hemophilus influenzae* in conjunction with *B. catarrhalis* persisted in three patients for 2-7 days despite treatment with ampicillin or amoxicillin, suggesting that the normal susceptibility of *H. influenzae* may be masked in the presence of beta-lactamase-producing *B. catarrhalis.*

The beta-lactamase produced by *B. catarrhalis* is a class IV enzyme similar to that from *Klebsiella* (see Chaps. 3 and 15).

E. *Hemophilus*

Ampicillin was effective in the 1960s against all forms of *H. influenzae,* invasive and noninvasive, and simplified the antibacterial management of meningitis in children, which previously required triple therapy with penicillin, chloramphenicol, and sulfonamides. This solution was short lived, however, for in the 1970s reports of resistance began to appear (55-66). According to statistics from the Centers for Disease Control, ampicillin-resistant *H. influenzae* strains are found in 22% of infections caused by *H. influenzae*, but the incidence varies widely according to geographical location (67). Introduction of the first-generation cephalosporins did not alleviate the problem; poor cerebrospinal fluid penetration precluded their use in invasive *H. influenzae* infections. Second- and third-generation cephalosporins have offered greater promise.

Cefamandole, a second-generation cephalosporin, was active in vitro, but numerous clinical failures in children were reported (65). Third-generation cephalosporin derivatives, in particular cefotaxime, have worked well against *H. influenzae* (31). In 1983 Kaplan et al. (66) reported on the use of the oxacephem moxalactam in 38 children with serious infections due to *H. influenzae* type b. Seven of the strains were ampicillin resistant. All of the children responded well to moxalactam.

Resistance to ampicillin in strains of *H. influenzae* type b occurs by production of beta-lactamase (12, 68). Genes coding for the beta-lactamase are carried on an R plasmid, and the beta-lactamase produced is the most common TEM variety (see Chap. 3).

F. Gram-Negative Bacilli

Gram-negative bacilli have steadily increased in importance as serious pathogens in hospitalized patients. As documented in a series of studies from Boston City Hospital, infections caused by *Escherichia coli, Klebsiella, Enterobacter, Proteus,* and *Pseudomonas aeruginosa* occurred at a rate of 12% of the total cases of bacteremia in 1935 but increased to 40% in 1969 (8).

With *E. coli* bimodal distibutions of MIC values were noted for all beta-lactam antibiotics tested against strains isolated between November 1965 and August 1966. A small proportion of these strains were highly resistant to the drugs. The incidence of resistant strains was higher in the group isolated from hospital-acquired infections than from those acquired in the community (8).

Klebsiella pneumoniae and *Enterobacter* (*Aerobacter*) isolated from patients at Boston City Hospital in 1964 were nearly always resistant to penicillins and cephalosporins when large inocula were used in the susceptibility tests, but with smaller inocula resistance to these drugs was less uniform (8). *Klebsiella* strains isolated in 1972 were about evenly divided between moderate and high resistance to penicillins. All were susceptible to cephalosporins. Current clinical isolates are highly susceptible to second- and third-generation cephalosporins, with the exception of occasional highly resistant strains (12, 28).

Enterobacter strains isolated in the same study at Boston City Hospital in 1972 were nearly all resistant to cephalosporins, but many showed some susceptibility to carbenicillin and related penicillins (8). Newer clinical isolates tested against the newest beta-lactam antibiotics show a high percentage of strains susceptible to third-generation cephalosporins (cefotaxime, cefoperazone), moxalactam, and piperacillin or mezlocillin, with the second-generation cephalosporins being less effective (12, 28, 67, 68).

Pseudomonas aeruginosa and *Proteus* species are resistant to many older penicillins, but the broad-spectrum penicillins and the third-generation cephalosporins have activity against many strains (11, 69, 70). These organisms have been noted to colonize in patients who receive antibiotics for infections caused by other organisms (8).

The resistance of the gram-negative bacilli to beta-lactam antibiotics arises from a combination of effects: lowered penetration to the target proteins, beta-lactamase inactivation of the drugs, and less affinity of the drugs for the target proteins. Many of the newer agents combine better penetration with high resistance to beta-lactamase. The effectiveness of the drug is therefore high.

In spite of the increased utility of newer beta-lactam antibiotics for infections caused by gram-negative bacilli, resistance of these drugs may continue to be a problem. For example, Murray et al. observed the development of cross-resistance in cephalosporins during antimicrobial therapy in one patient with multiple blood cultures positive for *Enterobacter cloacae* (71). Sanders and co-workers have found that many of the gram-negative bacteria that have been added to the spectrum of the third-generation cephalosporins possess inducible beta-lactamases (72, 73). Such enzymes have been demonstrated in genera such as *Enterobacter, Serratia,* and *Pseudomonas* (74). The impact of the presence of these organisms on the clinical incidence of resistance is yet to be fully assessed.

G. Anaerobic Bacteria

A retrospective review of the results of susceptibility testing of clinically significant anaerobes in 1977-1981 at the Mayo Clinic indicated an increase in resistance to penicillin in the "non-*fragilis*" *Bacteroides* in comparison with the results of two previous surveys (75). Additionally, some penicillin resistance was noted among clostridia other than *Clostridium perfringens*. Correlation of penicillin MIC values and beta-lactamase activity in isolates of non-*fragilis Bacteroides* indicated that this resistance was indeed beta-lactamase related; 59% (331 of 559) of the non-*fragilis Bacteroides* species tested at the Mayo Clinic were positive for beta-lactamase production. Although prior surveys had emphasized penicillin susceptibility among the non-*fragilis Bacteroides,* these studies reported MIC data alone; no attempt was made to measure beta-lactamase production. Beta-lactamase production sometimes occurs even on *Bacteroides* strains with low MIC values; for example, in the Mayo Clinic study 3 of 11 strains with MIC values less than or equal to 0.78 μg/ml penicillin produced beta-lactamase. The rapid determination of beta-lactamase production may be of greater significance than the precise MIC for the clinician in choosing appropriate effective antibiotic therapy (75).

IV. PROBLEMS WITH DETECTION OF ANTIBIOTIC RESISTANCE

In hospitals nonfastidious gram-negative bacilli, which are resistant, are particularly perplexing. These bacteria, which possess inducible beta-lactamases, also have chromosomally mediated cephalosporinases (see Chap. 3). The genera *Enterobacter, Serratia,* and *Pseudomonas* harbor these elements. When third-generation cephalosporins are used to treat infections caused by these microbes, these bacteria may develop wide resistance to beta-lactam antibiotics as a result of derepression or induction. Derepressed beta-lactamases may cause resistance to old beta-lactam antibiotics, as well as to several of the newer agents that are not susceptible to hydrolysis (72, 74).

Failure to detect resistance to beta-lactams in certain susceptibility tests used routinely in hospital bacteriology laboratories is commonplace (2). Testing of organisms producing beta-lactamase in agar or broth media is influenced by inoculum size. Either falsely susceptible or falsely resistant reports may result (2). Inappropriate therapeutic intervention as the result of failure to detect resistance may occur.

Kirby/Bauer disk diffusion tests have been criticized when used with organisms that produce beta-lactamase; nevertheless, with little modification they can be adapted and used effectively in documenting inducible beta-lactamases and indexing susceptibility (76).

Synergistic combinations of beta-lactam antimicrobials have been suggested as appropriate measures to gain broad antibiotic advantage as well as low toxicity, but the question of antibiotic antagonism among third-generation beta-lactams indicates the need for clinical trials for combination therapy (77, 79). Although stable to beta-lactamase, these drugs may facilitate induction of beta-lactamase (especially the chromosomally mediated enzymes of gram-negative bacilli), which results in the possibility that these agents act antagonistically against other beta-lactams.

It is important to weigh the use of third-generation cephalosporins as replacement therapy for older yet still effective antimicrobial agents. In addition to the high cost and microbiological risk involved the question of reliable susceptibility testing requires that we examine utilization of these antibiotics and the encumbent risk of encouraging multiply beta-lactam-resistant bacteria as nosocomial (hospital acquired) pathogens. The examination of these elements is critical in light of multiply drug-resistant bacterial epidemics within hospitals (80).

V. RESISTANCE AND ANTIBIOTIC USE: GEOGRAPHICAL DIFFERENCES

As a result of international commerce, immigration, and travel, resistant bacteria have been widely spread among countries. In many countries antibiotics are marketed as nonprescription drugs. Third-world nations spend in excess of twice the amount their industrialized counterparts do on drugs in relation to their total health budget. As a result of this free access to antimicrobial agents, as well as the introduction of antibiotics into animal feed, there appears to be a plethora of resistant pathogenic bacilli poised to proliferate and spread disease among human populations. The development of resistant strains of *Shigella flexneri* in Mexico, *Shigella dysenteriae, Salmonella typhi,* and other salmonellae may illustrate this potential. *Salmonella typhi* strains, which originated in Mexico and are resistant to chloramphenicol, have produced cases of typhoid fever in California.

Still further south in the Americas there is a documented transmittance of antibiotic-resistant pathogens from shellfish contaminated with untreated sewage to fishermen and consumers. In Brazil there exists a multiresistant *Salmon-*

ella typhimurium that slowly ferments lactose, as well as resistant strains of enteropathogenic bacteria. As a result, epidemic dysentery poses a major health problem in Mexico and Central and South America. Furthermore, *S. dysenteriae* type I exhibited resistance to ampicillin, streptomycin, sulfonamides, tetracycline, and chloramphenicol. By contrast, salmonellosis in the United States occurs with greater frequency than shigellosis. The proliferation of nontyphoidal salmonellae that are multiply resistant does not require therapeutic intervention in otherwise healthy individuals.

Growing antibiotic resistance among strains of *Salmonella* in the United States has been seen over the past 17 years. Since 1967 increases in resistance to streptomycin, sulfonamide, ampicillin, and kanamycin, in addition to chloramphenicol were seen. Elsewhere, isolates of *Salmonella* in a 6-year study in India were seen to show resistance to streptomycin, tetracycline, ampicillin, kanamycin, neomycin, chloramphenicol, and sulfadiazine.

The prevalence of bacterial resistance is substantially different between Europe and the United States (81). The incidence of resistance to specific antibiotics was approximately three times higher in Europe than in the United States, while the number of isolated strains resistant to six or more antibiotics was 14 times greater in Europe than in the United States.

While it is clear that experience in region-specific pathogens varies, international differences in preference of treatment modalities, environment, and antibiotic availability certainly contribute to the flux in resistant microbes. Further studies should be encouraged to document variance in rates, types, and treatments of infectious disease.

VI. DISCUSSION

The third-generation beta-lactam antibiotics are a welcome addition to an already large arsenal for battling pathogenic microbes. This group of drugs possesses a broader antimicrobial spectrum and enhanced pharmacokinetics, which minimize dosage frequency, and is well tolerated. These drugs are especially effective for difficult nosocomial infections, particularly in surgically or immunologically compromised patients (see Chap. 11).

With these admirable attributes comes the temptation to abandon caution with regard to their implementation. Judiciously applied, beta-lactam antibiotics are clearly an efficacious and safe means of controlling many obstreperous strains of microbes. However, prudence is strongly indicated as the means to avoid the selective encouragement of resistance to these agents, as well as increased costs in patient care. Clearly, the improper use of these agents results in the proliferation of resistant microbial strains and should serve as a warning, not only to clinicians but also to those involved in and responsible for the introduction of antimicrobial agents into the food chain, that such action is ultimately counterproductive and potentially dangerous.

Reliance on newer broad-spectrum beta-lactam treatment when conventional agents would suffice should obviously be avoided. Yet further steps should be taken to resolve and document issues of beta-lactam susceptibility and resistance in institutions and over wide geographical areas. There has been an unfortunate general tendency for those removed from the sphere of pathology and infectious disease to ignore the ramifications of the injudicious applications of antimicrobials until faced with near-catastrophic consequence. Education of those within and without the academic community could and should be implemented to obviate the misapplied or misguided use of beta-lactam antibiotics.

REFERENCES

1. J. F. Acar. The disc susceptibility test, in *Antibiotics in Laboratory Medicine* (V. Lorian, ed.), Williams and Wilkins, Baltimore, 1980, pp. 24–54.
2. L. D. Thrupp. Susceptibility testing of antibiotics in liquid media, in *Antibiotics in Laboratory Medicine* (V. Lorian, ed.), Williams and Wilkins, Baltimore, 1980, pp. 73–113.
3. H. C. Neu. Antibiotic inactivating enzymes and bacterial resistance, in *Antibiotics in Laboratory Medicine* (V. Lorian, ed.), Williams and Wilkins, Baltimore, 1980, pp. 454–473.
4. S. C. Edberg. In vitro antimicrobial susceptibility testing, in *Antibiotics and Infection* (S. C. Edberg and S. A. Berger, eds.), Churchill Livingstone, New York, 1983, pp. 211–223.
5. E. Steers, E. L. Folte, and B. S. Graves. Inocula replicating apparatus for routine testing of bacterial susceptibility. *Antibiot. Chemother., 9*:307–311 (1959).
6. A. L. Barry. Standardized disc diffusion methods for antimicrobic susceptibility testing of common rapid-growing bacterial pathogens, in *The Clinical Laboratory as an Aid in Chemotherapy of Infectious Disease* (A. Bondi, J. T. Bartola, and J. E. Prier, eds.), University Park Press, Baltimore, 1977, pp. 9–20.
7. A. Balows, C. T. Hall, and T. L. Gavan. Standardization and quality control of disc susceptibility testing in the United States, in *The Clinical Laboratory as an Aid in Chemotherapy of Infectious Disease* (A. Bondi, J. T. Bartola, and J. E. Prier, eds.), University Park Press, Baltimore, 1977, pp. 29–43.
8. M. Finland. Emergence of antibiotic resistance in hospitals, 1935–1975. *Rev. Infect. Dis., 1*:4–21 (1979).
9. G. P. Youmans. Staphylococci, in *The Biologic and Clinical Basis of Infectious Diseases* (G. P. Youmans, P. Y. Paterson, and H. M. Sommers, eds.), Saunders, Philadelphia, 1980, pp. 639–648.
10. T. C. Eickhoff. Antibiotics and nosocomial infections, in *Hospital Infections* (J. V. Bennett and P. S. Brachman, eds.), Little, Brown, Boston, 1979, pp. 195–221.
11. M. Finland. Changing patterns of susceptibility of common bacterial pathogens to antimicrobial agents. *Ann. Intern. Med., 76*:1009–1036 (1972).

12. A. Kucers and N. McK. Bennett. Penicillin G, in *The Use of Antibiotics,* 3rd ed., Heinemann, London, 1979, pp. 3-54.
13. M. A. Mufson. Pneumococcal infections. *J. Am. Med. Assoc., 246*:1942-1948 (1981).
14. P. C. Appelbaum, J. N. Scragg, A. J. Bowen, A. Bhamjee, A. F. Hallett, and R. C. Cooper. *Streptococcus pneumoniae* resistant to penicillin and chloramphenicol. *Lancet, 2*:995 (1977).
15. P. D. Meers and R. B. Matthews. Multiply resistant *pneumococcus. Lancet, 2*:219 (1974).
16. M. R. Jacobs, H. J. Koornhof, R. M. Robins-Browne, C. M. Stevenson, Z. A. Vermaak, I. Friedman, G. M. Miller, M. A. Witcomb, M. Isaäcson, J. I. Ward, and R. Austrian. Emergence of multiply resistant pneumococci. *N. Engl. J. Med., 299*:735-740 (1978).
17. Centers for Disease Control. Multiple-antibiotic resistance of pneumococci in South Africa. Epidemiologic notes and reports. *Morbid. Mortal. Week. Rep., 26*:285-286 (1977).
18. M. Gratten, S. Naraqi, and D. Hansman. High prevalence of penicillin-insensitive pneumococci in Port Moresby, Papua, New Guinea. *Lancet, 2*: 192-196 (1980).
19. M. A. Barry, D. E. Craven, and M. Finland. Serotypes of *Streptococcus pneumoniae* isolated from blood cultures at Boston City Hospital between 1979 and 1982. *J. Infect. Dis., 149*:449-452 (1984).
20. B. Tempest, J. P. Carney, and B. Eberle. Distribution of the sensitivities to penicillin of types of *Diplococcus pneumoniae* in an American Indian population. *J. Infect. Dis., 130*:67-79 (1974).
21. K. C. Anderson, M. J. Maurer, and A. S. Dajani. Pneumococci relatively resistant to penicillin: Prevalence survey in children. *J. Pediatr., 97*:939-941 (1980).
22. R. Williamson, S. Zighelboim, and A. Tomasz. Penicillin-binding proteins of penicillin-resistant and penicillin-tolerant *Streptococcus pneumoniae*, in *Beta-Lactam Antibiotics. Mode of Action, New Developments, and Future Prospects* (M. Salton and G. C. Shockman, eds.), Academic, New York, 1981, pp. 215-225.
23. G. H. Stollerman. Global changes in group A streptococcal diseases and strategies for their prevention. *Adv. Intern. Med., 27*:373-406 (1982).
24. R. Fujii. Consumption of antibiotics in Japan. *Chemotherapy, 25*:418 (1977).
25. K. S. Kim and B. F. Anthony. Penicillin tolerance in group B streptococci isolated from infected neonates. *J. Infect. Dis., 144*:411-419 (1981).
26. C. J. Baker. Group B streptococcal infections in neonates. *Pediatr. Rev., 1*: 5-14 (1979).
27. P. Y. Paterson. Central nervous system infection: General considerations, in *The Biologic and Clinical Basis of Infectious Diseases* (G. P. Youmans, P. Y. Paterson, and H. M. Sommers, eds.), Saunders, Philadelphia, 1980, pp. 583-595.

28. B. A. Atkinson. Species incidence, trends of susceptibility to antibiotics in the United States, and minimum inhibitory concentration, in *Antibiotics in Laboratory Medicine* (V. Lorian, ed.), Williams and Wilkins, Baltimore, 1980, pp. 607–722.
29. J. B. Cornett, B. E. Redman, and G. D. Shockman. *J. Bacteriol., 133*:631 (1978).
30. R. B. Sykes and N. H. Georgopapadakou. Bacterial resistance to beta-lactam antibiotics: An overview, in *Beta-Lactam Antibiotics. Mode of Action, New Developments, and Future Prospects* (M. Salton and G. D. Shockman, eds.), Academic, New York, 1981, pp. 199–214.
31. R. L. Thompson and A. J. Wright. Cephalosporin antibiotics. *Mayo Clin. Proc., 58*:79–87 (1983).
32. R. E. Dixon. Epidemiology of drug resistance in hospital, in *Drug Inactivating Enzymes and Antibiotic Resistance* (S. Mitsuhashi, L. Rosival, and V. Kremerg, eds.), Springer-Verlag, New York, 1975, pp. 349–360.
33. G. N. Rolinson. Celbenin-resistant staphylococci. *Br. Med. J., 1*:125 (1961).
34. M. P. Jevons. Celbenin-resistant staphylococci. *Br. Med. J., 1*:124 (1961).
35. F. H. Kayser. Methicillin-resistant *Staphylococci* 1965–75. *Lancet, 2*:650–653 (1975).
36. K. Rosendal, O. Jessen, M. W. Bentzon, and P. Bulow. Antibiotic policy and spread of *Staphylococcus aureus* strains in Danish hospitals, 1969–1974. *Acta Pathol. Microbiol. Scand. Sect. B, 85*:143–152 (1977).
37. G. A. J. Ayliffe, H. A. Lilly, and E. J. L. Lowbury. Decline of the hospital *Staphylococcus*? Incidence of multiresistant *Staphylococcus aureus* in three Birmingham hospitals. *Lancet, 1*:538–540 (1979).
38. D. L. Hahn and W. A. Baker. Penicillin G. Susceptibility of "rural" *Staphylococcus aureus* strains isolated in Denmark in 1979. *Acta Pathol. Microbiol. Scand. Sect. B, 89*:185–191 (1981).
39. M. McDonald, A. Hurse, and K. Sim. Methicillin-resistant *Staphylococcus aureus* bacteraemia. *Med. J. Aust., 2*:191–194 (1981).
40. G. Saroglou, M. Cromer, and A. L. Bisno. Methicillin-resistant *Staphylococcus aureus*: Interstate spread of nosocomial infections with emergence of gentamicin–methicillin resistant strains. *Infect. Control. 1*:81–89 (1980).
41. F. F. Barrett, R. F. McGehee, Jr., and M. Finland. Methicillin-resistant *Staphylococcus aureus* at Boston City Hospital. *New Engl. J. Med., 279*: 441–448 (1968).
42. R. S. Holzman, A. L. Florman, and M. Lyman. Gentamicin resistant and sensitive strains of *S. aureus*. Factors affecting colonization and virulence for infants in a special care nursery. *Am. J. Epidemiol., 112*:352–361 (1980).
43. P. J. Demuth, D. N. Gerding, and K. Crossley. *Staphylococcus aureus* bacteriuria. *Arch. Intern. Med., 139*:78–80 (1979).
44. C. C. Linnemann, Jr., M. Mason, P. Moore, and T. Korfhagen. Methicillin-resistant *Staphylococcus aureus*: Experience in a general hospital over four years. *Am. J. Epidemiol., 115*:941–950 (1982).

45. L. D. Sabath, C. D. Leaf, D. A. Gerstein, and M. Finland. Cell walls of methicillin-resistant *Staphylococcus aureus*. *Nature, 225*:1074 (1970).
46. F. H. Kayser, J. Wust, and P. Santanam. Genetic and molecular characterization of resistance determinants in methicillin resistant *Staphylococcus aureus*. *J. Med. Microbiol., 9*:137–148 (1976).
47. F. H. Kayser, J. Wust, and P. Corrodi. Transduction and elimination of resistance determinants in methicillin-resistant *Staphylococcus aureus*. *Antimicrob. Agents Chemother., 2*:217–223 (1972).
48. M. S. Cohen, M. H. Cooney, E. Blackman, and P. F. Sparling. *In vitro* antimicrobial susceptibility of penicillinase-producing and intrinsically resistant *Neisseria gonorrhoeae* strains. *Antimicrob. Agents Chemother., 24*:597–599 (1983).
49. W. M. McCormack. Penicillinase-producing *Neisseria gonorrhoeae*—A retrospective. *N. Engl. J. Med., 307*:438–439 (1982).
50. W. Rodriguez and A. K. Saz. Possible mechanism of decreased susceptibility of *Neisseria gonorrhoeae* to penicillin. *Antimicrob. Agents Chemother., 7*: 788 (1975).
51. J. L. Beebe, P. Ligeti, and T. J. Wlodkowski. Absence of penicillin-degrading enzymes in penicillin-resistant strains of *Neisseria gonorrhoeae*. *Antimicrob. Agents Chemother., 10*:179–181 (1976).
52. N. J. Slevin, J. Aitken, and P. E. Thornley. Clinical and microbiological features of *Branhamella catarrhalis* bronchopulmonary infections. *Lancet, 1*:782–783 (1984).
53. M. O. Tomeh, S. E. Starr, J. E. McGowna, P. M. Terry, and A. J. Nahmias. Ampicillin-resistant *Haemophilus influenzae* type B infection. *J. Am. Med. Assoc., 229*:295–304 (1974).
54. A. A. Medeiros and T. F. O'Brien. Ampicillin-resistant *Haemophilus influenzae* type B possessing a TEM-type β-lactamase but little permeability barrier to ampicillin. *Lancet, 1*:716–718 (1975).
55. A. L. Smith. Antibiotics and invasive *Haemophilus influenzae*. *New Engl. J. Med., 294*:1329–1331 (1976).
56. R. Schwartz, W. Rodriguez, W. Khan, and S. Ross. The increasing incidence of ampicillin-resistant *Haemophilus influenzae*. *J. Am. Med. Assoc., 239*: 320–323 (1978).
57. D. W. Scheifele. Ampicillin-resistant *Hemophilus influenzae* in Canada: Nationwide survey of hospital laboratories. *Can. Med. Assoc. J., 121*:198–202 (1979).
58. S. L. Katz. Ampicillin-resistant *Hemophilus influenzae* type B. A status report. *Pediatrics, 15*:6–8 (1979).
59. P. F. Sparling. Antibiotic resistant in *H. influenzae* and *N. gonorrhoeae*. *Hosp. Pract., 14*:55–61 (1979).
60. S. Simasathien, C. Duangmani, and P. Echeverria. *Haemophilus influenzae* type B resistance to ampicillin and chloramphenicol in an orphanage in Thailand. *Lancet, 1*:1214–1216 (1980).
61. D. W. Scheifele and S. J. Fussell. Frequency of ampicillin-resistant *Haemophilus parainfluenzae* in children. *J. Infect. Dis., 243*:495–498 (1981).

62. R. E. Markham, R. A. Insel, R. F. Betts, and R. G. Robertson. Cefamandole failure in ampicillin-resistant *Haemophilus influenzae* type B pneumonia. *South. Med. J., 74*:147–150 (1981).
63. R. H. Schwartz, R. I. Goldenberg, C. Park, and E. V. Soto. Systemic *Haemophilus influenzae* infections in a community hospital: Prevalence of ampicillin resistance. *South. Med. J., 74*:151–152 (1981).
64. H. A. Kilham and D. C. Dorman. Ampicillin-resistant *Haemophilus influenzae. Med. J. Aust., 1*:658 (1981).
65. E. A. Steinberg, G. D. Overturf, J. Wilkens, L. J. Baraff, J. M. Streng, and J. M. Lecdom. Failure of cafemandole in the treatment of meningitis due to *Haemophilus influenzae* type b. *J. Infect. Dis., Suppl. 137*:S180–S186 (1978).
66. S. L. Kaplan, E. O. Mason, Jr., S. I. Kvernland, E. M. Loiselle, and R. D. Feigin. Treatment of serious infections primarily due to *Haemophilus influenzae* type b in children. *Pediatrics, 71*:187–191 (1983).
67. C. Thornsberry and L. K. McDougal. Ampicillin-resistant *Haemophilus influenzae.* 1. Incidence, mechanism, and detection. *Postgrad. Med., 71*:133–145 (1982).
68. A. A. Medeiros and T. F. O'Brien. Ampicillin-resistant *Haemophilus influenzae* type B possessing a TEM-type-beta-lactamase but little permeability barrier to ampicillin. *Lancet, 1*:716–719 (1975).
69. J. H. Dabernat and C. Delmas. Comparative activity of cefotaxime and selected beta-lactam antibiotics against *Haemophilus influenzae* and aerobic gram-negative bacilli. *Rev. Infect. Dis., 4*:S401–S405 (1982).
70. K. P. Fu and H. C. Neu. Azlocillin and mezlocillin: New ureido penicillins. *Antimicrob. Agents Chemother., 13*:930–938 (1978).
71. P. R. Murray, G. G. Granich, D. J. Krogstad, and A. C. Niles. In vivo selection of resistant to multiple cephalosporins to *Enterobacter cloacae. J. Infect. Dis., 247*:590 (1983).
72. C. C. Saunders. Novel resistance selected by the new expanded-spectrum cephalosporins: A concern. *J. Infect. Dis., 147*:585–598 (1983).
73. T. D. Gootz, C. C. Sanders, and R. V. Goering. Resistance to cefamandole: Depression of beta-lactamases by cefoxitin and mutation in *Enterobacter cloacae. J. Infect. Dis., 146*:34–42 (1982).
74. C. C. Sanders. Inducible beta-lactamases and non-hydrolytic resistance mechanisms. *J. Antimicrob. Chemother., 13*:1–3 (1984).
75. R. S. Edson, J. E. Rosenblatt, D. T. Lee, and E. A. McVey. III. Recent experience with antimicrobial susceptibility of anaerobic bacteria. Increasing resistance to penicillin. *Mayo Clin. Proc., 57*:737–741 (1982).
76. K. S. Thomson, Z. A. Majglo, G. N. Pearce, and T. J. Regan. 3-Dimensional susceptibility testing of beta-lactam antibiotics. *J. Antimicrob. Chemother., 13*:45–54 (1984).
77. H. C. Neu. Combination of ceftizoxime with azlocillin mezlocillin, piperacillin, and ticarcillin. *J. Antimicrob. Chemother., Suppl. C, 10*:63–68 (1982).
78. R. C. Moellering, Jr., S. Wiley, and G. M. Eliopoulos. Synergism and an-

tagonism of ceftizoxime and other new cephalosporins. *J. Antimicrob. Chemother. Suppl. C, 10*:69–79 (1982).
79. M. A. Miller, M. Finan, and M. Yousuf. *In vitro* antagonisms by N-formin doyl thienamycin and cefoxitin of second and third generation cephalosporins in *Aeromonas hydrophila* and *Serratia marcescens*. *J. Antimicrob. Chemother., 11*:311–318 (1983).
80. D. L. Palmer. Epidemiology of antibiotic resistance. *J. Med., 11*:255–261 (1980).
81. T. F. O'Brien, J. F. Acar, A. A. Medeiros, R. A. Norton, F. Goldstein, and R. L. Kent. International comparison of prevalence of resistance to antibiotics. *J. Am. Med. Assoc., 239*:1518–1523 (1978).

5

Biosynthesis of Penicillins and Cephalosporins

SIR EDWARD P. ABRAHAM
Sir William Dunn School of Pathology, University of Oxford, Oxford, England

I. INTRODUCTION

A. Penicillin G and Penicillin V

In the course of a massive Anglo-American effort during World War II to make penicillin in quantity, determine its structure, and obtain it, if possible, by chemical synthesis, the British and American penicillins produced by fermentation of *Penicillium notatum* and *Penicillium chrysogenum* were found to differ. The former (penicillin F, 2-pentenylpenicillin) contained a hexenoyl side chain (R = $CH_3CH_2CH{=}CH{\cdot}CH_2$ in [1]), and the latter (penicillin G, benzylpenicillin) a

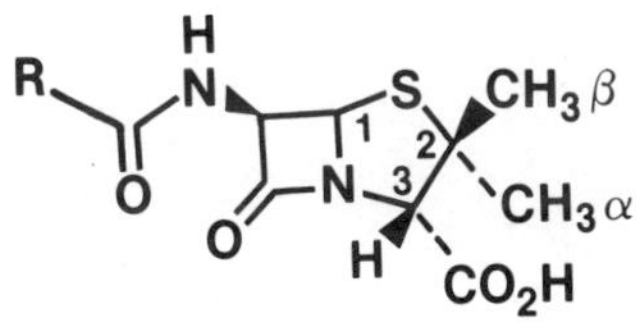

[1]

phenylacetyl side chain (R = $C_6H_5CH_2$ in [1]) (1,2).* This difference was traced to the incorporation of corn-steep liquor, containing derivatives of phenylacetic acid, into the American culture media. Subsequent studies showed that a variety of similar monosubstituted acetic acids could act as side chain pre-

*Publications on the biosynthesis of penicillins and cephalosporins are now so numerous that review articles have been cited for references to much of the research described in this chapter, but references to original papers have been given for some of the most recent work.

cursors of corresponding penicillins (3). None of the further penicillins obtained in this way were markedly superior to penicillin G in their antibacterial properties. However, penicillin V (phenoxymethylpenicillin), with a phenoxyacetyl side chain ($R = C_6H_5OCH_2$ in [1]), was relatively stable at a low pH. It survived in the presence of gastric acid and was effective when given by mouth.

Among the penicillins that have found long-lasting clinical use, only penicillin G and penicillin V are produced entirely by fermentation. Attempts to make penicillins by a commercially acceptable total synthesis have been unsuccessful, but semisynthesis, in which different side chains are coupled chemically with the penicillin nucleus, has been responsible for the production of new penicillins with a wider spectrum of activity.

The finding that a limited number of penicillins with different side chains could be produced by *P. chrysogenum* and that a transacylase could catalyze the exchange of the side chains of penicillins G and V with the penicillin nucleus provided the first definitive information about penicillin biosynthesis (4). This was followed by the demonstration, with isotopically labeled amino acids, that the ring system of the molecule is formed from L-cysteine and L-valine. Since penicillin has the D configuration at C-3 in the fragment derived from L-valine, a change in the configuration occurs at some stage in the biosynthetic pathway (3).

Two further observations that were relevant to the elucidation of this pathway were made in Japan in the early 1950s. One was that chemical assays gave higher values than antibacterial assays for the amount of penicillin in culture fluids from fermentations to which no side-chain precursor has been added. This led to the conclusion that a relatively inactive penicillin nucleus was present. The second observation was that an amidase (acylase) from *P. chrysogenum* could apparently remove the penicillin side chain to yield the nucleus. Toward the end of the decade independent research by members of Beecham Laboratories (5) led to the isolation of this compound in quantity and its characterization as 6-aminopenicillanic acid (6-APA, [2]).

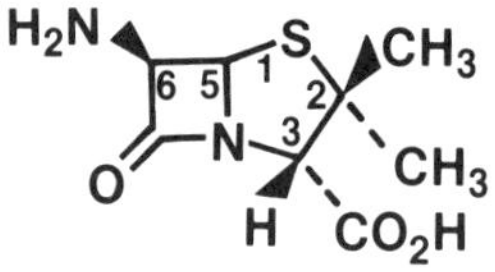

[2]

The question then arose as to whether 6-APA was an intermediate in penicillin biosynthesis.

B. Cephalosporin C

The discovery in Oxford that a Sardinian strain of *Cephalosporium acremonium* produced a hydrophilic penicillin with a new side chain (penicillin N) and that this penicillin was accompanied by a related beta-lactam antibiotic (cephalosporin C), with the same side chain but a different ring system (6,7), led to further understanding of penicillin biosynthesis. As was to be expected, L-cysteine and L-valine were precursors of the ring systems of penicillin N [3] and cephalo-

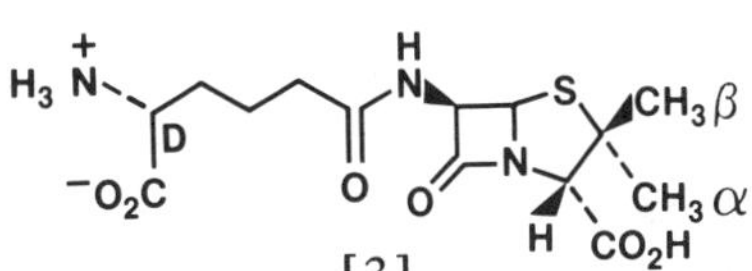

[3]

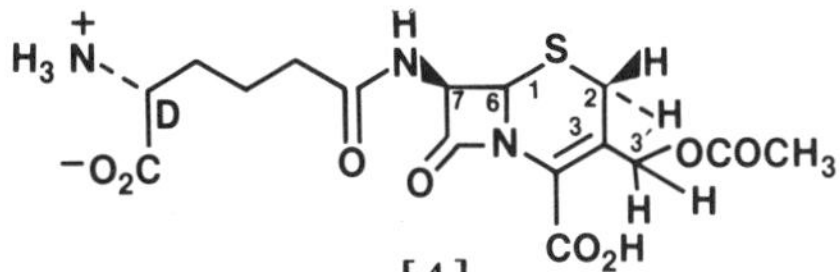

[4]

sporin C [4]. But the δ-(D-α-aminoadipyl) side chains of these compounds could not be varied by the addition of potential side-chain precursors to the fermentation. The *Cephalosporium* species, unlike *P. chrysogenum*, incorporated only α-aminoadipic acid into a penicillin and it produced little, if any, 6-APA. However, isopenicillin N, with a δ-(L-α-aminoadipyl) side chain, was later shown in the Beecham and Lilly laboratories to be produced by *P. chrysogenum.*

II. BIOSYNTHETIC PATHWAYS

Following the discovery of penicillin N, in 1960 the tripeptide δ-aminoadipylcysteinylvaline (ACV) was found to be present in small amounts in the mycelium of *P. chrysogenum* (8). The sequence of the amino acids in this peptide suggested that it might be a precursor of penicillin N and other penicillins. Later the same peptide was isolated from the mycelium of *C. acremonium* and its α-aminoadipic acid, cysteine, and valine residues [5] were shown to have the L,

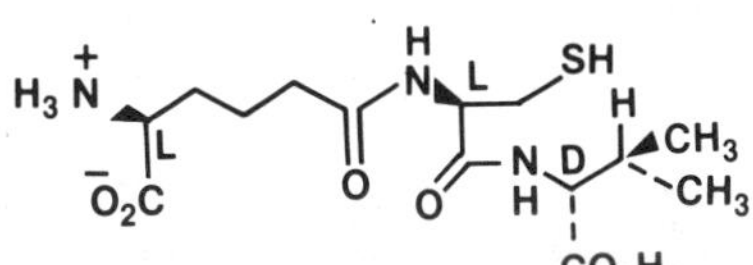

[5]

L, and D configurations, respectively (9).

A. Biosynthesis by Cell-Free Enzymes

Although the pattern of labeling from [^{14}C] valine of L,L,D-ACV and penicillin N in mycelial suspensions of *C. acremonium* was consistent with a precursor-product relationship, a direct demonstration of penicillin formation from the tripeptide required a cell-free system, since exogenous peptide was not transported into the mycelial cell. The first cell-free system in which the synthesis of a penicillin N-like substance from L,L,D-ACV could be detected was obtained by the osmotic lysis of protoplasts of *C. acremonium* (7). Later it was shown that a soluble enzyme responsible for this reaction could also be liberated by mechanical or ultrasonic disruption of the mycelium of *C. acremonium, P. chrysogenum,* and *Streptomyces clavuligerus* and could then be purified (10). The enzyme proved to be an iron-requiring oxygenase with a molecular weight of about 35,000. Its activity was greatly enhanced in the presence of dithiothreitol, ascorbate, and catalase. The product of the reaction it catalyzed, was isopenicillin N.

In the presence of isopenicillin N synthetase, the carbon skeleton of doubly labeled L,L,D-ACV is incorporated intact into isopenicillin N, with retention of the configuration of its three amino acid residues (11) and no exchange of its oxygen atoms (12). The formation of isopenicillin N can be followed by not only antibacterial assay but also recording changes in the nuclear magnetic resonance spectrum of the system (13) as the cyclization of the tripeptide proceeds. One mole of oxygen is absorbed per mole of penicillin formed (14).

Isopenicillin N has a central role in the biosynthesis of penicillin G and penicillin V by *P. chrysogenum* and of cephalosporin C and related compounds by *C. acremonium* and *Streoptomyces* spp. A labile acyltransferase has been found in extracts of *P. chrysogenum* that catalyzes the formation of penicillin G from 6-APA and also from isopenicillin N in the presence of phenylacetylcoenzyme A (15). In addition, preparations of this acyltransferase catalyze the hydrolytic removal of the side chains of penicillin V and (less readily) of isopenicillin N to yield 6-APA (15). It has been suggested that a single enzyme with multiple activities is involved in some of these reactions (16).

Further studies are required for the determination of the precise sequence of events in the last stage of penicillin biosynthesis in *P. chrysogenum*. But the results of experiments with cell-free systems are consistent with the hypothesis that isopenicillin N functions as a direct or indirect precursor of penicillin G and penicillin V. In *C. acremonium*, on the other hand, an epimerase converts some isopenicillin N into penicillin N and only the latter is excreted into the extracellular fluid (17).

The structural relationship of cephalosporin C [4] to penicillin N [3] raised the question as to whether the latter was a precursor of the former in *C. acremonium.* In 1976 it was shown that penicillin N was converted into a cephalosporin-like substance in a cell-free system obtained by lysis of protoplasts of the *Cephalosporium,* and this substance was later identified as deacetoxycephalosporin C (18). Like isopenicillin N synthetase, the enzyme which catalyzes the expansion of the thiazolidine to the dihydrothiazine is an oxygenase which requires ferrous iron and ascorbate for maximum activity. It differs from the synthetase, however, in also requiring α-ketoglutarate (19), and it thus belongs to a group of dioxygenases that utilize one atom of molecular oxygen for the oxidation of substrate and a second atom for a coupled oxidative conversion of α-ketoglutarate to succinate and carbon dioxide. The ring expansion enzyme has been separated from the isopenicillin N synthesis by ion exchange chromatography (20; B. Chakravarti and J. E. Baldwin, unpublished experiments).

Two further reactions, which lead finally to cephalosporin C, have been demonstrated in cell-free systems (15). Deacetoxycephalosporin C is first converted to deacetylcephalosporin C by oxidation of its methyl group at C-3 in the presence of an oxygenase which also requires ferrous iron, ascorbate, and α-ketoglutarate and may be similar to the ring expansion enzyme (21). The resulting hydroxyl group at C-3' is then acylated by acetyl coenzyme A.

In *Streptomyces* spp., including *S. clavuligerus* and *Streptomyces lipmanii*, a fourth oxidative reaction results in the introduction of a 7α-methoxy group into the cephalosporin molecule. The resulting products have been named cephamycins. The oxygen of the methoxyl group comes from molecular oxygen and the methyl from S-adenosylmethionine. Again, this reaction has been shown to be catalyzed in a cell-free system by an oxygenase requiring ferrous iron and α-ketoglutarate (15).

The biosynthetic pathways to penicillins and cephalosporins that have been constructed from the results of experiments with cell-free systems are summarized in Scheme 1. The frequency with which iron-requiring oxygenases are involved in stages of these pathways is notable.

Scheme 1

L-α-aminoadipic acid, L-cysteine, L-valine
↓
δ-(L-α-aminoadipyl)-L-cysteinyl-D-valine
↓
Isopenicillin N

P. chrysogenum ↙ ↘ *C. acremonium*

P. chrysogenum: Penicillin G, Penicillin V, 6-APA

C. acremonium: Penicillin N → Deacetoxycephalosporin C → Deacetylcephalosporin C → Cephalosporin C

B. Biosynthesis in Blocked Mutants

Several steps in the biosynthetic pathways are supported by the behavior of mutants of penicillin- or cephalosporin-producing organisms in which a step in the pathway is blocked. For example, lysine auxotrophs of *P. chrysogenum* blocked before α-aminoadipic acid (a precursor of lysine) failed to synthesize penicillin G when grown in the presence of lysine unless α-aminoadipic acid was added to the culture. This revealed an essential role for α-aminoadipic acid in the biosynthesis of penicillins which did not have an α-aminoadipyl side chain. Furthermore, mutants of both *P. chrysogenum* and *C. acremonium* that were unable to synthesize the tripeptide L,L,D-ACV failed to produce a penicillin (22).

The isolation of mutants of *C. acremonium* that could synthesize penicillin N but not cephalosporin C, and the failure to isolate cephalosporin C-producing organisms that synthesized no penicillin N, was consistent with the proposed conversion of penicillin N to cephalosporin C. Some cephalosporin C-negative mutants, however, formed deacetoxycephalosporin C but no deacetylcephalosporin C, and others produced small amounts of deacetylcephalosporin C but no cephalosporin C itself. These findings indicated that a pathway in the *Cephalosporium* sp. led from deacetoxycephalosporin C to cephalosporin C via deacetylcephalosporin C (22).

III. MECHANISMS AND SPECIFICITY OF BIOSYNTHETIC REACTIONS

A. Hypothetical Intermediates

Although the mechanisms of formation of the penicillin and cephalosporin ring systems have not been finally established, several hypothetical mechanisms have been excluded. Experiments with ^{3}H-labeled valine have shown that in the inversion of L-valine to form the D-valine residue of L,L,D-ACV and the cyclization of L,L,D-ACV to yield isopenicillin N there is no free α,β-dehydrovaline-containing intermediate. Similarly, no α, β-dehydrocysteine residue is involved in the closure of the beta-lactam ring (7).

Several compounds, in addition to those containing a dehydrovaline or dehydrocysteine residue, have been proposed as free intermediates in the biosynthesis of penicillins and cephalosporins. Thus it has been suggested that the valine residue of L,L,D-ACV is oxidized to a D-β-hydroxyvaline residue and that the resulting analog of ACV yields an intermediate "cyclic cysteinylvaline" containing a seven-membered thiazepinone ring [6]. This hypothesis was tested when the peptide analog and [6] were obtained by chemical synthesis. Neither compound was accepted as a substrate by a preparation of isopenicillin N synthetase (23).

An early suggestion that the formation of the penicillin ring system occurred in two discrete steps, the first being the closure of the beta-lactam ring, appeared to have experimental support when it was reported that the monocyclic beta-lactam [7] was formed from L,L,D-ACV in a protoplast lysate of *P. chryso-*

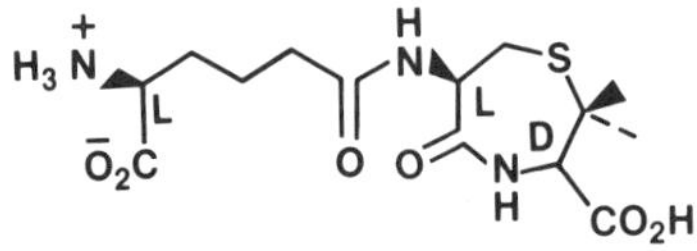

[6]

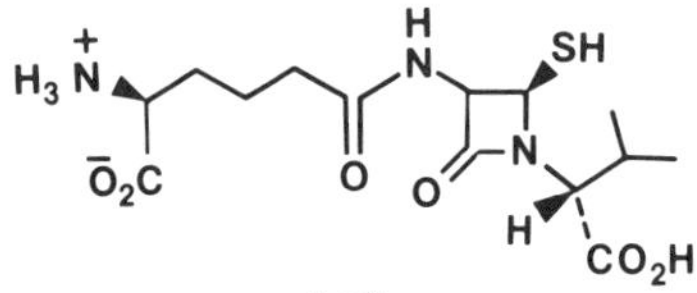

[7]

genum. But this claim could not be confirmed (24). Although the synthetic disulfide of the monocyclic compound was relatively stable, the thiol [7] was extremely unstable at pH 7 and above, having a lifetime of less than 3 min. No isopenicillin N was formed when isopenicillin N synthetase was incubated with the disulfide or with the latter reduced in situ with dithiothreitol. Nevertheless, the exclusion of a free intermediate does not eliminate the possibility that cyclization to an enzyme-bound monocyclic beta-lactam is the first step in the production of isopenicillin N from L,L,D-ACV. It may be that there is no intermediate in the cyclization or ring expansion reaction that is not enzyme bound.

B. Specificity of Biosynthetic Reactions

Although L,L,D-ACV is by far the best substrate found so far for isopenicillin synthetase, it is not the only substrate for the cell-free enzyme, and studies with analogs of this tripeptide have thrown further light on penicillin formation. The failure of the enzyme to cyclize phenylacetyl-L-cysteinyl-D-valine to penicillin G in significant yield is consistent with earlier indications that this and related peptides are not intermediates in penicillin biosynthesis by *P. chrysogenum.* But the synthetase catalyzes the conversion of adipyl-L-cysteinyl-D-valine to a penicillin with an adipyl side chain (25). This penicillin is known to be produced in fermentations of *P. chrysogenum* to which adipic acid has been added (26), but the stage at which adipic acid enters the biosynthetic pathway is at present uncertain. D,L,D-ACV is a substrate for the synthetase (although a very much poorer one than L,L,D-ACV) and is cyclized to penicillin N instead of isopenicillin N (25). There is no indication, however, of the synthesis of the D,L,D tripeptide by penicillin-producing organisms.

Changes in the cysteine residue of L,L,D-ACV yielded peptides that are neither substrates nor inhibitors of isopenicillin N synthetase. Examples are analogs of L,L,D-ACV containing an L-serine and and L-alanine residue, respectively, in place of L-cysteine. These peptides have been isolated from the fermentation fluid of *P. chrysogenum*, but they do not yield a nuclear analog of isopenicillin N with oxygen in place of sulfur and do not inhibit the formation of isopenicillin N from L,L,D-ACV. It appears that the thiol group of L,L,D-ACV is required for the binding of the peptide to the enzyme as well as for ring formation.

In contrast, analogs of L,L,D-ACV in which certain changes have been made in the D-valine residue are cyclized by isopenicillin N synthetase to yield corresponding penicillins (27,28). Examples are peptides in which D-valine has been replaced by D-isoleucine, D-allo-isoleucine, and D-α-aminobutyric acid. The penicillins from the latter two peptides have been reported to be acceptable to the ring expansion enzyme and to be convertible to the corresponding cephalosporins ([8] with $R = C_2H_5$ and $R = H$, respectively).

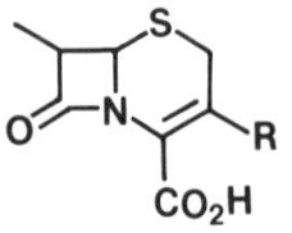

[8]

IV. STEREOCHEMISTRY AND MECHANISMS OF RING CLOSURE

The synthesis of chirally labeled [4-^{13}C] valines enabled it to be shown that the insertion of the cysteine sulfur at C-3 of the valine residue of L,L,D-ACV to form the thiazolidine ring of isopenicillin is stereospecific and occurs with retention of configuration. Carbon-13 nuclear magnetic resonance (NMR) studies showed that the ^{13}C of 3R-[4-^{13}C] valine [9] was incorporated exclusively into

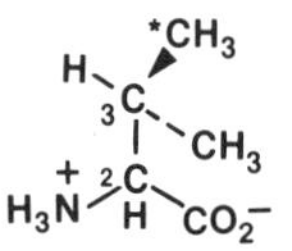

[9]

the β-methyl group of penicillin and the ^{13}C of 3S-[4-^{13}C] valine was incorporated exclusively into the α-methyl group [1]. The incorporation of the chiral gem-dimethyl group into cephalosporin C is also stereospecific, the α- and β-methyl groups of penicillin N becoming the exo- and endocyclic methylenes, respectively, of the cephalosporin (7). Further studies with methyl-deuterated valines showed that the methyl groups of valine remained intact during penicillin biosynthesis and that only one deuterium was lost from each methyl group during the ring expansion of penicillin N to cephalosporin C.

More recently, the synthesis of "chiral methyl valines," in which one hydrogen of each methyl group is replaced by tritium and one by deuterium, has made it possible to study the stereochemistry of the incorporation of the methyl groups into the methylene groups of cephalosporin C. Comparison of the ^{3}H-NMR spectrum of cephalosporin C derived from valine having the 3S-4R and 3R-4S configuration [10] with that from valine having the 3S-4S and 3R-4R configuration [11] indicated that the incorporation into the exocyclic methylene (C-3' in [4]) was stereospecific (29). On the other hand, the NMR signals obtained from tritium in the endocyclic methylene (C-2 in [4]) showed little

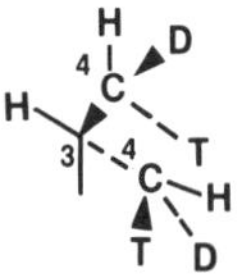

[10]

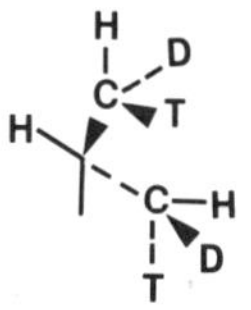

[11]

change when the configuration in the valine methyl groups was reversed and indicated that ^3H had been incorporated almost equally into the α- and β-positions [4]. It thus appears that "racemization" of a valine methyl group occurs during the ring expansion reaction.

The D-isoleucine analog of L,L,D-ACV yielded a penicillin with an α-methyl group and a β-ethyl group at C-2 instead of [3], whereas the D-allo-isoleucine analog (a much poorer substrate) gave a penicillin in which the positions of these two groups were reversed. Hence ring closure occurred with retention of configuration. With the D-α-aminobutyric acid analog the major product was a norpenicillin, with a β-methyl group and an α-hydrogen at C-2. In these cases, therefore, the most facile cyclization was that in which the larger group came to occupy the β-position.

Further information about the stereochemistry of the carbon–sulfur bond formation was obtained from the synthetic peptides in which C-terminal D-α-aminobutyric acid residues had one deuterium at C-3 and the 3R and 3S configuration, respectively (30). The ^1H-NMR spectra of the norpenicillins from these two peptides were identical and the penicillins yielded identical norpenicillanic acids on oxidative degradation. In each case the penicillin methyl group was in the β-position. Hence retention of configuration occurred in one case during C–S bond formation, and inversion in the other.

A minor product was detected during a study of the oxidative cyclization of δ-(L-α-aminoadipyl)-L-cysteinyl-D-α-aminobutyric acid into 2S-norisopenicillin N by a purified preparation of isopenicillin N synthetase having no ring expansion activity. This product was shown by ^1H-NMR data and by its degradation to homocysteic acid to contain a dihydrocephalosporin (cepham) ring system [12]. Thus the synthetase can bring about both a 5- and 6-ring closure from an

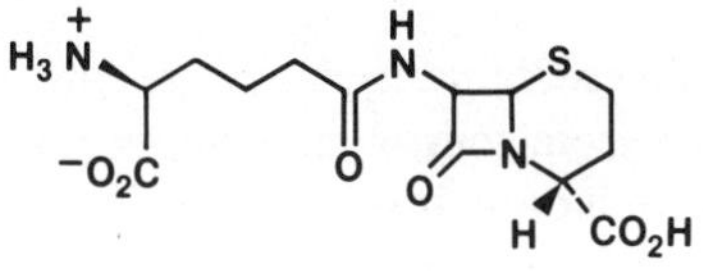

[12]

appropriate tripeptide precursor (31).

The structures of the compounds formed when the D-α-aminobutyric acid analog of L,L,D-ACV is a substrate for isopenicillin N synthetase appear to be consistent with the suggestion of a radical mechanism (32) for the formation of a C–S bond in penicillin biosynthesis. If ring closure to give isopenicillin from [13] were faster than rotation about the valine C2–C3 bond, the insertion of

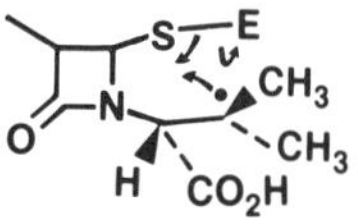

[13]

sulfur with retention of configuration would be expected. But a less sterically hindered radical from an α-aminobutyric acid residue might allow more rapid rotation and the formation of a norisopenicillin N with a single configuration preferred by the enzyme, irrespective of whether this required retention or inversion [14]. The exclusive formation of the radical $-\dot{C}(CH_3)_2$ from a valine

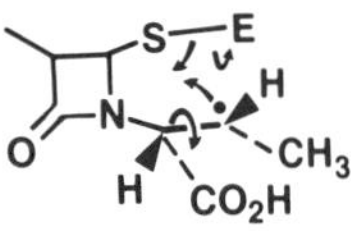

[14]

residue, but the formation $-CH_2-\dot{C}H_2$ as well as $-\dot{C}HCH_3$ from an α-aminobutyric acid residue, would account for the synthesis of a cepham in addition to a norpenicillin.

V. BIOSYNTHESIS AND RECOMBINANT DNA

Increases in the yields of penicillins and cephalosporins produced by fermentation have hitherto been obtained mainly by mutagenesis and the selection of mutant strains and by the introduction of new culture media (33). In the case of penicillins G and V the increase has been more than 20,000-fold since Fleming's observation of penicillin activity. Discoveries of new cephalosporins and other beta-lactam antibiotics produced by *Streptomyces* spp. and Eubacteria have come from systematic screening of wild strains for antibiotic production, aided in recent years by the availability of supersensitive test organisms. Much attention is now being given to the question of whether these essentially empirical procedures can be supplemented or replaced by more rational ones based on genetic engineering (22,34,35).

An increase in antibiotic yield might be achieved, in principle, by genetic changes which liberate the biosynthetic process from control mechanisms that restrict its rate or duration, or by the introduction of multiple copies of genes coding for enzymes. The mechanisms that control the biosynthesis of penicillins and cephalosporins are not yet understood at the level of transcription or translation, but some of them may lead to feedback inhibition. Thus the production of penicillin G in *P. chrysogenum* is inhibited by lysine, because lysine inhibits the biosynthesis of α-aminoadipic acid and thus that of the penicillin precursors (18).

In the prokaryotic *Streptomyces* substantial advances have been made in the techniques of gene cloning by the use of novel plasmid or phage DNA vectors that are taken up by protoplasts (35), and related techniques may become applicable to the eukaryotic *Penicullium* and *Cephalosporium* (36). Substantial numbers of genes are clearly involved in the production of penicillin G and cephalosporin C, since at least four and seven enzymes, respectively, are used to bring about the reactions on the biosynthetic pathways. A gene required for a specific biosynthetic step might be found in a gene library by the introduction of DNA fragments from an antibiotic-producing strain into a mutant blocked at a known stage, such as that leading from L,L,D-ACV to isopenicillin N. Clones carrying the gene would then be marked by their ability to produce antibiotic. Alternatively, the isolation of a specific enzyme and the determination of part, at least, of its amino acid sequence would reveal nucleotide sequences to be looked for in the corresponding structural gene. By this procedure the isopenicillin N synthetase gene has recently been cloned (37).

Another conceivable outcome of the application of recombinant DNA technology is the production of new penicillins or cephalosporins by new combinations of genes that have not been found in nature. *Penicillium chrysogenum* can produce penicillin G and 6-APA, but not cephalosporin C, whereas *C. acremonium* produces cephalosporins with an α-aminoadipyl side chain but no penicillin G or 6-APA. Both organisms produce isopenicillin N. If a gene responsible for the synthesis of a transacylase in the *Penicillium* were introduced into the *Cephalosporium* and continued to function, the latter organism might produce penicillin G, penicillin V, and 6-APA. A more interesting possibility would arise if the specificity of the acylase were low enough for cephalosporin C or its immediate precursors to be substrates. Cephalosporins with the side chains of penicillins G and V might then become accessible by fermentation. Here there is now evidence for the existence of an acylase with the required properties. But isopenicillin N synthetase can cyclize certain analogs of L,L,D-ACV, and small amounts of peptides structurally related to L,L,D-ACV are known to be produced by *Penicillium* and *Cephalosporium* fungi. Is it possible, therefore, for new penicillins to be obtained from mutants in which a normal amino acid precursor is not readily available for tripeptide synthesis? In one case at least this is so. A lysine auxotroph of *C. acremonium* that does not synthesize α-aminoadipic acid and therefore cannot make L,L,D-ACV produces a penicillin with an S-carboxymethyl-D-cysteinyl side chain when the L isomer of this amino acid (in which $-S-$ replaces one $-CH_2-$ in α-aminoadipic acid) is added to the culture medium (38).

Whether a lysine auxotroph can also synthesize a penicillin with an adipyl side chain in a medium containing adipic acid is apparently not yet known. In any event, other questions arise (22). Will microorganisms be found that do not produce isopenicillin N synthetase but which synthesize tripeptides that differ from L,L,D-ACV in the isopropyl portion of a D-valine residue? If so, could cloning of genes for the synthetase provide a source of new penicillins and cephalosporins? It can scarcely be doubted that genetic engineering will eventually contribute to a more rational approach to the discovery of new beta-lactam antibiotics of medical interest. But we can still only speculate on how and when this will come about.

REFERENCES

1. O. K. Behrens. Biosynthesis of penicillins, in *The Chemistry of Penicillin* (H. T. Clarke, J. R. Johnson, and Sir Robert Robinson, eds.), Princeton University Press, Princeton, N.J., 1949, p. 657.
2. E. P. Abraham. The chemistry of penicillin. Historical introduction, in *Antibiotics,* Vol. 2 (H. W. Florey, E. Chain, N. G. Heatley, M. A. Jennings, A. G. Sanders, E. P. Abraham, and M. E. Florey, eds.), Oxford University Press, London, 1949, p. 768.
3. H. R. V. Arnstein. The biosynthesis of penicillin and some other antibiotics. *Ann. Rep. Prog. Chem., 54*:339 (1957).
4. D. L. Preuss and M. J. Johnson. Penicillinacyltransferase in *Penicillium chrysogenum. J. Bacteriol., 94*:1502 (1967).
5. F. P. Doyle and J. H. C. Naylor. Penicillins and related structures, in *Advances in Drug Research,* Vol. 1 (N. J. Harper and A. B. Simmonds, eds.), Academic, London, 1964, p. 2.
6. E. P. Abraham and P. B. Loder. Cephalosporin C, in *Cephalosporins and Penicillins* (E. H. Flynn, ed.), Academic, New York, 1972, p. 2.
7. P. A. Fawcett and E. P. Abraham. Biosynthesis of penicillins and cephalosporins, in *Biosynthesis,* Vol. 4, Specialist Periodical Report, The Chemical Society, London, 1976, p. 248.
8. H. R. V. Arnstein, M. Artman, D. Morris, and E. J. Toms. Sulphur-containing amino acids and peptides in the mycelium of *Penicillium chrysogenum. Biochem. J., 76*:353 (1960).
9. P. B. Loder and E. P. Abraham. Isolation and nature of intracellular peptides from a cephalosporin C-producing *Cephalosporium* sp. *Biochem. J., 123*:471 (1971).
10. E. P. Abraham, J. A. Huddleston, G. S. Jayatilake, J. O'Sullivan, and R. L. White. Conversion of δ-(L-α-aminoadipyl)-L-cysteinyl-D-valine to isopenicillin N in cell free extracts of *Cephalosporium acremonium,* in *Recent Advances in the Chemistry of β-Lactam Antibiotics* (G. I. Gregory, ed.), Special Publication, The Royal Society of Chemistry, London, 1981, p. 125.
11. J. O'Sullivan, R. C. Bleaney, J. A. Huddleston, and E. P. Abraham. Incorporation of ^{3}H from δ-(L-α-amino[4,5-^{3}H]adipyl)-L-cysteinyl-D-[4,4-^{3}H]-valine into isopenicillin N. *Biochem. J., 184*:421 (1979).
12. R. M. Adlington, R. T. Aplin, J. E. Baldwin, L. D. Field, E.-M. M. John, Sir Edward Abraham, and R. L. White. Conversion of ^{17}O/^{18}O-labelled δ-(L-α-aminoadipyl)-L-cysteinyl-D-valine into ^{17}O/^{18}O-labelled isopenicillin N in a cell-free extract of *C. acremonium. J. Chem. Soc. Chem. Commun., 1982*:137 (1982).

13. J. E. Baldwin, B. L. Johnson, J. J. Usher, E. P. Abraham, J. A. Huddleston, and R. L. White. Direct n.m.r. observation of cell-free conversion of (L-α-amino-δ-adipyl)-L-cysteinyl-D-valine into isopenicillin N. *J. Chem. Soc. Chem. Commun., 1980*:1271 (1980).
14. R. L. White, E.-M. M. John, J. E. Baldwin, and E. P. Abraham. Stoichiometry of oxygen consumption in the biosynthesis of isopenicillin from a tripeptide. *Biochem. J., 203*:791 (1982).
15. E. P. Abraham and J. O'Sullivan. Biosynthesis of β-lactam antibiotics, in *Antibiotics,* Vol. 4 (J. W. Corcoran, ed.), Springer-Verlag, Berlin, 1981, p. 101.
16. B. Spencer and C. Maung. Multiple activities of penicillin acyl transferase of *Penicillium chrysogenum. Biochem. J., 118*:29P (1970).
17. G. S. Jayatilake, J. A. Huddleston, and E. P. Abraham. Conversion of isopenicillin N into penicillin N in cell-free extracts of *Cephalosporium acremonium. Biochem. J., 194*:645 (1981).
18. A. L. Demain and N. A. Solomon. Biosynthesis of β-lactam antibiotics, in *Antibiotics Containing the Beta-Lactam Structure* (A. L. Demain and N. A. Solomon, eds.), Springer-Verlag, Berlin, 1983, p. 189.
19. J. Kupka, Y.-Q. Shen, S. Wolfe, and A. L. Demain. Partial purification and properties of the α-ketoglutarate-linked ring expansion enzyme of β-lactam biosynthesis of *Cephalosporium acremonium. FEMS Microbiol. Lett., 16*:1 (1982).
20. J. Kupka, Y.-Q. Shen, S. Wolfe, and A. L. Demain. Studies on the ring-cyclisation and ring-expansion enzymes of β-lactam biosynthesis in *Cephalosporium acremonium. Can. J. Microbiol., 29*:488 (1983).
21. A. Scheidegger, M. T. Küenzi, and J. Nuesch. Partial purification and catalytic properties of a bifunctional enzyme in the biosynthetic pathway of β-lactams in *Cephalosporium acremonium. J. Antibiot., 37*:522 (1984).
21a. S. E. Jensen, D. W. S. Westlake, and S. Wolfe. Deacetoxycephalosporin C synthetase and deacetoxycephalosporin C hydroxylase are two separate enzymes in *Streptomyces clavuligerus. J. Antibiot., 38*:263 (1985).
22. S. W. Queener and N. Neuss. The biosynthesis of β-lactam antibiotics, in *Chemistry and Biology of β-Lactam Antibiotics,* Vol. 3 (R. B. Morin and M. Gorman, eds.), Academic, New York, 1982, p. 1.
23. G. Bahadur, J. E. Baldwin, T. Wan, M. Jung, E. P. Abraham, J. A. Huddleston, and R. L. White. On the proposed intermediacy of β-hydroxyvaline- and thiazepinone-containing peptides in penicillin biosynthesis. *J. Chem. Soc. Chem. Commun., 1981*:1146 (1981).
24. E. P. Abraham, R. M. Adlington, J. E. Baldwin, M. J. Crimmin, L. D. Field, G. S. Jayatilake, and R. L. White. Monocyclic β-lactam tripeptide, 1-(D-carboxy-2-methylpropyl)-3-L-(δ-L-2-aminoadipamido)-4-L-mercaptoazetidin-2-one, a putative intermediate in penicillin biosynthesis. *J. Chem. Soc. Chem. Commun., 1982*:1130 (1982).
25. G. S. Jayatilake, R. L. White, E. P. Abraham, and J. E. Baldwin. Unpublished experiments.
26. A. Ballio, F. Dentice di Accadia, M. Francesca, M. Pietro-Cancellieri, G. Morpurgo, G. Serlupi-Crescenzi, and G. Sermonti. Incorporation of α,ω-

dicarboxylic acids as side-chain precursors into the penicillin molecule. *Nature London, 185*:97 (1960).

27. G. A. Bahadur, J. E. Baldwin, J. J. Usher, E. P. Abraham, G. S. Jayatilake, and R. L. White. Cell-free biosynthesis of penicillins. Conversion of peptides into new β-lactam antibiotics. *J. Am. Chem. Soc., 103*:7650 (1981).
28. S. Wolfe. Studies related to β-lactam compounds, in *Current Trends in Organic Chemistry* (H. Nozaki, ed.), IUPAC, Pergamon, Oxford, 1983, p. 111.
29. C.-P. Pang, R. L. White, E. P. Abraham, D. H. G. Crout, M. Lutstorf, P. J. Morgan, and A. E. Derome. Stereochemistry of the incorporation of methyl groups into methylene groups in cephalosporin C. *Biochem. J. 222*:777 (1984).
30. J. E. Baldwin, E. P. Abraham, R. M. Adlington, J. A. Murphy and (in part) N. Green, H.-H. Ting, and J. J. Usher. Penicillin biosynthesis. On the stereochemistry of carbon-sulphur bond formation with modified substrates. *J. Chem. Soc. Chem. Commun., 1983*:1319 (1983).
31. J. E. Baldwin, E. P. Abraham, R. M. Adlington, B. Chakravarti, A. E. Derome, J. A. Murphy, and (in part) L. D. Field, N. Green, H.-H. Ting, and J. J. Usher. Penicillin biosynthesis. Dual pathways from a modified substrate. *J. Chem. Soc. Chem. Commun., 1983*:1317 (1983).
32. J. E. Baldwin and T. S. Wan. Penicillin biosynthesis. Retention of configuration at C-3 of valine during its incorporation into the Arnstein tripeptide. *Tetrahedron, 37*:1589 (1981).
33. R. P. Elander. Trends in the genetic improvement of antibiotic producing microorganisms, in *Trends in Antibiotic Research* (H. Umezawa, A. L. Demain, T. Hata, and C. R. Hutchinson, eds.), Japan Antibiotics Research Association, Tokyo, 1982, p. 16.
34. C. Ball. Genetics of β-lactam-producing fungi, in *Antibiotics Containing the Beta-Lactam Structure* (A. L. Demain and N. A. Solomon, eds.), Springer-Verlag, Berlin, 1983, p. 147.
35. D. A. Hopwood, M. J. Bibb, D. J. Bruton, K. F. Chater, J. S. Feitelson, and J. A. Gil. Cloning *Streptomyces* genes for antibiotic production. *Trends Biotechnol., 1*:1 (1983).
36. S. W. Queener, T. D. Ingolia, P. L. Skatrud, J. L. Chapman, and K. R. Kaster. A system for genetic transformation of *Cephalosporium acremonium. Microbiology - 1985*:468-472, 1985.
37. S. M. Samson, R. Belagaje, D. T. Blankenship, J. L. Chapman, D. Perry, P. L. Skatrud, R. M. VanFrank, E. P. Abraham, J. E. Baldwin, S. W. Queener, and T. D. Ingolia. Isolation, sequence determination and expression in *Escherichia coli* of isopenicillin N synthetase gene from *Cephalosporium acremonium.* Nature 311: , 1985.
38. H. Troonen, P. Roelants, and B. Boon. RIT2214. A new biosynthetic penicillin produced by a mutant of *Cephalosporium acremonium. J. Antibiot., 29*:1258 (1976).

6
Manufacture of Penicillins

DAVID A. LOWE
Bristol-Myers Company, Syracuse, New York

I. INTRODUCTION

In the past 40 years, penicillins have been developed from unstable, low-purity laboratory extracts into multiproduct, multinational, multi-billion-dollar industries, using the services of over 20,000 people in their direct manufacture. Today there is sufficient fermentation and production capacity worldwide to provide each individual on this planet with sufficient penicillin for one therapeutic treatment each year.

The market for penicillins has reached maturity in the developed countries, and future expansion will depend upon penetration into developing countries, which at the moment is restricted by currency exchange and low per capita income. With patent expiration and the increase in the availability of high-producing mutant strains and relevant manufacturing technology, developing countries should be able to establish their own processes.

Penicillin fermentation and semisynthetic penicillin manufacture are dominated presently by U.S. and European companies. In 1982 the United States produced 4.8 x 10^6 kg of fermented penicillin (30% of the total world production) and manufactured 0.94 x 10^6 kg of semisynthetic penicillins, or 18% of the world production (1,2). European companies dominate the manufacture of semisynthetic penicillins and their important intermediate 6-aminopenicillanic acid (6-APA). Worldwide, 9% of fermented penicillin G is converted by chemical ring expansion into the 7-aminodesacetoxycephem nucleus to manufacture oral cephalosporins. In 1975 only 2% of the bulk penicillin G volume was used for ring expansion (3).

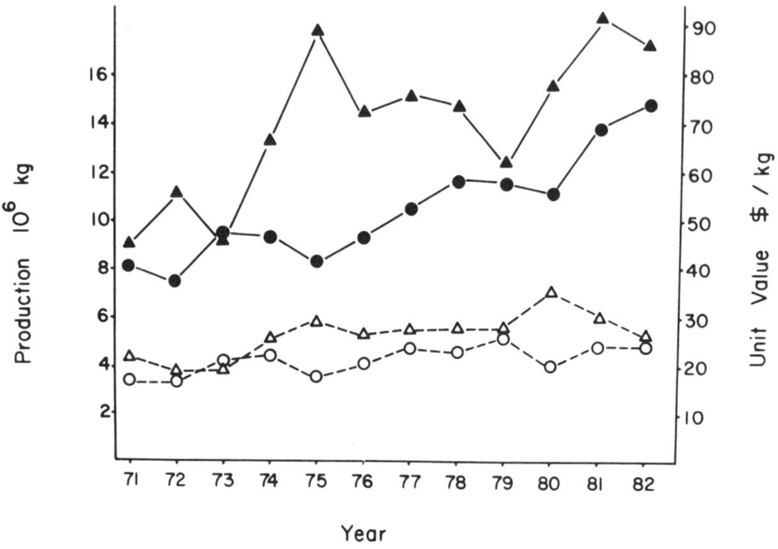

Figure 1 The U.S. manufacture of total antibiotics and penicillin: total antibiotics unit value (▲), total antibiotics production (●), penicillin unit value (△), and penicillin production (○).

Over the period 1971-1982 the volume of penicillin produced in the United States has remained fairly constant (Fig. 1). The unit value for penicillin during this period increased by 18%, compared to a 90% increase in the unit value of all manufactured antibiotics, with the latter figure reflecting a different product mix. Figure 1 demonstrates the sensitivity of antibiotic production to recessionary periods. However, unit value increases during these periods tend to support investors' concepts that the pharmaceutical industry is recession proof.

During the same 11-year period, semisynthetic penicillin sales have increased over 300%, with a unit value reduction of 45% (Fig. 2). The actual value reduction is greater than 80%, allowing for inflation.

Ampicillin, introduced in 1961, has dominated the sales of semisynthetic penicillins. With the expiration of the ampicillin patent, many generic forms of this antibiotic are available today. Ampicillin sales are static mainly owing to the increase in the sales of amoxicillin, introduced in 1971, a semisynthetic of similar structure to ampicillin but having better absorption and pharmacological properties. Amoxicillin should capture a major portion of future sales because of its recent patent expiration and its potential use in combination with the beta-lactamase inhibitor clavulanic acid.

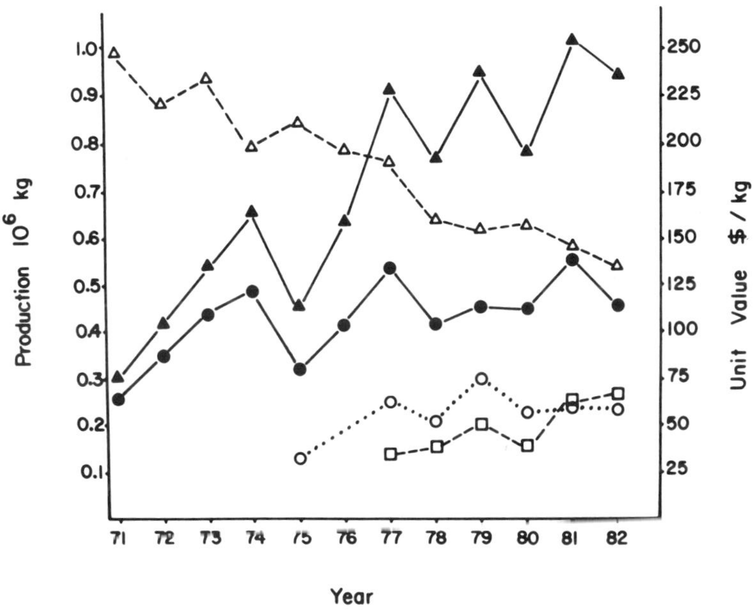

Figure 2 The U.S. manufacture of semisynthetic penicillins: total semisynthetic unit value (△), total semisynthetic production (▲), ampicillin production (●), amoxicillin production (□), and other semisynthetics production (○).

II. HISTORICAL PERSPECTIVE

The fermentation and marketing of penicillin G was the major process which enabled the pharmaceutical industry to become established. The cost effectiveness of penicillin G manufacture rapidly increased by the selection of highly productive mutant strains coupled to the optimization of fermentation and extraction processes. The fact that the form of the fermented penicillin can be directed by the addition of precursor, for example, phenylacetic acid as a precursor of penicillin G, stimulated searches for other suitable precursors (4). This work led to the identification of phenoxyacetic acid as a precursor of penicillin V, an acid-stable penicillin, a property useful for oral administration. Phenoxyacetic acid was less toxic than phenylacetic acid to the producing culture. Therefore the precursor can be batched into the starting medium (3), thereby eliminating the need to feed the more toxic phenylacetic acid throughout the fermentation cycle. This division into two precursored penicillins was also the result of industrial screening programs producing cultures that were superior in the production of either penicillin V or penicillin G. The choice of precursored penicillin caused

Table 1 Semisynthetic Penicillin Patents

Year	Penicillin	U.S. patent (or other)	Company
1960	Diphenicillin, methicillin	2,951,839	Beecham
1961	Ampicillin	2,985,648	Beecham
1961	Clometocillin	3,007,920	RIT
1961	Nafcillin	British patent # 880,400	Beecham
1963	Oxacillin	2,996,501	Beecham
1964	Azidocillin	3,293,242	Beecham
1964	Carbenicillin, ticarcillin	3,282,926	Beecham
1964	Amoxicillin	3,192,198	Beecham
1965	Cyclacillin	3,194,802	American Home Products
1965	Hetacillin	3,198,804	Bristol-Myers
1965	Penamecillin	3,250,679	Wyeth
1968	Carfecillin	3,853,849	Beecham
1969	Carindacillin	3,557,090	Pfizer
1969	Fubenicillin	3,479,339	Bristol-Myers
1969	Epicillin	3,485,819	Squibb
1969	Pivampicillin	3,660,575	Loevens
1970	Sulbenicillin	3,660,379	Takeda
1971	Amdinocillin	3,957,764	Loevens
1971	Azlocillin	3,933,795	Bayer
1972	Talampicillin	3,951,954	Yamanouchi
1973	Bacampicillin	3,873,521	Astra
1973	Apalcillin	3,864,329	Sumitomo
1976	Mezlocillin	3,972,869	Bayer
1976	Piperacillin	4,087,424	Toyama
1976	Temocillin	German patent # 2,600,866	Beecham
1978	Piridicillin	4,101,661	Warner-Lambert
1979	Furazlocillin	4,147,693	Bayer

further process polarizations with the advent of specific penicillin-splitting acylase enzymes and ring expansion chemistry.

By the mid-1950s the widespread use of penicillin G had caused an increase in the occurrence of penicillin-resistant microorganisms owing to their ability to produce penicillase. All naturally precursored penicillins were destroyed by penicillinase activity. However, this potentially dangerous situation was changed by the characterization and isolation of the penicillin nucleus 6-APA and the realization that it could be used to form a range of semisynthetic penicillins by simple chemical acylation. Several industrial systems were developed for the large-scale manufacture of 6-APA and its conversion to new penicillins. The penicillin nucleus could be made by direct fermentation by excluding precursor from penicillin fermentations; however, considerable 6-APA loss occurred owing to its chemical reaction with CO_2 to give 8-hydroxy-penicillic acid (5–7). In addition, 6-APA production was low and it was difficult to extract in high yield. Better commercial routes for 6-APA manufacture were developed by hydrolysis of the precursored penicillin by either chemical or enzymatic techniques (see later).

The availability of 6-APA stimulated a further expansion of the penicillin fermentation industry and the commercialization of the manufacture of semisynthetic penicillins to create an extensive range of antibiotics with properties of penicillinase resistance, altered pharmacological distribution, and a broad spectrum of activity, particularly against gram-negative bacteria.

Table 1 summarizes the chronological development of semisynthetic penicillins. Most of the clinically important derivatives were discovered in the 1960s. The patenting of new semisynthetic penicillins has now declined, mainly because of the rapid devlopment of cephalosporin antibiotics in the 1970s and the current interest in novel beta-lactam antibiotics such as the monobactams and carbapenems. The manufacture of the various classes of semisynthetic penicillins will be discussed later.

III. FERMENTATION OF PENICILLIN

Fleming's *Penicillium notatum* (8) discovered at St. Mary's Hospital in London and Thom's *Penicillium chrysogenum* discovered at Peoria (9) both produce a variety of structures containing the penicillin nucleus (Table 2). When fermented in a suitable medium in the absence of supplemented precursor, several natural penicillins are produced, namely, penicillin F, dihydropenicillin F, and penicillin K. Production of these natural penicillins is also stimulated by the presence of triglycerides or fatty acids in the medium. Absence of precursor in high-producing strains also leads to the synthesis of 6-APA and isopenicillin N. Medium supplementation with phenylacetic acid, phenylacetamide, or β-phenylethylamine stimulates the production of penicillin G. Behrens and co-workers (4) at Lilly concluded that compounds with a free methylene adjacent to their carboxylic

Table 2 Structures Containing the Penicillin Nucleus

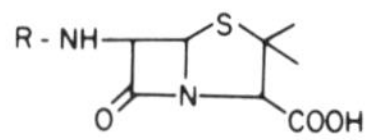

Name	R	Origin	Reference
6-aminopenicillanic acid	H-	without precursor	10
isopenicillin N	L-$NH_2(COOH)CH(CH_2)_3CO$-	without precursor / intermediate	11, 12
penicillin F	$CH_3CH_2CH=CH$-CH_2-CO-	natural penicillin	8
penicillin dihydro F	$CH_3(CH_2)_4$-CO-	natural penicillin	8
penicillin K	$CH_3(CH_2)_6$-CO-	natural penicillin	8
penicillin N	D-$NH_2(COOH)CH(CH_2)_3CO$-	Cephalosporium sp.	13, 14
penicillin G	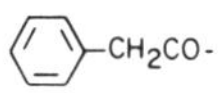	phenylacetic acid precursor	9
p-hydroxypenicillin G	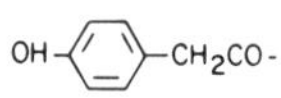	phenylacetic acid precursor	15
penicillin V	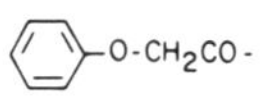	phenoxyacetic acid precursor	4
p-hydroxypenicillin V	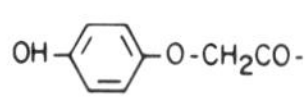	phenoxyacetic acid precursor	16
penicillin BT	$CH_3(CH_2)_3SCH_2CO$-	butylthioacetic acid precursor	17
penicillin O	$CH_2=CHCH_2SCH_2CO$-	allymercaptoacetic acid precursor	17
penicillin S	CH_3-C(Cl)$=CHCH_2SCH_2CO$-	γ-chlorocrotylmercaptoacetic acid precursor	18
RIT-2214	D-$NH_2(COOH)$-$CHCH_2$-S-CH_2CO-	carboxymethyl-L-cysteine added to blocked mutant	19

acid were essential for precursorability. Minor quantities of unwanted precursor-related penicillins can occur in penicillin G and V fermentations, namely, p-hydroxypenicillin G and p-hydroxypenicillin V resulting from the enzymic hydroxylation of the precursor. Strains have now been developed that lack these specific enzymes (16,20).

Penicillins have also been produced by other eukaryotic organisms, notably, *Aspergillus* (21), *Malbranchea* (22), *Cephalosporium* (23–28), *Emericellopsis* (29–32), *Paecilomyces* (33), *Epidermophyton* (34), *Trichophyton* (34), *Anixiopsis* (35), *Diheterospora* (36), *Scopulariopsis* (36), and *Spiroidium* (35). Penicillin N has been produced by prokaryotic *Streptomycetes* (37). None of these microorganisms has been used for the industrial production of penicillins; however, detailed genetic studies have been described in *Aspergillus* 38,39). *Cephalosporium acremonium* and *Streptomyces* species are used industrially for the manufacture of cephalosporin and cephamycin antibiotics.

A. Strain Improvement

Over the past 30 years individual pharmaceutical companies have carried out extensive mutation and selection programs to screen for mutant cultures of *P. chrysogenum* with higher productivities. These independent programs have created a wide variety of subspecies, each unique in its ability to perform optimally in its specific manufacturing environment. Strain improvement programs are considered proprietary information. However, some details have been made available in the reviews by Elander (40,41). Panlabs, Inc., has had a nonexclusive penicillin strain development program in operation for many years (3,20). All of today's industrial strains were derived ultimately from the Wisconsin Q-176 and Wisconsin 51-20 improved strains (42).

Mutations in *P. chrysogenum* are generally induced by ultraviolet (UV) radiation or N-methyl-N′-nitro-N-nitrosoguanidine (NTG). The former has the advantage of being cleaner to use and avoids the handling of potent carcinogenic material. However, NTG has an extremely high mutagenic effect with relatively low kill and its mechanism of mutagenesis complements that of UV radiation (43). Combinations of these treatments can also be effective.

Emphasis in strain improvement has been directed toward titer increase, with secondary emphasis on mycelial vigor and sporulation and germination efficiency. The latter properties are important for strain preservation and inoculum propagation. Initially selection techniques were empirical, relying on the use of large numbers to identify positive mutations. However, more rational screening procedures are now considered to be more effective. Such techniques are based on known or probable biochemical mechanisms and many can be adapted to agar prescreen technology (32,44). Typical selection techniques are summarized in Table 3. Today's cultures are capable of producing in excess of 30 mg/ml penicillin G (45,46).

B. Strain Maintenance

Highly mutated industrial strains have inherent genetic instabilities, and it is of prime importance to maintain both primary stock cultures and working cultures under conditions where phenotypic changes are minimized. This normally entails storage at the temperature of the gaseous (-167°C) or liquid (-196°C) phase of nitrogen (41). Long-term preservation procedures used at Bristol-Myers have been reported (41). Squibb (59) reported the storage of *P. chrysogenum* for 3

Table 3 Biochemical Characteristics and Selection Techniques

	References
Resistance to toxic side-chain precursor	47
Resistance to amino acid analogs	41, 48–50
Resistance to sulfur analogs	40, 49
Selection for better germination	20
Auxotroph reversion	49
Removal of phenylacetic acid oxidase	20
Reduction of p-hydroxypenicillin V	16
Parasexual recombination	51
Accumulation of intracellular sulfate	52
Increased assimilation of carbohydrate and precursor	53
Glucose catabolite repression	54
Levels of acetohydroxy acid synthetase	55
Levels of acyltransferase	56
Lysine feedback control of homocitrate synthetase	57
Recombination of biochemically blocked mutants	58

years in liquid nitrogen with no loss in conidial viability and minimal loss in productivity.

C. Fermentation Development

Companies involved in penicillin production generally have development groups whose responsibilities are to generate new strains with improved productivities, develop new processes to take advantages of new raw materials or modern control and fermentation concepts, and trouble-shoot production-specific problems. At the laboratory stage such operations, of necessity, rely on the use of shake flask fermentations to evaluate new strains and culture conditions. Analytical services have to be available to assay for antibiotic production and for other required analyses. Successful shake flask culture conditions are transferred to a pilot plant to scale up to a stirred tank process for thorough evaluation before recommendation for production trials. Scale-up studies are the most exacting and demanding of development skills and the most critical in the development of successful new strains and culture conditions.

1. Shaken Flask Culture

Shaken cultures in erlenmeyer flasks of 125–500 ml total volume are suitable for primary and secondary strain evaluation and for preliminary media and fermentation development. Mutants from selection programs can be conveniently grown on agar slants to provide surface spores that can be maintained at +4°C for several weeks. If longer storage is required, the spores are removed aseptically and stored in the presence of cryoprotective agents at -70°C or -196°C. Suitable aliquots from these primary stocks are used to start an inoculum stage, that is, cultured in a medium specifically designed to give high germination and vigorous vegetative growth. Portions of this seed stage are then inoculated into a production-stage shake flask that contains a medium designed to provide limited carbohydrate utilization, which is inducive of penicillin synthesis. Lactose is commonly used, as its hydrolysis by β-galactosidase activity in *P. chrysogenum* is limited. Many alternative feeding systems have been devised to replace lactose (60,61), but their general use has not been adopted. Typical shake flask production media are summarized in Table 4.

Current shake flask conditions use oil and greater concentrations of lactose, additional nitrogen sources, as well as supplements of nonmetabolizable buffers such as morpholinopropane sulfonic acid (MOPS). Fermentation conditions are run to express both maximum production and fast production rates. There is a trend to higher shaking rates to facilitate better oxygen transfer. Humidity is controlled to avoid undue evaporation. Flask openings are covered with paper or cloth disks to afford better aeration and to allow use of in-cycle nutrient/precursor addition. In penicillin V fermentations phenoxyacetic acid can be used up to 1% concentration in the starting medium without growth inhibition. In penicillin G fermentations lower starting concentrations of phenylacetic acid are used owing to the toxicity of this precursor and in-cycle shots are necessary to provide a constant precursor supply. Alternatively, the less toxic derivatives phenylacetamide, β-phenylethylamine, and the phenyl-n-alkanes (64) can be used.

Replication is necessary to reduce inherent biological variability. Replicate flasks can either be assayed separately or combined together before assay for penicillin. The former is preferred but requires considerably more analytical work. Replicate conditions can also be used in media or fermentation development studies, although factorial studies and surface response analysis can be used as an alternative (65).

2. Penicillin Assay

Microbiological bioassay can be used, particularly as a preliminary assay, but such techniques are labor intensive and lack the precision at the high dilutions

Table 4 Typical Media for Shake Flask Culture of *P. Chrysogenum*

Component	Quantity (g/liter)	Reference
Lactose	35	62
Glucose	10	
Corn-steep solids	35	
KH_2PO_4	4	
$CaCO_3$	10	
Vegetable oil	2.5	
Lactose	50	63
Corn-steep solids	30	
Phenylacetic acid	Added daily up to 1 g/liter	
Lactose	20	63
Pharmamedia[a]	10	
$CaCO_3$	5	
KH_2PO_4	3	
$(NH_4)_2SO_4$	5	
$MgSO_4 \cdot 7H_2O$	0.5	
Soybean oil	2	
Polypropylene glycol	0.25	
Lactose	40	3
Corn-steep solids	20	
$NaNO_3$	3	
KH_2PO_4	0.5	
$MgSO_4 \cdot 7H_2O$	0.25	
$CaCO_3$	4	
Phenylethylamine	2.5	

[a]Traders Oil Mill Company.

required with today's high producers. Automated assays such as Technicon have been used extensively over the past 20 years using hydroxylamine (66) or penicillanic acid (67) detection. Over the past 10 years the use of high-pressure liquid chromatography (HPLC) has become common, using reverse-phase C18 columns and UV detection (68). High-pressure liquid chromatography has the advantage of high accuracy and good precision and can give excellent quantitative results for penicillin, precursor, and side products (69,70). Analytical departments are now using automated or semiautomated systems to improve the productivity and accuracy of their measurements. Laboratory robots, such as the Zymate from the Zymark Company (71), are now capable of sample preparation, for example, automated weighing, diluting, mixing, and filtering. Such machines even have their own automated injection station for HPLC analysis. The majority of HPLC manufacturers supply automated sample injection systems together with automated data acquisition, which can greatly facilitate sample throughput by running unattended overnight.

3. Pilot Plant

All promising laboratory strains and conditions are further studied in a pilot plant department which has a wide variety of stirred tank vessels of similar configuration, though at a reduced scale, to production tanks. Here standard operating conditions can be run to assess the performance of new strains under normal conditions. The vessels are normally highly instrumented and computerized. Divergencies from normal can be easily assessed for further process optimization. Similar analyses can be applied to medium development. Pilot plant vessels are also suitable for trials of new analytical devices, pumps, valves, and sterility techniques, where run failures are of no consequence. In this regard the pilot plant works as a service to the production department to evaluate conditions and systems which may be too risky to run on a manufacturing scale. Modern pilot plants have considerable computerized data handling for monitoring and analysis (72) and are ideal for the development of current bioengineering optimization concepts.

D. Inoculum Preparation

To serve a manufacturing fermentation system on a daily basis, it is essential to make working stocks of the current production culture of sufficient size and number to initiate a propagation sequence that terminates in the production vessel. All stocks should be stored at −196°C. Owing to the inherent instability of highly mutated cultures and the probability of spontaneous back-mutation at a frequency of 1×10^{-8}, it is necessary to reduce the number of nuclear divisions to a minimum in this propagation series. The number of cellular divisions required to develop a single spore, through frozen stocks, into a large production vessel is in the range 1×10^{20}-10^{22}.

The main purpose of inoculum buildup is to ensure the uniform, rapid development of cell mass to a volume large enough to provide a seed culture to initiate fast growth and maximum penicillin production in the production vessels. Aliquots of spores are used to inoculate suitable growth media in shaken culture, which after a period of incubation are used to inoculate larger shaken containers or small shaken tanks. In general, inoculum volume will represent 2-10% of the total culture volume. The process is repeated until sufficient volume is attained. The medium used for such propagation is similar across all stages and usually consists of corn-steep liquor and an easily fermentable carbohydrate such as glucose. Calcium carbonate is used to buffer the system against low pH values. Ammonium sulfate and other inorganic salts may be required for optimum growth.

As an alternative buildup, an intermediate sporulation cycle can be used to generate a greater number of growth centers for subsequent seed development. This is achieved normally by inoculating a semisolid mixture of cracked corn and supplemented nutrients with a vegetative growth to provide a large surface area for growth and sporulation. The spores are then dislodged by shaking with a suitable liquid, and the suspension can be either stored or used directly to inoculate a seed stage at a comparatively low cross-volume.

Aseptic conditions are used throughout these procedures and cultures are routinely sampled to detect any foreign contamination, usually by transfer of part of the whole broth into a clear nutrient broth that, after 12-18 hr of incubation at 30-37°C, is observed for turbidity. Semiautomated monitoring equipment has been reported (73).

Special attention is taken for the growth of the last seed stage, which is used to inoculate the production tank. Conditions for uniform growth and mycelial vigor have to be developed to ensure maximum performance in the production fermentor. Exit gas CO_2, pH values, sugar analysis, and centrifuged sediment volumes are typically measured to assess the optimum time for transfer. A holding period may be required owing to schedule problems, and broth chilling may be employed to maintain seed quality. Typical seed buildup protocols are summarized in Figure 3.

E. Production Fermentation

Vessels of 30,000-200,000 liters are used for penicillin fermentation. Agitation is provided by turbine impellers at a power input of 1-4 W/liter. Volumetric oxygen uptake rates of a rapidly growing *Penicillium* culture can attain 0.4-0.8 mmol/liter per minute (3) and it is necessary to supply air at rates of 0.5-1.0 vol/vol per minute. Compressed air is normally sterilized by using depth filters

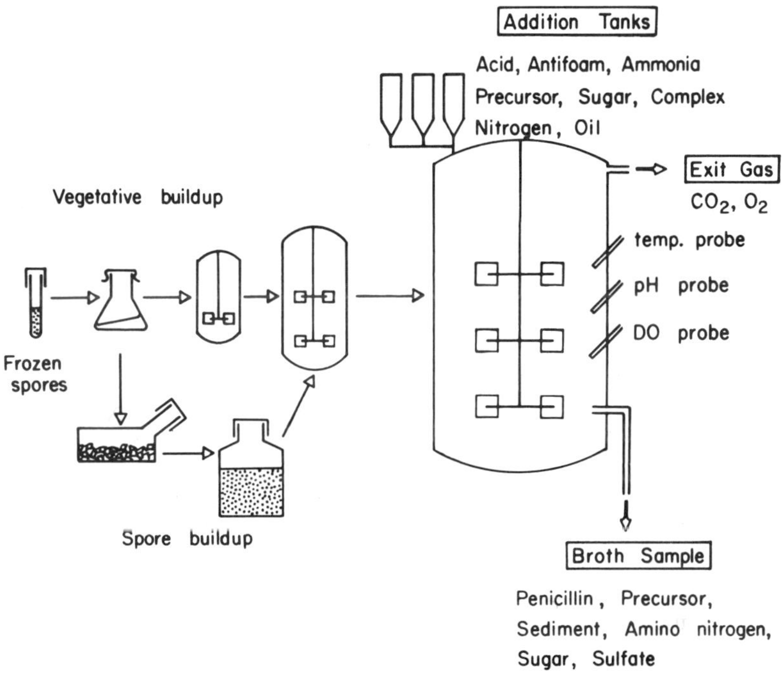

Figure 3 Seed buildup protocols.

packed with fiberglass; however, the use of hydrophobic absolute cartridge filters is now becoming popular (74,75). Small tanks can be cooled adequately by external water-circulated jackets, but larger tanks have to be cooled by internal coils containing chilled brine.

The fermentation medium can be sterilized either in the fermentation tank itself or in a dedicated sterilization vessel. In either case a more concentrated form of the medium is sterilized. Membrane-filtered water can be used to dilute the concentrated mass. Alternatively, continuous high-temperature, short-time (HTST) sterilization can be used. This method of sterilization is considered to be more energy efficient and is less likely to cause detrimental heat effects. For further details on fermentation equipment design operation and control the reader is referred to more specific reviews (76–79).

Fermentation media compositions are generally regarded as proprietory but are based typically on corn-steep liquor and/or a high-protein vegetable meal to make available complex nitrogen and inorganic salts to provide extra nitrogen and the necessary sulfate. Small quantities of lactose, sucrose, glucose, dextrin, or oil are batched into the starting medium to initiate rapid early growth. However, the majority of the carbohydrate is supplied by feeding glucose, sucrose, corn syrup, or some other similar carbon source throughout the fermentation at predetermined rates to provide a limited but sustained growth during the early stages of the fermentation, and restricted growth during the latter stage to allow for maximum penicillin production. Typical raw material requirements are corn-steep solids, 22 g/liter; $(NH_4)_2SO_4$, 10 g/liter; KH_2PO_4, 3 g/liter; sodium phenyl acetate, 16 g/liter; and glucose (or equivalent), 280 g/liter (46). Foaming is controlled by the addition of vegetable oil or an antifoam agent such as polypropylene glycol. Because of the feeding of sugar solutions, volume expansion can be very high and miniharvest schedules can be used to obtain high productivity rates.

The fermentation environment inside the tanks is controlled either by using in situ sensors or by sampling the broth and manually measuring the necessary parameters. In situ, on-line analysis can easily be applied to pH, dissolved oxygen, and exit gas CO_2 by the use of the appropriate probes and analytical instruments. On-line analysis is necessary to operate feedback control of the fermentation broth. Monitoring of pH enables the fermentations to be run at predetermined pH profiles, the actual pH being adjusted by addition of acid, as sulfuric acid, and alkali, as ammonia gas bled into the air input line. Dissolved oxygen can be used to regulate the air flow in order to use the minimum amount of air necessary to maintain predetermined dissolved oxygen levels. Exit gas analysis, by infrared for CO_2 or mass spectrometry for CO_2, O_2, H_2O, and N_2, can provide metabolic information to regulate the feed rates. Periodic broth sampling is always necessary to determine concentrations of soluble penicillin, precursor, sulfate, amino nitrogen, and carbohydrate and dry cell weight. Such values can be used to regulate the addition of precursor, ammonia, or sulfate and to provide detailed fermentation patterns which can be recorded for retrospective analysis.

Considerable effort both in industry and in university research has been directed toward the various relationships between mycelial growth, metabolic pathways, nutrient assimilation, and penicillin production. Descriptions of these analyses were summarized in 1978 (3). Recent topics are summarized in Table 5.

Today's industrial fermentations are concerned with obtaining the highest penicillin productivities related to minimum capital, raw material, labor, and service outlays. The economics of penicillin fermentation have been reviewed by Swartz (46). Considerable cost savings can be obtained by using the least expensive raw materials provided that titers are not reduced. Today agricultural crop prices are extremely variable owing to both political and climatic conditions far beyond the control of the fermentation industry, and considerable effort is directed toward developing fermentations that can effectively use a variety of raw materials.

Table 5 Bioengineering Studies on Penicillin Fermentations

Topic	References
Conversion yields for sugar to penicillin	45
Carbon and nitrogen limitations on growth and penicillin formation	80, 81
Quantitative physiology, specific uptake rates for sugar, NH_3, PO_4, SO_4	82, 83
Enzyme electrodes and thermistor analyses	84–86
Growth modeling and on-line monitoring for process optimization	87–90
Use of pelleted growth in specific reactors	91–93
Filtration probe sensor	94
Automation and computer control	95, 96
Cycling dissolved oxygen tension	97

IV. RECOVERY OF PENICILLINS

A. Treatment of Harvest Broth

Penicillin has only limited stability in fermentation broth, and some unavoidable degradation occurs during the fermentation cycle. Instability is caused by both enzymic and chemical degradation to penicilloic acid. Extracellular "penicillinase-type" enzyme activity has been characterized in high-producing strains (98). To obtain maximum penicillin recovery from the fermentation broth, it is necessary to reduce these degradative activities as quickly as possible before downstream processing. This can be accomplished by lowering the pH to 4–5 and reducing the temperature to below 10°C prior to harvesting. Fast temperature reduction is not possible in large fermentation batches, and temperatures can be reduced quickly by passage through efficient heat exchangers on transit to surge tanks. Low temperature and low pH can also reduce the effects of bacterial contamination in the nonsterile downstream processes. Penicillinase-producing bacteria can rapidly destroy penicillin during processing.

B. Solvent Extraction

The monocarboxylic acid function of penicillin is convenient for extraction into solvent at acidic pH values. Penicillin G has only a short half-life below pH 3.0, and therefore solvent extraction and reextraction to a neutral pH or salt form has to be rapid and is conveniently accomplished by continuous countercurrent, multistage centrifugal extractors such as those described by Podbielniak (99). Penicillin V is acid stable but is handled in a similar manner. Whole broth extractions can be accomplished by Podbielniak extractors, although product quality may be lower. Normally, whole broths are filtered prior to extraction (100) on high-capacity rotary vacuum filters. String filters or precoat filters can be used, depending upon the mycelial nature of the broth. In either case the mycelial mat is washed with sufficient water to remove most of the residual penicillin while on the filter. Penicillins G and V are normally extracted into amyl acetate or butyl acetate below 5°C at pH 2.5-3.0. Improved recoveries have been reported with the use of a second water-miscible solvent such as ethanol or butanol to give extraction efficiencies of 88% (101). Extraction efficiencies of penicillin G into butyl acetate have been discussed by Zhukovskaya (102), who suggested an optimum performance at pH 3.0 with a five- to seven-fold concentration. Operation of multistage extractors has been adequately reviewed by Queener and Swartz (3) from several literature sources (103,104).

Carbon treatment of the penicillin in organic solvent is used if the final product specifications dictate the removal of pigments and other impurities. Normally such treatments are bypassed for the production of a cruder penicillin product as would be used in 6-APA manufacture. In either case the penicillin is precipitated from the concentrated organic solvent as the sodium or potassium salt by the addition of a concentrated solution of the alkali acetate (3). The crystals are collected in a basket centrifuge or by filtration, washed, and predried with anhydrous alcohols, which can also remove some color. The crystals are finally dried over warm air under vacuum. These procedures can be carried out on horizontal belt filters or in rotary driers.

C. Direct Acid Precipitation

Penicillin V, because of its acid stability, can be precipitated directly from broth filtrates by the addition of dilute sulfuric acid to pH 2.0 (105). Impurities in the penicillin V acid can be removed by dissolution of the acid in organic solvent and direct precipitation of the salt by the addition of alkali acetate or alkali 2-ethyl hexanoate or by extraction into neutral aqueous solutions and precipitation by organic solvent addition. Direct precipitation reduces the use of organic solvents, which can have a significant cost impact on the final product.

Table 6 U.S. Manufacturers' Trade Names for Fermented Penicillins

Penicillin type	Trade name (manufacturer)
Penicillin G – benzathine salt	Bicillin (Wyeth), Permapen (Pfizer)
Penicillin G – potassium salt	Pfizerpen G (Pfizer), SK-Penicillin (Smith Kline and French)
Penicillin G – procaine salt	Cystacillin (Squibb), Duracillin (Lilly), Wycillin (Wyeth)
Penicillin V – potassium salt	Betapen VK (Bristol-Myers), Pen-Vee (Wyeth), Pfizerpen VK (Pfizer), Robicillin VK (Robins), SK-Penicillin VK (Smith Kline and French), V-Cillin K (Lilly)

Source: Ref. 107.

D. Finishing

All penicillins used in medicine are subject to rigorous production and testing controls under the regulations of the Federal Drug Administration (FDA) as published in the *Federal Register* (106). The purification of penicillin and semisynthetic penicillins as bulk commodity chemicals is controlled by the nature of these substances and the respective federal regulations. Final preparation for a parenteral dosage form involves procedures for sterilization and the removal of pyrogens and particulate matter.

Finished products are subject to tests for identity and potency, that is, HPLC, color reaction, optical spectra, nuclear magnetic resonance, quality and purity, water content, pH-specific rotation, and safety (contamination, pyrogens). Dosage forms and the potency of penicillins are expressed in terms of weight. The standard unit of penicillin G was established in 1944 and represents the penicillin activity contained in 0.6 μg of a master standard of crystalline sodium penicillin G: 1 mg of pure penicillin G sodium salt equals 1667 units.

In 1982, 1.2×10^6 kg of fermented penicillin was sold in the United States in its various salt forms (1). The manufacturers of these various forms are listed in Table 6.

V. 6-AMINOPENICILLANIC ACID

A. Chemical Hydrolysis

The chemical hydrolysis of penicillins (Fig. 4) involves the protection of the C-3 carboxyl group of penicillin by reaction in methylene chloride with silyl reagents

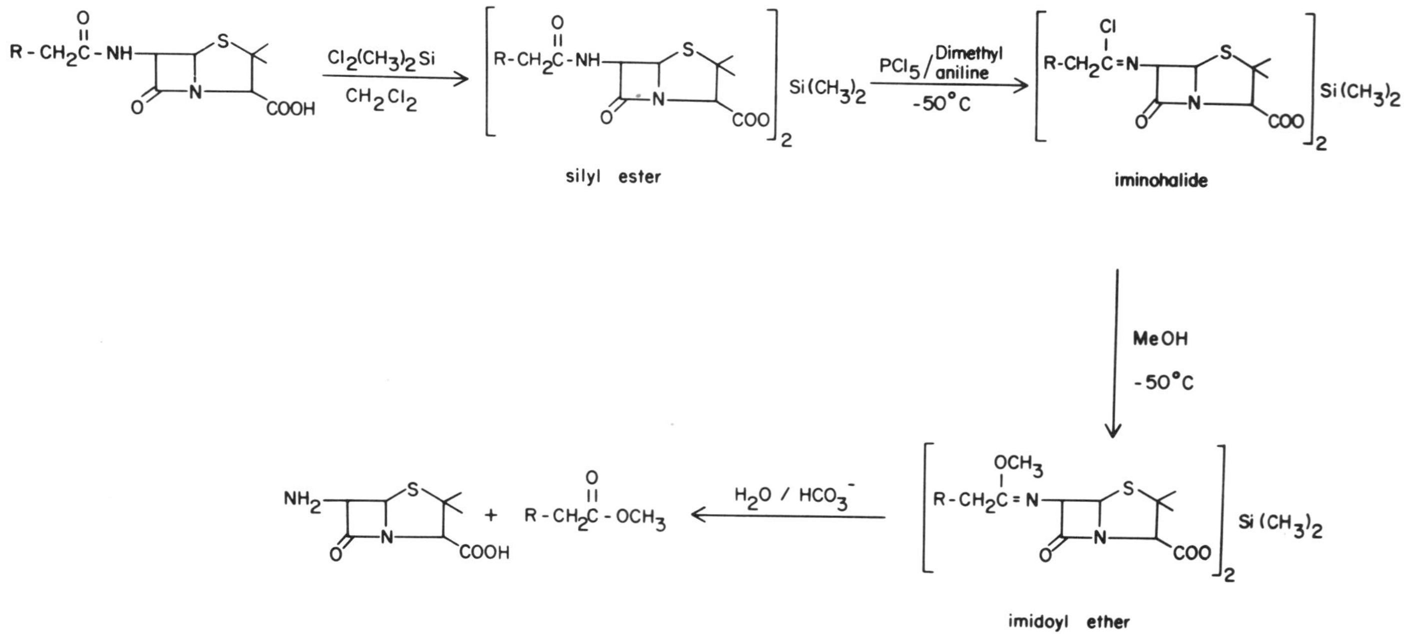

Figure 4 Chemical hydrolysis of penicillins G and V.

such as dimethyldichlorosilane to form the silyl ester. Analogous tin derivatives (108), anhydrides (109), or phosphate esters (110) can be used. The ester is reacted with phosphorous pentachloride to form the iminohalide at a temperature of -50°C in the presence of hydrogen chloride acceptors such as pyridine or dimethylaniline. Alcohol is added to the reaction to hydrolyze the silyl ester and form the imidoyl ether intermediate, which, upon addition of water and a bicarbonate salt, yields 6-APA, which is precipitated as the free acid at pH 4.0 at 0–5°C. The 6-APA can be recovered at yields as high as 95% with 95% purity (111). These yields are probably somewhat unrealistic for large-scale manufacture.

B. Enzymic Hydrolysis

Owing to the increasingly high cost of solvents and the ease of immobilization of enzymes and enzyme-containing microorganisms, the enzymic hydrolysis of penicillins is now the major method of 6-APA manufacture. Enzymic hydrolysis has none of the disadvantages of chemical splitting, the latter process using solvents, high energy for refrigeration, toxic reactants, and toxic and hazardous side products, with associated poor environmental impact and low side-chain recovery. Modern enzymic hydrolysis processes involve the reuse of immobilized enzyme catalysts hundreds of times under mild pH and temperature conditions. Details of such industrial processes are generally not available for publication owing to the proprietary nature of the information.

A full description of the use of microorganisms and their enzymes for the production of 6-APA is beyond the scope of this chapter and the reader should consult current review articles (112–116).

1. Source of Microbial Enzymes

There are a great variety of known sources of penicillin-splitting enzymes, here to be termed penicillin acylases. They can generally be grouped into three classes: penicillin G acylases, penicillin V acylases, and D-α-aminobenzylpenicillin acylases.

Penicillin G acylases are found mainly in prokaryotes, with *Escherichia coli* and *Bacillus* strains being the most frequently studied. Other microbial sources include *Acetobacter* (117), *Achromobacter* (118), *Aerobacter* (119), *Aeromonas* (117), *Alcaligenes* (120), *Arthrobacter* (121), *Azotobacter* (122), *Bacillus* (123, 124), *Beneckea* (118), *Bordetella* (125), *Brevibacterium* (126), *Clostridium* (127), *Corynebacterium* (128), *Escherichia* (129–133), *Flavobacterium* (128), *Kluyvera* (34), *Micrococcus* (119,125), *Mycobacterium* (119), *Nocardia* (120, 125), *Proteus* (128,135), *Pseudomonas* (117,125,135), *Rhodopseudomonas* (135), *Streptomyces* (120,136), *Streptosporangium* (137), *Thiobacillus* (138), and *Xanthomonas* (117).

Penicillin V acylases occur mainly in eukaryotes, and sources include *Absidia* (139), *Alternaria* (140), *Aspergillus* (141), *Botrytis* (140), *Bovista* (142), *Candida* (139), *Cephalosporium* (143,144), *Cryptococcus* (121), *Debaryomyces* (139), *Emericellopsis* (146), *Endomycopsis* (139), *Endothia* (139), *Epidermophyton* (134), *Fusarium* (146–149), *Gibberella* (150), *Leptosphaerulina* (151), *Malbranchea* (152), *Penicillium* (140,141), *Phidomyces* (151), *Piricularia* (139), *Pleurotus* (153), *Pseudofusarium* (154), *Rhizopus* (139), *Rhodotorula* (155), *Robillarda* (151), *Sclerotinia* (139), *Schizophyllum* (139), *Thermoascus* (156), *Torulopsis* (139,141), *Trichophyton* (34,141), *Trichosporon* (140), and *Wickerhamia* (139).

Penicillin V acylases have also been isolated from several bacterial sources, namely, *Achromobacter* (157), *Acinetobacter* (116), *Bacillus* (158), *Erwinia* (159), *Micrococcus* (134), *Nocardia* (134), *Pseudomonas* (116), and *Streptomyces* (160).

D-α-Aminobenzylpenicillin acylase activity has only been detected in *Pseudomonas* (161,162). Penicillin G and V sulfoxides (154), tetrazoles (121), and dimethyl-silane esters (163) can serve as acylase substrates to yield 6-APA on hydrolysis.

2. Use of Free Cells and Cell-Free Enzyme Extracts

The hydrolysis of penicillin to 6-APA can be conveniently carried out with washed suspensions of active cells. Washed intact cells and mycelium (34,129, 134,140,145,157), acetone-dried cells (164), lyophilized cells (128), and fungal spores (149) have been used as catalytic sources. Such preparations can be reused only a limited number of times. Cells can be collected by centrifugation or filtration with a filter aid, but generally their operational life is short and their lysis can cause recovery problems and reduce product purity. Whole-cell preparations typically have low enzyme-specific activity and can contain several unwanted enzymes, such as penicillinase and proteases. Yields of 6-APA are relatively low and of poor quality and color stability. Some of these limitations can be removed by using soluble cell-free enzyme systems. Purification procedures can remove interfering enzyme activities and, in addition, can concentrate and increase the specific activity of the enzyme. Use of the crude cell-free extracts (147), purified intracellular enzyme activity (116,142,159,145), and purified extracellular activities (123) have been reported. Purified enzymes can provide shorter reaction times, thus reducing product degradation and yielding cleaner reactions. However, their reuse is limited. The relatively high cost resulting from the various purification procedures and process losses necessitate their reuse in commercial 6-APA manufacture. Typical penicillin acylase molecular weights are in the range 60,000–80,000 and they can be recovered by ultrafiltration.

However, the slow rates of ultrafiltration and the high capital expense of the membranes have restricted the further development of this approach for the large-scale production of 6-APA. Development of improved membranes capable of withstanding higher pressures and with resistance to fouling could stimulate future use of soluble acylase enzymes.

Penicillin acylases from a wide range of microorganisms have been immobilized by many techniques. Immobilization systems for both penicillin V acylases and penicillin G acylases have been summarized recently (115). Immobilization of a sufficiently purified enzyme enables the catalyst to be used many times and facilitates the convenient removal of enzyme from the product. Similar approaches can be taken with whole cells and obviate the need for enzyme purification. However, the crude nature of the enzyme material with its low specific activity can result in lower 6-APA yields compared to immobilized enzymes. There is an obvious trade-off between the cost of manufacture of the enzyme catalyst and the recovery and purity requirements for the product.

3. Reactor Design

Typically the form of the enzyme will dictate the reactor design. Whole free cells and cell-free enzyme can be most conveniently used in a stirred tank reactor. Temperatures of the reaction are normally a compromise between enzyme rate, enzyme stability, and product stability and are generally between 30 and 37°C. Hydrolyses are carried out at the pH optimum of the enzyme, which can range from 5.5 for *Erwinia* to 9.0 for *Micrococcus*, but typical pH hydrolysis optima range from 7.5 to 8.0. The pH of the reaction has to be maintained constant by the addition of alkali. The rate of alkali addition can be conveniently used to monitor the hydrolysis. Fiber-supported acylases (133,166) are carried out in columns used in a recirculated mode. Particle- and resin-immobilized enzyme forms have been studied in a variety of batch and column reactors in single or recirculated mode and in multistage recirculated modes (167–169). Kinetic behavior and process optimization for such reactors have been studied for *E. coli*-derived penicillin G acylases (170,171) and for penicillin V acylases (172, 173). Approximately 60% of the 6-APA produced today is by enzymic hydrolysis. Current immobilized enzymes are capable of producing 100–250 kg of 6-APA per kilogram of immobilized catalyst. Thus 3 x 10^6 kg of 6-APA are produced annually from 15,000–30,000 kg of immobilized enzyme (174). 6-Aminopenicillanic acid is produced by Beecham, Bristol-Myers, Fermenta AB, and Pfizer in the United States, by Antibioticos, Astra, Bayer, Beecham, Biochemie, Gist-Brocades, and Glaxo in Europe, by Kyowa Hakko in Japan, and by Beecham and Yung Jin Pharmaceuticals in the Far East.

VI. SIDE-CHAIN SYNTHESIS

A. D-Phenylglycine and Related Amino Acids

1. Chemical Synthesis and Resolution

D(-)-Phenylglycine is required for the manufacture of ampicillin and related derivatives. The racemic DL-phenylglycine can be synthesized by either of two routes, namely, using the Strecker synthesis from benzaldehyde,

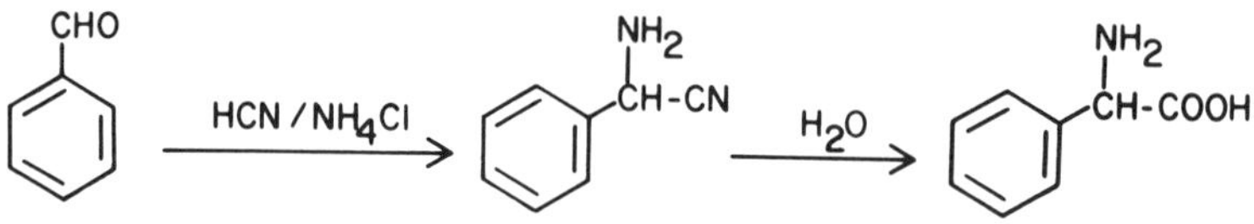

(1)

or from phenylacetic acid,

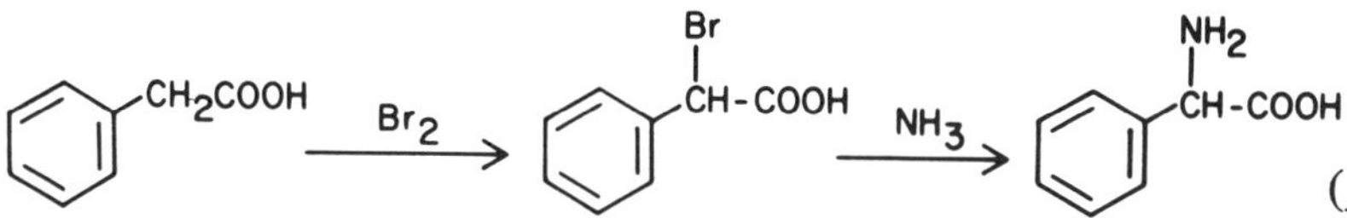

(2)

Optical resolution occurs by precipitating the D(-)-acid with D(-)-camphorsulfonic acid or a tartaric acid. The unprecipitated L isomer is racemized with caustic to recycle to the first stage. D(-)-Dihydrophenylglycine, required for the manufacture of epicillin, is manufactured by reducing D(-)-phenylglycine in liquid ammonia:

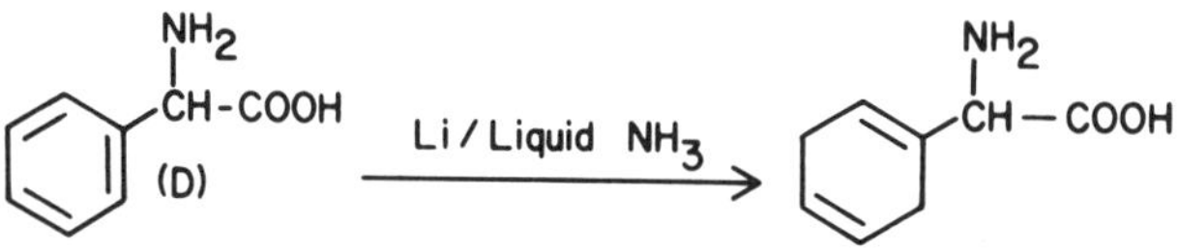

(3)

D(-)-para-Hydroxyphenylglycine is used as an intermediate in amoxicillin manufacture. It can be synthesized from anisaldehyde by the Strecker process or from phenol and glyoxylic acid:

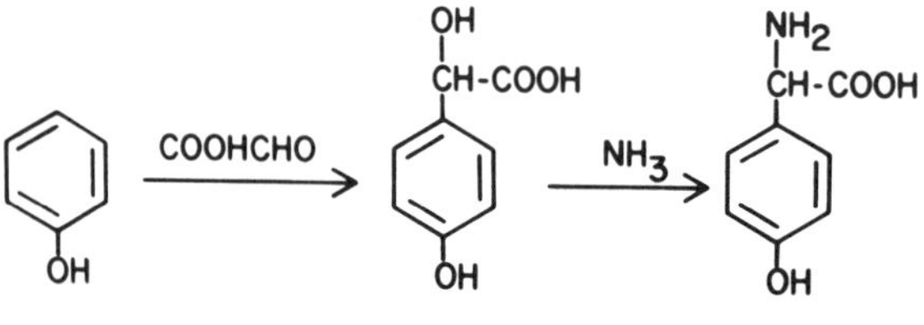

(4)

2. Enzymic Resolution

Microbial enzymes can be used for the resolution of phenylglycine and p-hydroxyphenylglycine. Penicillin G acylase immobilized on XAD7 has been described by Savidge et al. (175) to purge the L isomer of N-phenylacetyl-DL-p-hydroxyphenylglycine; the unhydrolyzed D(-) derivative can be recovered by solvent extraction and chemical hydrolysis:

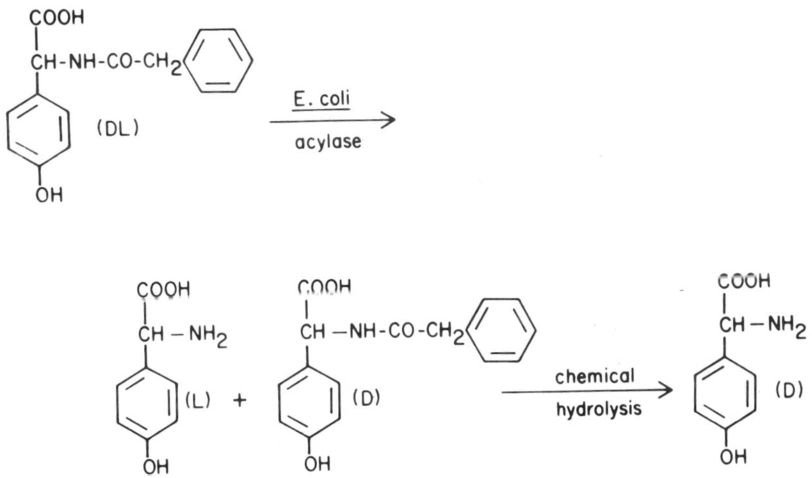

(5)

In similar types of reactions, *Pseudomonas putida* amidase specific for L(+)-phenylglycine amide and a protease, "subtilisin," specific for N-acetyl-L(+)-phenylglycine can be used to resolve phenylglycine stereoisomers (115). However, in the above cases the D derivative has to be hydrolyzed chemically.

Specific D(-)-amino acid acylases from *Streptomyces* spp. (176) can yield D(-)-phenylglycine directly from N-acetyl-DL-phenylglycine. The unreacted L isomer can be easily recycled by chemical racemization. Similarly, a *Pseudomonas* with a D-hydantoinase (115) can be used to specifically hydrolyze DL-p-hydroxyphenylhydantoin to a D(-)-carbamoyl derivative which is subsequently chemically hydrolyzed to the required D(-)-p-hydroxyphenylglycine. A more convenient process has been developed from the isolation of a strain of *Agrobacterium radiobacter* which has D(-)-carbamoylase activity in addition to a D(-)-hydantoinase (177):

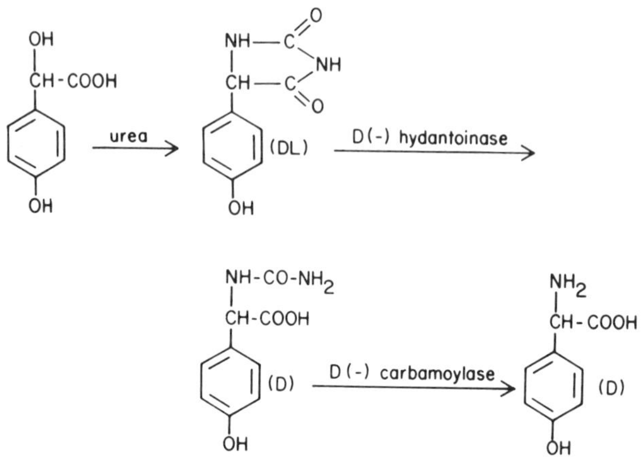

(6)

The L(+)-hydantoin is recycled by chemical racemization.

B. Methylisoxazole Carboxylic Acids

These side chains are required for the synthesis of oxacillin and the related haloderivatives cloxacillin, dicloxacillin, and flucloxacillin. The substrate benzaldehyde (oxacillin) or appropriate substituted benzaldehyde is modified by the type reactions

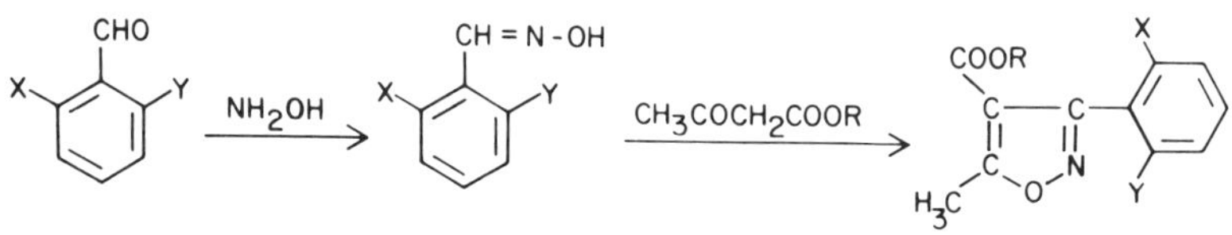

(7)

C. 3-Thiophenemalonic Acid

This side chain is used for the manufacture of ticarcillin and temocillin. 3-Substituted thiophene derivatives are difficult to synthesize owing to the relative unreactive nature of the 3-position. 3-Bromothiophene can be reacted with malonitrile by the type reaction

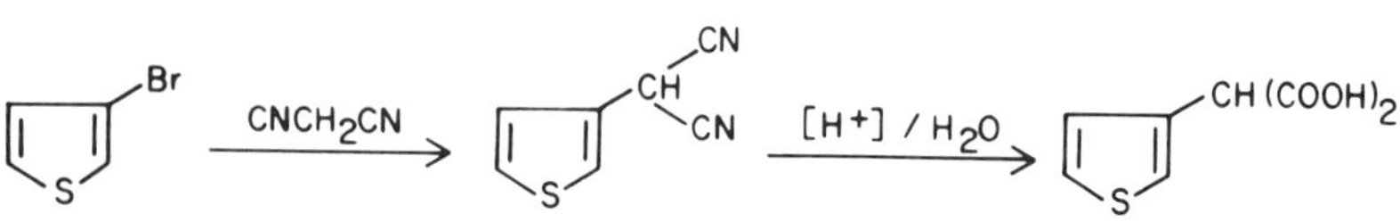

(8)

VII. SYNTHESIS OF SEMISYNTHETIC PENICILLINS

Figures for the production and sales of semisynthetic penicillins are difficult to assess owing to intercompany sales, particularly of intermediates and various third-party-licensed manufacturing agreements. Table 7 lists U.S. manufacturers' trade names for semisynthetic penicillins available by prescription (107).

Chemical acylation reactions used in the manufacture of semisynthetic penicillins have been reviewed by several authors (3,178). Information concerning the manufacture of the various semisynthetic penicillins is strictly proprietary. However, general methodologies can be obtained from the patent literature, although one must accept the limitations of drawing practical information from such sources.

Table 7 U.S. Manufacturers' Trade Names for Semisynthetic Penicillins

Penicillin type	Trade name (manufacturer)
Amoxicillin	Amoxil (Beecham), Larotid (Roche), Polymox (Bristol-Myers), Trimox (Squibb), Wymox (Wyeth), Utimox (Parke Davis)
Ampicillin	Amcill (Parke Davis), Omnipen (Wyeth), Pfizer Pen A (Pfizer), Polycillin (Bristol-Myers), SK-Ampicillin (Smith Kline and French), Principen (Squibb)
Azlocillin	Azlin (Miles)
Becampicillin	Spectrobid (Roerig)
Carbenicillin	Geopen (Roerig), Geocillin (Roerig)
Cloxacillin	Tegopen (Bristol-Myers)
Cyclacillin	Cyclapen-W (Wyeth)
Dicloxacillin	Dynapen (Bristol-Myers), Pathocil (Wyeth)
Hetacillin	Versapen (Bristol-Myers)
Methicillin	Staphcillin (Bristol-Myers)
Mezlocillin	Mezlin (Miles)
Nafcillin	Nafcil (Bristol-Myers), Unipen (Wyeth)
Oxacillin	Prostaphlin (Bristol-Myers)
Piperacillin	Pipracil (Lederle)
Tricarcillin	Ticar (Beecham)

Source: Ref. 107.

A. D-Aminobenzylpenicillin and Related Penicillins

The structures of ampicillin and related compounds are listed in Table 8. Ampicillin is prepared by reacting D(-)-phenylglycine with ethylacetoacetate to block the amine group followed by reaction with pivaloylchloride and triethylamine to form the mixed anhydride. The mixed anhydride is reacted with 6-APA and deblocked to yield ampicillin (179):

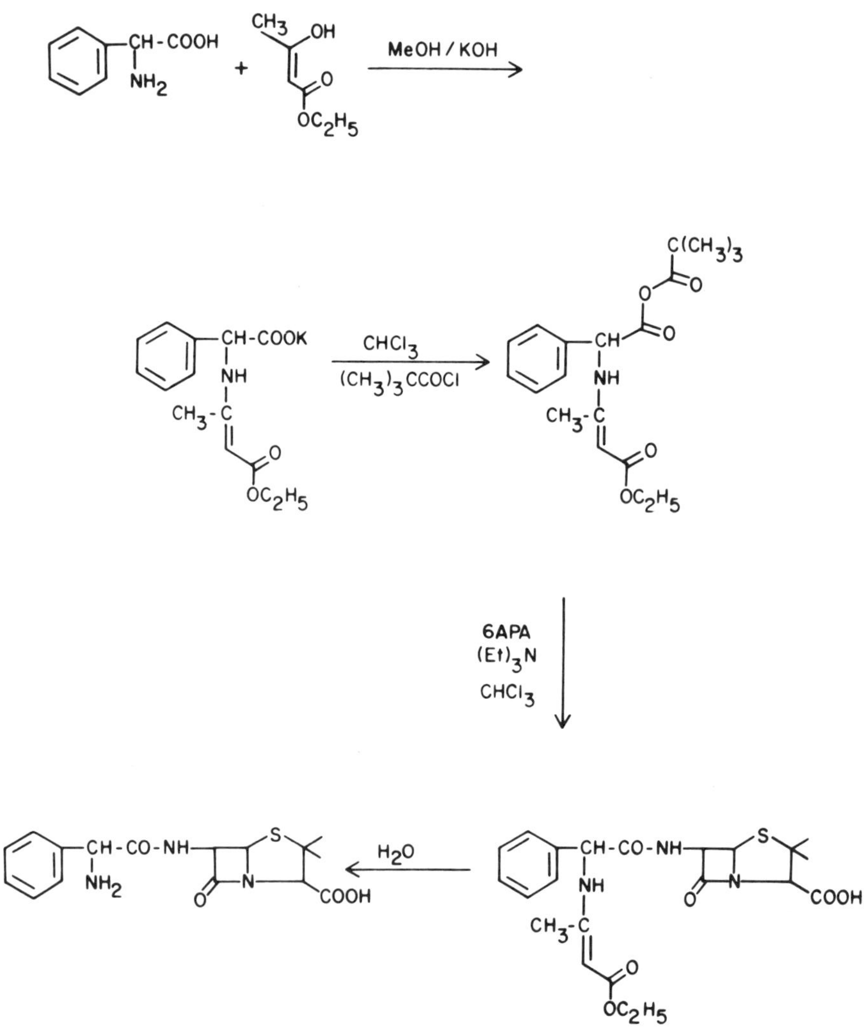

(9)

Table 8

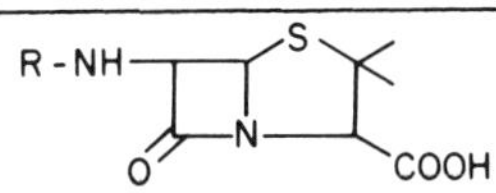

R	
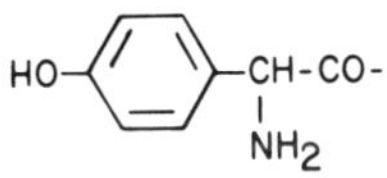	Amoxicillin
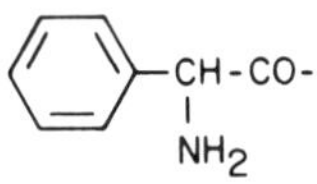	Ampicillin
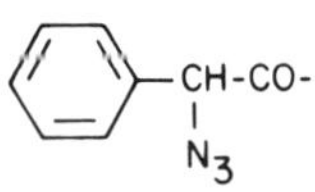	Azidocillin
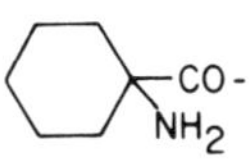	Cyclacillin
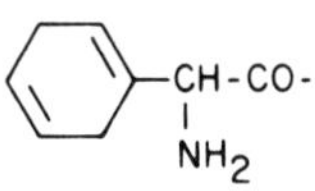	Epicillin
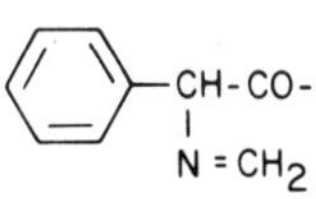	Metampicillin
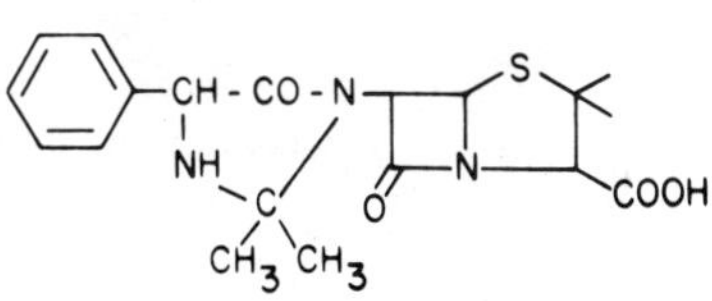	Hetacillin

Table 9

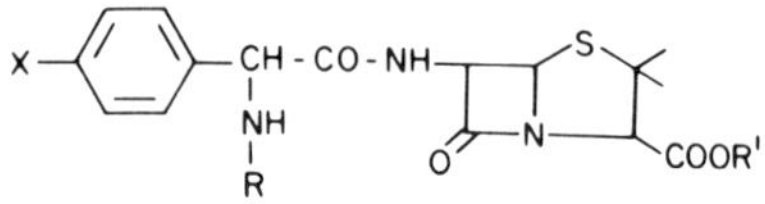

α-amino derivatives: R	X	R'	
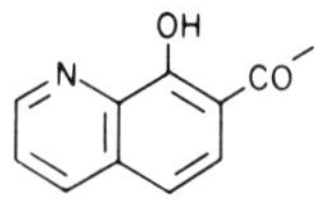	H	H	Apalcillin
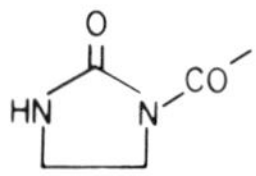	H	H	Azlocillin
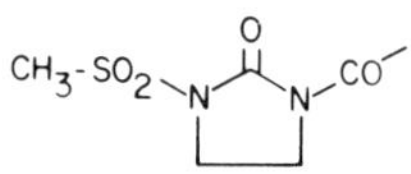	H	H	Mezlocillin
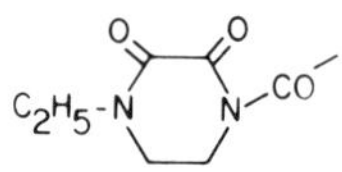	H	H	Piperacillin
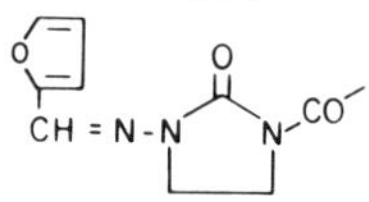	OH	H	Furazlocillin
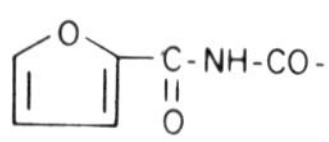	H	H	Furbenicillin
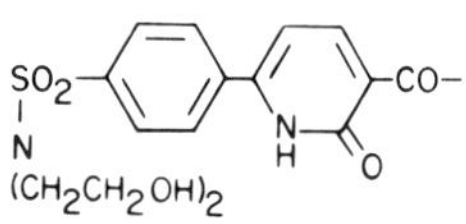	H	H	Piridicillin
3-carboxylic acid derivatives			
H	H	$-CH(CH_3)OCOCH_2CH_3$	Bacampicillin
H	H	$-CH_2OCOC(CH_3)_3$	Pivampicillin
H	H	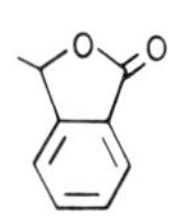	Talampicillin

Ampicillin can also be synthesized by reacting the chloride hydrochloride of D(-)-phenylglycine directly with 6-APA silyl ester (180) in the presence of a hydrogen chloride acceptor such as dimethylaniline or acetamide. Amoxicillin is prepared by similar methodologies to those developed for ampicillin.

Cyclacillin and epicillin are prepared by routes similar to those for ampicillin, using the appropriate side chain.

Azidocillin is prepared by reacting 6-APA with the α-azido acid chloride in acetone (181).

Ampicillin and related structures have been derivatized into several pre-ampicillin forms (Table 9). Such forms are absorbed more quickly but are subsequently hydrolyzed in vivo to ampicillin, where they exhibit the same antimicrobial spectrum. Hetacillin is prepared by reacting ampicillin with acetone (182,183).

Pivampicillin, talampicillin, and bacampicillin are esters formed from the penam 3-carboxylic acid. Pivampicillin is prepared by reacting 6-APA with pivaloyloxychloromethane followed by a mixed anhydride acylation with blocked D(-)-phenylglycine as in Eq. (9):

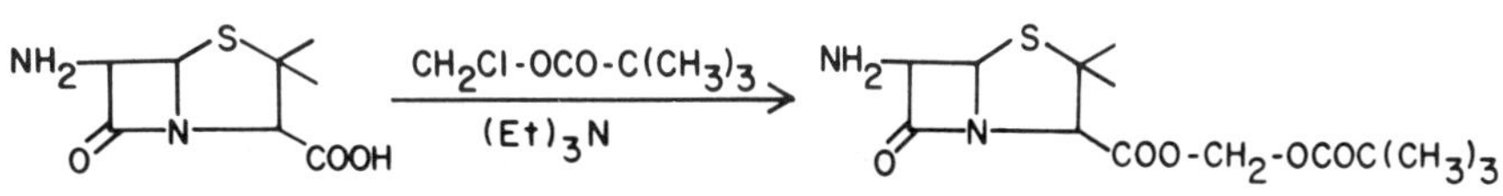

(10)

Talampicillin and bacampicillin are made in a similar manner, using the appropriate chlorinated esterifying agent to yield the 1-oxo-1,3-dihydroisobenzofuranyl and ethoxycarbonyloxyethyl esters, respectively.

Acylation of the α-amino group of ampicillin has generated many new semisynthetics possessing improved pharmacodynamic properties and effectiveness against ampicillin-resistant strains (Table 9).

The parent penicillin, that is, ampicillin or amoxicillin, is the starting material for the manufacture of these α-amino-substituted compounds. The synthesis of piperacillin can be used as an example.

Typically ampicillin is initially silylated with trimethylsilyl chloride in the presence of triethylamine. The silyl-protected ampicillin is then acylated with 4-ethyl-2,3-dioxo-1-piperazinocarbonyl chloride to form the silyl-protected piperacillin, which is subsequently hydrolyzed with n-butanol to yield the free acid:

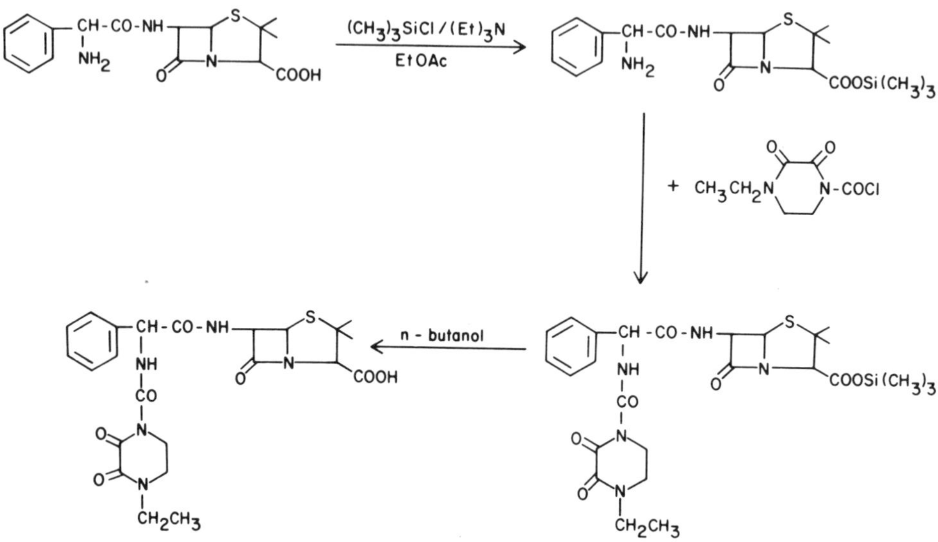

(11)

B. α-Carboxypenicillins and Derivatives

Semisynthetic penicillins of this type (Table 10) form an important chemotherapeutic group because of their activity against gram-negative microorganisms that are not inhibited by ampicillin. They are particularly active against *Pseudomonas* and *Proteus* species. Carbenicillin is the parent type; however, its acid instability requires parenteral administration. Carbenicillin is prepared by reacting phenylmalonyl dichloride with the trimethylsilyl-protected form of 6-APA in methylene chloride; silyl groups are then removed by aqueous NaOH hydrolysis:

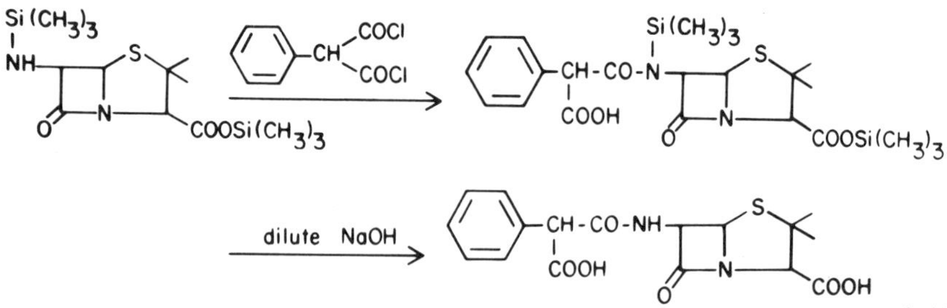

(12)

Ticarcillin and temocillin can be made in a similar manner using thienylmalonyl dichloride.

Table 10

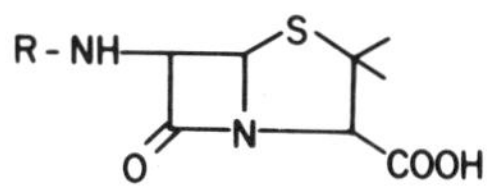

R	
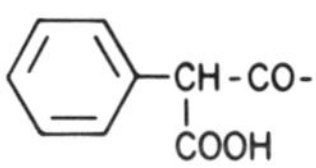	Carbenicillin
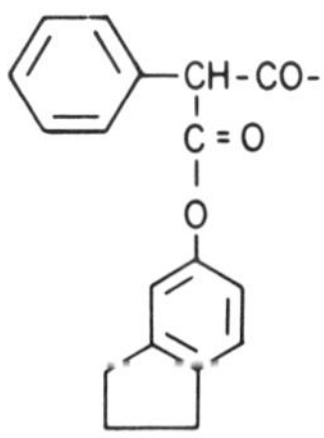	Carindacillin
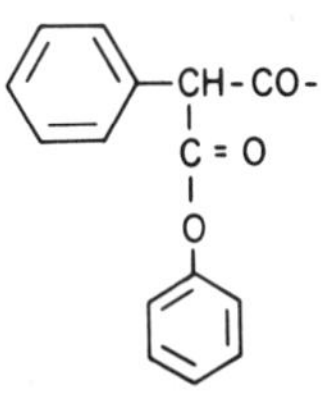	Carfecillin
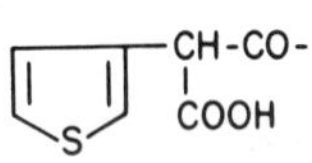	Ticarcillin
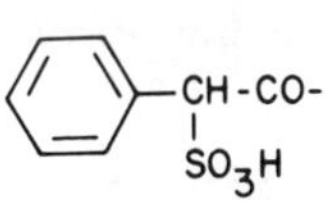	Sulbenicillin
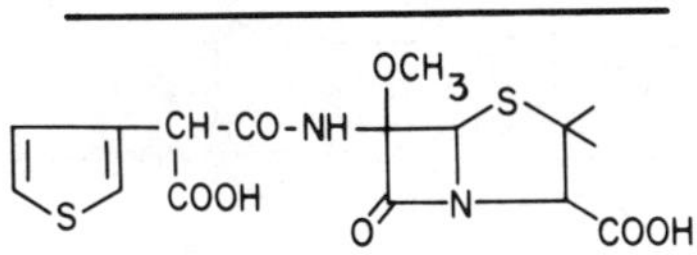	Temocillin

Sulbenicillin is produced by reaching D(-)-α-sulfophenyl acetyl chloride with silylated 6-APA (184).

The α-carboxy esters of carbenicillin, for example, carindacillin and carfecillin, are acid stable and suitable for oral administration. The esters are hydrolyzed to the parent carbenicillin in vivo.

Carindacillin is prepared by converting the phenylmalonyl dichloride to its ketene, which is then reacted with 5-indanol to produce the corresponding ester:

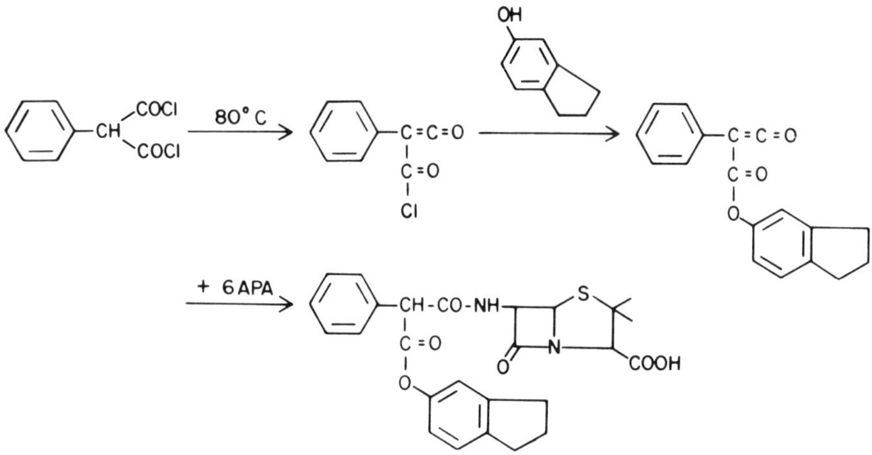

(13)

The ester is then reacted with an equimolar concentration of the triethylamine salt of 6-APA to give carindacillin.

C. Ortho-Substituted Aryl Acid Penicillins

Methicillin and nafcillin (Table 11) can be prepared by typically reacting the trimethylsilyl ester of 6-APA with the acid chloride or mixed anhydride of the appropriate halo-substituted aryl acid (185):

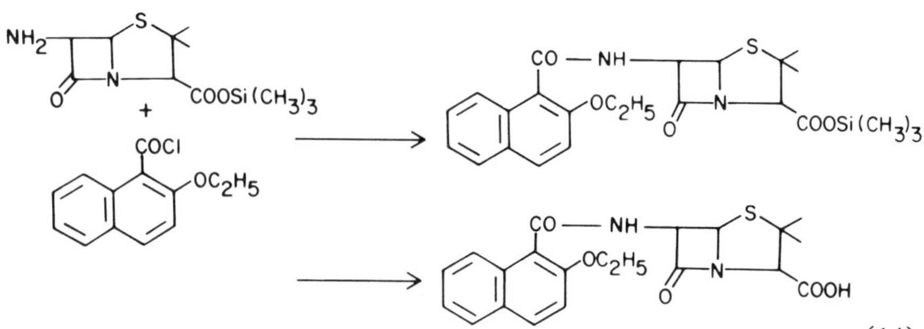

(14)

Table 11

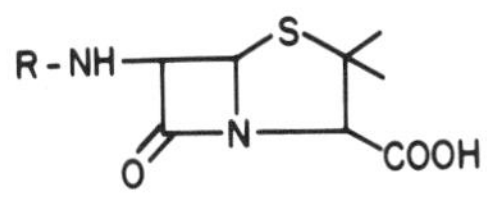

R	
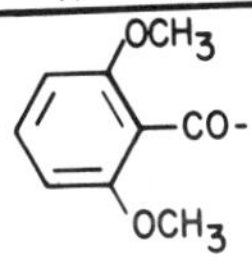	Methicillin
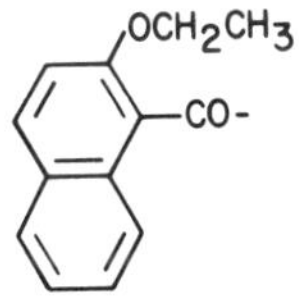	Nafcillin
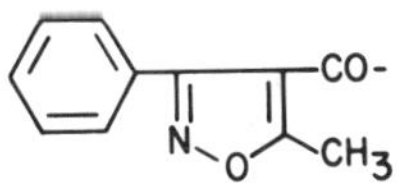	Oxacillin
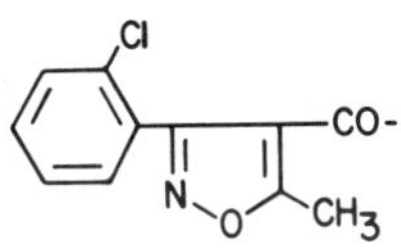	Cloxacillin
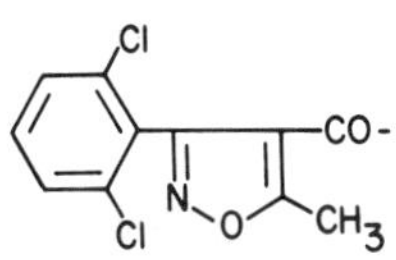	Dicloxacillin
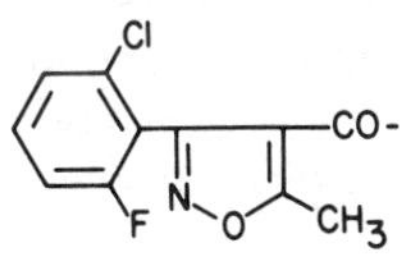	Floxacillin

Methicillin and nafcillin are both resistant to staphylococcal penicillinase activity and can be used in the treatment of penicillin G-resistant staphylococcal and related infections. Nafcillin is unusual among penicillins in being excreted primarily in the bile.

D. Isoxazolyl Penicillins

Oxacillin, cloxacillin, dicloxacillin, and floxacillin (Table 11) exhibit high resistance to penicillinase activity. They are more acid stable than methicillin and can therefore be used orally to combat penicillinase-producing staphylococcal infections.

Isoxazolyl penicillins can be prepared by several routes. In preparations analogous to the manufacture of methicillin [Eq. (14)] the acid chloride of the corresponding isoxazole can be reacted directly with the silyl ester of 6-APA. Alternatively, 6-APA can be reacted directly with 2-butynoylchloride and then condensed with the appropriate phenylnitrile oxide (186):

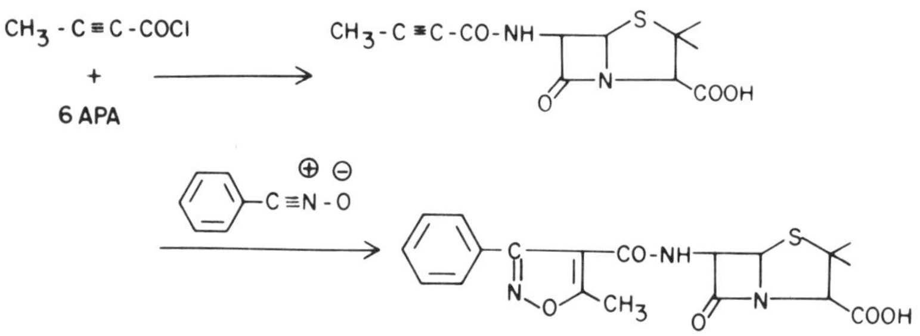

(15)

E. Enzymic Synthesis

Many bacterial penicillin acylase enzymes have been reported to be reversible, particularly at low pH values. Such activity has been demonstrated in *E. coli* (129,187), *Alcaligenes faecalis* (119), and *Kluyvera citrophila* (188). For optimum yield esters of the various substituted carboxylic acid side chains are used, typically the methyl ester. Enzyme systems have been used to make ampicillin (117,118,127,134,138,188), amoxicillin (189,190), carbenicillin (191), and isoxazoyl penicillins (192,193).

The specific D-α-aminobenzyl penicillin acylase from *Pseudomonas melanogenum* (161) can also be used as an ampicillin acylase. It has also been used in combination with an acylase from *K. citrophila* which hydrolyzes penicillin G to 6-APA and phenylacetic acid to react the released 6-APA with D(-)-phenylglycine to form ampicillin (161).

REFERENCES

1. *Synthetic Organic Chemicals, United States Production and Sales,* U.S. International Trade Commission Publication, U.S. Government Printing Office, Washington, D.C., 1982.
2. *Semisynthetic Penicillins and Cephalosporins – Intermediates, Side-Chains, Auxiliary Chemicals: World Markets and Economics,* EcoPlan International, Paris, 1980.

3. S. Queener and R. Swartz. Penicillins: Biosynthetic and semisynthetic, in *Economic Microbiology*, Vol. 3 (A. H. Rose, ed.), Academic, New York, 1978, p. 35-122.
4. O. K. Behrens. Biosynthesis of penicillins, in *The Chemistry of Penicillins* (H. T. Clarke, J. R. Johnson, and R. Robinson, eds.), Princeton University Press, Princeton, N.J., 1949, p. 657-679.
5. F. R. Batchelor, D. Garrard, and J. H. C. Nayler. Action of carbon dioxide on 6-amino-penicillanic acid. *Nature London, 191*:910 (1961).
6. A. Ballio, E. B. Chain, F. Dentice DiAccadia, M. Mauri, K. Rauer, M. J. Schlesinger, and S. Schlesinger. Identification of a compound related to 6-APA, isolated from a culture of *Penicillium chrysogenum. Nature London, 191*:909 (1961).
7. D. A. Johnson and G. A. Hardcastle. Reaction of 6-aminopenicillanic acid with carbon dioxide. *J. Am. Chem. Soc., 83*:3534 (1961).
8. H. W. Florey, E. B. Chain, N. G. Heatley, M. A. Jennings, A. G. Sanders, E. P. Abraham, and M. E. Florey. Penicillins, in *Antibiotics,* Vol. 2, Oxford University Press, London, 1949, p. 631-1293.
9. A. J. Moyer and R. D. Coghill. Penicillin X. Effect of phenylacetic acid on penicillin production. *J. Bacteriol., 53*:329-341 (1946).
10. F. R. Batchelor, F. P. Doyle, J. H. C. Nayler, and G. N. Rolinson. Synthesis of penicillin: 6-Aminopenicillanic acid in penicillin fermentations. *Nature London, 183*:257 (1959).
11. E. H. Flynn, M. H. McCormick, M. C. Stamper, H. DeValeria, and C. W. Godzeski. A new natural penicillin from *Penicillium chrysogenum. J. Am. Chem. Soc., 84*:4594 (1962).
12. M. Cole and F. R. Batchelor. Aminoadipyl penicillin in penicillin fermentations. *Nature London, 198*:383 (1963).
13. B. H. Olson, J. C. Jennings, and A. J. Junek. Separation of synnematin into components A and B by paper chromatography. *Science, 117*:76-78 (1953).
14. K. Crawford, N. G. Heatley, P. F. Boyd, C. W. Hale, B. K. Kelley, G. A. Miller, and N. Smith. Antibiotic production by a species of *Cephalosporium. J. Gen. Microbiol., 6*:41-59 (1952).
15. K. B. Raper and D. I. Fennel. The production of penicillin X in submerged culture. *J. Bacteriol., 51*:761 (1946).
16. L. T. Chang, D. T. Terasaka, and R. P. Elander. Protoplast fusion in industrial fungi. *Dev. Ind. Microbiol., 23*:21 (1982).
17. O. K. Behrens, J. Corse, J. P. Edwards, L. Garrison, R. G. Jones, Q. F. Soper, F. R. VanAbeele, and C. W. Whitehead. Biosynthesis of penicillins IV. New crystalline biosynthetic penicillins. *J. Biol. Chem., 175*:793 (1948).
18. J. H. Ford, H. A. Nelson, W. H. DeVries, and R. Hanson. γ-Chlorocrotylmercaptoacetic acid and γ-chlorocrotylmercaptomethylpenicillin. *J. Am. Chem. Soc., 70*:3522 (1948).
19. P. Troonen, P. Roelants, and B. Boon. RIT 2214, a new biosynthetic penicillin produced by a mutant of *Cephalosporium acremonium. J. Antibiot., 29*:1258 (1976).

20. J. Lein. Strain development with non-recombinant DNA technologies. *ASM News, 49*:576 (1983).
21. E. L. Dulaney. Penicillin production by the *Aspergillus nidulans* group. *Mycologia, 39*:570 (1947).
22. L. J. Rode, J. W. Foster, and V. T. Schuhardt. Penicillin production by a thermophilic fungus. *J. Bacteriol., 53*:565 (1947).
23. G. Brotzu. Ricerche su di un nuova antibiotico. Lavori dell'Istituto d'Igiene di Caliari, 1948, p. 1–11.
24. R. Y. Gottshall, J. M. Roberts, L. M. Portwood, and J. C. Jennings. Synnematin: An antibiotic produced by *Tilachlidium. Proc. Soc. Exp. Biol. Med., 76*:307 (1951).
25. J. M. Roberts. Antibiotics produced by a species of *Cephalosporium,* with a description of a new species. *Mycologia, 44*:292 (1952).
26. G. G. F. Newton and E. P. Abraham. Isolation of penicillanic acid and D-aminoadipic acid from cephalosporin N. *Nature London, 172*:395 (1953).
27. E. P. Abraham, G. G. F. Newton, and C. W. Hale. Purification and some properties of cephalosporin N, a new penicillin. *Biochem. J., 58*:94 (1954).
28. R. S. Sukapure and M. J. Thirumalachar. Studies on *Cephalosporium* species from India. *Mycologia, 55*:563 (1963).
29. J. H. Grosklags and M. E. Swift. The perfect stage of an antibiotic-producing *Cephalosporium. Mycologia, 49*:305 (1957).
30. B. K. Bhuyan and M. J. Johnson. Chemically defined media for synnematin production. *J. Bacteriol., 76*:376 (1958).
31. F. Kavanagh, D. Tunin, and G. Wild. Antibiotics formed by a species of *Emericellopsis. Mycologia, 50*:370 (1958).
32. R. P. Elander, J. F. Stauffer, and M. P. Backus. Antibiotic production by various species and varieties of *Emericellopsis* and *Cephalosporium,* in *Antimicrobial Agents Annual – 1960* (P. Gray, B. Tabenkin, and S. G. Bradley, eds.), Plenum, New York, 1961, p. 91–102.
33. M. A. Pisano and E. M. Velozzi. Production of cephalosporin C by *Paecilomyces persicinus* P-10. *Antimicrob. Agents Chemother., 6*:447 (1974).
34. J. Uri, G. Valer, and I. Bekesi. Production of 6-amino penicillanic acid by dermatophytes. *Nature London, 200*:896 (1963).
35. K. Kitano, K. Kintaka, S. Suzuki, K. Katamoto, K. Nara, and Y. Nakao. Screening of microorganisms capable of producing β-lactam antibiotics. *J. Ferment. Technol., 53*:327 (1975).
36. C. E. Higgens, R. L. Hamill, T. H. Sands, M. M. Hoehn, N. E. Davis, R. Nagarajan, and L. D. Boeck. The occurrence of deacetoxycephalosporin C in fungi and streptomycetes. *J. Antibiot., 27*:298 (1974).
37. I. M. Miller, E. O. Stapley, and L. Chaiet. Production of synnematin B by a member of the genus *Streptomyces. Bacteriol. Proc.,* A49:32 (1962).
38. M. J. Merrick. The inheritance of penicillin titer in crosses between lines of *Aspergillus nidulans* selected for increased productivity. *J. Gen. Microbiol., 91*:287 (1975).
39. J. F. Makins, G. Holt, and K. D. MacDonald. The genetic location of three mutations impairing penicillin production in *Aspergillus nidulans. J. Gen. Microbiol., 129*:3027 (1983).

40. R. P. Elander. Mutations affecting antibiotic synthesis in fungi producing β-lactam antibiotics, in *Genetics of Industrial Microorganisms* (O. K. Sebek and A. I. Laskin, eds.), American Society for Microbiology, Washington, D.C., 1979, p. 21–35.
41. R. P. Elander. Strain improvement and preservation of β-lactam-producing microorganisms, in *Antibiotics Containing the β-Lactam Structure* (A. L. Demain and N. A. Solomon, eds.), Springer-Verlag, New York, 1983, p. 97.
42. D. A. Lowe and R. P. Elander. Contributions of mycology to the antibiotic industry. *Mycologia, 75*:361–373 (1983).
43. C. Ball. The genetics of *Penicillium chrysogenum. Prog. Ind. Microbiol., 12*:47 (1973).
44. C. Ball and M. P. McGonagle. Development and evaluation of a potency index screen for detecting mutants of *Penicillium chrysogenum* having increased penicillin yield. *J. Appl. Bacteriol., 45*:67 (1978).
45. C. L. Cooney. Conversion yields in penicillin production: Theory *vs.* practice. *Proc. Biochem., 14*:31 (1979).
46. R. W. Swartz. The use of economic analysis of penicillin G manufacturing costs in establishing priorities for fermentation process improvement. *Annu. Rep. Ferment. Processes, 3*:75 (1979).
47. S. Fuska and F. Welwardova. Selection of productive strains of *Penicillium chrysogenum. Biologia, 24*:691 (1969).
48. C. G. Friedrich and A. L. Demain. Effects of lysine analogs on *Penicillium chrysogenum. Appl. Environ. Microbiol., 34*:706 (1977).
49. R. P. Elander and L. T. Chang. Microbial culture selection, in *Microbiology Technology,* Vol. 2, 2nd ed. (H. Peppler and D. Perlman, eds.), Academic, New York, 1979, p. 243–302.
50. L. T. Chang and R. P. Elander. Rational selection for improved productivity in strains of *Acremonium chrysogenum* Gams. *Dev. Ind. Microbiol., 20*:367 (1979).
51. G. Sermonti. Parasexuality, in *Genetics of Antibiotic-Producing Microorganisms,* Wiley, London, 1969, p. 175–228.
52. I. H. Segel and M. J. Johnson. Accumulation of intracellular sulfate by *Penicillium chrysogenum. J. Bacteriol., 81*:91 (1961).
53. C. H. Pan, L. Hepler, and R. P. Elander. Control of pH and carbohydrate addition in the penicillin fermentation. *Dev. Ind. Microbiol., 13*:103 (1972).
54. G. Revilla, J. M. Luengo, J. R. Villanueva, and J. F. Martin. Carbon catabolite repression of penicillin biosynthesis, in *Advances in Biotechnology,* Vol. 3 (C. Vezina and K. Singh, eds.), Pergamon, Toronto, 1981, p. 155–160.
55. S. A. Goulden and F. W. Chattaway. End-product control of acetohydroxy acid synthetase by valine in *Penicillium chrysogenum* Q-176 and a high penicillin yielding mutant. *J. Gen. Microbiol., 59*:111 (1969).
56. D. L. Preuss and M. J. Johnson. Penicillin acyltransferase in *Penicillium chrysogenum. J. Bacteriol., 94*:1502 (1967).
57. A. L. Demain and P. S. Masurekar. Lysine inhibition of in vivo homocitrate synthesis in *Penicillium chrysogenum. J. Gen. Microbiol., 82*:143 (1974).
58. C. Ball. Genetics in the development of the penicillin process, in *Antibiotics*

and Other Secondary Metabolites (R. Hutter, T. Leisinger, J. Nuesch, and W. Wehrli, eds.), Academic, New York, 1978, p. 165-176.
59. K. F. Fortney and R. W. Thoma. Stabilization of culture productivity. *Dev. Ind. Microbiol., 18*:319 (1977).
60. S. J. Pirt. The diffusion capsule, a novel device for the addition of a solute at a constant rate to a liquid medium. *Biochem. J., 121*:293 (1971).
61. J. S. Shultz and P. Gerhardt. Dialysis culture of microorganisms: Design, theory, and results. *Bacteriol. Rev., 33*:1 (1969).
62. C. T. Calam. Starting investigational and production cultures. *Proc. Biochem., 11*:7 (1976).
63. D. W. Zabriskie, W. B. Armiger, D. H. Phillips, and P. A. Albano. Fermentation media formulations, in *Traders Guide to Fermentation Media Formulations,* Traders Oil Mill Co., Fort Worth, Texas, 1980, p. 2-41.
64. L. J. Szarka. The use of different 1-phenyl-n-alkanes for benzyl penicillin biosynthesis by *Penicillium chrysogenum. Adv. Biotechnol., 3*:167 (1981).
65. L. E. McDaniel, E. G. Bailey, S. Ethiraj, and H. P. Andrews. Application of response surface optimization techniques to polyene macrolide fermentation studies in shake flasks. *Dev. Ind. Microbiol., 17*:91 (1976).
66. G. E. Boxer and P. M. Everett. Colorimetric determination of benzyl penicillin. *Anal. Chem., 21*:670 (1949).
67. H. Bundgaard and K. Ilver. A new spectrophotometric method for the determination of penicillins. *J. Pharm. Pharmacol., 24*:790 (1972).
68. R. D. Miller and N. Neuss. High performance liquid chromatography of β-lactam antibiotics, in *Antibiotics Containing the Beta-Lactam Structure,* (A. L. Demain and N. A. Solomon, eds.), Springer-Verlag, New York, 1983, p. 301-328.
69. R. D. Miller and N. Nuess. High performance liquid chromatography of natural products, part II. Direct biological correlation of components in the fermentation broth. *J. Antibiot., 31*:1132 (1978).
70. R. L. Hussey, W. G. Mascher, and A. L. Lagu. Determination of ρ-hydroxypenicillin V, ρ-hydroxyphenoxyacetic acid, phenoxyacetic acid, and penicillin V in production fermentation broth. *J. Chromatogr., 268*:120 (1983).
71. Zymark Corporation, Zymark Center, Hopkington, Mass.
72. L. Bowski, C. R. Perley, and J. M. West. A minicomputer system for analyzing and reporting pilot plant fermentor data. *Biotech. Bioeng., 25*:1237-1250 (1983).
73. J. McLaughlin, C. F. Bruno, and T. Forrest. A rapid method for detecting bacterial contamination in the presence of *Penicillium* and *Streptomyces* antibiotic fermentations. *Biotechnol. Bioeng., 25*:1229 (1983).
74. C. F. Bruno and L. A. Szabo. Fermentation air filtration upgrading by use of membrane cartridge filters. *Biotechnol. Bioeng., 25*:1223 (1983).
75. C. A. Perkowski. Fermentation process air filtration via cartridge filters. *Biotechnol. Bioeng., 25*:1215 (1983).
76. J. W. Richards. *Introduction to Industrial Sterilization,* Academic, New York, 1968.
77. S. Aiba, A. E. Humphrey, and N. F. Mills. *Biochemical Engineering,* 2nd ed., Academic, New York, 1973.

78. *Fermentation and Biochemical Engineering Handbook* (H. C. Vogel, ed.), Noyes, Park Ridge, N.J., 1983.
79. D. G. Mou. Biochemical engineering and β-lactam antibiotic production, in *Antibiotics Containing Beta-Lactam Structure* (A. L. Demain and N. A. Solomon, eds.), Springer-Verlag, New York, 1983, p. 255–284.
80. J. R. Court and S. J. Pirt. Carbon and nitrogen limited growth of *Penicillium chrysogenum* in fed batch culture: The optimal ammonium ion concentration for penicillin production. *J. Chem. Technol. Biotechnol., 31*:235–240 (1981).
81. S. Sanchez, L. Paniagua, R. C. Mateos, F. Lara, and J. Mora. Nitrogen regulation of penicillin G biosynthesis in *Penicillium chrysogenum. Adv. Biotechnol., 3*:147 (1981).
82. J. S. Lee, K. C. Shin, H. S. Yang, and D. D. Y. Ryu. Effects of carbon sources and other process variables in fed-batch fermentations of penicillin. *Misaengmul Hakhoe Chi, 16*:21 (1978).
83. D. D. Y. Ryu and J. Hospodka. Quantitative physiology of *Penicillium chrysogenum* in penicillin fermentation. *Biotechnol. Bioeng., 22*:289 (1980).
84. S. O. Enfors and H. Nilsson. Design and response characteristics of an enzyme electrode for measurement of penicillin in fermentation broth. *Enzyme Microb. Technol., 1*:260 (1979).
85. B. Mattiasson, B. Danielsson, F. Winquist, H. Nilsson, and K. Mosbach. Enzyme thermistor analysis of penicillin in standard solutions and in fermentation broth. *Appl. Environ. Microbiol., 41*:903 (1981).
86. J. W. Hewetson, T. H. Jong, and P. P. Gray. Use of an immobilized penicillinase electrode in the monitoring of the penicillin fermentation. *Biotechnol. Bioeng. Symp., 9*:125 (1979).
87. J. J. Heijnen, J. A. Roels, and A. H. Stouthamer. Application of balancing methods in modeling the penicillin fermentation. *Biotechnol. Bioeng., 21*:2175 (1979).
88. V. F. Lubentsov, N. R. Yusupbekov, A. V. Babayants, and G. T. Kuz'minova. Dynamic models of fermentation in penicillin manufacture. *Khim. Farm. Zh., 16*:483 (1982).
89. D. G. Mou and C. L. Cooney. Growth monitoring and control through computer aided on-line mass balancing in a fed-batch penicillin fermentation. *Biotechnol. Bioeng., 25*:225 (1983).
90. R. K. Bajpai and M. Reuss. A mechanistic model for penicillin production. *J. Chem. Technol. Biotechnol., 30*:332 (1980).
91. B. Koenig, C. Seewald, and K. Schnegerl. Stategies for penicillin fermentation. *Chem. Ing. Tech., 53*:891 (1981).
92. B. Koenig, K. Schuegerl, and C. Seewald. Stategies for penicillin fermentation in tower-loop reactors. *Biotechnol. Bioeng., 24*:259 (1982).
93. J. C. Van Suijdam, H. Hols, and N. W. F. Kossen. Unstructured model for growth of mycelial pellets in submerged cultures. *Biotechnol. Bioeng., 24*: 177 (1984).
94. E. Nestaas and D. I. C. Wang. A new sensor, the "filtration probe" for quantitative characterization of penicillin fermentation. Part III. An automatically operating probe. *Biotechnol. Bioeng., 25*:1981 (1983).

95. S. K. Basu and V. C. Vora. Automation in penicillin fermentation. *Hind. Antibiot. Bull., 24*:97 (1982).
96. I. Nelligan and C. T. Calam. Optimal control of penicillin production using a mini-computer. *Biotech. Lett., 5*:561 (1983).
97. F. Vardar and M. D. Lilly. Effect of cycling dissolved oxygen concentrations on product formation in penicillin fermentations. *Eur. J. Appl. Microbiol. Biotechnol., 14*:203 (1982).
98. S. W. Lee, K. C. Hur, K. S. Lee, and W. S. Kim. Extracellular production of β-lactamase by *Penicillium chrysogenum. Han'gu Kyum. Chi, 8*:63–68 (1980).
99. W. J. Podbielniak, H. R. Kaiser, and G. J. Ziegenhorn. The history of penicillin production. *Chem. Eng. Symp. Ser., 66*:44 (1970).
100. I. Berkovitch. Painless computer control at penicillin plant. *Proc. Eng.,* p. 95 (1976).
101. J. Kliment, A. Daucik, and M. Hudec. Isolation of pure phenoxymethylpenicillin or benzylpenicillin. Czech patent # CS 191,597 (1981).
102. S. A. Zhukovskaya. Selection of effective conditions for penicillin extraction. *Khim. Farm. Zh., 6*:42 (1972).
103. D. B. Todd. Improving performance of centrifugal extractors. *Chem. Eng., 79*:153 (1972).
104. D. B. Todd and G. R. Davies. Centrifugal pharmaceutical extractors. *Filtr. Sep.,* Nov./Dec., *10*:663–666 (1973).
105. J. M. Edmundowicz and E. E. Allanson. Non-extractive penicillin V recovery process. U.S. patent # 4,354,971 (1982).
106. *Code of Federal Registrations,* U.S. Government Printing Office, Washington, D.C.
107. *Physician's Desk Reference,* 37th ed., Medical Economics, Oradell, N.J., 1983.
108. A. Pereira da Luz. 6-Aminopenicillanic acid derivatives. Austrian patent # 322,101 (1975).
109. R. R. Chauvette. Use of mixed anhydride protecting group in cleaving acyl groups from cephalosporins and penicillins. U.S. patent # 3,839,328 (1974).
110. J. H. Seustedt. Process for preparation of 6-aminopenicillanic acid. U.S. patent # 3,896,110 (1975).
111. F. M. Huber, R. R. Chauvette, and B. G. Jackson. Preparative methods for 7-aminocephalosporanic acid and 6-aminopenicillanic acid, in *Cephalosporins and Penicillins: Chemistry and Biology* (E. H. Flynn, ed.), Academic, New York, 1972, p. 27–73.
112. T. A. Savidge and M. Cole. Penicillin acylase (bacterial). *Methods Enzymol., 43*:705 (1975).
113. E. J. Vandamme. Enzymes involved in β-lactam antibiotic biosynthesis. *Adv. Appl. Microbiol., 21*:89 (1977).
114. E. J. Vandamme. Penicillin acylases and beta-lactamases, in *Economic Microbiology,* Vol. 5 (A. H. Rose, ed.), Academic, New York, 1980, p. 467–522.

115. E. J. Vandamme. Immobilized enzyme and cell technology to produce peptide antibiotics, in *Enzyme Technology* (R. M. Lafferty, ed.), Springer-Verlag, New York, 1983, p. 237–270.
116. D. A. Lowe, G. Romancik, and R. P. Elander. Penicillin acylases: A review of existing enzymes and the isolation of a new bacterial penicillin V acylase. *Dev. Ind. Microbiol., 22*:163 (1981).
117. T. Takahashi and M. I. Sono. Microbiological production of aminopenicillins. German patent # 2,163,792 (1972).
118. T. Fujii, K. Matsumoto, and T. Matsuda. α-Aminopenicillin and cephalosporin production by *Achromobacter* or *Beneckea.* Japanese patent # 124,288 (1974).
119. C. A. Claridge, A. Gourevitch, and J. Lein. Bacterial penicillin amidases. *Nature London, 187*:237 (1960).
120. J. Chibata, T. Tosa, and T. Sato. Manufacture of 6-aminopenicillanic acid by immobilized penicillin amidase-containing microorganisms. German patent # 2,414,128 (1974).
121. J. J. Hamsher. Enzymatic deacylation of benzyl- and phenoxymethylpenicillin tetrazoles. U.S. patent # 3,905,868 (1975).
122. H. Takeda, I. Matsumoto, M. Tomiyasu, and T. Kawakami. Aminopenicillin derivatives. Japanese patent # 89,595 (1975).
123. D. Chiang and R. E. Bennett. Purification and properties of penicillin amidase from *Bacillus megaterium. J. Bacteriol., 93*:302 (1967).
124. B. J. Abbott. Preparation of pharmaceutical compounds by immobilized enzymes and cells. *Adv. Appl. Microbiol., 20*:203 (1976).
125. H. T. Huang, A. R. English, T. A. Seto, G. M. Shull, and B. A. Sobin. Enzymatic hydrolysis of the side chain of penicillins. *J. Am. Chem. Soc., 82*: 3790 (1960).
126. T. Nara, M. Misawa, and M. Okaji. Process for the preparation of α-aminobenzyl penicillin. Japanese patent # 7,757 (1976).
127. R. Aries. Semisynthetic penicillins. French patent # 2,188,608 (1974).
128. H. T. Huang, T. A. Seto, and G. M. Shull. Distribution and substrate specificity of benzylpenicillin acylases. *Appl. Microbiol., 11*:1 (1963).
129. G. N. Rolinson, F. R. Batchelor, D. Buterworth, J. Cameron-Wood, M. Cole, G. C. Eustace, V. Hart, M. Richards, and E. B. Chain. Formation of 6-aminopenicillanic acid from penicillin by enzymatic hydrolysis. *Nature London, 187*:236 (1960).
130. T. Sato, T. Tosa, and I. Chibata. Continuous production of 6-aminopenicillanic acid from penicillin by immobilized microbial cells. *Eur. J. Appl. Microbiol., 2*:153 (1976).
131. K. Bauer, W. Kaufmann, and G. A. Ludwig. A simplified determination of penicillin amidase from *Escherichia coli. H. S. Z. Physiol. Chem., 352*: 1723 (1971).
132. M. Cole and R. S. Sutherland. The role of penicillin acylase in the resistance of gram-negative bacteria to penicillins. *J. Gen. Microbiol., 42*:354 (1966).
133. W. Marconi, F. Bartoli, F. Cerere, G. Galli, and F. Morisi. Synthesis of

penicillins and cephalosporins by penicillin amidase entrapped in fiber. *Agr. Biol. Chem., 39*:277 (1975).
134. T. Nara, M. Misawa, R. Okachi, and M. Yamamoto. Enzymatic synthesis of D(-)-α-aminobenzyl penicillin. *Agric. Biol. Chem., 35*:1676 (1971).
135. R. Okachi and T. Nara. Penicillin acylase of *Pseudomonas melanogenum* KY 3987. *Agric. Biol. Chem., 37*:2797 (1973).
136. L. J. Heuser, C. Chiang, and C. Francis. Method for the production of 6-Aminopenicillanic acid. U.S. patent # 3,446,705 (1969).
137. T. Yamaguchi, T. Furumai, K. Tani, and N. Matsuzawa. 6-Aminopenicillanic acid. Japanese patent # 20,393 (1974).
138. H. Takeda, I. Matsumoto, M. Tomiyasu, M. Naito, T. Kawakami, and K. Matsuda. Enzymatic production of antibiotics. Japanese patent # 117,990 (1975).
139. T. Nara and M. Misawa. 6-Aminopenicillanic acid. Japanese patent # 02,759 (1975).
140. F. R. Batchelor, E. B. Chain, M. Richards, and G. N. Rolinson. 6-Aminopenicillanic acid. Part VI. Formation of 6-aminopenicillanic acid from penicillin by enzymic hydrolysis. *Proc. R. Soc. Ser. B., 154*:522 (1961).
141. M. Cole. Formation of 6-aminopenicillanic acid, penicillins and penicillin acylases by various fungi. *Appl. Microbiol., 14*:98 (1966).
142. W. J. Schnieder and M. Rohr. Purification and properties of penicillin acylase of *Bovista plumbea. Biochim. Biophys. Acta, 452*:177 (1976).
143. T. Nara and M. Misawa. 6-Aminopenicillanic acid. Japanese patent # 46,080 (1974).
144. D. W. Dennen, C. C. Allen, and D. D. Carver. Arylamidase of *Cephalosporium acremonium* and its specificity for cephalosporin C. *Appl. Microbiol., 21*:907 (1971).
145. M. Cole and G. N. Robinson. 6-Aminopenicillanic acid. Part II. Formation of 6-aminopenicillanic acid by *Emericellopsis minima* (Stakl) and related fungi. *Proc. R. Soc. Ser. B, 154*:490 (1961).
146. F. Baumann, R. Brunner, and M. Rohr. The substrate specificity of penicillin amidase from *Fusarium semitectum. H. S. Z. Physiol. Chem., 352*:853 (1971).
147. H. Vanderhaeghe, M. Claesen, A. Vlietinck, and G. Parmentier. Specificity of penicillin acylase of *Fusarium* and of *Penicillium chrysogenum. Appl. Microbiol., 16*:1557 (1968).
148. S. B. Thadhani, P. S. Borkar, and S. Ramachandran. Structural requirements of inducer for the formation of penicillin acylase in *Fusarium* sp. *Biochem. J., 128*:49 (1972).
149. K. Singh, S. N. Seghal, and D. Vezina. Hydrolysis of phenoxymethyl penicillin into 6-aminopenicillanic acid with spores of *Fusarium. Appl. Microbiol., 17*:643 (1969).
150. I. Vasilescu, M. Vociu, R. Voinescu, R. Birladeanu, E. Sasarman, and I. Rafiroiu. The synthesis of 6-aminopenicillanic acid by enzymatic hydrolysis of phenoxymethylpenicillin, in *Antibiotics* (M. Herold and Z. Gabriel, eds.), Butterworths, London, 1966, p. 518–520.

151. E. Kondo and T. Mitsugi. New process for the preparation of 6-aminopenicillanic acid. U.S. patent # 3,926,728 (1975).
152. K. Kitano, Y. Fujisawa, K. Katamoto, K. Nara, and Y. Nakao. Occurrence of 7-(4-carboxybutanamido)-cephalosporin compounds in the culture broth of some strains of the genus *Cephalosporium*. *J. Ferment. Technol., 54*: 712–719 (1976).
153. E. Brandl. The kinetics of penicillin amidase. *H. S. Z. Physiol. Chem., 342*: 86 (1965).
154. E. Kondo, T. Mitsugi, and T. Matsushima. Process for preparing 6-aminopenicillanic acid. U.S. patent # 3,915,801 (1975).
155. E. J. Vandamme and J. P. Voets. Some aspects of penicillin V acylase produced by *Rhodotorula glutinis var glutinis. Z. Allg. Mikrobiol., 13*:701 (1973).
156. K. Kitano, K. Kintaka, K. Katamoto, K. Nara, and Y. Nakao. Occurrence of 6-aminopenicillanic acid in culture broths of strains belonging to the genera *Thermoascus, Gymnoscus, Polypaecilum,* and *Malbranchea. J. Ferment. Technol., 53*:339 (1975).
157. M. Cole. Properties of the penicillin deacylase enzyme. *Nature London, 203*:519 (1964).
158. F. Carlsen and C. Emborg. *Bacillus sphaericus* V-penicillin acylase. I Fermentation. *Biotechnol. Lett., 3*:375 (1981).
159. E. J. Vandamme and J. P. Voets. Properties of the purified penicillin V acylase of *Erwinia aroideae. Experientia, 31*:140 (1975).
160. M. H. Weiner. Penicillin intermediate. U.S. patent # 3,616,223 (1971).
161. R. Okachi, F. Kato, Y. Miyamura, and T. Nara. Selection of *Pseudomonas melanogenum* KY3987 as a new ampicillin-producing bacteria. *Agric. Biol. Chem., 37*:1953 (1973).
162. M. Shimizu, T. Masuike, H. Fjuita, K. Kimura, R. Okachi, and T. Nara. Search for microorganisms producing cephalosporin acylase and enzymatic synthesis of cephalosporins. *Agric. Biol. Chem., 39*:1225–1232 (1975).
163. E. Zukowski and K. Skrzypkowska. 6-Aminopenicillanic acid. Polish patent # 70,336 (1974).
164. D. L. Pruess and M. J. Johnson. Enzymatic deacylation of S^{35}-benzylpenicillin. *J. Bacteriol., 90*:380–383 (1965).
165. G. Greco, F. Veronese, R. Largajolli, and L. Gianfreda. Purified penicillin acylase performance in a stabilized ultrafiltration membrane reactor. *Eur. J. Appl. Microbiol. Biotechnol., 18*:333 (1983).
166. F. Giacobbe, A. Iasonna, and F. Cecer. Production of 6-APA in the penicillin G fermentation plant by using fiber-entrapped penicillin amidase. *Enzyme Eng., 4*:245 (1978).
167. S. W. Carleysmith and M. D. Lilly. Deacylation of benzylpenicillin by immobilized penicillin acylase in a continuous four-stage stirred-tank reactor. *Biotechnol. Bioeng., 21*:1057 (1979).
168. J. M. Park, C. Y. Choi, B. L. Seong, and M. H. Han. Effect of mass transfer in a recirculation batch reactor system for immobilized penicillin amidase. *Biotechnol. Bioeng., 24*:2215 (1982).

169. J. M. Park, C. Y. Choi, B. L. Seong, and M. H. Han. The production of 6-APA by a multistage tubular reactor packed with immobilized penicillin amidase. *Biotechnol. Bioeng., 24*:1623 (1982).
170. S. W. Carleysmith, P. Dunhill, and M. D. Lilly. Kinetic behavior of immobilized penicillin acylase. *Biotechnol. Bioeng., 22*:735 (1980).
171. S. B. Lee and D. D. Y. Ryu. Reaction kinetics and mechanisms of penicillin amidase: A comparative study by computer stimulation. *Enzyme Microb. Technol., 4*:35 (1982).
172. S. Gestrelius. Immobilized penicillin acylase for production of 6-APA from penicillin V. *Enzyme Eng., 5*:439 (1980).
173. P. Haagensen, L. G. Karlsen, J. Petersen, and J. Villadsen. The kinetics of penicillin V deacylation on an immobilized enzyme. *Biotechnol. Bioeng., 25*:1873 (1983).
174. P. B. Poulsen. European and American trends in the industrial application of immobilized biocatalysts. *Enzyme Microb. Technol., 3*:271 (1981).
175. T. A. Savidge, L. W. Powell, and M. D. Lilly. Enzymes. U.S. patent # 1,357,317 (1974).
176. M. Sugie and H. Suzuki. Optical resolution of DL-amino acids with D-amino acylase of *Streptomyces. Agric. Biol. Chem., 49*:1089 (1980).
177. R. Olivieri, E. Fascetti, L. Angelini, and L. Degen. Enzymatic conversion of N-carbamoyl-D-amino acids to D-amino acids. *Enzyme Microb. Technol., 1*:201 (1979).
178. G. V. Kaiser and S. Kukolja. Modification of the β-lactam system, in *Cephalosporins and Penicillins: Chemistry and Biology* (E. H. Flynn, ed.), Academic, New York, 1972, p. 74–133.
179. E. Dane and T. Dockner. Synthese von 6-D-α-amino-phenylacetylamino Penicillansaure umter verwendung von β-Dicarbonyl-verbindungen als Aminoschutzgruppen. *Chem. Ber., 98*:789 (1965).
180. C. A. Robinson. Process for producing α-amino penicillin intermediates. U.S. patent # 3,678,037 (1972).
181. G. Ekstrom, A. Gomez-Revilla, R. Mallberg, H. Thelin, and B. Sjoberg. Semi-synthetic penicillins, III, Aminopenicillins via azidopenicillins. *Acta Chem. Scand., 19*:281 (1965).
182. G. A. Hardacstle, D. A. Johnson, C. A. Panetla, A. I. Scott, and S. A. Sutherland. The preparation and structure of hetacillin. *J. Org. Chem., 31*:897 (1966).
183. R. Sutherland and O. Robinson. Laboratory and pharmeceutical studies in man with hetacillin and ampicillin. *Br. Med. J., 2*:804 (1967).
184. S. Morimoto, H. Nomura, T. Ishiguro, T. Fugono, and K. Maeda. Semi-synthetic β-lactam antibiotics. Part I. Acylation of 6-aminopenicillanic acid with activated derivatives of α-sulfophenylacetic acid. *J. Med. Chem., 15*:1105 (1972).
185. K. W. Glombitza. Acylierung der 6-Aminopenicillansaure in wasserfreiem Medium. Justus Liebigs Annalen der Chemie. *Liebigs Ann. Chem., 673*: 166–170 (1964).
186. S. A. Lisac. 4-(3-Phenyl-5-Methyl)-isoxazolylcarbonylpenicillin preparation by reaction of 6-APA with tetrolic acid chloride and then with phenyl

nitrile oxide. Japanese patent # 48,684 (1976).
187. D. A. Self, G. Kay, M. D. Lilly, and P. Dunhill. The conversion of penicillin G to 6-aminopenicillanic acid using an insoluble derivative of penicillin amidase. *Biotechnol. Bioeng., 11*:337 (1969).
188. T. Nara, R. Okachi, and H. Misawa. Enzymatic synthesis of D(-)-α-amino benzylpenicillin by *Kluyvera citrophila. J. Antibiot., 24*:321 (1971).
189. K. Kato, K. Kawahara, T. Takahashi, and S. Igarasi. Enzymic synthesis of amoxicillin by the cell-bound α-amino acid ester hydrolase of *Xanthomonas citri. Agric. Biol. Chem., 44*:821 (1980).
190. M. Cole. Process for preparing penicillins. U.S. patent # 1,367,342 (1974).
191. T. Fujii, Y. Shibuya, and T. Yamaguchi. α-Carboxybenzylpenicillin. Japanese patent # 42,892 (1974).
192. T. Kamogashira, W. Miyazaki, M. Niinobe, and T. Dohi. Enzymic acylation of 6-Aminopenicillanic acid. Japanese patent # 29,586 (1972).
193. P. S. Delin, B. A. Ekstrom, B. O. H. Sjoberg, K. H. Thelin, and L. S. Narthorst-Westfeld. Water-insoluble penicillin acylase. German patent # 1,966,428 (1972).

7

Pharmacology and Pharmacokinetics of Penicillins

JOHN F. QUAY and RICHARD F. BERGSTROM
Lilly Research Laboratories, Eli Lilly and Company, Indianapolis, Indiana

I. INTRODUCTION

The purpose of this review is to summarize and update the pharmacokinetics of the penicillin antibiotics in humans. We will attempt to describe and quantify the absorption, distribution, biotransformation, and excretion of penicillins of proven clinical value. To make the treatment as general and as standard as possible, we have used throughout the pharmacokinetic symbols and definitions published by the American College of Clinical Pharmacology (1). Error values are quoted as standard deviations. In some cases this approach required reinterpretation of symbols and conversion of units from the original literature sources. Data obtained from studies in experimental animals are presented only where important processes are not elucidated by data from available clinical studies, and the animal data are identified in each instance as to the species of origin. Unless otherwise stated, all clinical data were obtained from experiments in healthy volunteers.

Many reviews of the pharmacokinetic behavior of penicillins have appeared in recent years. Different aspects of the behavior of penicillins in vivo have been highlighted by different authors. Barza and Weinstein (2) and Bergan (5) have emphasized the clinical applications of knowledge of penicillin pharmacokinetics. Prince and Neu described the utility of the newer penicillins in clinical pediatric practice (3). Metabolic reactions of the penicillin antibiotics have been reviewed exhaustively by Kwan and Rogers (4). Bergan has published extensive comparisons of plasma kinetics of penicillin antibiotics after administration by a variety of routes (5). Relationships between chemical structure and pharmacokinetics characteristics of beta-lactam antibiotics were explored by Webber and Wheeler (6).

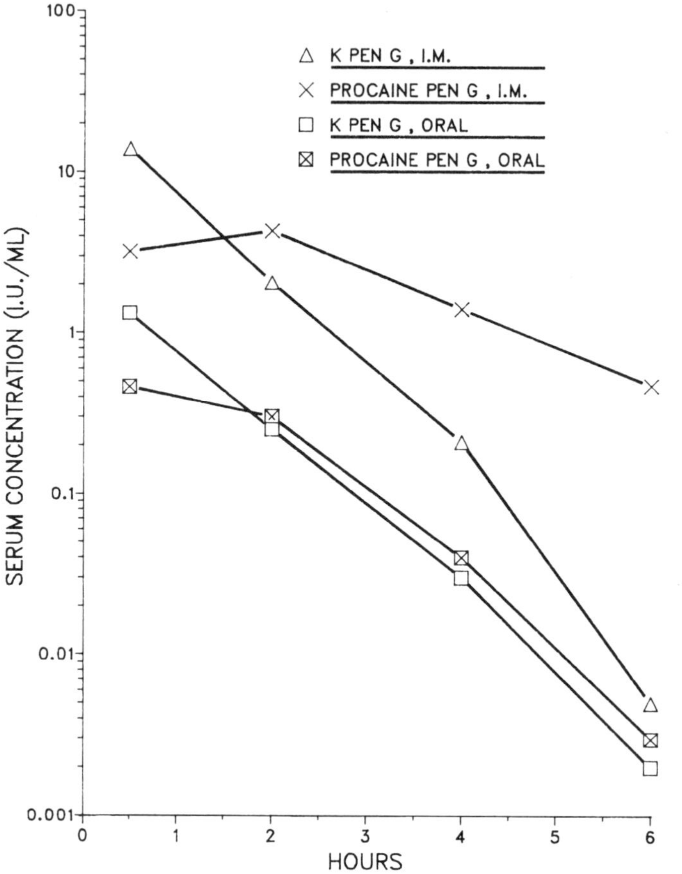

Figure 1 Mean serum antibacterial activity in children after administration of single doses of 10,000 units/lb penicillin G. (Redrawn from Ref. 9.)

II. EARLY PENICILLINS

A. Penicillin G

Because of the exquisite sensitivity of streptococci to the inhibitory effect of penicillin G, the oldest member of the penicillin family, this antibiotic remains today a widely used agent. Absorption of penicillin G (see Table 2 in Chap. 6 for the structure) after oral administration is limited and variable owing to chemical instability in the acid milieu of the stomach (7,8). As shown in Figure 1, peroral administration of penicillin G as the soluble potassium salt or as the relatively insoluble procaine salt results in lower serum concentrations of antibacterial activity than does intramuscular administration of the same salts (9). Prolonged absorption of penicillin G from a depot of procaine penicillin G at an intramuscular injection site produces lower peak serum concentrations and long-lasting low serum levels (10,11). Benzathine salts of penicillin G have been used in this way to maintain detectable serum penicillin concentrations for periods of up to 3 weeks after a single injection (12). However, the two insoluble salts given to children individually or in combination do not reliably maintain detectable antibacterial activity in serum beyond 10 days (13).

Following intravenous administration of a 500-mg dose, penicillin G was reported to be about 50% bound to plasma proteins. After the distribution phase the concentration in serum declined with a half-life of 45 min and 46% of the activity was excreted in the urine (14). Following constant infusion, the total serum clearance was 477 ± 58 ml/min, the renal clearance was 466 ml/min, and the volume of distribution (VD_{SS}) was 22 liters (15).

Penicillin G penetrates rapidly into skin blister fluid and persists longer in inflammatory exudates than in noninflammatory fluid (16). In patients with latent syphilis and normal meninges, little penicillin G penetrates into cerebrospinal fluid. Probenecid elevates both serum and cerebrospinal fluid levels of penicillin G by inhibiting the secretion of penicillin G anion by the choroid plexus and renal tubules (17-20). As shown in Table 1, probenecid alters the two-compartment model characteristics of penicillin G. Changes in penicillin G distribution and kinetics wrought by probenecid are extensive and interactive (21). Other drugs, such as phenylbutazone, sulfipyrazone, acetylsalicylic acid, sulfaphenazole, and indomethacin, also increase the serum half-life of penicillin G (22). Following intravenous administration of penicillin G in cancer patients, free drug

Table 1 Effect of Probenecid on Mean Parameters of a Two-Compartment Model of Penicillin G in Five Patients

Parameter[a]	Control	Probenecid
K_{12} (hr^{-1})	0.93	1.57
K_{21} (hr^{-1})	1.43	2.60
K_{10} (hr^{-1})	2.59	1.21
V_C (liters)	9.72	8.52
$100/F_C$	39.7	63.7
F_T/F_C	1.7	0.62

[a]V_C = volume of central compartment, F_C = fraction of drug in central compartment, and F_T = fraction of drug in tissue compartment.
Source: Data from Ref. 21.

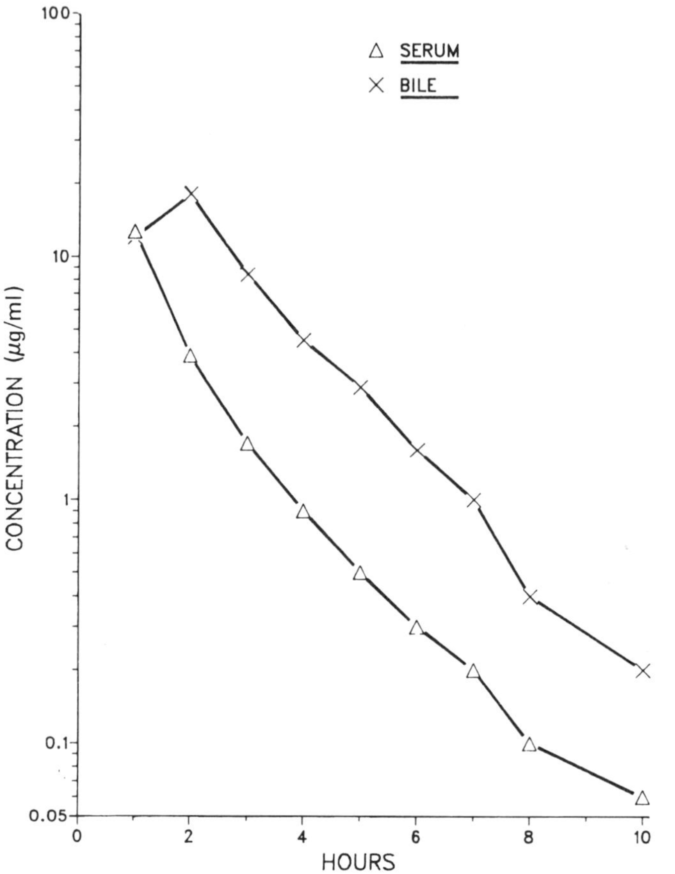

Figure 2 Mean concentration of penicillin G in the serum and bile of 10 choles-cystectomized patients after intravenous administration of single 599-mg doses of penicillin G. (Redrawn from Ref. 27.)

concentrations in thoracic duct lymph and serum coincided (23). A recent report has indicated that penicillin G penetration into cerebrospinal fluid in neonates is much more extensive than in adults (24).

In vitro and in vivo penicillin G breaks down to benzylpenicilloic acid. After intramuscular doses of 300 mg, 19% appeared in urine as penicilloic acid and 66% as unchanged penicillin G. Less than 1% appeared in urine as 6-aminopenicillanic acid (25). Rapid renal elimination of penicillin G severely limits serum drug levels produced by slow release from depot formulations. Eagle and Newman found that the renal clearance of penicillin G was three- to fourfold larger than the glomerular filtration rate (26). Thus renal excretion of penicillin G occurs primarily by secretion. The antibiotic has been measured in the bile of T-tube patients (Fig. 2); only 0.12% of the dose was excreted by this route (26). In patients with severe renal impairment serum concentrations of penicillin G are elevated after a standard dose, but hemodialysis reduces the serum half-life toward normal values (28). Serum and blister fluid concentrations of penicillin G are also extended in patients with compromised renal excretory function: geriatric patients, premature infants, and patients with kwashiorkor (protein deficiency) (29-31).

B. Penicillin V

Penicillin V and penicillin G possess similar antibacterial spectra, but penicillin V is more stable in acidic gastric secretions. Together with the adequate lipid solubility of the un-ionized form and the good aqueous solubility of the potassium salt, the improved acid stability made penicillin V the first reliable oral penicillin (32-34). The superiority of potassium penicillin V over insoluble salts of penicillin G for oral adminstration is illustrated in Figure 3. After intravenous administration penicillin V and penicillin G have similar kinetics but the serum half-life of penicillin V is slightly shorter (Fig. 4) (35). Therefore the higher serum concentrations of penicillin V after peroral administration provide direct evidence of the improved peripheral bioavailability of penicillin V.

In vivo studies of various salts and formulations of penicillin V have revealed significant differences in bioavailability. Bergan and co-workers found that the bioavailability of penicillin V from 16 oral formulations was, in general, higher from solutions and solid dosage forms of the potassium salt, and lower from suspensions of poorly soluble salts such as benzathine penicillin V (36). However, suspensions of calcium and potassium salts of penicillin V were bioequivalent (37). Sweetening agents used in formulating solutions can alter penicillin V bioavailability, and penicillin V is less available from an oil suspension of the calcium salt than from a tablet formulation of this salt (38,39). Oral absorption of penicillin V is also reduced when the dose is given with a meal or milk (40,41).

In a crossover study with adult male subjects Josefsson and Bergan found that graded oral doses of potassium penicillin V produced peak serum penicillin concentrations that were not proportional to the dose. However, the areas under the serum concentration versus time curve (AUC) were linearly related to the dose (42). Urinary excretion of antibacterial activity apparently declined from 43 to 37% of the dose as the amount given was increased from 400 to 3000 mg. The serum half-life also appeared to increase with dose. Dimmling and co-workers found, to the contrary, that both AUC and urinary excretion of orally administered penicillin V were linear with dose (43).

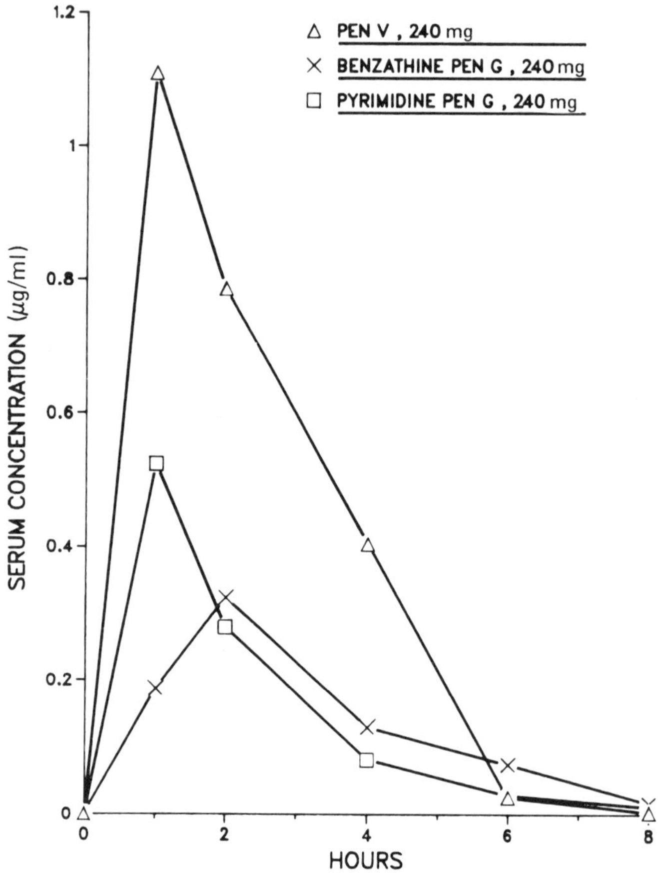

Figure 3 Mean serum concentrations of penicillins in 16–17 subjects after oral administration of single 400,000-unit doses of penicillins. (Redrawn from Ref. 34.)

Penicillin V penetrated tonsillar tissue to a peak concentration of 0.6 μg/g at a time when the serum concentration was 2.6 μg/ml. Concurrently the ratio of penicillin V concentrations in skin window fluid to serum was 24% (44,45). Tissue penetration of penicillin V is constrained by moderate (69–78%) binding to plasma proteins (44–46).

Approximately 45% of a peroral dose of potassium penicillin V labeled with ^{35}S was absorbed in the upper small intestine of male subjects. Fecal radioactivity accounted for 32% of the dose and urinary radioactivity was 40%. Unchanged

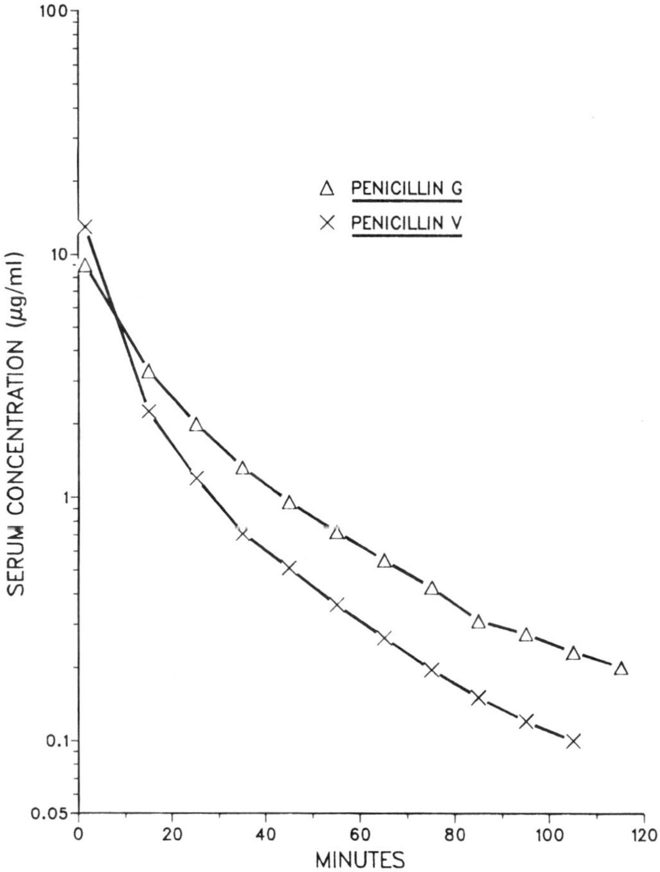

Figure 4 Serum concentrations of penicillins in a single subject after intravenous administration of a single 100-mg dose of penicillin G or penicillin V. (Redrawn from Ref. 35.)

drug accounted for 60% of the fraction of radioactivity in urine, penicilloic acid accounted for 20%, and less than 5%, if any, was present as p-hydroxypenicillin V (47). However, the parahydroxylated metabolite does, in fact, appear in human urine (48). In a separate study 34% of an oral dose was excreted in the urine as the penicilloic acid and 26% was excreted as parent antibiotic (25). Those results show that the peripheral bioavailability of penicillin V is limited by both incomplete absorption and instability.

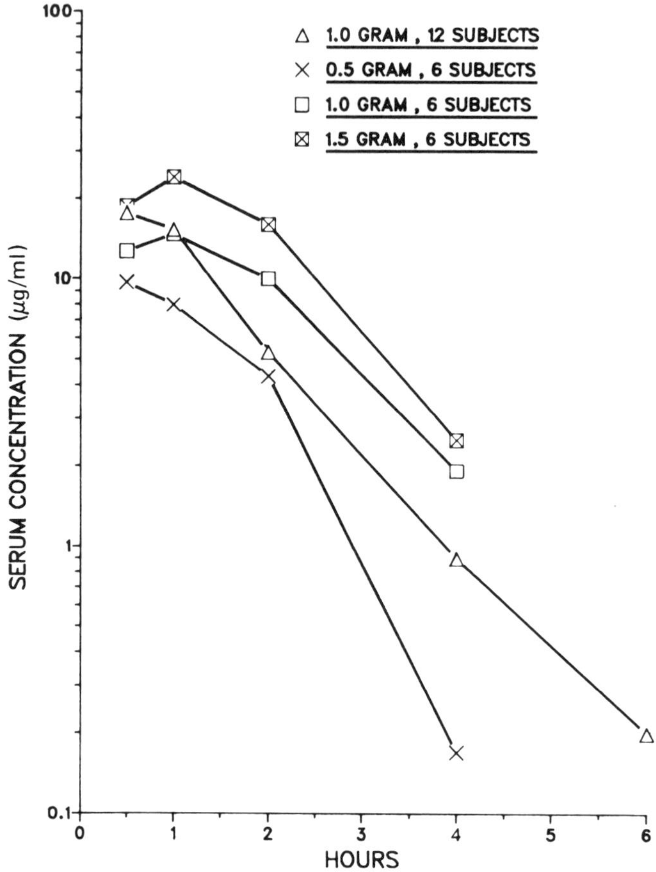

Figure 5 Mean total (bound plus free) serum concentration of methicillin after oral administration of graded doses of methicillin. (Redrawn from Refs. 51 and 52).

III. ANTISTAPHYLOCOCCAL PENICILLINS

A. Methicillin

Methicillin was the first penicillin modification (see Table 11 of Chap. 6) to have useful resistance to hydrolysis by the beta-lactamase of *Staphylococcus aureus.* The acid lability and relatively low lipid solubility of methicillin combine to limit its oral absorption (49,50). However, after intramuscular administration of a range of doses, absorption is essentially complete (51,52). Typical plasma concentration versus time data are shown in Figure 5. When 500 mg of radioactive methicillin was given intramuscularly, 75% of the dose appeared in the urine unchanged and 7% appeared as the penicilloic acid derivative (25). No microbiologically active metabolites have been observed (53).

The binding of methicillin to protein components is 37% in human plasma, 35% in serum, and essentially zero in thoracic duct lymph (54). Kunin has pointed out that, by virtue of its low binding, methicillin provides higher serum concentrations of unbound drug per unit dose than the other antistaphylococcal penicillins (55).

Results of a multitude of studies have confirmed the observation that the coadministration of probenecid and methicillin provides serum levels of methicillin significantly higher than those achieved with methicillin alone (51,56–58). Bile obtained from T-tube patients given intramuscular 1-g doses contained a maximum of 3.2 μg/ml of methicillin, accounting for less than 0.1% of the dose (59).

B. Nafcillin

Nafcillin (see Table 11 of Chap. 6 for structure) is very lipid soluble and highly bound to serum proteins. These attributes influence its pharmacokinetic behavior in humans. Oral absorption of 0.5- and 1.0-g doses of sodium nafcillin yields low and erratic serum concentrations (60,61), due, in part, to a substantial first-pass effect. Better availability has been achieved with oral dosage forms consisting of either the free acid or the sodium salt buffered with calcium carbonate. Food taken before the drug reduces the peripheral bioavailability of nafcillin from all formulations (62).

Serum concentrations of nafcillin are higher and more prolonged in neonates than in older children or adults (63–65). In premature infants weighing less than 2.5 kg, intravenous nafcillin produced the following one-compartment model parameters: $K_{10} = 0.204\ hr^{-1}$, $V_C = 326$ ml/kg, Cl = 1.07 ml/min per kilogram body weight (66). In older children Feldman et al. reported corresponding values of $K_{10} = 0.912\ hr^{-1}$, $V_C = 893$ ml/kg, Cl = 595 ml/min per 1.73 m^2 (67).

Nafcillin has poor penetration into the cerebrospinal fluid (CSF) of patients with normal meninges. The peak concentration in CSF was reached 2 hr after a 42-mg/kg intravenous bolus, and at this time the CSF/serum ratio was 0.01 (68). Nafcillin is also excluded from the eye. Nafcillin distributes widely into many other tissues, reaching peak tissue/serum ratios of 0.6–3.0 (55,69), even though nafcillin is 90% bound to serum proteins.

In dogs, and presumably in humans, hepatic clearance is an important route for excretion of nafcillin, and bile/serum concentration ratios may reach 500 (70,71). In adults with normal hepatic function but impaired renal function, high-dose nafcillin kinetics were the same as in normal adults, and the serum half-life was unchanged by hemodialysis (72). In a similar population of patients,

Table 2 Selected Physical and Pharmcokinetic Parameters of the Isoxazolyl Penicillins

Parameter	Dose (g)	Route of Administration	Oxacillin
log P_u [a]			2.31
Serum binding			94
			93
AUC[b]	0.5	Oral	521
	1.0	Oral	732 ± 225
	0.5	i.m.	1038 ± 93
Urine excretion (%)	1.0	Oral	20.6 ± 5.1
	0.5	i.m.	39.5 ± 9.9
	0.7	i.v.	56
Plasma half-life (min)	0.75	i.v.	23
Renal clearance (ml/min)	0.75	i.v.	227
	4.6	i.v.	–
Extrarenal clearance (ml/min)	4.6	i.v.	–
Urine excretion (%)	0.5	Oral	16.9 ± 13.2[c]
			16.1 ± 13.3[d]

[a]P_u = Octanol/water partition coefficient of un-ionized form.
[b]Area under the plasma concentration versus time curve (μg·min/ml).
[c]As active drug.
[d]As the penicilloic acid.

decreased renal clearance of nafcillin was partly compensated by increased nonrenal clearance (73).

The serum half-life of nafcillin was 1.02 hr in subjects with normal hepatic function, 1.23 hr in cirrhotic patients, and 1.73 hr in patients with biliary obstruction (74). A significant reduction in VD_{SS} was also manifest in these patients. During continuous infusion in normal subjects the renal clearance of nafcillin was observed to be 160 ml/min per 1.73 m^2 when the total plasma clearance was 410 ml/min per 1.73 m^2 (75). Oral administration of probenecid elevates nafcillin plasma concentration after intramuscular or intravenous doses of the antibiotic (60,76,77). This result is probably mediated by a combination of effects of probenecid on renal secretion, hepatic clearance, hepatic blood flow, and the distribution volume of nafcillin.

Cloxacillin	Dicloxacillin	Flucloxacillin	Number of patients	References
2.43	2.61	2.91		49
95	98	–	–	55
94	97	95	–	78
1116	2481	1802	>11	78
1722 ± 465	2271 ± 520	–	6	55
–	1209 ± 192	–	6	55
30.7 ± 7.4	36.2 ± 9.9	–	6	55, 79
–	39.2 ± 5.4	–	6	55, 79
62	73	–	4	79
25	43	66	4	80, 81
162	114	–	4	80
102 ± 22	67 ± 16	88 ± 20	7	82, 117
51 ± 14	43 ± 12	35 ± 17	7	82, 83
38.1 ± 17.9[c]	32.9 ± 20.0[c]	40.6 ± 30.1[c]	6	25
11.1 ± 12.9[d]	3.8 ± 7.6[d]	3.7 ± 5.1[d]	6	25

IV. ISOXAZOLYL PENICILLINS

Structures of four isoxazolyl penicillins (oxacillin, cloxacillin, dicloxacillin, and flucloxacillin) are shown in Table 11 of Chap. 6. These antibiotics all share the properties of resistance to staphylococcal beta-lactamase, acid stability, and high plasma protein binding. Physical and pharmacokinetic properties of these penicillins are compared in Table 2. The octanol/water partition coefficient increases in the following order: oxacillin<cloxacillin<dicloxacillin<flucloxacillin. The plasma half-lives and the percent absorbed after oral dosing increase in parallel. Conversely, renal plasma clearance declines in the same rank order. Compared with penicillin G, penicillin V, methicillin, and nafcillin, the isoxazolyl penicillins are all more extensively and reliably absorbed by the oral route; however,

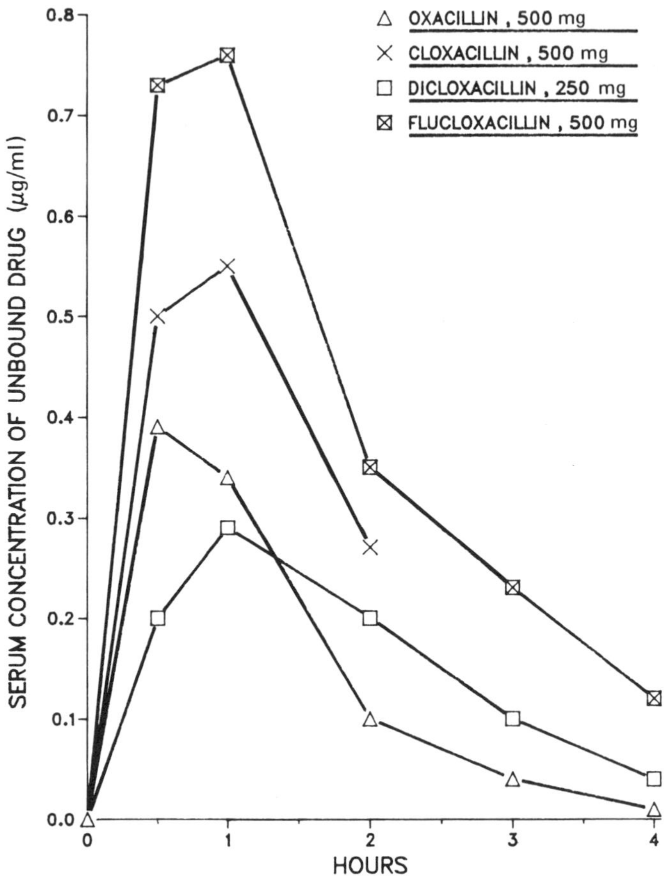

Figure 6 Mean serum concentrations of free drug in 25–122 subjects after oral administration of single doses of isoxazolyl penicillins. (Redrawn from Ref. 78.)

because of their affinity for plasma proteins, the circulating levels of free drug are low (Fig. 6).

A. Oxacillin

Conventional pharmacokinetic analysis of the time course of plasma and urine concentrations of antibacterial activity after doses of the isoxazolyl penicillins and especially after oxacillin is confounded by the appearance of active metabolites (53,84,85). Following an oral dose of 2 g of oxacillin, 21% of the antimicrobial activity against *Sarcina lutea* in an 8-hr pooled urine sample was found to reside in a metabolite more hydrophilic than oxacillin. In both rats and humans the active metabolite in urine is produced by metabolic hydroxylation of the 5-methyl group of the isoxazole ring system (86,87). The 5-hydroxymethyl metabolite is then degraded to the inactive penicilloic acid derivative (88). When 500 mg of oxacillin was given orally, 27.4% was excreted in the urine as oxacillin, 16% as 5-hydroxymethyl oxacillin, 22.2% as the penicilloic acid of oxacillin, and 22.4% as the penicilloic acid of the 5-hydroxymethyl oxacillin (89). Corresponding mean residence times for these compounds in the body were 1.76, 3.79, 2.04, and 3.89 hr, respectively.

Bordt and co-workers were unable to find antibacterial activity in fat or mammary gland tissue after an intravenous infusion of 2 g of oxacillin (90). Oxacillin penetrates cortical bone and synovial fluid erratically (91). Tissue/serum ratios of oxacillin activity in excised tissues during the period of 30–45 min after a 2-g dose given intravenously were as follows: artery, 0.13; vein, 0.08; muscle, 0.076; fascia, 0.076; fat, 0.082; skin, 0.056; nerve, 0.073 (92). In dogs oxacillin is 36% bound in thoracic duct lymph, suggesting that total tissue fluid concentrations might exceed the free drug concentrations in serum (54). Oxacillin penetrates efficiently into tissue fluid in the periprosthetic space after hip joint replacement (93).

Simultaneous administration of oxacillin with ampicillin, mezlocillin, or carbenicillin elevated serum concentrations and depressed elimination rates for each pair of antibiotics (94).

B. Cloxacillin

Following an intravenous dose of ^{35}S-labeled cloxacillin, 82% of the radioactivity appeared in urine and 11% in the feces. After oral dosing 54% appeared in urine and 33% in feces (95). At 90 min 90% of the ^{35}S in urine was unchanged drug, but thereafter the percentage declined with time. At 4 and 7 hr postdose, 20% of the radioactivity in bile was unchanged drug. Penicilloic and penilloic acids accounted for most of the microbiologically inactive metabolites.

Cloxacillin penetrates synovial joint fluid in patients with osteo- and rheumatoid arthritis until unbound drug concentrations in the synovium are similar to those in the serum (96). Cloxacillin also penetrates spongy and cortical bone tissue (97). In patients devoid of kidney function, probenecid reduces the rate of elimination of cloxacillin and dicloxacillin without altering the volume of distribution (98). These results suggest that these antibiotics are eliminated by some extrarenal anion secretory process that is inhibited by probenecid.

C. Dicloxacillin

Antibacterial activity against *S. lutea* found in an 8-hr cumulative urine sample after a 2-g peroral dose of dicloxacillin is 85% parent drug and 15% metabolite, which is essentially the same pattern found with cloxacillin (85). The metabolite was first identified in rat urine as the 5-hydroxymethyl derivative and it has recently also been identified in humans (86,88). In rats the ^{35}S label from dicloxacillin appears as follows in bile: 10% as unchanged drug, 20% as 5-hydroxymethyl dicloxacillin, and 70% as inactive metabolites (99). In humans only 3.8% of a 500-mg peroral dose is excreted in urine as the penicilloic acid derivative (25).

The beta-phase disappearance of dicloxacillin activity from the plasma of patients with severe renal dysfunction is only moderately slower than the disappearance from the plasma of normal subjects, and hemodialysis is without effect (83,100,101). Coadministration of sulfaethidole and dicloxacillin increases the total plasma concentration as well as the extravascular distribution of dicloxacillin (102). Distribution volumes of dicloxacillin are much smaller than those of oxacillin, suggesting that, in general, dicloxacillin penetrates tissues less readily (103).

Following the peroral administration of 62.5- to 520-mg doses of dicloxacillin to fasted subjects, the bioavailability of the drug, based on plasma antibacterial activity, was between 63 and 83% for both capsule and suspension formulations (104).

D. Flucloxacillin

In humans flucloxacillin is partially converted to a microbiologically active metabolite that accounts for 10% of the activity in an 8-hr pooled urine (85). Like dicloxacillin, very little (3.7%) of the dose of flucloxacillin is converted to the penicilloic acid derivative (25). Plasma half-lives of flucloxacillin and hydroxyflucloxacillin are similar, even though the renal clearance of the hydroxylated derivative is higher (105,106).

Penetration of flucloxacillin into synovial effusion fluid is slow and unpredictable (107). Penetration into trabecular, cancellous, and compact bone after parenteral injection is slow but has been judged adequate for antistaphylococcal prophylaxis during hip and knee surgery (108–110). After a 500-mg intramuscular dose, flucloxacillin concentrations in lung parenchyma, cardiac muscle, and cardiac valve tissue reached 7–36% of the concomitant serum levels, but no activity was found in pericardial fluid (111). Wise and co-workers have shown that amoxycillin and other antibiotics with low protein binding penetrate into cantharides blister fluid much better than flucloxacillin (81). However, owing to excellent absorption, slow elimination, and modest binding compared to the other members of the group, flucloxacillin appears to possess the best tissue kinetics of any of the isoxazolyl penicillins (78,82,112).

The plasma half-life of flucloxacillin is significantly increased by coadministration of probenecid or piperacillin, owing to inhibition of renal tubular secretion (113,114). Amoxycillin, however, does not influence flucloxacillin pharmacokinetics (115).

V. AMINOPENICILLINS

Ampicillin differs from penicillin G only by the substitution of an amino group for a hydrogen at the α-position in the side chain (see Tables 2 and 8 of Chap. 6). The amino group confers acid stability, pharmacokinetic advantages, and an expanded gram-negative antibacterial spectrum, but not resistance to beta-lactamases (116). In aqueous solution ampicillin, like all of the aminopenicillins and aminocephalosporins, is charged at any pH. Distribution between aqueous buffer and octanol greatly favors the aqueous phase, independent of pH in the range 3.0–7.9 (117). Nevertheless, orally administered ampicillin is moderately well absorbed in humans (118,119). The mechanisms of the efficient absorption of the aminopenicillins has been explored by a number of investigators using rat intestine both in vivo and in vitro (120–126,214–220). None of these authors have reported evidence for active transport of ampicillin. However, the closely related aminopenicillins cyclacillin and amoxicillin are absorbed by concentration-dependent and temperature-dependent mechanisms. These processes are perturbed by metabolic inhibitors and are competitively inhibited by certain aminocephalosporins and dipeptides. These characteristics are all consistent with the behavior of known intestinal active solute transport pathways and inconsistent with diffusive processes. Tsuji and Yamana have reviewed the various mechanisms by which the intestinal absorption of beta-lactam antibiotics proceeds (127). Table 3 compares the pharmacokinetic parameters of ampicillin, bacampicillin, and pivampicillin.

A. Ampicillin

Judged by the AUC and the cumulative amount of activity excreted in urine, the peroral bioavailability of ampicillin trihydrate is lower in fed than in fasted subjects (132-135). However, absorption in subjects is not affected by bed rest (136). Bioavailability differs among some commercial brands of ampicillin trihydrate, and none are as available as formulations of the anhydrate (137,138). The bioavailability of the soluble potassium salt is also superior to that of the trihydrate (139,140). Judged by both AUC and peak plasma concentrations, the oral availability of ampicillin decreases as the dose is increased (141). Bioavailability considerations are especially important for ampicillin, because increased absorption yields not only more effective therapy but also a decreased incidence of lower gastrointestinal side effects (142).

Following oral administration, peak ampicillin concentrations in bronchial secretions or aqueous humour are 5–10% of concomitant serum concentrations

Table 3 Single-Dose Pharmacokinetics of Ampicillin and Prodrugs After Oral Administration[a]

Drug	Dose (mg)	Number of subjects	K_a (hr^{-1})	K_{10} (hr^{-1})	$t_{1/2}$ (hr)
Ampicillin	500	13	0.88 ± 0.31	0.77 ± 0.13	0.91 ± 0.20
Pivampicillin	700	13	1.82 ± 0.68	0.71 ± 0.08	0.98 ± 0.16
Ampicillin	278	11	0.99 ± 0.21	0.66 ± 0.14	1.09 ± 0.21
Bacampicillin	400	11	2.25 ± 1.23	1.03 ± 0.30	0.75 ± 0.24
Pivampicillin	398	11	1.16 ± 0.22	0.75 ± 0.15	0.96 ± 0.21
Bacampicillin	800	10	1.80 ± 0.43	0.694 ± 0.0133	1.04 ± 0.22
Bacampicillin	1200	10	1.07 ± 0.62	0.604 ± 0.117	1.18 ± 0.21
Bacampicillin	1800	10	2.09 ± 0.58	0.479 ± 0.113	0.50 ± 0.11
Bacampicillin	800	10	1.4 ± 0.51	0.776 ± 0.115	0.91 ± 0.14
Ampicillin	495	5			
Bacampicillin	808	5			
Pivampicillin	702	5			

[a]Listed values are means ± SD; K_a = first-order absorption rate constant, K_{10} = first-order elimination rate constant, $t_{1/2}$ = elimination half-life, C_{max} = maximum concentration of ampicillin in plasma; and AUC = area under the plasma concentration versus time curve.

(143,144). Concentrations are also low in sputum (3.2%), oviduct mucosa (2.5%), saliva (0.8%), and tears (0.6%), expressed as percent of serum concentration (145-147). Ampicillin penetrates erythrocytes and nasal secretions but reaches only 10% of serum levels (148,149). The concentration of ampicillin in synovial fluid is 70% of serum levels and in both bronchial tissue biopsies and peritoneal fluid from patients with pelvic inflammatory disease may exceed 50% (96,150,151). In the CSF of adults with bacterial meningitis, ampicillin reaches CSF/serum ratios of 0.43 and 0.40% after intramuscular and intravenous administration, respectively (152). In children with meningitis the ratio is 0.58% at 3 hr after large intravenous doses (153). Ratios of ampicillin levels in skin window fluids to levels in serum reach 0.47% after 1-g oral doses, 0.32% after 2-g oral doses, and 0.51% after 1-g intravenous doses (45,154,155). Concentrations in pleural fluid achieve 77%, in peritoneal fluid 92%, and in thoracic duct lymph 85% of serum concentrations (23,156,157). In skin blister fluid the area under the concentration versus time curve (AUC) was equal to the AUC in serum (158). The ratio of the AUC in tissue fluid to the AUC in serum was defined by Sjovall as the partition index (159). If appropriate data are collected, this index

C_{max} (μg/ml)	AUC (μg·hr/ml)	Percent of dose in urine	Bioavailability (%)	Reference
3.64 ± 1.67	12.4 ± 5.2	33.6 ± 7.7		118
6.49 ± 1.58	16.7 ± 4.0	47.5 ± 12.6		118
3.70 ± 1.25	10.3 ± 2.9	44.6 ± 14.8		128
3.27 ± 1.63	15.5 ± 3.6	71.5 ± 10.5		128
7.14 ± 1.33	15.2 ± 3.0	64.7 ± 19.1		128
9.50 ± 0.65	30.3 ± 13.1	71		129
12.1 ± 0.7	52.5 ± 31.4	68		129
15.8 ± 1.2	61.5 ± 29.1	73		129
11.1 ± 4.6	35.1 ± 8.8		37 ± 22	130
6.7 ± 2.1	16.6 ± 2.8	46.6 ± 12.6	55.3 ± 17.8	131
13.5 ± 2.9	28.9 ± 2.7	63.5 ± 5.1	83.3 ± 13.5	131
10.2 ± 1.6	25.9 ± 2.9	69.8 ± 15.7	36.8 ± 22.0	131

provides a convenient way to compare the penetrations of different antibiotics into various physiological compartments. In general, the partition index for ampicillin is low in fluids elaborated by epithelial cell systems, except for the intestinal and renal epithelia, with their specialized transport processes. In sharp contrast, because of its low plasma binding, the partition index for ampicillin is high in fluids formed by filtration of plasma.

Nishida et al. first described a microbiologically active metabolite of ampicillin in human urine that was later identified as a Schiff base of ampicillin with acetaldehyde (160,161). An active metabolite that chromatographed as penicillin G was also observed in the urine of subjects given ampicillin (162). Following oral doses of [^{35}S] ampicillin, 44% of the radioactivity appeared in urine. Of this portion, 87% was unchanged drug and 7% was a single inactive metabolite (163). Uno et al. reported that 29% of an oral dose was excreted in the urine unchanged, 4.3% was excreted as the penicilloic acid derivative, and 2.0% as the penamaldic acid derivative (164). A somewhat larger fraction, 10% of an oral dose, was found both by Cole et al. and Graber et al. to be excreted as the penicilloic acid derivative (25,84). Ampicillin is apparently not hydroxylated by hu-

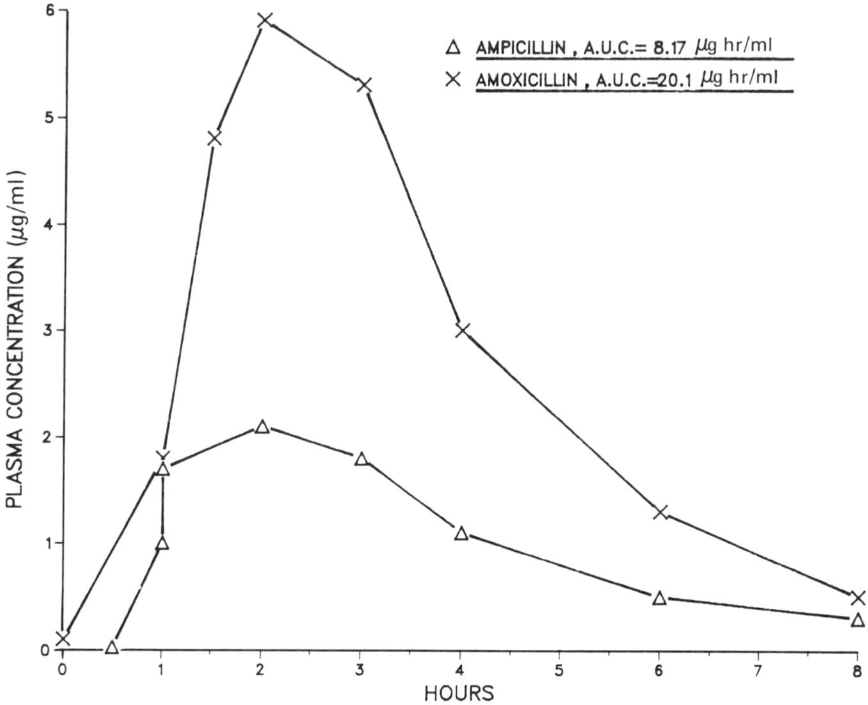

Figure 7 Mean plasma concentrations of ampicillin or amoxicillin in eight subjects after oral administration of single 500-mg doses of ampicillin or amoxicillin. (Redrawn from Ref. 266.)

mans, and the other active metabolites are formed in insufficient quantities to disturb pharmacokinetic evaluations based on determinations of antibacterial activity in body fluids (53,165,166).

Ampicillin is primarily excreted via the kidneys. Excretion of antibacterial activity in the urine of male subjects accounted for 77-88% of intravenous doses, 68% of intramuscular doses, and 40% of oral doses of either the anhydrous or trihydrate form (167). In these studies the renal clearance of ampicillin averaged 260 ml/min, independent of peak plasma ampicillin levels up to 10 μg/ml. The adult glomerular filtration rate is about 125 ml/min; therefore the observed clearance indicates that secretion of ampicillin by the renal tubules contributes significantly to the renal excretory rate. Ehrnebo et al., who found 73% of a 471-mg dose of ampicillin in the urine of male subjects and a mean renal clearance of 206 ml/min, reached the same conclusion (131). Probenecid increases

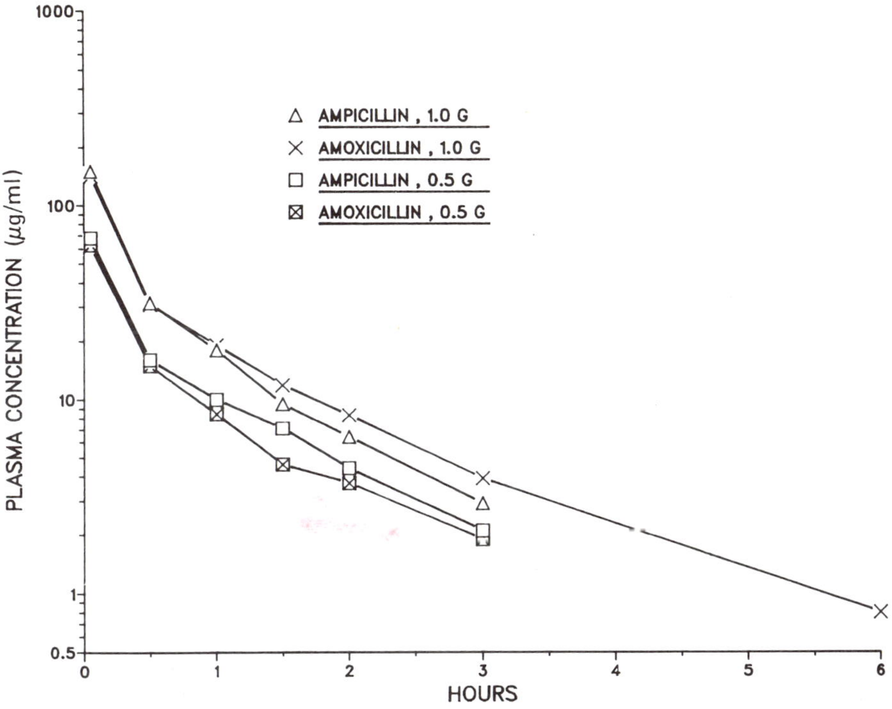

Figure 8 Mean plasma concentrations of ampicillin or amoxicillin in six subjects after intravenous administration of single doses of ampicillin or amoxicillin. (Redrawn from Ref. 207.)

serum concentrations of ampicillin by reducing both tubular secretion and the volume of distribution of the antibiotic (76).

Renal clearance of ampicillin by pregnant women in the first and second trimester increases to 330 ml/min as renal blood flow rises. Clearance then declines to normal in the third trimester and postpartum periods (168–170). In patients with 10% or less of normal renal function, the serum half-life of ampicillin approaches 10 hr (171). Renal clearance is also reduced in cirrhotic patients, but metabolic clearance is elevated (172). In elderly subjects plasma clearance is less than in younger subjects owing to decreased renal function (173). Ampicillin concentrations in T-tube bile of adult females given 250- to 500-mg oral doses ranged from less than 1 to 5 μg/ml and accounted for about 0.1% of the dose (174,175).

Table 4 Intravenous Pharmacokinetics of Ampicillin and Amoxicillin in Normal Human Subjects[a]

Drug	Dose (mg)	Number of subjects	K_{10} (hr^{-1})	K_{12} (hr^{-1})	K_{21} (hr^{-1})	λ^1 (hr^{-1})
Amoxicillin	250	8	1.43 ± 0.21	1.29 ± 0.67	1.94 ± 0.73	3.99 ± 1.30
Amoxicillin	1000	4	1.41 ± 0.32	0.690 ± 0.504	1.13 ± 0.63	2.66 ± 1.22
Amoxicillin	500	9	1.16 ± 0.37	0.92 ± 0.85	1.99 ± 0.99	3.40 ± 1.88
Amoxicillin	b	7	2.22 ± 0.50	1.67 ± 0.67	1.41 ± 0.26	
Amoxicillin	250	8	2.65	3.05	2.76	5.90
Amoxicillin	500	8	1.68	1.43	1.64	4.04
Amoxicillin	1000	8	1.50	0.70	1.22	2.72
Ampicillin	471	5	2.33 ± 0.50	2.29 ± 2.87	2.46 ± 1.05	6.06 ± 4.39
Ampicillin	250	6	2.0	1.7	1.6	4.6
Ampicillin	556	10	2.45 ± 0.70	1.72 ± 0.78	1.57 ± 0.27	4.24 ± 1.27

[a]Listed values are means ± SD; K_{10} = first-order elimination rate constant, K_{12} = first-order transfer rate constant from control to peripheral compartment, K_{21} = first-order transfer rate constant from peripheral to central compartment, λ^1 = fastest hybrid disposition rate constant, λ^2 = shortest hybrid disposition rate constant, V_C = volume of central compartment, V_2 = volume of distribution during terminal phase, VD_{SS} = volume of distribution at steady state, and Cl = total body clearance of drug from plasma.

[b]Calculated for a 10-mg/kg dose from data obtained with 250-, 500-, and 1000-mg doses.

Table 5 Single-Dose Pharmacokinetics of Ampicillin After Oral Administration[a]

Dose (mg)	Number of subjects	K_a (hr^{-1})	K_{10} (hr^{-1})	$t_{1/2}$ (hr)
291	11	1.12 ± 0.29	0.76 ± 0.17	0.95 ± 0.20
500	12	1.70 ± 0.35	0.82 ± 0.05	0.88 ± 0.05
500	8	3.0 ± 0.36	0.48 ± 0.06	1.5 ± 0.17
250	8	1.08 ± 0.86	0.68 ± 0.17	
500	9	1.02 ± 0.15	0.73 ± 0.17	1.00 ± 0.28
500	16	0.80 ± 0.21	0.69 ± 0.12	

[a]Listed values are means ± SD; K_a = first-order absorption rate constant, K_{10} = first-order elimination rate constant, $t_{1/2}$ = elimination half-life, C_{max} = maximum concentration of ampicillin in plasma, and AUC = area under the plasma concentration versus time curve.

λ^2 (hr^{-1})	V_C (liter/kg)	V_2	VD_{SS} (liter/kg)	Cl (liter/kg)	AUC (μg hr/ml)	Ref.
0.692 ± 0.141	0.187 ± 0.048		0.311 ± 0.088	0.264 ± 0.025		179
0.588 ± 0.203	0.190 ± 0.075	0.466 ± 0.149	0.294 ± 0.093	0.260 ± 0.103		184
0.68 ± 0.16	0.178 ± 0.038	0.304 ± 0.081	0.252 ± 0.060	0.200 ± 0.504	37.0 ± 9.7	178
	0.093 ± 0.023		0.193 ± 0.027			185
2.55	0.17		0.29	0.32		180
0.72	0.22		0.46	0.32		
0.79	0.22		0.49	0.34		
1.02 ± 0.102	0.10 ± 0.030	0.228 ± 0.040		0.232 ± 0.040	29.6 ± 4.7	131
0.69	0.14	0.39		0.27	13.3	103
0.610 ± 0.080		0.336 ± 0.076	0.191 ± 0.073			130

C_{max} (μg/ml)	AUC (μg hr/ml)	Percent of dose in urine	Bioavailability (%)	Ref.
7.68 ± 2.74	17.7 ± 4.1	73.5 ± 9.4		128
8.2 ± 0.9	19.4 ± 1.3	68 ± 46	51 ± 5	191
	11.4 ± 1.1	65		194
	9.17 ± 1.69		89 ± 13	179
10.4	27.4 ± 3.1	43 ± 9.5	77 ± 17	178
8.9 ± 2.3	30.5 ± 5.9	47.1 ± 22		133

B. Amoxicillin

The activities of ampicillin and amoxicillin (see Table 8 of Chap. 6) are essentially equivalent against a wide spectrum of pathogenic bacteria (176,177). After the ingestion of equivalent doses of the two antibiotics, however, their behavior differs. In adult subjects amoxicillin is better absorbed in the small intestine than ampicillin. Typical values for the bioavailability of amoxicillin range from 65 to 93%, compared to 48-89% for ampicillin (Table 5) (147,178-180,234). A comparable difference also occurs in infants and children (181,182). The absorption advantage of amoxicillin is not predictable from ionization states in aqueous solution, which are practically identical at physiological pH values, or from oil-water distributions which would favor passive permeation of ampicillin (124,183). Rather, the absorption advantage of amoxicillin must reside in its affinity for the membrane-mediated process by which aminopenicillins penetrate the cells of the intestinal epithelium. Plasma concentrations of amoxicillin and ampicillin after oral and intravenous administration are compared in Figures 7 and 8. More detailed pharmacokinetic analyses of the two drugs are presented in Table 4.

Amoxicillin absorption is not significantly impaired if the dose is taken with or following food (133,183,186); however, absorption is reduced in bed-fast patients and delayed in ambulatory patients after recovery from vagotomy and pyloroplasty (187,188). Pharmacokinetic parameters of orally administered amoxicillin from several independent studies are compared in Table 5.

In combination with clavulanic acid, an inhibitor of beta-lactamase, amoxicillin successfully treats infections caused by organisms otherwise resistant to its action because of production of this enzyme. The manufacture, pharmacokinetics (189-192), activity spectrum, and clinical use of this combination (193) are reviewed in Chapter 15.

Metabolic conversion of amoxicillin in humans to microbiologically active products has not been observed (84,162,165). After oral administration of amoxicillin, 59% of the dose was excreted in urine as unchanged drug, 16% as the penicilloic acid, and 7% as the penamaldic acid derivative (164). Graber et al. found that 73% of the dose was excreted unchanged and 19% was excreted as the penicilloic acid (84).

Both amoxicillin and ampicillin in the circulation are about 17% bound to plasma proteins (195,196). The weak binding has little influence on tissue penetration of either antibiotic. The oral absorption advantage that amoxicillin possesses over equivalent doses of ampicillin provides higher plasma concentrations of amoxicillin and consequently slightly higher amounts of amoxicillin than ampicillin in skin window fluids, sputum, and bronchial secretions (143, 145,154,159). After intravenous administration, plasma concentrations of amoxicillin and ampicillin are similar (see Fig. 8) and both drugs penetrate into CSF through normal and inflamed meninges equally well (153,197,198).

Amoxicillin penetrates gingival tissue and produces a tissue/serum ratio of 0.50; middle ear effusion fluid serum ratio is 0.60 (199,200). Amoxicillin reportedly reaches higher ratios in sputum after intramuscular administration, 0.35, than after oral administration, 0.04–0.06 (201,202). Penetration into sputum increased with increasing purulence during primary infections in some studies, but was independent of purulence in others (203,204). In children given intramuscular amoxicillin, CSF/serum ratios reached 0.05–0.10 (205). The tissue distribution and therapeutic efficacy of amoxicillin in localized infections have been extensively reviewed by Brogden et al. (206,207).

Elimination of amoxicillin from the body proceeds principally by renal processes. From 54 to 73% of oral doses of amoxicillin appeared in the urine of normal subjects of both sexes (176,208–210). Slightly more, 75–80%, was excreted in urine after intravenous administration of single 250-, 500-, or 1000-mg doses (211). In this study the mean renal clearance of amoxicillin in eight male subjects was 276 ± 37 ml/min during a period when the glomerular filtration rate, estimated by clearance of endogenous creatinine, was 120 ± 8.5 ml/min. It is therefore reasonable that probenecid significantly elevates amoxicillin concentrations in serum and CSF while reducing urinary excretion (208,212,213). In patients with renal failure terminal plasma half-life values are between 7 and 21 hr but can be lowered to 2.3–2.8 hr by hemodialysis (184,214,215). Half-lives are also extended in elderly patients, leading to elevated AUC values after oral doses (216,217).

After administration of intravenous amoxicillin, concentrations in gallbladder bile, T-tube bile, and bile aspirated through a tube placed in the intestinal lumen typically reach approximately 50% of concurrent concentrations in plasma, and the terminal half-lives in plasma and bile are comparable (218,219). Clearly the hepatic extraction, biliary excretion, and intestinal reabsorption (enterohepatic recycling) of unchanged drug play minor roles in the disposition of amoxicillin.

VI. ESTER PRODRUGS OF AMINOPENICILLINS

Labile esters of the carboxyl group of ampicillin have been developed into useful prodrugs with significant oral absorption advantages over the parent antibiotic. The most useful oral esters of ampicillin are pivampicillin, the pivaloyloxymethyl ester; bacampicillin, the ethoxy carbonyloxyethyl ester; and talampicillin, the phthalidyl ester. These structures are shown in Table 9 of Chap. 6. Sarpicillin and sarmoxicillin, methoxymethyl esters of the condensation products of ampicillin or amoxicillin, respectively, with acetone, are briefly discussed in this section.

All of these prodrugs are more water soluble than ampicillin at pH 3–5 and are more lipid soluble at any pH (220,221). Owing to perturbation of the intes-

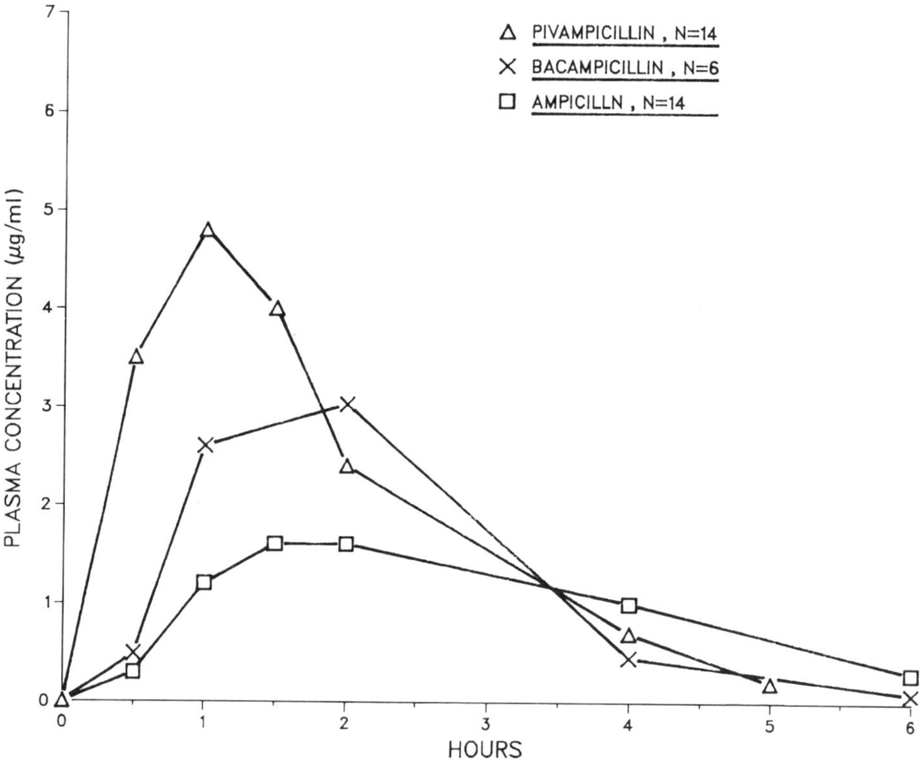

Figure 9 Mean plasma concentrations of ampicillin after oral administration of single 250-mg equivalent doses of ampicillin, pivampicillin, or bacampicillin. (Redrawn from Refs. 134 and 267.)

tinal microflora by unabsorbed antibiotic, diarrhea often follows peroral use of ampicillin. Use of the ester prodrugs has reduced the frequency of diarrhea at the expense of an increased frequency of upper gastrointestinal distress (222, 223). The plasma concentrations of ampicillin tend to be lower after oral administration of a single 250-mg dose of ampicillin than after an equivalent dose of bacampicillin or of pivampicillin (Fig. 9).

A. Pivampicillin

In aqueous solution pivampicillin is hydrolyzed to ampicillin, pivalic acid, and formaldehyde. The reaction is slow in aqueous buffers at physiological pH values, but is catalyzed by nonspecific esterases present in the intestinal mucosa, liver, and blood (224). After oral administration of ^{35}S-labeled pivampicillin,

84% of the radioactivity was lost in the urine and 9% in the feces. Hydrolysis occurred before, during, and after absorption (225).

Peak plasma concentrations of ampicillin after oral doses of pivampicillin hydrochloride range from two- to threefold higher than those achieved with ampicillin (134,135,224,226). Most investigators have concurred that absorption of ampicillin from pivampicillin is unchanged or moderately enhanced in fed subjects (134,135,227). However, opposite results have also been obtained, possibly owing to widely divergent feeding protocols (228). The frequency of upper gastrointestinal distress is reduced when pivampicillin hydrochloride is taken following meals or when it is replaced by the sparingly soluble pivampicillin base (229,230,232).

Excretion of antibacterial activity in urine after oral administration of single doses of pivampicillin accounts for about 70% of the amount of ampicillin given, independent of dose size from 125 to 1500 mg (231).

In postoperative patients the bioavailability of ampicillin from pivampicillin capsules has been found to be unexpectedly low and variable (232). In newborn infants the absorption advantage of pivampicillin over ampicillin is less evident than in older children and adults (233–235).

B. Bacampicillin

Nonspecific esterases in serum and intestinal tissue hydrolyze bacampicillin to ampicillin, acetaldehyde, carbon dioxide, and ethanol. Absorption of ^{35}S-labeled drug is rapid and extensive in the upper gastrointestinal tract, with 80% of the radioactivity excreted in urine and 14% in feces (225). Judged by AUC and urinary excretion, the oral bioavailability of ampicillin in adults from doses of bacampicillin ranges from 130 to 180% of that from equivalent oral doses of ampicillin itself and slightly exceeds the availability from intramuscular doses of ampicillin (130,221,236,237). In crossover comparisons with amoxicillin, bacampicillin typically provides slightly higher peak plasma concentrations with less intrasubject variability (238,239). Two commercial formulations of bacampicillin were bioequivalent, and in a separate study absorption was unaffected by the ingestion of food (240,241).

Comparisons of tolerance of bacampicillin HCl and pivampicillin in outpatient populations have indicated that pivampicillin base produced more frequent side effects when the drugs were prescribed with special instructions, but that the frequency of side effects from the two drugs was equal when the patients were instructed to take the doses with food (242,243). Bacampicillin appears to have a slightly greater absorption advantage over ampicillin in infants and children than in adults (244,245).

High plasma concentrations of ampicillin obtained after oral administration of modest doses of bacampicillin produce, in turn, improved ampicillin concentrations in those tissue fluids into which ampicillin permeates rapidly, such as skin window and skin blister fluids (16,45,147,155,246). The same relationships hold true for penetration of ampicillin into pleural fluids, lung tissue, and middle ear effusions from patients with otitis media (247-251). On the other hand, adequate penetration of ampicillin into refractory compartments such as sinus and bronchial secretions can be ensured only by the prescription of large (800-1200 mg three times per day) doses of bacampicillin (150,252-254). Extensive considerations of ampicillin tissue distribution after bacampicillin administration can be found in separate reviews by Sjovall (159) and Craig (255). Neu has recently reviewed the human pharmacokinetics of bacampicillin (256).

C. Talampicillin

Talampicillin hydrolyzes to ampicillin and phthaldehydic acid. Hydrolysis of talampicillin in 2% blood and in liver homogenate proceeds faster than the hydrolysis of pivampicillin (257). In vivo the inactive phthaldehydic acid is further metabolized to α-hydroxy-o-toluic acid and excreted in the urine (258,259). In humans urinary excretion of ampicillin activity is about twice as great after oral talampicillin as after oral ampicillin (260-262). The administration of talampicillin with food delays the absorption of ampicillin but does not reduce the amount absorbed (261).

The bioavailabilities of ampicillin from orally administered talampicillin and bacampicillin have been compared. Sjovall and co-workers, in a study employing 10 male volunteers, concluded that bacampicillin provided more absorbed ampicillin per unit dose of ampicillin than did talampicillin (263). Mazzei and co-workers, in a crossover study with 16 women, found no difference in bioavailability of ampicillin from bacampicillin or talampicillin (264). Ampicillin concentrations in the serum of six Oriental subjects given equimolar doses of bacampicillin, talampicillin, and ampicillin were highest for bacampicillin and lowest for ampicillin (265) (Fig. 10).

D. Sarpicillin

Sarpicillin is the lipid-soluble methoxymethyl ester of hetacillin. In rabbits intravenous sarpicillin produced higher concentrations of antibacterial activity in the CSF than did intravenous ampicillin (268). In dogs the same pattern was observed in prostatic fluid (269). In humans oral sarpicillin produced detectable concentrations of both ampicillin and sarpicillin in plasma and of ampicillin in saliva, suggesting that this ester is incompletely hydrolyzed during the absorption process (270).

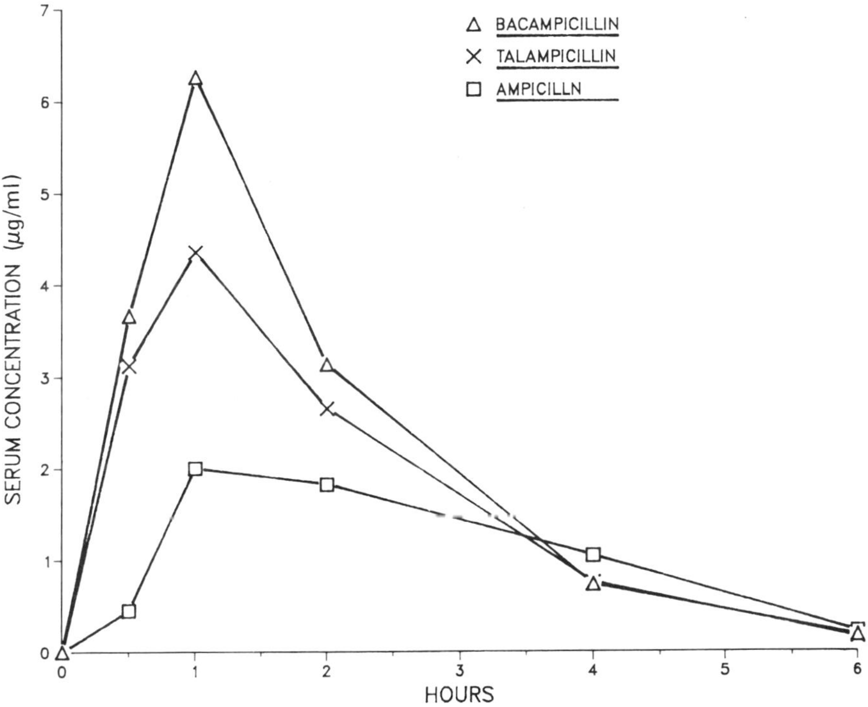

Figure 10 Mean serum ampicillin concentration in six subjects in a crossover study after oral administration of single 250-mg doses of ampicillin as ampicillin, talampicillin, or bacampicillin. (Redrawn from Ref. 265.)

E. Sarmoxicillin

Sarmoxicillin is the lipid-soluble methoxymethyl ester of hetamoxicillin. Incomplete hydrolysis of sarmoxicillin during absorption allows detection of the intact ester in the systemic circulation after oral administration and causes reduced maximum plasma concentrations of amoxicillin as well as increased persistance of amoxicillin in plasma (271).

F. Sultamicillin

This prodrug is a diester of ampicillin and sulbactam with formaldehyde hydrate. Sulbactam is penicilloic acid sulfone, an inhibitor of many bacterial beta-lactamase enzymes. Following oral administration of sultamicillin, equimolar amounts of ampicillin and sulbactam are released during the absorptive process.

Both in the presence and absence of probenecid the plasma half-lives of the constituent drugs are similar to each other (272).

The bioavailability of the two constituent drugs from single oral doses of sultamicillin exceeded 80%; thus sultamicillin is an efficient prodrug (273). After repeated doses of sultamicillin excellent absorption of ampicillin was maintained; nevertheless, diarrhea of varying severity appeared (274). Davies et al. confirmed these results in patients with flare-ups of chronic bronchitis and concluded that sultamicillin should be evaluated further for treatment of infections caused by beta-lactamase-producing bacteria (275).

VII. EXPANDED-SPECTRUM PENICILLINS

In recent years the new penicillin antibiotics that have been developed possess greater antibacterial activity against a wider spectrum of microorganisms. These expanded-spectrum penicillins include the acylureidopenicillins. The structures of these extended-spectrum drugs are shown in Table 9 of Chapter 6.

A. Azlocillin

Azlocillin is an acylureidopenicillin with a wide spectrum of antibacterial activity. Azlocillin is only administered parenterally (intravenously or intramuscularly), as the bioavailability after oral administration is poor (less than 60%). Bioavailability after intramuscular injection is 100% (276). The apparent volume of distribution is about 0.20 liter/kg, with a mean of 14 liter, suggesting that azlocillin distributes into extracellular fluid (277). The volume of distribution is expanded (0.26-0.55 liter/kg) in burn patients (278). Protein binding is about 28% in normal subjects and slightly lower in uremic patients (279).

The pharmacokinetics of azlocillin are dose dependent or capacity limited, that is, the plasma concentrations increase more than a proportional amount for increased dosage (Fig. 11). The dose-dependent kinetics of azlocillin result in a prolonged half-life and decreased total body clearance as the dose is increased (280). The half-life was 0.89, 0.98, and 1.5 hr and the total body clearance was 12.0, 9.2, and 6.4 liter/hr for doses of 1, 2, and 5 g administered as 5-min intravenous bolus injections. Similar results were obtained by other investigators who infused doses of 5 and 10 g (281).

Approximately 60% of the dose is excreted in the urine in subjects with normal renal function and the kinetics are dependent upon renal function (279). The half-life is prolonged and the clearance is reduced for patients with impaired renal function (282). A dosage nomogram has been developed for patients with renal insufficiency (283).

Hemodialysis shortens the half-life of azlocillin, and a supplemental dose after the completion of dialysis is recommended (284). Peritoneal dialysis is less effective in removing the antibiotic (285).

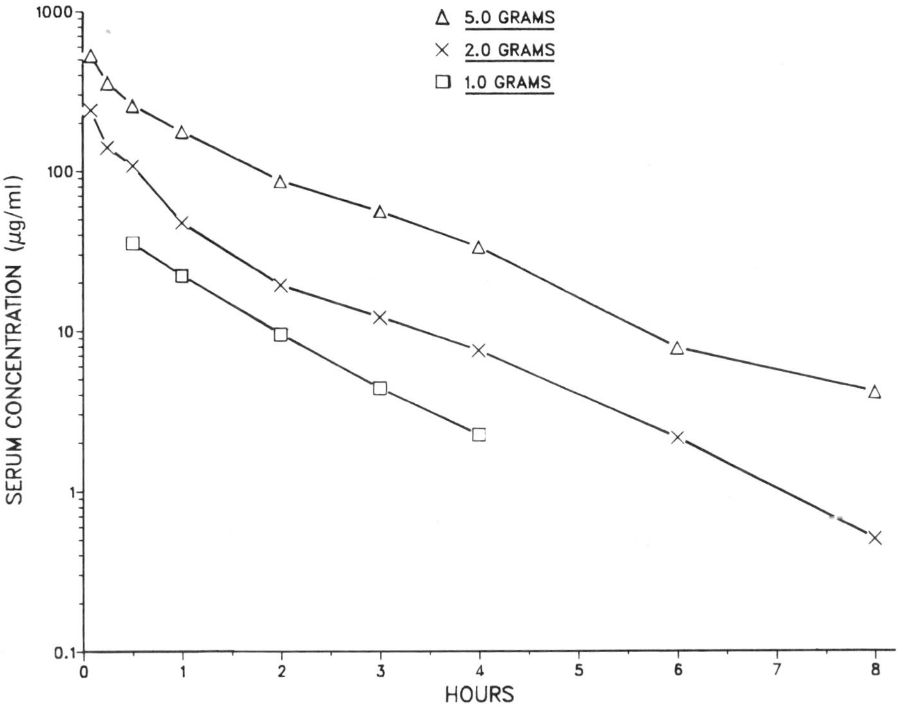

Figure 11 Mean serum concentrations of azlocillin activity after intravenous administration of single graded doses.

Azlocillin is excreted in the bile, with 0.2-7.5% of the dose appearing in 8 hr in T-tube patients (286). Comparison of the biliary excretion of azlocillin and mezlocillin using marker dilution techniques showed that the biliary excretion of azlocillin (1-7% of dose) is significantly less than the biliary excretion of mezlocillin (24-51% of dose) (287).

The half-life is prolonged in newborn and infants less than 3 months old, but approaches that of an adult in school-aged children (288).

B. Carbenicillin

Carbenicillin, one of the oldest and most extensively studied benzylpenicillins, has excellent activity against gram-negative pathogens which produce beta-lactamase, including *Pseudomonas aeruginosa.* The disodium salt of carbenicillin is administered parenterally (intramuscularly or intravenously) because the compound is not well absorbed from the gastrointestinal tract.

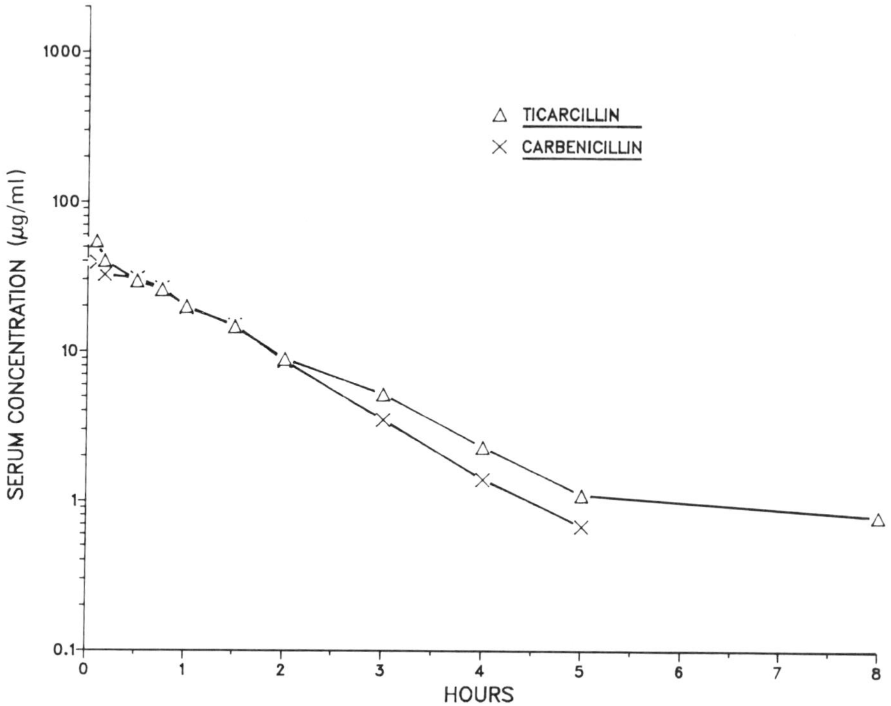

Figure 12 Mean serum concentrations of carbenicillin and ticarcillin after 30-min intravenous infusions of single 2-g doses to 10 subjects. (Data from Ref. 299).

The clinical pharmacology of carbenicillin was described in the literature as early as 1967–1968 (289,290). Plasma concentrations of carbenicillin contrasted against ticarcillin are shown in Figure 12. The volume of distribution of carbenicillin is 16–22% of body weight. Carbenicillin is about 50% bound to plasma proteins as determined by ultrafiltration (291). The intestinal fluid concentrations of carbenicillin are lower but parallel to plasma concentrations, as demonstrated in studies of blister fluid by a number of investigators (292,293). Nevertheless, the degree of penetration into such fluid provides concentrations exceeding the minimal inhibitory concentrations for many important pathogens.

The elimination half-life for carbenicillin ranges from 0.75 to 1.3 hr in normal adults, with approximately 80% of a dose being excreted in the urine unchanged (289). Therefore the elimination half-life is significantly prolonged by renal impairment (294) or administration of probenecid (295). For example, in patients with severe renal failure the half-life ranged from 8 to 24 hr. Hemodialysis or peritoneal dialysis shortens the half-life (294). The half-life is also prolonged in neonates and premature infants (296,297). The pharmacokinetics of carbenicillin are similar to that of ticarcillin and piperacillin (298,299).

C. Furazlocillin

Therapeutic results with furazlocillin, a semisynthetic acylureidopenicillin, are good, but a relatively high number of adverse effects have been associated with its clinical use (300). As is true for the other penicillins of this class, furazlocillin is administered parenterally (intramuscularly or intravenously). The protein binding of furazlocillin is 65%, independent of concentration over the range 50-400 μg/ml (301).

The pharmacokinetics of furazlocillin are nonlinear and dose dependent. Dose-normalized serum concentration versus time curves and the percent excreted per hour in the urine after 2- and 4-g doses were not superimposable (301). The half-life is longer than observed for mezlocillin, ranging from 1.0 to 3.0 hr in subjects with normal renal function (300,301). The apparent volume of distribution is about 18–20% of body weight.

The renal elimination of the drug is less than that observed for other penicillins of this class, as shown by a direct comparison with mezlocillin (300). Only 25–30% of the dose is excreted in the urine (300,302). The renal clearance of furazlocillin, 80 ml/min, is linear and dose dependent but accounts for only a small part of the total serum clearance of the drug, which is dose dependent and nonlinear (300,301).

Nonrenal elimination, which averages about 70% of the dose, is primarily metabolic, as only a small fraction of the dose (0.1%) is excreted in the bile. This nonrenal elimination accounts for the nonlinear kinetics of the drug, resulting in decreased nonrenal clearance after larger doses. Furazlocillin is metabolized differently than many penicillins. Hydrolysis of furazlocillin to an inactive penicilloic acid derivative is not the major metabolic route but, rather, a large fraction of the dose is metabolized to unknown compounds (290).

The kinetics of furazlocillin are not dependent upon posture (300). Further work is necessary, however, to establish the kinetics of this compound in special populations such as patients with impaired renal function and geriatric and neonatal patients.

D. Mecillinam

Mecillinam (amdinocillin) is a 6-amidinopenicillanic acid derivative that possesses good activity against many clinically relevant gram-negative organisms but relatively poor activity against gram-positive bacteria. This penicillin has a novel effect on cell wall synthesis, causing a ballooning of the bacterial cells (303). Mecillinam must be administered parenterally (intramuscularly or intravenously)

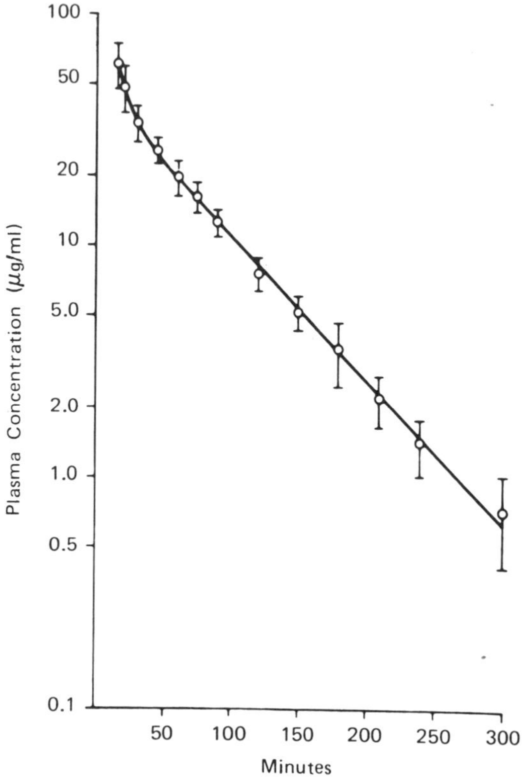

Figure 13 Mean plasma concentrations ± SD of mecillinam activity after 10-min intravenous infusions of single 10-mg/kg doses to 12 subjects. (Data from Ref. 308.)

because it is not well absorbed orally (304). Several esters of mecillinam have been tested and were found to improve its oral absorption (304,305).

The penetration of mecillinam into the CSF has been investigated (306,307). Mecillinam, as with other penicillins, penetrates the noninflamed meninges poorly but penetration across the blood-brain barrier for two patients with suspected meningitis was significantly higher. The CSF levels decline much more slowly than the plasma levels of mecillinam (306).

Following a 15-min intravenous infusion of 10 mg/kg in normal subjects, plasma concentrations of mecillinam exhibit a biphasic decline (Fig. 13). The terminal half-life is 0.85-0.9 hr, with an apparent VD_{SS} of 0.23 liter/kg and a plasma clearance of 245 ml/min (303,308,309). Renal excretion of mecillinam is the major elimination pathway, with 70% of the dose excreted unchanged in the urine (308,309). Renal clearance is 175 ml/min, approximately twice the clearance of creatinine, suggesting net tubular secretion (308).

Mecillinam is also excreted in the bile. Patients given an 800-mg intramuscular dose 1 hr preoperatively had common bile duct biliary concentrations ranging from 5 to 100 μg/ml, with a mean concentration of 50 μg/ml. The biliary concentrations were significantly reduced in patients with nonfunctional gallbladders and were inversely correlated with serum bilirubin in jaundiced patients (310).

Multiple-dose administration of 10 mg/kg every 4 hr for six doses did not result in accumulation of drug in plasma in normal volunteers (309); however, the half-life is prolonged in renally impaired patients, ranging from 4.4 to 7.6 hr in patients with a creatinine clearance of less than 20 ml/min (311,312). The urine recovery of mecillinam is reduced in patients with impaired renal function and also by the coadministration of probenecid (312,308). Patients with severe renal impairment should have their dosage reduced appropriately.

In a crossover study in normal subjects mecillinam (10 mg/kg) exhibited higher mean plasma concentrations, a longer half-life (1.6 hr), and reduced plasma clearance (225 ml/min) when given concurrently with cephalothin (15 mg/kg) (307). These changes, however, were not statistically significant and the clinical significance of such changes has not been evaluated.

E. Mezlocillin

Mezlocillin is administered parenterally (intravenously or intramuscularly) and is rapidly absorbed after intramuscular injection. The apparent volume of distribution in normal volunteers is about 14 liters (20% of body weight, i.e., nearly equivalent to the extracellular fluid volume) (313). Penetration into CSF is low but is increased when the meninges are inflamed. Good penetration into bronchial secretions has been demonstrated in tracheostomized patients (5-g dose), with peak concentrations ranging from 10 to 20 μg/ml and levels exceeding 1.5 μg/ml for 6 hr (314). Penetration into pleural effusion fluid has also been demonstrated (315).

The elimination of mezlocillin is dose dependent and exhibits nonlinear kinetics. The plasma levels achieved after 1, 2, and 5 g administered as 5-min infusions are not proportional to dose (Fig. 14). The half-life in normal subjects ranges from 0.7 to 0.9 hr, but is prolonged by renal impairment and following high dosage (316,317).

About 60-70% of the dose is excreted in the urine, so that the rate of elimination is dependent on renal function and is decreased by probenecid (318,319). Figure 15 shows both the dose dependency and the effect of renal impairment on mezlocillin clearance (320). Dosage adjustments based upon creatinine clearance are recommended for patients with severe renal impairment (321).

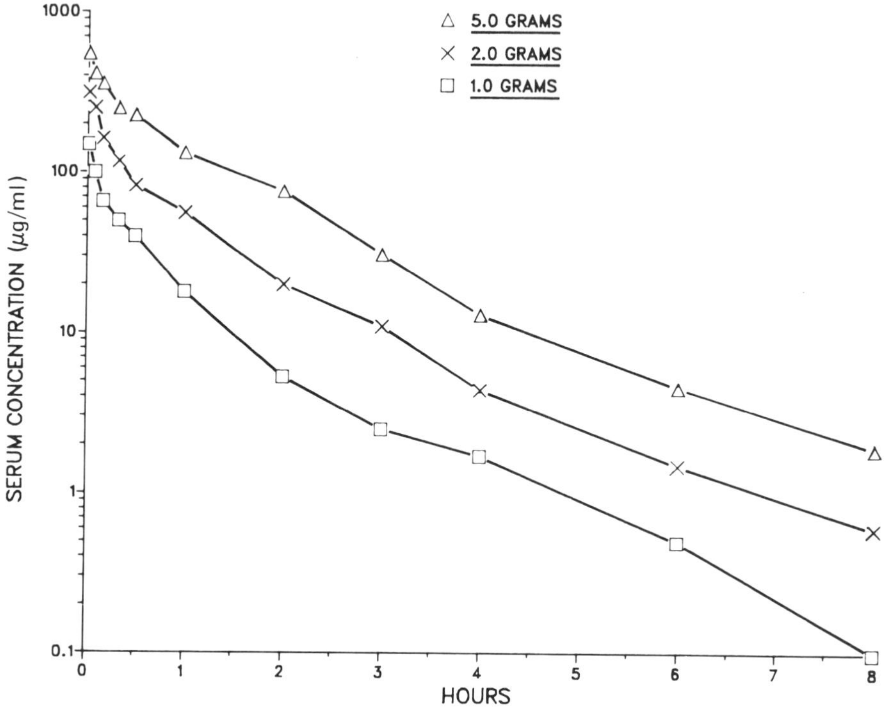

Figure 14 Mean serum concentrations of mezlocillin activity after intravenous administration of single graded doses.

In general, the dose should be one-half normal in patients with a creatinine clearance of less than 25 ml/min, and reduced to one-third normal for patients having creatinine clearances less than 10 ml/min. Hemodialysis removes mezlocillin effectively (322). Approximately 18% of the dose was recovered in 4 hr of dialysis. Other investigators have demonstrated that hemodialysis shortens the half-life of mezlocillin but that peritoneal dialysis has little overall effect (323).

Biliary excretion of mezlocillin is significant and is much greater than a number of other beta-lactam antibiotics (324,325). In cholecystectomized patients, mezlocillin excreted in the bile (collected from T-tube drainage) accounted for 2.6% of the dose (324), although other investigators have shown that up to 25% of the dose was excreted in the bile (326).

Correspondingly, nonrenal elimination of mezlocillin plays a substantial role in total body clearance, and hepatic insufficiency prolongs the half-life of mezlocillin (327). Patients with marked hepatic impairment should be given only 50% of the normal adult dose.

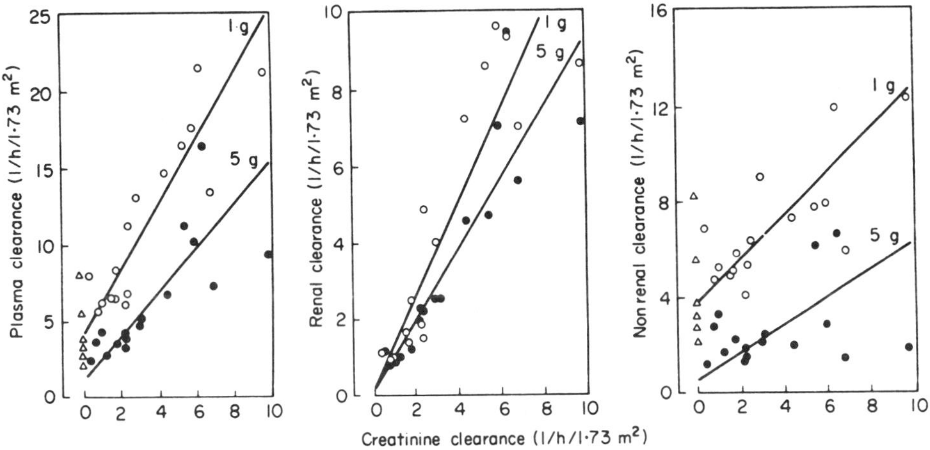

Figure 15 Relationship between clearances of mezlocillin and creatinine in normal (○, 1-g dose; ●, 5-g dose) and hemodialysis (△, 1-g dose) patients. (Reproduced with permission from Ref. 320. Copyright 1982 by the British Society for Antimicrobial Chemotherapy.)

In newborn the half-life of mezlocillin is prolonged and the dosage should be reduced (328). The half-life in infants less than 7 days old was 4.3 hr, whereas the half-life was 2.5 hr for those 7 days and older.

F. Piperacillin

Piperacillin is a semisynthetic aminobenzylpenicillin with broad antimicrobial activity against many gram-positive and gram-negative bacteria, including *Pseudomonas.* Resistance of clinical isolates as well as adverse reactions, including leukopenia and nephrotoxicity, have been reported (329). Piperacillin must be given parenterally (intramuscularly or intravenously) because it is not well absorbed when administered orally (330). It is approximately 22% bound to serum proteins and is primarily excreted unchanged in urine and bile (330).

Piperacillin penetrates skeletal muscle and adipose tissues (331,332). Significant CSF levels are achieved in patients with meningitis (333).

In subjects with normal renal function piperacillin exhibits dose-dependent pharmacokinetics, characterized by a decreasing plasma clearance, decreasing volume of distribution, and prolonged half-life as the dosage of piperacillin is increased (Fig. 16) (334,335). The dose dependency may be mediated by saturable renal tubular secretion (336). In normal volunteers the half-life increased from 0.9 to 1.2 hr and the plasma clearance decreased from 224 to 135 ml/min following intravenous bolus administration of single 15- and 60-mg/kg doses (336).

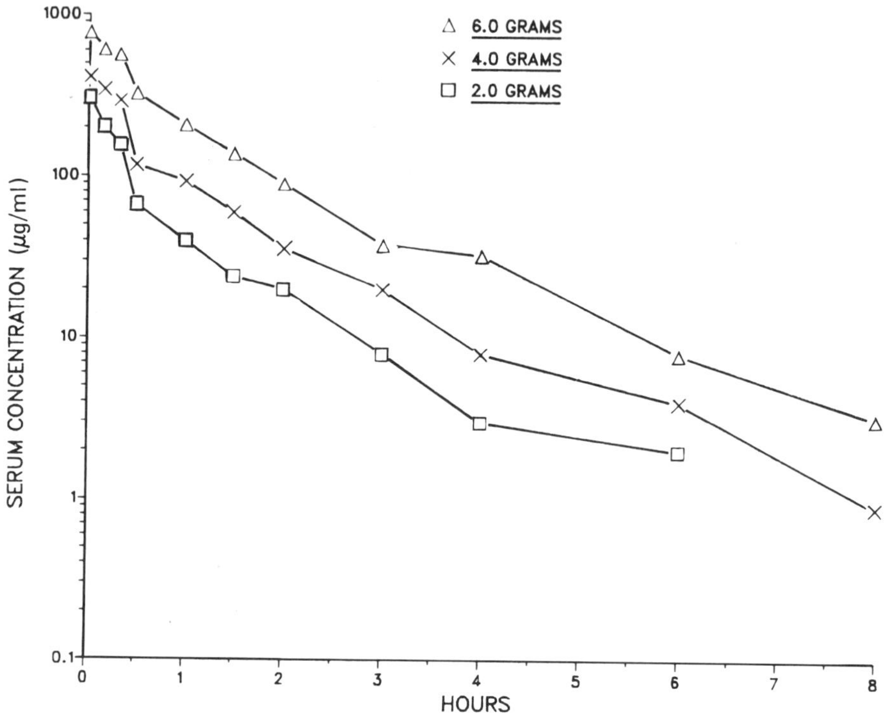

Figure 16 Mean serum concentrations of piperacillin activity after intravenous administration of single graded doses.

Piperacillin elimination is prolonged in patients with impaired renal function, resulting in a three- to fivefold increase in the half-life, 80% reduction of plasma clearance, and decreased renal clearances (336). Although piperacillin undergoes significant nonrenal clearance, including biliary excretion (337,338), a dosage reduction based on creatinine clearance is recommended in patients with severe renal impairment (336,339,340). The half-life during hemodialysis is shortened (341–343), but the necessity of dose supplementation after hemodialysis is controversial.

Liver impairment prolongs the half-life (341). Coadministration of probenecid results in higher serum levels and prolongs the half-life by 30% (344). The half-life of piperacillin is also extended during cardiopulmonary bypass surgery (331).

Piperacillin kinetics change with age. In the newborn the half-life is two to four times that of the adult (345), but in preadolescent children the half-life of piperacillin is shorter than in adults: 47 min for infants 1-6 months old and 29 min for children 6 months to 12 years old (346,347).

G. Ticarcillin

Ticarcillin and carbenicillin are structurally similar, ticarcillin having a 3-thienyl moiety in place of the benzene ring of carbenicillin (Table 10, Chap. 6). Both antibiotics have two ionizable carboxyl groups and exist principally as lipid-insoluble dianions at the pH of most body fluids. As a consequence of their similar structures, ticarcillin and carbenicillin, in general, have similar antibacterial spectra and pharmacokinetics (see Fig. 12). In particular, however, ticarcillin is somewhat more active than carbenicillin against most strains of *P. aeruginosa,* has a slightly longer terminal half-life in plasma (72 versus 66 min), and is less completely excreted in urine after an intravenous infusion (299,348,349).

Following oral administration, only 2.8% of a 500-mg dose of ticarcillin appears in the urine. After intramuscular administration of single 1-g doses 83% was excreted by the same route (350,351). Judged by the ratio of areas under the curve, the intramuscular dose was 86% as bioavailable as the intravenous dose (352). Coadministration of probenecid with ticarcillin slightly increases the plasma half-life of the antibiotic, slows urine excretion, and increases the volume of distribution (295,298,353).

Ticarcillin and carbenicillin penetrate equally into skin window fluid to reach a concentration of 22% of concomitant serum concentrations 2 hr after 30-min infusions of 3-g doses (292). On the other hand, Findlay et al. found that ticarcillin penetrated cantharides blister fluid to a greater extent than carbenicillin after 1-g doses administered as intravenous boluses (293).

Tissue/serum ratios of ticarcillin ranged from 0.17 to 0.30 in the endometrium, fallopian tube, ovary, and myometrium after 30-min intravenous infusions of 5-g doses in patients undergoing preparation for gynecological surgery (354). In patients admitted for abdominal surgery ratios reached 0.28 in muscle tissue and 0.22 in fat after intravenous bolus administrations of 5-g doses (355). From the fluid/serum AUC ratio the ticarcillin penetration index for cantharides blister fluid is 73% following intravenous bolus doses of 3 g together with 200 mg of the beta-lactamase inhibitor clavulanic acid (356).

Excretion of carbon-14 in urine accounted for 95% of a 5-g intravenous bolus of labeled ticarcillin, and 3.0% appeared in feces (353). Unchanged ticarcillin accounted for 96% of the urinary radioactivity and the remainder presumably was the corresponding penicilloic acid. Ticarcillin persists longer in the plasma of neonates (half-life, 5 hr) than in the plasma of 1- to 8-week-old infants (half-life, 2 hr). A dosage schedule for ticarcillin in pediatric patients has been proposed to adjust for these changes (357). In patients with chronic renal failure the ticarcillin half-life is increased to 8.8–11 hr but reverts to 4.9 hr with hemodialysis (358).

VIII. ORAL ESTERS OF EXPANDED-SPECTRUM PENICILLINS

A. Carindacillin

The indanyl ester of the side-chain α-carboxyl group of carbenicillin, known as carindacillin (Table 10, Chap. 6) is more lipophilic and less susceptible to degradation under acidic conditions than the parent molecule (358). Like carfecillin, but unlike prodrugs of other penicillins, carindacillin possesses intrinsic antibacterial activity and small amounts of the unhydrolyzed ester appear in serum after oral administration (359). The indanol moiety released by intestinal and hepatic esterases is excreted in urine as glucuronide and sulfate conjugates; the carbenicillin released is principally excreted in urine unchanged.

Peak plasma concentrations of carbenicillin achieved after oral administration of carindacillin were shown to be formulation dependent, reaching 2.5 μg/ml after capsules, 10 μg/ml after solutions, and 12 μg/ml after tablets containing glycine or sodium citrate as excipients. Using moment analysis, Tanigawara et al. found that 69% of a 0.5-g oral dose of carindacillin was absorbed in fasting subjects; after larger doses absorption appeared to be capacity limited (361). Diarrhea was a frequent (10 out of 15 cases) side effect following repeated oral administration of 8 g of carindacillin per day (360).

B. Carfecillin

Carfecillin, like carindacillin, is an ester of the α-carboxyl group of carbenicillin. On hydrolysis carfecillin, the phenyl ester, yields carbenicillin and phenol. In vivo the phenol is conjugated to form glucuronide or sulfate derivatives and excreted in the urine. Compared to carindacillin, carfecillin is slightly more resistant to enzymatic hydrolysis by hepatic esterases and slightly more labile to hydrolysis in homogeneous solution (362,363). Wilkinson and co-workers measured peak mean plasma carbenicillin concentrations of 5.1 μg/ml after oral administration of single 1.0-g doses and 3 μg/ml after single 0.5-g doses (364). Graber et al. found higher peak plasma concentrations, 15 μg/ml after single 1.0-g doses (365). Both groups concluded that carfecillin provided carbenicillin absorption that was adequate for the treatment of urinary tract infections but inadequate for the treatment of septicemia. About 43% of oral doses ranging from 0.5 to 1.5 g of carfecillin was absorbed and transferred into the systemic circulation as carbenicillin and 40% of the dose was excreted in urine (361).

C. Pivmecillinam

The prodrug pivmecillinam is the pivaloyloxymethyl ester of mecillinam. The pivaloyloxymethyl ester of ampicillin, pivampicillin, was discussed earlier. According to early reports, absorption of mecillinam into the systemic circulation improved from a few percent of the dose after orally administered mecillinam to a range of 65-75% of the dose after pivmecillinam (366,367). Others found lower bioavailability of mecillinam, 38-45%, from orally administered pivmecillinam (368). Oral capsules, tablets, and solutions of the soluble hydrochloride salt are bioequivalent, and absorption of mecillinam from capsules of pivmecillinam is slightly delayed but not reduced after a standard breakfast (369,370). Plasma concentrations of mecillinam after oral pivmecillinam doses are slightly reduced by bed rest and significantly elevated by pretreatment with probenecid (371). A new tablet of pivmecillinam, formulated with microcrystalline cellulose for rapid disperson, has been claimed to provide greater systemic bioavailability of mecillinam than the conventional tablet, as well as reduced propensity for gastric irritation (372).

D. Bacmecillinam

Bacmecillinam is a recently introduced active ester of mecillinam. This 1-thioxycarbonyloxyethyl ester is rapidly hydrolyzed to acetaldehyde, ethanol, carbon dioxide, and mecillinam by nonspecific tissue esterases. After oral dosing of 244 mg of bacmecillinam the unhydrolyzed ester reaches concentrations of only 2.5 ng/ml in blood (373). In two crossover studies bacampicillin has appeared to be a more efficient oral prodrug than pivmecillinam, judged by peak plasma mecillinam levels, AUC, or urinary recovery of antibacterial activity (374,375). In these studies the AUC increased linearly with increased oral doses of bacmecillinam. Bacmecillinam administered with bacampicillin as an oral tablet yielded plasma and lymph concentrations of mecillinam and ampicillin that were close to the optimal ratios needed to obtain synergistic activity of the two agents in vitro (376).

REFERENCES

1. L. Allen, K. Kimura, J. MacKichan, and W. A. Ritschel. Manual of symbols, equations and definitions in pharmacokinetics. *J. Clin. Pharmacol. 22*:15-235 (1982).
2. M. Barza and L. Weinstein. Pharmacokinetics of the penicillins in man. *Clin. Pharmacokin., 1*:297-308 (1976).
3. A. S. Prince and H. S. Neu. New penicillins and their use in pediatrics. *Pediatr. Clin. North Am., 30*:3-16 (1983).

4. K. C. Kwan and J. D. Rogers. Pharmacokinetics of β-lactam antibiotics, in *Antibiotics Containing the Beta-Lactam Structure II*, 247–370 (A. L. Demain and N. A. Solomon, eds.), Springer-Verlag, Berlin, 1983.
5. T. Bergan. Penicillins. *Antibiot. Chemother. Pharmacokinet., 25*:1–222 (1978).
6. J. A. Webber and W. J. Wheeler. Antimicrobial and pharmacokinetic properties of newer penicillins and cephalosporins, in *Chemistry and Biology of β-Lactam Antibiotics*, Vol. 1 (R. B. Morin and M. Gorman, eds.), Academic, New York, pp. 372–427, 1982.
7. C. G. McCarthy and M. Finland. Absorption and excretion of four penicillins. *N. Engl. J. Med., 263*:315–326 (1960).
8. F. B. Peck, Jr., and R. S. Griffith. Comparative clinical laboratory studies of penicillin V and penicillin G. *Antibiot. Annu.*, 506–509 (1956).
9. N. N. Huang and R. H. High. Comparison of serum levels following the administration of oral and parenteral preparations of penicillin to infants and children of various age groups. *J. Pediatr., 42*:657–668 (1953).
10. W. P. Boger, J. E. Oritt, H. L. Israel, and H. F. Flippin. Procaine penicillin G in oil. *Am. J. Med. Sci., 215*:250–256 (1948).
11. N. P. Sullivan, A. T. Symmes, H. C. Miller, and H. W. Rhodehamel, Jr. A new penicillin for prolonged blood levels. *Science, 107*:169–170 (1948).
12. W. Elias, A. H. Price, and H. J. Merrion. N,N'-Dibenzylethylenediamine penicillin: A new repository form of penicillin. *Antibiot. Chemother., 1*: 491–498 (1951).
13. C. M. Ginsburg, G. H. McCracken, Jr., and T. C. Zweighaft. Serum penicillin concentrations after intramuscular administration of benzathine penicillin G in children. *Pediatrics, 69*:452–454 (1982).
14. C. M. Kunin. Serum binding, distribution and excretion of four penicillin analogues following intravenous injection in man. *Proc. Soc. Exp. Biol. Med., 107*:337–341 (1961).
15. C. Simon, J. Vock, and V. Malerczyk. Zur Blutspiegelkinetik bei hochdosierter parenteraler Penicillin-G Therapie. *Dtsch. Med. Wochenschr., 96*: 1393–1399 (1971).
16. A. Schreiner, K. B. Hellum, A. Diganes, and I. Bergman. Transfer of penicillin G and ampicillin into human skin blisters induced by suction. *Scand. J. Infect. Dis. Suppl., 14*:233–237 (1978).
17. J. Ducas and H. G. Robson. Cerebrospinal fluid penicillin levels during therapy for latent syphilis. *J. Am. Med. Assoc., 246*:2583–2584 (1981).
18. E. M. C. Dunlop, S. S. Al-Egaily, and E. T. Houang. Penicillin levels in blood and CSF achieved by treatment of syphilis. *J. Am. Med. Assoc., 241*: 2538–2540 (1979).
19. R. A. Fishman. Active transport and the blood–brain barrier to penicillin and related organic acids. *Trans. Am. Neurol. Assoc., 89*:51–55 (1964).
20. D. Goldmeier and P. M. Waterworth. Penetration of penicillin into the cerebrospinal fluid of patients with latent syphilis. *Pharmatherapeutica, 3*:14–17 (1981).

21. M. Gibaldi, D. Davidson, M. E. Plaut, and M. A. Schwartz. Modification of penicillin distribution and elimination by probenecid. *Int. Z. Klin. Pharmakol. Ther. Toxicol., 3*:182–189 (1970).
22. J. Kampmann, J. M. Hansen, K. Siersboeck-Nielsen, and H. Laursen. Effect of some drugs on penicillin half-life in blood. *Clin. Pharmacol. Ther., 13*: 516–519 (1972).
23. A. Lithander, B. O. A. Werner, and L. O. Forsgren. Passage of benzylpenicillin and ampicillin into the thoracic duct lymph after intravenous injection in man. *Antimicrob. Agents Chemother.*, 366–372 (1968).
24. M. E. Speer, E. O. Mason, and J. T. Scharnberg. Cerebrospinal fluid concentrations of aqueous procaine penicillin G in the neonate. *Pediatrics, 67*: 387–388 (1981).
25. M. Cole, M. D. Kenig, and V. Hewitt. Metabolism of penicillins to penicilloic acids and 6-aminopenicillanic acid in man and its significance in assessing penicillin absorption. *Antimicrob. Agents Chemother., 3*:463–468 (1973).
26. H. Eagle and E. Newman. The renal clearance of penicillins F, G, K, and X in rabbits and man. *J. Clin. Invest., 26*:903–918 (1947).
27. J. M. Brogard, M. Pinget, M. Doffoel, M. Adloff, and J. Lavillaureix. Evaluation of the biliary excretion of penicillin G. *Chemotherapy, 25*:129–139 (1979).
28. J. L. Lefrock and B. R. Smith. Antimicrobials in renal impairment. *Am. Fam. Physician, 25*:201–205 (1982).
29. E. Leikola and K. O. Vartia. On penicillin levels in young and geriatric subjects. *J. Gerontol., 12*:48–52 (1957).
30. H. L. Barnett, H. McNamara, S. Schultz, and R. Tompsett. Renal clearances of sodium penicillin G, procaine penicillin G, and inulin in infants and children. *Pediatrics, 3*:418–421 (1949).
31. N. Buchanan, R. Robinson, H. S. Koornhof, and C. Eyberg. Penicillin pharmacokinetics in kwashiorkor. *Am. J. Clin. Nutr., 32*:2233–2236 (1979).
32. W. W. Wright, A. Kirshbaum, B. Arret, L. E. Putnam, and H. Welch. Serum concentrations and urinary excretion following oral administration of penicillin V and comparison with penicillin G. *Antibiot. Med., 1*:490–495 (1955).
33. F. B. Peck, Jr., and R. S. Griffith. Comparative clinical laboratory studies of potassium penicillin V with acid penicillin V. *Antibiotics Annual 1957–1958*, 1004–1011 (1958).
34. A. C. White, R. A. Couch, F. Foster, J. Calloway, W. Hunter, and V. Knight. Absorption and antimicrobial activity of penicillin V (phenoxymethyl penicillin), in *Antibiotics Annual 1955-1956*, 490–501, 1956.
35. N. G. Heatley. Comparative serum concentration and excretion experiments with benzyl penicillin (G) and phenoxymethyl penicillin (V) on a single subject. *Antibiot. Med., 2*:33–41 (1956).
36. T. Bergan, B. P. Berdal, and V. Holm. Relative bioavailability of phenoxymethylpenicillin preparations in a crossover study. *Acta Pharmacol. Toxi-*

col., 38:308–320 (1976).

37. K. Soininen, H. Allonen, and J. Posti. Bioavailability of pediatric mixtures containing phenoxymethylpenicillin calcium or potassium salt. *J. Int. Med. Res., 10*:379–382 (1982).
38. M. Eriksson, P. Bolme, and Y. Finkel. The influence of the sweetening agent on the oral absorption of penicillin V. *Acta Pharmacol. Toxicol., 52*:75–77 (1983).
39. P. Bolme and M. Eriksson. Absorption of phenoxymethylpenicillin in children. *Scand. J. Infect. Dis., 10*:223–227 (1978).
40. Y. Finkel, P. Bolme, and M. Eriksson. The effect of food on the oral absorption of penicillin V preparations in children. *Acta Pharmacol. Toxicol., 49*: 301–304 (1981).
41. G. H. McCracken, C. M. Ginsburg, J. C. Clahsen, and M. L. Thomas. Pharmacological evaluation of orally administered antibiotics in infants and children: Effect of feeding on bioavailability. *Pediatrics, 62*:738–743 (1978).
42. K. Josefsson and T. Bergan. Pharmacokinetics of phenoxymethyl penicillin in volunteers. *Chemotherapy, 28*:241–246 (1982).
43. T. Dimmling, H. G. Bredehorst, and E. V. Elst. Bioavailability of various preparations and doses of penicillin V. *Eur. J. Clin. Pharmacol., 10*:55–58 (1976).
44. S. E. Holm and C. Ekedahl. Comparative study of the penetration of penicillin V and cefadroxil into tonsils in man. *J. Antimicrob. Chemother. Suppl. B, 10*:121–123 (1982).
45. J. S. Tan, S. J. Salstrom, and T. M. File, Jr. Levels of antibiotic in human blood and interstitial fluid after oral administration of bacampicillin or phenoxymethylpenicillin and intravenous administration of amoxicillin or ampicillin. *Rev. Infect. Dis., 3*:121–124 (1981).
46. I. M. Rollo. Physiological disposition of some semisynthetic penicillins. *Can. J. Physiol. Pharmacol., 50*:986–998 (1972).
47. K. Hellstrom, A. Rosen, and A. Swahn. Absorption and decomposition of potassium ^{35}S-phenoxymethyl penicillin. *Clin. Pharmacol. Ther., 16*:826–833 (1974).
48. H. Vanderhaeghe, G. Parmentier, and E. Evrard. Identification of p-hydroxyphenoxymethyl penicillin as a metabolite of phenoxymethyl penicillin. *Nature, 200*:891 (1963).
49. A. Tsuji, O. Kubo, E. Miyamoto, and T. Yamana. Physiochemical properties of β-lactam antibiotics: Oil–water distribution. *J. Pharm. Sci., 66*: 1675–1679 (1977).
50. L. D. Sabath, B. Postic, and M. Finland. Laboratory studies on methicillin. *Am. J. Med. Sci., 244*:484–500 (1962).
51. C. E. Roberts, J. D. Allen, and W. M. M. Kirby. Laboratory and clinical studies of penicillin X-1497. *Clin. Pharmacol. Ther., 2*:70–79 (1961).
52. E. T. Knudsen and G. N. Rolinson. Absorption and excretion of a new antibiotic (BRL 1241). *Br. Med. J., 2*:700–703 (1960).

53. G. N. Rolinson and F. R. Batchelor. Penicillin metabolites. *Antimicrob. Agents Chemother.*, 654–660 (1962).
54. W. F. Verwey, H. R. Williams, Jr., and C. Kalsow. Penetration of chemotherapeutic agents into tissues. *Antimicrob. Agents Chemother.*, 1016–1024 (1965).
55. C. M. Kunin. Clinical pharmacology of the new penicillins. *Clin. Pharmacol. Ther.*, *7*:166–179 (1966).
56. F. H. Stevenson and K. J. Harrison. "Celbenin" and probenecid. *Br. Med. J.*, *2*:1596 (1960).
57. A. H. Douthwaite, J. A. P. Trafford, D. A. F. McGill, and I. E. Evans. Methicillin. *Br. Med. J.*, *2*:6–8 (1961).
58. W. R. Henderson, J. Carleton, and M. Hamburger. The effect of probenecid upon serum levels of methicillin. *Am. J. Med. Sci.*, *243*:489–495 (1962).
59. G. C. Henegar, M. Silverman, R. J. Gardner, J. C. Kukral, and F. W. Preston. Excretion of methicillin in human bile. *Antimicrob. Agents Chemother.*, 348–351 (1961).
60. A. C. Whitehouse, J. G. Morgan, J. Schumacher, and M. Hamburger. Blood levels and antistaphylococcal titers produced in human subjects by a penicillinase-resistant penicillin, nafcillin, compared with similar penicillins. *Antimicrob. Agents Chemother.*, 385–392 (1962).
61. J. O. Klein and M. Finland. Nafcillin: Antibacterial action *in vitro* and absorption and excretion in normal young men. *Am. J. Med. Sci.*, *246*:10–26 (1963).
62. C. Watanakunakorn. Absorption of orally administered nafcillin in normal healthy volunteers. *Antimicrob. Agents Chemother.*, *11*:1007–1009 (1977).
63. W. J. O'Conner, G. H. Warren, P. S. Mandala, L. S. Edrada, and S. B. Rosenman. Serum concentrations of nafcillin in newborn infants and children. *Antimicrob. Agents Chemother.*, 188–191 (1964).
64. W. J. O'Conner, G. H. Warren, L. S. Edrada, P. S. Mandala, and S. B. Rosenman. Serum concentrations of sodium nafcillin in infants during the perinatal period. *Antimicrob. Agents Chemother.*, 220–222 (1965).
65. M. Grossman and W. Ticknor. Serum levels of ampicillin, cephalothin, cloxacillin, and nafcillin in the newborn infant. *Antimicrob. Agents Chemother.*, 214–219 (1965).
66. W. Banner, Jr., W. M. Gooch III, G. Burckart, and S. B. Korones. Pharmacokinetics of nafcillin in infants with low birth weights. *Antimicrob. Agents Chemother.*, *17*:691–694 (1980).
67. W. E. Feldman, J. D. Nelson, and L. R. Stanberry. Clinical and pharmacokinetic evaluation of nafcillin in infants and children. *J. Pediatr.*, *93*:1029–1033 (1978).
68. B. E. Fossieck, J. G. Kane, C. R. Diaz, and R. H. Parker. Nafcillin entry into cerebrospinal fluid. *Antimicrob. Agents Chemother.*, *11*:965–967 (1977).
69. H. L. Nunes, C. C. Pecora, K. Judy, S. B. Rosenman, G. H. Warren, and C. M. Martin. Turnovers and distribution of nafcillin in tissues and body fluids of surgical patients. *Antimicrob. Agents Chemother.*, 237–249 (1964).
70. S. S. Walkenstein, R. Wiser, E. LeBoutillier, C. Gudmundsen, and H. Kim-

mel. Absorption, metabolism, and excretion of the semisynthetic penicillin 6-(2-ethoxy-1-naphthamido)penicillanic acid (nafcillin). *J. Pharm. Sci., 52*: 763–767 (1963).

71. M. Barza, J. Brusch, M. G. Bergeron, O. Kemmetsu, and L. Weinstein. Extraction of antibiotics from the circulation by liver and kidney: Effect of probenecid. *J. Infect. Dis., 131*:S86–S97 (1975).
72. C. R. Diaz, J. G. Kane, R. H. Parker, and F. R. Pelsor. Pharmacokinetics of nafcillin in patients with renal failure. *Antimicrob. Agents Chemother., 12*:98–101 (1977).
73. M. Rudnick, G. Morrison, B. Walker, and I. Singer. Renal failure, hemodialysis and nafcillin kinetics. *Chin. Pharmacol. Ther., 20*:413–423 (1976).
74. J. P. Marshall, W. B. Salt, R. O. Elam, G. R. Wilkinson, and S. Schenker. Disposition of nafcillin in patients with cirrhosis and extrahepatic biliary obstruction. *Gastroenterology, 73*:1383–1392 (1977).
75. A. C. Kind, T. E. Tupasi, H. C. Standiford, and W. M. M. Kirby. Mechanisms responsible for plasma levels of nafcillin lower than those of oxacillin. *Arch. Intern. Med., 125*:685–690 (1970).
76. M. Gibaldi and M. A. Schwartz. Apparent effect of probenecid on the distribution of penicillins in man. *Clin. Pharmacol. Ther., 9*:345–349 (1968).
77. E. S. Waller, M. A. Sharanevych, and G. J. Yakatan. The effect of probenecid on nafcillin disposition. *J. Clin. Pharmacol., 22*:482–489 (1982).
78. R. Sutherland, E. A. P. Croydon, and G. N. Rolinson. Flucloxacillin, a new isoxazolyl penicillin, compared with oxacillin, cloxacillin, and dicloxacillin. *Br. Med. J., 4*:455–460 (1970).
79. C. M. Kunin. Therapeutic implications of serum protein binding of the new semisynthetic penicillins. *Antimicrob. Agents Chemother.*, 1025–1034 (1965).
80. J. E. Rosenblatt, A. C. Kind, J. L. Brodie, and W. M. M. Kirby. Mechanisms responsible for the blood level differences of isoxazolyl penicillins. *Arch. Intern. Med., 121*:345–348 (1968).
81. R. Wise, A. P. Gillett, B. Cadge, S. R. Durham, and S. Baker. The influence of protein binding upon tissue fluid levels of six β-lactam antibiotics. *J. Infect. Dis., 142*:77–82 (1980).
82. E. H. Nauta and H. Mattie. Pharmacokinetics of flucloxacillin and cloxacillin in healthy subjects and patients on chronic intermittent haemodialysis. *Br. J. Clin. Pharmacol., 2*:111–121 (1975).
83. E. H. Nauta and H. Mattie. Dicloxacillin and cloxacillin: Pharmacokinetics in healthy and hemodialysis subjects. *Clin. Pharmacol. Ther., 20*:98–108 (1976).
84. H. Graber, T. Perenyi, M. Arr, and E. Ludwig. On human biotransformation of some penicillins. *Int. J. Clin. Pharmacol., 14*:284–289 (1976).
85. H. H. W. Thijssen and H. Mattie. Active metabolites of isoxazolylpenicillins in humans. *Antimicrob. Agents Chemother., 10*:441–446 (1976).
86. H. H. W. Thijssen. Identification of the active metabolites of the isoxazolylpenicillins by means of mass spectrometry. *J. Antibiot., 32*:1033–1037 (1979).

87. Y. Murai, T. Nakagawa, and T. Uno. GC–MS identification of active metabolite of oxacillin in man. *Chem. Pharm. Bull., 28*:362–364 (1980).
88. Y. Murai, T. Nakagawa, K. Yamaoka, and T. Uno. Comparative pharmacokinetics of metabolism and urinary excretion of isoxazolylpenicillins in man. *Chem. Pharm. Bull., 31*:3292–3301 (1983).
89. Y. Murai, T. Nakagawa, K. Yamaoka, and T. Uno. High performance liquid chromatographic analysis and pharmacokinetic investigation of oxacillin and its metabolites in man. *Chem. Pharm. Bull., 29*:3290–3297 (1981).
90. J. Bordt, H. Wagner, and D. Adam. Mezlocillin and oxacillin concentrations in serum, mammary gland, and fat, in *Current Chemotherapy and Immunotherapy 1*:651–652, (P. Periti and G. G. Grassi, eds.), American Society for Microbiology, Washington, D.C., 1982.
91. R. H. Fitzgerald, Jr., P. J. Kelly, R. J. Snyder, and J. A. Washington II. Penetration of methicillin, oxacillin and cephalothin into bone and synovial tissues. *Antimicrob. Agents Chemother., 14*:723–726 (1978).
92. B. Steckmeier, D. Adam, A. Schaudig, and M. Zimmermann. Concentrations of mezlocillin and oxacillin in vessel walls and other tissues during vascular surgery. *Drugs Exp. Clin. Res., 9*:133–137 (1983).
93. D. H. Wittmann, J. Fedder, and H. H. Schassan. Influence of protein binding on tissue fluid concentrations of isoxaloyl- and acylureidopenicillins, in *Current Chemotherapy and Immunotherapy 1*:652–654, (P. Periti and G. G. Grassi, eds.), American Society for Microbiology, Washington, D.C., (1982).
94. V. D. Adam, W. Bauer, B. Seitz, and I. Voigt. Pharmacokinetische untersuchungen mit Breitspektrum-Penicillin/oxacillin-Kombinationen bei freiwilligen Probanden. *Arzneim. Forsch., 29*:1769–1804 (1979).
95. K. Hellstrom, A. Rosen, and A. Swahn. Fate of oral ^{35}S-cloxacillin in man. *Eur. J. Clin. Pharmacol., 7*:125–131 (1974).
96. A. Howell, R. Sutherland, and G. N. Rolinson. Effect of protein binding on levels of ampicillin and cloxacillin in synovial fluid. *Clin. Pharmacol. Ther., 13*:724–732 (1972).
97. J. Sirot, R. Lopitaux, C. Dumont, J. J. Delisle, S. Rampon, and R. Cluzel. Diffusion de la cloxacilline dans le tissu osseux humain aprés administration par voie orale. *Pathol. Biol. Sem. Hop., 30*:332–335 (1982).
98. E. H. Nauta, H. Mattie, and W. R. O. Goslings. Effect of probenecid on the apparent volume of distribution and elimination of cloxacillin. *Antimicrob. Agents Chemother., 6*:300–303 (1974).
99. D. R. Van Harken, C. W. Dixon, and J. M. Essery. An active metabolite of dicloxacillin. *Pharmacologist, 12*:220 (1970).
100. T. W. Williams, Jr., S. A. Lawson, M. I. Brook, E. M. Ory, and R. O. Morgan. Effect of hemodialysis on dicloxacillin concentration in plasma. *Antimicrob. Agents Chemother.,* 767–769 (1967).
101. R. V. McCloskey and C. P. Hayes, Jr. Plasma levels of dicloxacillin in oliguric patients and the effect of hemodialysis. *Antimicrob. Agents Chemother.,* 770–772 (1967).
102. K. A. Desante, L. W. Dittert, S. Stavchansky, and J. T. Doluisio. Influence

102. K. A. Desante, L. W. Dittert, S. Stavchansky, and J. T. Doluisio. Influence of sulfaethidole on the human pharmacokinetics of dicloxacillin. *J. Clin. Pharmacol., 20*:534-542 (1980).
103. L. W. Dittert, W. O. Griffen, Jr., J. C. LaPiana, E. J. Shainfield, and J. T. Doluisio. Pharmacokinetic interpretation of penicillin levels in serum and urine after intravenous administration. *Antimicrob. Agents Chemother.,* 42–48 (1969).
104. J. T. Doluisio, J. C. LaPiana, G. R. Wilkinson, and L. W. Dittert. Pharmacokinetic interpretation of dicloxacillin levels in serum after extravascular administration. *Antimicrob. Agents Chemother.,* 49–55 (1969).
105. H. H. W. Thijssen and J. Wolters. The metabolic disposition of flucloxacillin in patients with impaired kidney function. *Eur. J. Clin. Pharmacol., 22*:429–434 (1982).
106. H. H. W. Thijssen. Analysis of isoxazloyl penicillins and their metabolites in body fluids by high-performance liquid chromatography. *J. Chromatogr., 183*:339–345 (1980).
107. M. A. Sattar, S. P. Barrett, and M. I. D. Cawley. Concentrations of some antibiotics in synovial-fluid after oral administration, with special reference to anti-staphylococcal activity. *Ann. Rheum. Dis., 42*:67–74 (1983).
108. P. F. Unsworth, F. W. Heatley, and I. Phillips. Flucloxacillin in bone. *J. Clin. Pathol., 31*:705–711 (1978).
109. S. Holm and S. E. Larsson. The penetration of flucloxacillin into cortical and cancellous bone during arthroplasty of the knee. *Int. Orthop., 6*:243–247 (1982).
110. J. P. Pollard, S. P. F. Hughes, M. J. Evans, J. E. Scott, and M. K. D. Benson. Concentration of flucloxacillin in femoral head and joint capsule in total hip replacement. *J. Antimicrob. Chemother., 5*:721–726 (1979).
111. I. J. Kiss, E. Farago, A. Gomory, and J. Szamaranszky. Investigations on the flucloxacillin levels in human serum, lung tissue, pericardial fluid, and heart tissue. *Int. J. Clin. Pharmacol. Ther. Toxicol., 18*:405–411 (1980).
112. G. P. Bodey, C. Vellejos, and D. Stewart. Flucloxacillin: A new semisynthetic isoxazolyl penicillin. *Clin. Pharmacol. Ther., 13*:512–515 (1972).
113. S. A. Hedstrom and G. Kahlmeter. Dicloxacillin and flucloxacillin twice daily with probenecid in staphylococcal infections. *Scand. J. Infect. Dis., 12*:221–225 (1980).
114. D. Adam, A. Neiss, and U. Kisslinger. Pharmacokinetics of flucloxacillin in the presence of piperacillin, in *Current Chemotherapy and Immunotherapy 1*:706–708, (P. Periti and G. G. Grassi, eds.), American Society for Microbiology, Washington, D.C., (1982).
115. D. Adam, P. Koeppe, and H. D. Heilmann. Pharmacokinetics of amoxicillin and flucloxacillin following the simultaneous intravenous administration of 4 g and 1 g, respectively. *Infection, 11*:150–154 (1983).
116. H. C. Neu. New broad-spectrum penicillins. *Drugs, 9*:81–87 (1975).
117. C. F. Carney and A. R. Hurwitz. pH partition behaviour of ampicillin. *J. Pharm. Sci., 66*:294–295 (1977).
118. H. Lode, P. Janisch, G. Kupper, and H. Weuta. Comparative clinical

pharmacology of three ampicillins and amoxicillin administered orally. *J. Infect. Dis, Suppl. 129*:S156–S168 (1974).

119. I. A. Mikhail, D. C. Kent, K. Sorensen, W. R. Sanborn, and J. Smith. Concentrations of ampicillin and chloramphenicol in the serum of patients with acute salmonella enteric fever. *Antimicrob. Agents Chemother., 2*: 336–339 (1972).

120. S. C. Penzotti, Jr., and J. W. Poole. Transport mechanisms of β-lactam antibiotics across everted rat gut. *J. Pharm. Sci., 63*:1803–1806 (1974).

121. C. Dixon and L. W. Mizen. Absorption of amino penicillins from everted rat intestine. *J. Physiol., 269*:549–559 (1977).

122. A. Tsuji, E. Nakashima, I. Kagami, N. Honjo, and T. Yamana. Effect of dose-concentration on the absorption of amoxicillin and ampicillin from the rat intestine. *J. Pharm. Pharmacol., 29*:707–708 (1977).

123. A. Tsuji, E. Nakashima, I. Kagami, T. Asano, R. Nakashima, and T. Yamana. Kinetics of Michaelis–Menten absorption of amino-penicillins in rats. *J. Pharm. Pharmacol., 30*:508–509 (1978).

124. A. Tsuji, E. Nakashima, I. Kagami, and T. Yamana. Intestinal absorption mechanisms of amphoteric β-lactam antibiotics. I: Comparative absorption and evidence for saturable transport of amino-β-lactam antibiotics by *in situ* rat small intestine. *J. Pharm. Sci., 70*:768–772 (1981).

125. K. Miyazaki, K. Ohtani, K. Umeniwa, and T. Arita. Intestinal absorption of several β-lactam antibiotics. III. Competitive inhibition behaviour among zwitterionic β-lactam antibiotics in the rat intestinal absorption. *J. Pharm. Dynam., 5*:555–563 (1982).

126. E. Nakashima, H. Mizuo, A. Tsuji, and T. Yamana. Carrier-mediated transport mechanism in the rat intestinal absorption of amino-β lactam antibiotics. *J. Pharm. Dynam., 6*:93 (1983).

127. A. Tsuji and T. Yamana. Gastrointestinal absorption of β-lactam antibiotics, in *Beta-Lactam Antibiotics 235*:258, (S. Mitsuhashi, ed.), Japan Scientific, Tokyo, and Springer-Verlag, Berlin, (1981).

128. J. Sjovall, L. Magni, and T. Bergan. Pharmacokinetics of bacampicillin compared with those of ampicillin, pivampicillin and amoxycillin. *Antimicrob. Agents Chemother., 13*:90–96 (1978).

129. P. C. Braga, F. Fraschini, G. Ceccarelli, F. Scaglione, and G. Scarpazza. Clinical pharmacokinetic evaluation of bacampicillin. *Clin. Ther., 4*:32–42 (1981).

130. T. Bergan. Pharmacokinetic comparison of oral bacampicillin and parenteral ampicillin. *Antimicrob. Agents Chemother., 13*:971–974 (1978).

131. M. Ehrnebo, S.-O. Nilsson, and L. O. Boreus. Pharmacokinetics of ampicillin and its prodrugs bacampicillin and pivampicillin in man. *J. Pharmacokinet. Biopharm., 7*:429–451 (1979).

132. H. C. Neu. In vitro activity and human pharmacology of amoxicillin. *J. Infect. Dis., Suppl. 129*:S123–S131 (1974).

133. F. N. Eshelman and D. A. Spyker. Pharmacokinetics of amoxicillin and ampicillin: Crossover study of the effect of food. *Antimicrob. Agents Chemother., 14*:539–543 (1978).

134. E. L. Foltz, J. W. West, I. H. Breslow, and H. Wallick. Clinical pharmacology of pivampicillin. *Antimicrob. Agents Chemother.*, 442–454 (1970).
135. M. C. Jordan, J. B. deMaine, and W. M. M. Kirby. Clinical pharmacology of pivampicillin as compared with ampicillin. *Antimicrob. Agents Chemother.*, 438–441 (1970).
136. J. Miranda, L. M. P. Pereira, and B. J. Vakil. Pharmacokinetics of ampicillin during ambulation and recumbency. *Curr. Ther. Res.*, *32*:936–940 (1982).
137. A. A. Ali. Comparative bioavailability of 8 brands of ampicillin. *Int. J. Pharm.*, *7*:301–306 (1981).
138. H. M. Ali and A. Farouk. Comparative studies on the bioavailability of ampicillin anhydrate and trihydrate. *Int. J. Pharm.*, *9*:239–243 (1981).
139. S. Kaumeier, E. Kisslinger, and A. Neiss. Pharmacokinetics of potassium ampicillin. *Arzneim. Forsch.*, *30*:1019–1021 (1980).
140. G. Hitzenberger and I. Jaschek. Comparative studies on the absorption of ampicillin trihydrate and potassium ampicillin. *Int. J. Clin. Pharmacol.*, *9*:114–119 (1974).
141. J. Sjovall. Dose dependence in human absorption of aminopenicillins. *Infection 7, (Suppl.) 5*:S458–S462 (1979).
142. F. Nordbring. Review of the side effects of aminopenicillins. *Infection 7 (Suppl.) 5*:S503–S506 (1979).
143. E. Bergogne-Berezin, C. Morel, Y. Benard, G. Berthelot, and H. Kafe. Pharmacokinetic study of β-lactam antibiotics in bronchial secretions. *Scand. J. Infect. Dis. Suppl.*, *14*:267–272 (1978).
144. H. J. H. Keshavan, N. K. Gurbani, V. Batra, P. C. Dandiya, and R. G. Sharma. Availability of ampicillin in biological fluids. *Indian J. Med. Res.*, *72*:920–922 (1980).
145. B. Davies and F. Maesen. Serum and sputum antibiotic levels after ampicillin, amoxycillin and bacampicillin in chronic bronchitis patients. *Infection 7, Suppl. 5*:S465–S468 (1979).
146. C. Brihmer and J. Brundin. Levels of ampicillin and doxycycline in human oviduct mucosa and serum. *Acta Obstet. Gynecol. Scand.*, *62*:231–234 (1983).
147. C. Simon, V. Malerczyk, and M. Klaus. Absorption of bacampicillin and ampicillin and penetration into body fluids (skin blister fluid, saliva, tears) in healthy volunteers. *Scand. J. Infect. Dis. Suppl.*, *14*:228–232 (1978).
148. M. Ehrnebo. Distribution of ampicillin in human whole blood. *J. Pharm. Pharmacol.*, *30*:730–731 (1978).
149. W. Giebel, K.-H. Schonleber, H. Breuninger, and U. Ullman. A comparison of the pharmacokinetics in serum and nasal secretions after oral bacampicillin and ampicillin. *Scand. J. Infect. Dis. Suppl.*, *14*:285–287 (1978).
150. P. T. Mannisto, U. Repo, and M. Malkki. Ampicillin concentrations in serum and bronchial mucosa after ampicillin and bacampicillin. *J. Antimicrob. Chemother.*, *5*:236–238 (1979).
151. M. Onsrud, T. Bergan, and H. Gjonnaess. Antibiotic levels in plasma and peritoneal fluid after administration of amoxicillin, ampicillin and bacam-

picillin during pelvic inflammatory disease, in *Current Chemotherapy and Immunotherapy 1*:139–140, (P. Periti and G. G. Grassi, eds.), American Society for Microbiology, Washington, D.C., 1982.

152. I. A. Mikhail, J. E. Sippel, N. I. Girgis, and M. W. Yassin. Cerebrospinal fluid and serum ampicillin levels in bacterial meningitis patients after intravenous and intramuscular administration. *Scand. J. Infect. Dis., 13*:237–238 (1981).
153. G. Pesnel, F. Squinazi, S. Lemerle-Gruson, C. Lassale, P. Geslin, and P. H. Reinhert. Diffusion méningée de l'amoxicilline intraveineuse au cours des méningites aiguës de l'enfant. *Med. Mal. Infect., 13*:300–304 (1983).
154. J. S. Tan, T. Bannister, and J. P. Phair. Levels of amoxicillin and ampicillin in human serum and interstitial fluid. *J. Infect. Dis. Suppl., 129*:S146–S148 (1974).
155. J. S. Tan and S.-J. Salstrom. Bacampicillin, ampicillin, cephalothin and cephapirin levels in human blood and interstitial fluid. *Antimicrob. Agents Chemother., 15*:510–512 (1979).
156. D. A. Taryle, J. T. Good, Jr., E. J. Morgan III, L. B. Reller, and S. H. Sahn. Antibiotic concentrations in human parapneumonic effusions. *J. Antimicrob. Chemother., 7*:171–177 (1981).
157. R. Wise, I. A. Donovan, J. M. Andrews, J. Drumm, and S. Bennett. Penetration of sulbactam and ampicillin into peritoneal fluid. *Antimicrob. Agents Chemother., 24*:290–292 (1983).
158. R. M. Brown, R. Wise, J. M. Andrews, and J. Hancox. Comparative pharmacokinetics and tissue penetration of sulbactam and ampicillin after concurrently intravenous administration. *Antimicrob. Agents Chemother., 21*:565–567 (1982).
159. J. Sjovall. Tissue levels after administration of bacampicillin: A prodrug of ampicillin, and comparisons with other aminopenicillins: A review. *J. Antimicrob. Chemother. Suppl. C, 8*:41–58 (1981).
160. M. Nishida, T. Murakawa, Y. Mine, S. Fukuda, Y. Kono, and Y. Sueda. Studies on the formation and activity of the transformation product of ampicillin. *J. Antibiot., 24*:641–646 (1971).
161. T. Murakawa, Y. Kono, and M. Nishida. Studies on the formation and activity of the transformation product of ampicillin. II. *J. Antibiot., 25*:421–426 (1972).
162. U. Ullmann and W. Wurst, Antibacterial active components in human urine after administration of penicillins. *Infection, 7*:187–189 (1979).
163. A. Swahn. On the absorption and metabolism of ^{35}S-ampicillin. *Eur. J. Clin. Pharmacol., 9*:117–124 (1975).
164. T. Uno, M. Masada, K. Yamaoka, and T. Nakagawa. High performance liquid chromatographic determination and pharmacokinetic investigation of amino-penicillins and their metabolites in man. *Chem. Pharm. Bull., 29*:1957–1968 (1981).
165. M. Cole and B. Ridley. Absence of bioactive metabolites of ampicillin and amoxicillin in man. *J. Antimicrob. Chemother., 4*:580–582 (1978).
166. H. M. Ali, A. Farouk, S. A. H. Khalil, and M. A. El-Nakeeb. Correlation

between microbiological and chemical assay of ampicillin in bioequivalence studies in man. *Int. J. Pharm.*, *9*:233–238 (1981).
167. J. C. K. Loo, E. L. Foltz, H. Wallick, and K. W. Kwan. Pharmacokinetics of pivampicillin and ampicillin in man. *Clin. Pharmacol. Ther.*, *16*:35–43 (1974).
168. A. Philipson. Pharmacokinetics of antibiotics in pregnancy and labour. *Clin. Pharmacokin.*, *4*:297–309 (1979).
169. R. T. Kubacka, H. E. Johnstone, H. S. I. Tan, P. D. Reeme, and S. A. Myre. Intravenous ampicillin pharmacokinetics in the third trimester of pregnancy. *Ther. Drug Mon.*, *5*:55–60 (1983).
170. B. M. Assael, M. L. Como, M. Miraglia, G. Pardi, and F. Sereni. Ampicillin kinetics in pregnancy. *Br. J. Clin. Pharmacol.*, *8*:286–288 (1979).
171. A. Whelton. Antibiotic pharmacokinetics and clinical application in renal insufficiency. *Med. Clin. North Am.*, *66*:267–281 (1982).
172. G. P. Lewis and W. J. Jusko. Pharmacokinetics of ampicillin in cirrhosis. *Clin. Pharmacol. Ther.*, *18*:475–484 (1975).
173. E. J. Triggs, J. M. Johnson, and B. Learoyd. Absorption and disposition of ampicillin in the elderly. *Eur. J. Clin. Pharmacol.*, *18*:195–198 (1980).
174. G. Acocella, R. Mattiussi, F. B. Nicolis, R. Pallanza, and L. T. Tenconi. Biliary excretion of antibiotics in man. *Gut*, *9*:536–545 (1968).
175. V. C. Simon, V. Malerczyk, G. Zierott, K. Lehmann, and U. Thiesen. Blut-, Harn- und Gallaspiegel von Ampicillin bie Intravenoser Dauerinfusion. *Arzneim. Forsch.*, *25*:654–656 (1975).
176. G. P. Bodey and J. Nance. Amoxicillin: In vitro and pharmacological studies. *Antimicrob. Agents Chemother.*, *1*:358–362 (1972).
177. H. C. Neu. Summary of Symposium on Amoxicillin. *J. Infect. Dis. Suppl.*, *129*:S272–S274 (1974).
178. A. Arancibia, J. Guttmann, G. Gonzalez, and C. Gonzalez. Absorption and disposition kinetics of amoxicillin in normal human subjects. *Antimicrob. Agents Chemother.*, *17*:199–202 (1980).
179. D. Zarowny, R. Ogilvie, D. Tamblyn, C. Macleod, and J. Ruedy. Pharmacokinetics of amoxicillin. *Clin. Pharmacol. Ther.*, *16*:1045–1051 (1974).
180. D. A. Spyker, R. J. Rugloski, R. L. Vann, and W. M. O'Brien. Pharmacokinetics of amoxicillin: Dose dependence after intravenous, oral, and intramuscular administration. *Antimicrob. Agents Chemother.*, *11*:132–141 (1977).
181. C. M. Ginsburg, G. H. McCracken, Jr., M. L. Thomas, and J. Clahsen. Comparative pharmacokinetics of amoxicillin and ampicillin in infants and children. *Pediatrics*, *64*:627–631 (1979).
182. K. F. Kerrebijn and M. F. Michel. Amoxycillin (BRL2333) in children. *Chemother. Suppl.*, *18*:92–96 (1973).
183. G. N. Rolinson. Laboratory evaluation of amoxicillin. *J. Infect. Dis. Suppl.*, *129*:139–145 (1974).
184. A. Arancibia, M. T. Droguett, G. Fuentes, G. Gonzalez, C. Gonzalez, S. Thambo, and G. Palombo. Pharmacokinetics of amoxicillin in subjects with normal and impaired renal function. *Int. J. Clin. Pharmacol. Ther. Toxicol.*, *20*:447–453 (1982).

185. A. Dalhoff and P. Koeppe. Comparative pharmacokinetic analysis of amoxycillin using open two- and three-compartment models. *Eur. J. Clin. Pharmacol.*, *22*:273–279 (1982).
186. D. H. Staniforth, R. J. Lillystone, and D. Jackson. Effect of food on the bioavailability and tolerance of clavulanic acid/amoxicillin combination. *J. Antimicrob. Chemother.*, *10*:131–139 (1982).
187. M. S. Roberts and M. J. Denton. Effect of posture and sleep on pharmacokinetics. I. Amoxycillin. *Eur. J. Clin. Pharmacol.*, *18*:175–183 (1980).
188. I. D. Farrell, A. P. Ball, G. Brookes, P. G. Davey, T. J. Muscroft, and I. Gonda. The absorption of amoxycillin after gastric surgery. *J. Antimicrob. Chemother.*, *7*:110–111 (1981).
189. A. P. Ball, A. M. Geddes, P. G. Davey, I. D. Farrell, and G. R. Brookes. Clavulanic acid and amoxycillin: A clinical, bacteriological and pharmacological study. *Lancet*, *1*:620–628 (1980).
190. J. D. Nelson, H. Kusmiesz, and S. Shelton. Pharmacokinetics of potassium clavulanate in combination with amoxicillin in pediatric patients. *Antimicrob. Agents Chemother.*, *21*:681–682 (1982).
191. D. Adam, I. D. Visser, and P. Koeppe. Pharmacokinetics of amoxicillin and clavulanic acid administered alone and in combination. *Antimicrob. Agents Chemother.*, *22*:353–357 (1982).
192. U. B. Schaad, P. A. Casey, and D. L. Cooper. Single-dose pharmacokinetics of intravenous clavulanic acid with amoxicillin in pediatric patients. *Antimicrob. Agents Chemother.*, *23*:252–255 (1983).
193. R. N. Brogdon, A. Carmine, R. C. Heel, P. A. Morley, T. M. Speight, and G. S. Avery. Amoxycillin/clavulanic acid: A review of its antibacterial activity, pharmacokinetics and therapeutic use. *Drugs*, *22*:337–362 (1981).
194. V. C. Simon and W. Toeller. Amoxycillin, ein neues Aminobenzylpenicillin. *Arzneim. Forsch.*, *24*:181–184 (1974).
195. K. Sato, M. Fukui, Y. Araki, M. Takahashi, S. Tamura, and H. Takahira. Microbiological and pharmacokinetic studies on a new synthetic penicillin, amoxycillin. *Chemotherapy*, *21*:1383–1387 (1973).
196. R. Sutherland and G. N. Rolinson. α-Amino-p-hydroxybenzylpenicillin (BRL2333), a new semisynthetic penicillin: In vitro evaluation. *Antimicrob. Agents Chemother.*, 411–415 (1971).
197. N. Clumeck, J. P. Thys, R. Vanhoot, M. D. Vanderlinden, J. P. Butzler, and E. Yourassowsky. Amoxicillin entry into human cerebrospinal fluid: Comparison with ampicillin. *Antimicrob. Agents Chemother.*, *14*:531–532 (1978).
198. L. S. Strausbaugh, N. I. Girgis, I. A. Mikhail, D. C. Edman, W. F. Miner, and M. W. Yassin. Penetration of amoxicillin into cerebrospinal fluid. *Antimicrob. Agents Chemother.*, *14*:899–902 (1978).
199. Y. Akimoto, T. Shibata, K. Kaneko, A. Fujii, and T. Tamura. Amoxicillin concentrations in human serum and gingiva following a single oral administration. *IRCS Med. Sci. Biochem.*, *11*:359–360 (1983).
200. P. J. Krause, N. J. Owens, C. H. Nightingale, J. J. Klimek, W. B. Lehmann, and R. Quintiliani. Penetration of amoxicillin, cefaclor, erythromycin-sulfisoxazole and trimethoprim-sulfamethoxazole into the middle ear

fluid of patients with chronic serous otitis media. *J. Infect. Dis., 145*:815–821 (1982).
201. E. Toma and L. Paun. Amoxycillin for parenteral use: A pharmacological and clinical evaluation. *J. Int. Med. Res., 7*:535–538 (1979).
202. R. W. Light and F. A. Wyle. Serum and sputum levels of amoxicillin and cephalexin. *Curr. Ther. Res., 33*:436–443 (1983).
203. S. M. Stewart, I. M. E. Anderson, G. R. Jones, and M. A. Calder. Amoxycillin levels in sputum, serum and saliva. *Thorax, 29*:110–112 (1974).
204. J. R. May and A. Ingold. Amoxicillin in the treatment of infections of the lower respiratory tract. *J. Infect. Dis. Suppl., 129*:S189–S193 (1974).
205. F. Denis, M. Cadoz, M. Mounier, M. Prince-David, S. M'Boup, O. Diouf, and I. Diopmar. Concentrations rachidiennes de l'amoxicilline au cours des méningites purulentes de l'enfant. *Pathol. Biol. Sem. Hop., 31*:308–310 (1983).
206. R. N. Brogden, T. M. Speight, and G. S. Avery. Amoxycillin: A review of its antibacterial and pharmacokinetic properties and therapeutic use. *Drugs, 9*:88–140 (1975).
207. R. N. Brogden, R. C. Heel, T. M. Speight, and G. S. Avery. Amoxycillin injectable: A review of its antibacterial spectrum, pharmacokinetic properties and therapeutic use. *Drugs, 18*:169–184 (1979).
208. H. C. Neu and E. B. Winshell. Pharmacological studies of 6[D(–)] α-amino-p-hydroxyphenylacetamido] penicillanic acid in humans. *Antimicrob. Agents Chemother.*, 423–426 (1971).
209. E. A. P. Croydon and R. Sutherland. α-Amino-p-hydroxybenzyl penicillin (BRL 2333), a new semisynthetic penicillin: Absorption and excretion in man. *Antimicrob. Agents Chemother.*, 427–430 (1971).
210. R. C. Gordon, C. Regamey, and W. M. M. Kirby. Comparative clinical pharmacology of amoxicillin and ampicillin administered orally. *Antimicrob. Agents Chemother., 1*:504–507 (1972).
211. S. A. Hill, K. H. Jones, and L. J. Lees. Pharmacokinetics of parenterally administered amoxycillin. *J. Infect., 2*:320–332 (1980).
212. R. Barbhaiya, R. N. Thin, P. Turner, and J. Wadsworth. Clinical pharmacological studies of amoxycillin: Effect of probenecid. *Br. J. Vener. Dis., 55*:211–213 (1979).
213. J. C. Craft, W. E. Feldman, and J. D. Nelson. Clinicopharmacological evaluation of amoxicillin and probenecid against bacterial meningitis. *Antimicrob. Agents Chemother., 16*:346–352 (1979).
214. J. Sabto, P. Carson, and T. Morgan. Evaluation of amoxycillin – A new semisynthetic penicillin. *Med. J. Aust., 11*:537–540 (1973).
215. E. L. Francke, G. B. Appel, and H. C. Neu. Kinetics of intravenous amoxicillin in patients on long-term dialysis. *Clin. Pharmacol. Ther., 26*:31–35 (1979).
216. P. Ball, T. Barford, J. Gilbert, T. Johnson, and M. Mitchard. Prolonged serum elimination half-life of amoxicillin in the elderly. *J. Antimicrob. Chemother., 4*:385–386 (1978).
217. R. Schafer, G. Witkowski, G. Hoffken, P. Koeppe, and H. Lode. Bioavaila-

bility of oral antibiotics in geriatric patients, in *Current Chemotherapy and Immunotherapy 1*:137–138, (P. Periti and G. G. Grassi, eds.), American Society for Microbiology, Washington, D. C., 1982.
218. P. Chelvan, J. M. T. Hamilton-Miller, and W. Brumfitt. Pharmacokinetics of parenteral amoxycillin, biliary excretion and effect of renal failure. *J. Antimicrob. Chemother., 5*:232–233 (1979).
219. D. P. Maudgal, J. D. Maxwell, L. J. Lees, and R. N. Wild. Biliary excretion of amoxycillin and ceftriaxone after intravenous administration in man. *Br. J. Clin. Pharmacol., 14*:213–217 (1982).
220. B. Ekstrom. The prodrug principle applied to antibiotics. *Drugs Exp. Clin. Res., 7*:269–276 (1981).
221. K. Miyazaki, O. Ogino, M. Nakano, and T. Arita. Intestinal absorption mechanisms of ampicillin derivatives in rats. *Chem. Pharm. Bull., 25*:246–252 (1977).
222. T. Bergan. Aminopenicillins: Concluding remarks. *Infection 7, Suppl. 5*: S507–S513 (1979).
223. H. Hey, T. J. Medalen, O. M. Molstad, and K. Stokholm. A clinical evaluation of the tolerance to pivampicillin tablets. *Infection, 5*:22–25 (1977).
224. W. V. Daehne, W. O. Godtfredsen, K. Roholt, and L. Tybring. Pivampicillin, a new orally active ampicillin ester. *Antimicrob. Agents Chemother.*, 431–437 (1971).
225. A. Swahn. Gastrointestinal absorption and metabolism of two ^{35}S-labelled ampicillin esters. *Eur. J. Clin. Pharmacol., 9*:299–306 (1976).
226. L. Verbist. Triple crossover study on absorption and excretion of ampicillin, pivampicillin and amoxycillin. *Antimicrob. Agents Chemother., 6*:588–593 (1974).
227. K. Roholt, B. Nielsen, and E. Kristensen. Clinical pharmacology of pivampicillin. *Antimicrob. Agents Chemother., 6*:563–571 (1974).
228. C. A. Fernandez, J. P. Menezes, and J. Ximenes. The effect of food on the absorption of pivampicillin and a comparison with the absorption of ampicillin potassium. *J. Int. Med. Res., 1*:530–533 (1973).
229. W. Brumfitt, I. Franklin, L. Hayek, and R. Pursell. Treatment of urinary tract infection with pivampicillin. *Scand. J. Infect. Dis., 5*:59–65 (1973).
230. H. Hey, P. Matzen, J. T. Andersen, E. Didriksen, and B. Nielsen. A gastroscopic and pharmacological study of the disintegration time and absorption of pivampicillin capsules and tablets. *Br. J. Clin. Pharmacol., 8*:237–242 (1979).
231. V. H. Knothe, B. Lauer, and V. Fabricius. Ampicillin, pivampicillin and amoxicillin. *Arzneim. Forsch., 24*:951–955 (1974).
232. M. W. Kunst and H. Mattie. Absorption of pivampicillin in postoperative patients. *Antimicrob. Agents Chemother., 8*:11–14 (1975).
233. W. Marget, F. Dascher, and K. Unertl. Investigations in pivampicillin treatment in newborns and infants. *Infection, 1*:41–46 (1973).
234. G. Lonnerholm, S. Bengtsson, and U. Ewald. Oral pivampicillin and amoxycillin in newborn infants. *Scand. J. Infect. Dis., 14*:127–130 (1982).
235. M. Eriksson and P. Bolme. The oral absorption of ampicillin, pivampi-

cillin and amoxycillin in infants and children. *Acta Pharmacol. Toxicol.*, *49*:38–42 (1981).
236. L. Magni, B. Sjoberg, J. Sjovall, and J. Wessman. Clinical pharmacological studies with bacampicillin, in *Chemotherapy* (J. D. Williams and A. M. Geddes, eds.), Plenum, New York, 1976, pp. 109–114.
237. M. Rozencweig, M. Staquet, and J. Klastersky. Antibacterial activity and pharmacokinetics of bacampicillin and ampicillin. *Clin. Pharmacol. Ther.*, *19*:593–597 (1976).
238. K. Nakagawa, K. Watanabe, Y. Kawaguchi, T. Suzuki, and M. Koyama. Laboratory and clinical studies on bacampicillin. *Chemotherapy, 27S-4*: 105–108 (1979).
239. L. Okolicsahyi, M. Venuti, R. Orlando, G. Benoni, M. T. Dorigo, T. Berti, M. Serembe, A. Porro, and G. Vettori. Pharmacokinetics of bacampicillin and amoxicillin in humans: A comparative multicentre study. *Drugs Exp. Clin. Res.*, *7*:725–730 (1981).
240. H. M. Ali. Bioequivalence studies on two brands of bacampicillin. *Int. J. Pharm.*, *9*:91–95 (1981).
241. H. M. Ali. The effect of Sudanese food and chloroquine on the bioavailability of ampicillin from bacampicillin tablets. *Int. J. Pharm.*, *9*:185–190 (1981).
242. A. Koldestam, S. Olsson, and L. Berglund. A double-blind comparison of the clinical tolerance of bacampicillin and pivampicillin. *Infection 7, Suppl. 5*:S495–S498 (1979).
243. N. Hjorst, K. Renmarker, B. Rosberg, P.-A. Skog, and H. Hey. Tolerance of two ampicillin esters: A comparison of pivampicillin and bacampicillin. *Pharmatherapeutica, 3*:398–404 (1983).
244. C. M. Ginsburg, G. H. McCracken, Jr., J. Clahsen, and T. Zweighaft. Comparative pharmacokinetics of bacampicillin and ampicillin suspensions in infants and children. *Rev. Infect. Dis.*, *3*:117–120 (1981).
245. G. M. McCracken, Jr. A comparison of the pharmacokinetics of bacampicillin, ampicillin, amoxicillin and cyclacillin. Oral administration in infants and children. *Bull. N.Y. Acad. Med.*, *59*:468–476 (1983).
246. A. Schreiner, T. Bergan, K. B. Hellum, and A. Digranes. Pharmacokinetics of ampicillin in serum and in dermal suction blisters after oral administration of bacampicillin. *Rev. Infect. Dis.*, *3*:125–131 (1981).
247. W. Bronsveld, J. Stam, and D. M. MacLaren. Concentration of ampicillin in pleural fluid and serum after single and repetitive doses of bacampicillin. *Scand. J. Infect. Dis., Suppl. 14*:274–278 (1978).
248. F. D. Daschner, E. Gier, H. Lentzen, D. Kaiser, and P. Bamberg. Penetration into the pleural fluid after bacampicillin and amoxycillin. *J. Antimicrob. Chemother.*, *7*:585–588 (1981).
249. D. Hallstrom, O. Keyrilainen, and H. Markkula. Ampicillin concentration in normal and pathological lung tissues after oral administration of bacampicillin. *Infection 7, Suppl. 5*:S469–S471 (1979).
250. S. Virtanen and E. A. Lahikainen. Ampicillin concentrations in middle ear effusions in acute otitis media after administration of bacampicillin. *Infection 7, Suppl. 5*:S472–S474 (1979).

251. H.-K. C. Kim, C. D. Bluestone, M. M. Blatter, K. S. Reisinger, F. P. Wucher, D. D. Rohn, P. H. Fall, K. Digaudio, and L. Rebholz. Comparison of bacampicillin and amoxicillin in acute otitis media with effusion. *Bull. N.Y. Acad. Med., 59*:515-523 (1983).
252. E. Bergogne-Berezin, G. Berthelot, H. Kafe, and C. Morel. Penetration of ampicillin into human bronchial secretions. *Infection 7, Suppl. 5*:S463-S464 (1979).
253. M. Sorri, K. Jokinen, and E. Peltomaki. A pharmacokinetic study of bacampicillin in patients with chronic maxillary sinusitis. *Infection 7, Suppl. 5*: S475-S477 (1979).
254. M. Sorri, E. Peltomaki, and K. Jokinen. Bacampicillin in acute maxillary sinusitis: Concentration in sinus secretion and clinical effect. *Scand. J. Infect. Dis., 13*:277-280 (1981).
255. W. A. Craig. Pharmacokinetics of bacampicillin tablets in adults. *Bull. N.Y. Acad. Med., 59*:457-467 (1983).
256. H. C. Neu. The pharmacokinetics of bacampicillin. *Rev. Infect. Dis., 3*: 110-116 (1981).
257. J. P. Clayton, M. Cole, S. W. Elson, and H. Ferres. BRL.8988 (talampicillin), a well-absorbed oral form of ampicillin. *Antimicrob. Agents Chemother., 5*:670-671 (1974).
258. Y. Shiobara, A. Tachibana, H. Sasaki, T. Watnabe, and T. Sado. Phthalydyl D-α-aminobenzylpenicillinate hydrochloride (PC-183), a new orally active ampicillin ester. *J. Antibiot., 27*:665-673 (1974).
259. D. J. Jeffery, K. H. Jones, and P. F. Langley. The metabolism of talampicillin in rat, dog and man. *Xenobiotica, 8*:419-427 (1978).
260. P. J. Wilkinson, A. L. Thomas, D. S. Reeves, and J. Symonds. Pharmacological and clinical studies with talampicillin, an ester of ampicillin, in *Chemotherapy* (J. D. Williams and A. M. Geddes, eds.), Plenum, New York, 1976, pp. 31-36.
261. K. H. Jones, P. F. Langley, and L. S. Lees. Bioavailability and metabolism of talampicillin. *Chemotherapy, 24*:217-226 (1978).
262. J. M. T. Hamilton-Miller and W. Brumfitt. The bioavailability of four different commercially available brands of ampicillin compared with that of talampicillin. *J. Antimicrob. Chemother., 5*:699-704 (1979).
263. J. Sjovall, L. Magni, and E. Vinnars. Bioavailability of bacampicillin and talampicillin, two oral prodrugs of ampicillin. *Antimicrob. Agents Chemother., 20*:837-838 (1981).
264. T. Mazzei, M. Ciuffi, E. Mini, and M. Bonazza. Comparative human pharmacokinetics of bacampicillin and talampicillin. *Drugs Exp. Clin. Res., 7*:479-483 (1981).
265. F. Miki, T. Asai, K. Kubo, M. Kawai, K. Takamatsu, and M. Kohno. Fundamental and clinical studies on bacampicillin. *Chemotherapy, 27S-4*: 132-142 (1979).
266. T. G. Vitti, M. J. Gurwith, and A. R. Ronald. Pharmacologic studies of amoxicillin in nonfasting adults. *J. Infect. Dis. Suppl., 129*:S149-S153 (1974).

267. K. Mashimo, O. Kunii, K. Fukaya, K. Yamato, K. Iwata, and H. Goto. Basic and clinical studies on bacampicillin. *Chemotherapia, 27S-4*:92–99 (1979).
268. J. A. Bodine, L. S. Strausbaugh, and M. A. Sande. Ampicillin and an ester in experimental *Hemophilus influenzae* meningitis. *Clin. Pharmacol. Ther., 20*:727–732 (1976).
269. T. B. Kjaer, P. G. Welling, and P. O. Madsen. Pharmacokinetics of ampicillin and methoxymethyl ester of hetacillin in dogs. *J. Pharm. Sci., 66*: 345–347 (1977).
270. S. Stavchansky, R. S. Pearlman, D. R. Van Harnen, R. D. Smyth, G. H. Hottendorf, A. Martin, J. Newburger, and L. W. Schneider. Evaluation of the bioavailability of sarpicillin, the methoxymethyl ester of hetacillin, in humans. *J. Pharm. Sci., 73*:169–173 (1984).
271. R. D. Smyth, M. Pfeffer, D. R. Van Harnen, A. Cohen, and G. H. Hottendorf. Human pharmacokinetics and disposition of sarmoxicillin, a lipophilic amoxicillin prodrug. *Antimicrob. Agents Chemother., 19*:1004–1012 (1981).
272. A. M. Emmerson, D. A. Cox, and L. S. Lees. Pharmacokinetics of sulbactam and ampicillin following oral-administration of sulfamicillin with probenecid. *Eur. J. Clin. Microbiol., 2*:340–344 (1983).
273. H. J. Rogers, I. D. Bradbrook, P. J. Morrison, R. G. Spector, D. A. Cox, and L. S. Lees. Pharmacokinetics and bioavailability of sulfamicillin estimated by high performance liquid chromatography. *J. Antimicrob. Chemother., 11*:435–445 (1983).
274. S. Hartley and R. Wise. A three-way crossover study to compare the pharmacokinetics and acceptability of sultamicillin at two base levels with that of ampicillin. *J. Antimicrob. Chemother., 10*:49–55 (1982).
275. B. I. Davies, F. P. V. Maesen, and J. A. van Noord. Clinical, bacteriological and pharmacokinetic results from an open trial of sultamicillin in patients with acute exacerbations of chronic bronchitis. *J. Antimicrob. Chemother., 13*:161–170 (1984).
276. T. Bergan and G. Sorensen. Pharmacokinetics of azidocillin in healthy adults. *Arzneim. Forsch., 30*:2185–2191 (1980).
277. A. Leroy, G. Humbert, and J. P. Fillastre. Pharmacokinetics of azlocillin in healthy subjects. *Scand. J. Infect. Dis. Suppl., 29*:49–54 (1981).
278. H. B. Drugeon, M. Pannier, and A. L. Courtieu. Pharmacokinetics of azlocillin in burned patients. *Curr. Chemother. Immunother., 1*:643–645 (1982).
279. P. Fiegel and K. Becker. Pharmacokinetics of azlocillin in persons with normal and impaired renal functions. *Antimicrob. Agents Chemother., 14*:288–291 (1978).
280. T. Bergan, S. B. Thorsteinsson, and I. Steingrimmson. Dose-dependent pharmacokinetics of azlocillin compared to mezlocillin. *Chemotherapy, 28*:160–170 (1982).
281. P. Spring and F. Follath. Dose-dependent elimination of azlocillin in healthy volunteers. *Curr. Chemother. Immunother., 1*:640–642 (1982).

282. A. Leroy, G. Humbert, M. Godin, and J. P. Fillastre. Pharmacokinetics of azlocillin in subjects with normal and impaired renal function. *Antimicrob. Agents Chemother., 17*:344–349 (1980).
283. A. Whelton, R. L. Stout, and F. A. Delgado. An azlocillin dosing nomogram for renal insufficiency. *J. Antimicrob. Chemother. Suppl. B, 11*:97–99 (1983).
284. J. M. Aletta, E. F. Francke, and H. C. Neu. Intravenous azlocillin kinetics in patients on long-term hemodialysis. *Clin. Pharmacol. Ther., 27*:563–566 (1980).
285. A. Whelton, R. L. Stout, and F. A. Delgado. Azlocillin kinetics during extracorporeal hemodialysis and perotoneal dialysis. *J. Antimicrob. Chemother. Suppl. B, 11*:89–95 (1983).
286. V. Gundert-Remy and E. Weber. Elimination of azlocillin in patients with biliary T-tube drainage. *Eur. J. Clin. Pharmacol., 22*:435–439 (1982).
287. V. Gundert-Remy, F. Frohnapfel, W. Jourdan, E. Weber, and A. Stiehl. Estimation of biliary excretion of ureidopenicillins in healthy volunteers using marker dilution technique. *Br. J. Clin. Pharmacol., 13*:795–801 (1982).
288. L. Weingartner, V. Sitka, R. Patsch, and H. H. Thiemann. Azlocillin and mezlocillin: Pharmacokinetic studies in children. *Curr. Chemother. Immunother., 1*:642–643 (1982).
289. O. P. W. Robinson. Human pharmacology of carbenicillin, a semisynthetic penicillin active against *Pseudomonas aeruginosa. Antimicrob. Agents Chemother.*, 614–618 (1967).
290. C. B. Smith and M. Finland. Carbenicillin: Activity in vitro and absorption and excretion in normal young men. *Appl. Microbiol., 16*:1753–1760 (1968).
291. H. C. Standiford, A. C. Kind, and W. M. M. Kirby. Laboratory and clinical studies of carbenicillin against gram-negative bacilli. *Antimicrob. Agents Chemother.*:286–291 (1968).
292. J. S. Tan and S. J. Salstrom. Levels of carbenicillin, ticarcillin, cephalothin, cefazolin, cefamandole, gentamicin, tobramycin, and amikacin in human serum and interstitial fluid. *Antimicrob. Agents Chemother., 11*:698–700 (1977).
293. C. D. Findlay, R. Wise, J. E. Allcock, and S. R. Durham. The tissue penetration, as measured by a blister technique, and pharmacokinetics of cefsulodin compared with carbenicillin and ticarcillin. *J. Antimicrob. Chemother.,* 7:637–642 (1981).
294. J. B. Eastwood and J. R. Curtis. Carbenicillin administration in patients with severe renal failure. *Br. Med. J., 1*:486–487 (1968).
295. L. J. Lees and R. Horton. Serum concentrations and urinary excretion in man after intravenous administration of ticarcillin and carbenicillin. *Prog. Chemother.*, 552–557 (1974).
296. C. D. Morehead, S. Shelton, H. Kusmiesz, and J. D. Nelson. Pharmacokinetics of carbenicillin in neonates of normal and low birth weight. *Antimicrob. Agents Chemother., 11*:267–271 (1972).
297. H. Yoskioka, M. Takimoto, T. Shimizu, and H. Haga. Pharmacokinetics

of intramuscular carbenicillin in the newborn. *Infection, 7*:27–29 (1979).

298. R. D. Libke, J. T. Clarke, E. D. Ralph, R. P. Luthy, and W. M. M. Kirby. Ticarcillin vs carbenicillin: Clinical pharmacokinetics. *Clin. Pharmacol. Ther., 17*:441-446 (1975).
299. B. R. Meyers, S. Z. Hirschman, L. Strougo, and E. Srulevitch. Comparative study of piperacillin, ticarcillin, and carbenicillin pharmacokinetics. *Antimicrob. Agents Chemother., 17*:608–611 (1980).
300. H. Lode, W. Tomas, P. Koeppe, and J. Wagner. Clinical pharmacology of a new ureidopenicillin: Bay k 4999, *Chemotherapy, 26*:81–90 (1980).
301. P. H. Hinderling, U. Gundert-Remy, D. Forster, and W. Gau. The pharmacokinetics of furazlocillin in healthy humans. *J. Pharmacokin. Biopharm., 11*:5-30 (1983).
302. R. Wise, B. Cadge, A. P. Gillett, A. Bhamjee, R. Livingston, P. G. Welling, and D. P. Thornhill. Pharmacokinetics of Bay k 4999, a new broad-spectrum penicillin. *Antimicrob. Agents Chemother., 15*:670–673 (1979).
303. B. R. Meyers, J. Jacobson, J. Masci, E. Srulevitch, and S. Z. Hirschman. Pharmacokinetics of amdinocillin in healthy adults. *Antimicrob. Agents Chemother., 23*:827–830 (1983).
304. K. Josefsson, T. Bergan, L. Magni, B. G. Pring, and D. Westerlund. Pharmacokinetics of bacmecillinam and pivmecillinam in volunteers. *Eur. J. Clin. Pharmacol., 23*:249–252 (1982).
305. H. Hey, H. J. Frederiksen, and J. T. Andersen. Gastroscopic and pharmacokinetics evaluation of a new pivmecillinam tablet. *Eur. J. Clin. Pharmacol., 22*:63–69 (1982).
306. O. Garborg. Mecillinam in cerebrospinal fluid in children. *Clin. Pharmacokinet., 6*:475–479 (1981).
307. J. G. Gambertoglio, S. L. Barriere, E. T. Lin, and J. E. Conte, Jr. Amdinocillin pharmacokinetics: Simultaneous administration with cephalothin and cerebrospinal fluid penetration. *Am. J. Med., 75*:54–59 (1983).
308. J. G. Gambertoglio, S. L. Barriere, E. T. Lin, and J. E. Conte, Jr. Pharmacokinetics of mecillinam in healthy subjects. *Antimicrob. Agents Chemother., 18*:952–956 (1980).
309. S. L. Barriere, J. G. Gambertoglio, E. T. Lin, and J. E. Conte, Jr. Multiple-dose pharmacokinetics of amdinocillin in healthy volunteers. *Antimicrob. Agents Chemother., 21*:54–57 (1982).
310. M. M. Hares, A. Hegarty, J. Tomkyns, D. W. Burdon, and M. R. B. Keighley. A study of the biliary excretion of mecillinam in patients with biliary disease. *J. Antimicrob. Chemother., 9*:217–222 (1982).
311. P. L. Svarva and T. Wessel-Aas. Serum levels of mecillinam in patients with severely impaired renal function. *Scand. J. Infect. Dis., 12*:303–305 (1980).
312. M. Ekberg, T. Denneberg, S. Larsson, and I. Juhlin. Pharmacokinetics and therapeutic studies of pivmecillinam in patients with normal and impaired renal function. *Scand. J. Infect. Dis., 10*:127–133 (1978).
313. S. J. Pancoast and H. C. Neu. Kinetics of mezlocillin and carbenicillin. *Clin. Pharmacol. Ther., 24*:108–116 (1978).

314. E. Bergogne-Berezin, P. Even, J. Pierre, and P. Reynaud. Pharmacokinetics of mezlocillin in bronchial secretions. *Infection, 8*:210–214 (1980).
315. J. Welter, D. H. Wittmann, and H. H. Schassan. Pharmacokinetics investigation of the penetration of mezlocillin into the pleural fluid. *Int. J. Clin. Pharm. Res., 2*:265–268 (1982).
316. G. R. Aronoff, R. S. Sloan, R. A. Stanish, and N. S. Fineberg. Mezlocillin dose dependent elimination kinetics in renal impairment. *Eur. J. Clin. Pharmacol., 21*:505–509 (1982).
317. T. Bergan. Review of the pharmacokinetics of mezlocillin. *J. Antimicrob. Chemother. Suppl. C, 11*:1–16 (1983).
318. T. Bergan. Pharmacokinetics of mezlocillin in healthy volunteers. *Antimicrob. Agents Chemother., 14*:801–806 (1978).
319. L. Verbist, T. B. Tjandramaga, R. Verbesselt, and P. J. De Schepper. Mezlocillin pharmacokinetics. Comparison with ampicillin and influence of probenecid. *Arzneim. Forsch., 29*:1962–1966 (1979).
320. A. Mangione, D. M. Janicke, F. D. Boudinot, R. M. Schultz, and W. J. Jusko. Dose-dependent pharmacokinetics of mezlocillin in subjects with normal and impaired renal function. *J. Antimicrob. Chemother. Suppl. A, 9*:81–85 (1982).
321. G. R. Aronoff, R. S. Sloan, F. C. Luft, R. L. Nelson, D. R. Maxwell, and S. A. Kleit. Mezlocillin pharmacokinetics in renal impairment. *Clin. Pharmacol. Ther., 28*:523–528 (1980).
322. E. Francke, S. Mehta, H. C. Neu, and G. B. Appel. Kinetics of intravenous mezlocillin in chronic hemodialysis patients. *Clin. Pharmacol. Ther., 26*: 228–231 (1979).
323. D. Kampf, R. Schurig, K. Weihermuller, and D. Forster. Effects on impaired renal function, hemodialysis, and peritoneal dialysis on the pharmacokinetics of mezlocillin. *Antimicrob. Agents Chemother., 18*:81–87 (1980).
324. J. M. Brogard, F. Comte, J. P. Arnaud, and J. Lavillaureix. Mezlocillin, serum and biliary concentrations level prediction with use of pharmacokinetics. *Drugs Exp. Clin. Res., 7*:277–285 (1981).
325. F. Comte, J. M. Brogard, J. Kopferschmitt, M. Dorner, and J. Lavillaureix. Excrétion biliare comparative de la mezlocilline et de 12 autres beta-lactamines. *Nouv. Presse Med., 11*:353–360 (1982).
326. U. Gundert-Remy, D. Forster, P. Schacht, and E. Weber. Kinetics of mezlocillin in patients with biliary T-tube drainage. *J. Antimicrob. Chemother. Suppl. A, 9*:65–75 (1982).
327. C. M. Bunke, G. R. Aronoff, M. E. Brier, R. S. Sloan, and F. C. Luft. Mezlocillin kinetics in hepatic insufficiency. *Clin. Pharmacol. Ther., 33*: 73–76 (1983).
328. T. Rubio, F. Wirth, and E. Karotkin. Pharmacokinetic studies of mezlocillin in newborn infants. *J. Antimicrob. Chemother. Suppl. A, 9*:241–244 (1982).
329. L. J. Eron, R. I. Goldenberg, D. M. Poretz, and C. H. Park. Piperacillin therapy for pseudomonas infections. *S. Med. J., 76*:859–862 (1983).
330. T. B. Tjandramaga, A. Mullie, R. Verbesselt, P. J. De Schepper, and L.

Verbist. Piperacillin: Human pharmacokinetics after intravenous and intramuscular administration. *Antimicrob. Agents Chemother., 14*:829–837 (1978).

331. F. D. Daschner, M. Just, G. Spillner, and V. Schlosser. Penetration of piperacillin into cardiac valves, subcutaneous and muscle tissue of patients undergoing open-heart surgery. *J. Antimicrob. Chemother., 9*:489–492 (1982).
332. J. Russo, Jr., M. I. B. Thompson, M. E. Russo, B. A. Saxon, J. M. Matsen, F. G. Moody, and L. F. Rikkers. Piperacillin distribution into bile, gallbladder wall, abdominal skeletal muscle, and adipose tissue in surgical patients. *Antimicrob. Agents Chemother., 22*:488–492 (1982).
333. G. M. Dickinson, D. G. Droller, R. L. Greenman, and T. F. Hoffman. Clinical evaluation of piperacillin with observations on penetrability into cerebrospinal fluid. *Antimicrob. Agents Chemother., 20*:481–486 (1981).
334. T. Bergan and J. D. Williams. Dose dependence of piperacillin pharmacokinetics. *Chemotherapy, 28*:153–159 (1982).
335. V. K. Batra, J. A. Morrison, K. C. Lasseter, and V. A. Joy. Piperacillin kinetics. *Clin. Pharmacol. Ther., 26*:41–53 (1979).
336. G. R. Aronoff, R. S. Sloan, M. E. Brier, and F. C. Luft. The effect of piperacillin dose on elimination kinetics in renal impairment. *Eur. J. Clin. Pharmacol., 24*:543–547 (1983).
337. J. A. Giron, B. R. Meyers, and S. Z. Hirschman. Biliary concentrations of piperacillin in patients undergoing cholecystectomy. *Antimicrob. Agents Chemother., 19*:309–311 (1981).
338. E. W. Taylor, V. Poxon, J. Alexander-Williams, and D. Jackson. Biliary excretion of piperacillin. *J. Int. Med. Res., 11*:28–31 (1983).
339. P. G. Welling, W. A. Craig, R. W. Bundtzen, F. W. Kwok, A. U. Gerber, and P. O. Madsen. Pharmacokinetics of piperacillin in subjects with various degrees of renal function. *Antimicrob. Agents Chemother., 23*:881–887 (1983).
340. M. I. B. Thompson, M. E. Russo, J. A. Matsen, and E. Atkin-Thor. Piperacillin pharmacokinetics in subjects with chronic renal failure. *Antimicrob. Agents Chemother., 19*:450–453 (1981).
341. P. J. De Schepper, T. B. Tjandramaga, A. Mullie, R. Verbesselt, A. van Hecken, R. Verberckmoes, and L. Verbist. Comparative pharmacokinetics of piperacillin in normals and in patients with renal failure. *J. Antimicrob. Chemother., 16*:49–57 (1982).
342. E. L. Franke, G. B. Appel, and H. C. Neu. Pharmacokinetics of intravenous piperacillin in patients undergoing chronic hemodialysis. *Antimicrob. Agents Chemother. 9, Suppl. B*:788–791 (1979).
343. J. A. Giron, B. R. Meyers, S. Z. Hirschman, and E. Srulevitch. Pharmacokinetics of piperacillin in patients with moderate renal failure and in patients undergoing hemodialysis. *Antimicrob. Agents Chemother., 19*:279–283 (1981).
344. M. A. L. Evans, P. Wilson, T. Leung, and J. D. Williams. Pharmacokinetics of piperacillin following intravenous administration. *J. Antimicrob. Chemother., 4*:255–261 (1978).

345. T. Rubio, F. H. Wirth, Jr., and E. H. Karotkin. Pharmacokinetics of piperacillin in newborn infants, in *Current Chemotherapy and Immunotherapy 1*: (P. Periti and G. G. Grassi, eds.), 677–679. American Society for Microbiology, Washington, D.C., (1982).
346. C. B. Wilson, J. R. Koup, K. E. Opheim, L. A. Adelman, J. Levy, T. L. Stull, C. Clausen, and A. L. Smith. Piperacillin pharmacokinetics in pediatric patients. *Antimicrob. Agents Chemother., 22*:442–447 (1982).
347. M. C. Thirumoorthi, B. I. Asmar, J. A. Buckley, R. O. Bollinger, R. E. Kauffman, and A. S. Dajani. Pharmacokinetics of intravenously administered piperacillin in preadolescent children. *J. Pediatr., 102*:941-946 (1983).
348. H. C. Neu and G. J. Garvey. Comparative in vitro activity and clinical pharmacology of ticarcillin and carbenicillin. *Antimicrob. Agents Chemother., 8*:457–462 (1975).
349. R. N. Brogden, R. C. Heel, T. M. Speight, and G. S. Avery. Ticarcillin: A review of its pharmacological properties and therapeutic efficacy. *Drugs, 20*:325–352 (1980).
350. R. Sutherland and P. J. Wise. α-Carboxy-3-thienylmethyl penicillin (BRL 2288), a new semisynthetic penicillin: Absorption and excretion in man. *Antimicrob. Agents Chemother., 2*:402–406 (1971).
351. V. Rodriguez, J. Inagaki, and G. P. Bodey. Clinical pharmacology of ticarcillin. *Antimicrob. Agents Chemother., 4*:31–36 (1973).
352. A. Gouyette, M. D. Kitzis, J. Guibert, and J. F. Acar. Pharmacokinetics and bioavailability of intramuscular preparation of ticarcillin. *J. Antimicrob. Chemother., 10*:419–425 (1982).
353. B. E. Davies, M. J. Humphrey, P. F. Langley, L. Lees, B. Legg, and G. A. Wadds. Pharmacokinetics of ticarcillin in man. *Eur. J. Clin. Pharmacol., 23*:167–172 (1982).
354. D. von Kobyletzki, A. Dalhoff, H. Lindemeyer, and C. A. Primavesi. Ticarcillin serum and tissue concentrations in gynecology and obstetrics. *Infection, 11*:144–149 (1983).
355. F. D. Daschner, G. Thoma, H. Langmaack, and A. Dalhoff. Ticarcillin concentrations in serum, muscle, and fat after a single intravenous injection. *Antimicrob. Agents Chemother., 17*:738–739 (1980).
356. S. Bennett, R. Wise, D. Weston, and J. Dent. Pharmacokinetics and tissue penetration of ticarcillin combined with clavulanic acid. *Antimicrob. Agents Chemother., 23*:831–834 (1983).
357. J. D. Nelson, H. Kusmiesz, S. Sheton, and E. Woodman. Clinical pharmacology and efficacy of ticarcillin in infants and children. *Pediatrics, 61*: 858–863 (1978).
358. K. Butler, A. R. English, B. Briggs, E. Gralla, R. B. Stebbins, and D. C. Hobbs. Indanyl carbenicillin: Chemistry and laboratory studies with a new semisynthetic penicillin. *J. Infect. Dis. Suppl., 127*:S97–S104 (1973).
359. K. Butler, A. R. English, A. K. Knirsch, and J. J. Korst. Metabolism and laboratory studies with indanyl carbenicillin. *Del. Med. J., 43*:336-375 (1971).
360. A. K. Knirsch, D. C. Hobbs, and J. J. Korst. Pharmacokinetics, toleration and safety of indanyl carbenicillin in man. *J. Infect. Dis. Suppl., 127*: S105–S110 (1973).

361. Y. Tanigawara, K. Yamaoka, T. Nakagawa, and T. Uno. Absorption kinetics of carbenicillin phenyl sodium and carbenicillin indanyl sodium in man. *Chem. Pharm. Bull., 30*:2174–2180 (1982).
362. J. P. Clayton, M. Cole, S. W. Elson, K. D. Hardy, L. W. Mizen, and R. Sutherland. Preparation, hydrolysis, and oral absorption of α-carboxy esters of carbenicillin. *J. Med. Chem., 18*:172–177 (1975).
363. R. Labia and A. Kazmierczak. Study of the physico-chemical properties of carfecillin. *Drugs Exp. Clin. Res., 8*:21–25 (1982).
364. P. J. Wilkinson, D. S. Reeves, R. Wise, and J. T. Allen. Volunteer and clinical studies with carfecillin: A new orally administered ester of carbenicillin. *Br. Med. J., 2*:250–252 (1975).
365. H. Graber, L. Benesch, M. Arr, and T. Magyar. Pharmacokinetic and clinical studies with carfecillin. *Int. J. Clin. Pharmacol., 16*:59–62 (1978).
366. F. Lund, K. Roholt, L. Tybring, and W. O. Godtfredsen. Mecillinam and pivmecillinam – New beta-lactam antibiotics with high activity against gram-negative bacilli, in *Chemotherapy*, Vol. 5 (J. D. Williams and A. M. Geddes, eds.), Plenum, New York, 1976, pp. 159–165.
367. M. Mitchard, J. Andrews, M. J. Kendall, and R. Wise. Mecillinam serum levels following intravenous injection: A comparison with pivmecillinam. *J. Antimicrob. Chemother. Suppl. B, 3*:83–88 (1977).
368. H. C. Neu, S. Srinivasan, E. L. Francke, C. Ortiz-Neu, and J. G. Christenson. Pharmacokinetics of amdinocillin and pivamdinocillin in normal volunteers. *Am. J. Med., 75*:60–64 (1983).
369. K. Roholt. Pharmacokinetic studies with mecillinam and pivmecillinam. *J. Antimicrob. Chemother. Suppl. B, 3*:71–81 (1977).
370. R. L. Parsons, G. A. Hossack, and G. M. Paddock. Pharmacokinetics of pivmecillinam. *Br. J. Clin. Pharmacol., 4*:267–273 (1977).
371. J. Andrews, M. J. Kendall, and M. Mitchard. Factors influencing the absorption and disposition of mecillinam and pivmecillinam in man. *Br. J. Clin. Pharmacol., 3*:627–632 (1976).
372. H. Hey, H. J. Frederiksen, and J. T. Andersen. Gastroscopic and pharmacokinetic evaluation of a new pivmecillinam tablet. *Eur. J. Clin. Pharmacol., 22*:63–69 (1982).
373. D. Westerlund, B. Pettersson, and J. Carlqvist. Determination of bacmecillinam, an amdinocillin prodrug, in human and canine whole blood by reserved-phase liquid chromatography. *J. Pharm. Sci., 71*:1148–1151 (1982).
374. K. Josefsson, T. Bergan, L. Magni, B. G. Pring, and D. Westerlund. Pharmacokinetics of bacmecillinam and pivmecillinam in volunteers. *Eur. J. Clin. Pharmacol., 23*:249–252 (1982).
375. J. O. Lernestedt, B. G. Pring, and D. Westerlund. Comparative clinical pharmacology of bacmecillinam along or in combination with bacampicillin and of pivmecillinam. *Curr. Chemother. Infect. Dis., 1*:314–316 (1980).
376. T. Bergan, A. Engeset, W. Olszewski, and R. Solberg. Pharmacokinetics of bacampicillin and bacmecillinam in plasma and peripheral lymph. *Lymphology, 12*:85–94 (1979).

PART 2
PENICILLINS

8

Clinical Applications of Penicillins

GEORGE M. ELIOPOULOS
New England Deaconess Hospital, Boston, Massachusetts

I. INTRODUCTION

Detailed information concerning the in vitro activity and pharmacokinetic properties of antimicrobial agents is necessary for their rational clinical use, but such data may not be sufficient for the design of optimal therapeutic regimens. The ultimate success or failure of any antibiotic treatment course will depend upon a number of additional factors, including the precise nature of the pathophysiological process, the biological characteristics of the pathogenic organism, and the ability of the patient's host-defense mechanisms to respond appropriately against bacterial invasion.

Antimicrobial therapy in an individual patient remains largely an empirical endeavor. Rarely is it possible in everyday clinical practice to obtain measurements of serum levels of the penicillins as a guide to proper treatment. Whether acceptable drug levels are attained at the actual site of infection would, in any case, be influenced by several variables, including the adequacy of regional blood flow, the presence or absence of visceral obstruction, and the extent of devitalized tissue at the infected focus. In patients with meningitis or endocarditis or in granulocytopenic patients, it is generally agreed that bactericidal antibiotic concentrations at the site of infection are essential to successful outcome. However, in most other circumstances, what antibiotic levels are necessary and for what period of time such levels must be maintained remain largely unanswered questions, since it appears that in some circumstances even subinhibitory penicillin concentrations may exert a beneficial effect, depending upon the integrity of host-defense systems (1) and also the identity of the pathogenic bacterium (2, 3).

The decision to select a particular antibiotic regimen for an individual patient is therefore heavily dependent upon its prior record of efficacy and safety under similar clinical conditions. This chapter intends to review the clinical use of the penicillins, with attention not only to their effectiveness in selected infections but also to potential adverse reactions which may compromise their use.

II. SPECIFIC AGENTS

A. Natural Penicillins

1. Penicillin G

After 40 years of clinical use, penicillin G (benzylpenicillin) continues to be an important and frequently used antibiotic. Although increasing resistance to the drug has appeared in several bacterial species in the years since its introduction, many important pathogens remain exquisitely susceptible to penicillin.

No drug has proven superior to penicillin G in the treatment of infections caused by penicillin-susceptible streptococci. For example, this drug continues to be the antibiotic of choice in patients with serious pneumococcal infections such as meningitis (4), where it is used in doses of approximately 20 million units daily in adults with normal renal function because of the need to penetrate the blood-brain barrier. Doses of this magnitude are unnecessary in the treatment of uncomplicated pneumococcal pneumonia and are more apt than lower doses to be associated with superinfections and other adverse reactions (5). Most pneumococci isolated in the United States remain highly susceptible to penicillin G, but strains which are resistant or relatively resistant to the drug were identified in South Africa and have been responsible for sporadic infections in the United States (6). Susceptibility to penicillin should be determined for all pneumococci isolated from blood or cerebrospinal fluid, since penicillin may be ineffective against infections caused by resistant strains.

Penicillin-susceptible streptococci remain the most common cause of native valve endocarditis. Although some clinicians prefer to add an aminoglycoside to penicillin during all or part of the treatment course in order to exploit the possibility of bactericidal synergism between these agents against *viridans* streptococci (7), treatment of endocarditis due to these organisms with high-dose penicillin alone for 4 weeks or longer results in high cure rates and avoids the potential toxicities of an aminoglycoside (8). In adults with streptococcal endocarditis penicillin G is usually employed at doses of 12 million to 24 million units daily. The dose may be adjusted in an attempt to attain serum bactericidal titers of 1:8 or higher at the nadir of serum penicillin levels. Because strains of *viridans* streptococci which are resistant to penicillin have been described (9), the susceptibility to penicillin of isolates causing endocarditis should always be determined. Enterococci not only are more resistant to penicillin than other commonly encountered streptococci but also are frequently tolerant to the lethal effect of cell wall-active antibiotics. Treatment of enterococcal endocarditis requires that penicillin be used in combination with an aminoglycoside in order to achieve effective killing of these organisms (7).

It would be difficult to compile a complete list of infections against which penicillin G has proven effective. The drug has been successfully employed against infections caused by group A (and other) streptococci, gonococci, non-beta-lactamase-producing staphylococci, spirochetes, and actinomyces, among others. Penicillin G is the antibiotic of choice in the treatment of clostridial gas gangrene. Doses of penicillin in these situations vary widely with the severity and site of the infectious process. Penicillin G is frequently used in the treatment of mixed aerobic-anaerobic infections due to oral flora, including head and neck infections and pleuropulmonary infections caused by aspiration of oral secretions. The recently recognized increasing resistance to penicillin G among *Bacteroides* species other than *Bacteroides fragilis* (10) suggests that the usefulness of penicillin against mixed infections due to oral flora may diminish in the future. Already there is some evidence that clindamycin may be more effective than penicillin in the treatment of anaerobic lung abscess (11).

Procaine Penicillin G. This preparation for intramuscular injection is used when modest serum levels of penicillin G are needed over a period of several hours. Doses of 600,000 units twice daily are as effective as intravenous doses of 20 million units of aqueous penicillin G daily in the treatment of uncomplicated pneumococcal pneumonia (5). Procaine penicillin in doses of 1.2 million units every 6 hr in combination with streptomycin has been successfully employed in 2-week regimens for the treatment of endocarditis due to highly susceptible streptococci (12). Procaine penicillin G, 4.8 million units, together with probenecid to delay urinary excretion of the drug, is curative in approximately 97% of patients with uncomplicated urogenital infection due to penicillin-susceptible *Neisseria gonorrhoeae* (13). This regimen is preferred to oral therapy for anorectal gonorrhea in men and in pharyngeal gonococcal infection. Procaine penicillin G together with aqueous penicillin G has been recommended as prophylaxis against bacterial endocarditis in patients with underlying valvular disease who are undergoing dental work or surgical procedures of the upper respiratory tract (14).

Benzathine Penicillin G. The slow absorption of penicillin following the intramuscular administration of benzathine penicillin results in low serum levels of the antibiotic over a prolonged period of time. The usefulness of this preparation is therefore limited to situations in which the organism is exquisitely susceptible to penicillin and when prolonged antibiotic therapy is required. Benzathine penicillin is highly effective in the treatment of streptococcal pharyngitis, where an important goal is to eradicate the organism in an attempt to prevent sequelae (15). Continuous prophylaxis against streptococcal upper respiratory tract infections is also indicated to prevent recurrent attacks of rheumatic fever in patients who have recovered from one episode of the disease. Benzathine penicillin, 1.2 million units every 4 weeks, is considered to be the most effective agent for this purpose, although alternative regimens may be better tolerated by patients (16). Recurrent streptococcal cellulitis and lymphangitis may be disabling in some patients with chronic disease of the lymphatic vessels. Benzathine penicillin in doses used for the prevention of rheumatic fever appears to be effective in preventing recurrent streptococcal infections in these patients (17).

Benzathine penicillin has been widely employed in the treatment of syphilis (18). While it is highly effective against most forms of the disease, benzathine penicillin is no longer considered optimal for therapy of neurosyphilis. In some patients treated with this formulation adequate cerebrospinal fluid levels of penicillin are not achieved (19) and treatment failures have occurred (20).

2. Penicillin V

Although the in vitro activities of penicillin V (phenoxymethylpenicillin) are not identical to those of penicillin G, they are comparable against most streptococci. Because of better systemic absorption following oral administration of penicillin V, this drug is often preferred to penicillin G for oral therapy. Penicillin V is effective in the treatment of upper respiratory tract infections or infections of the skin due to penicillin-susceptible streptococci. The usual dose of penicillin V employed in adults is 250-500 mg four times daily. Following administration of a 500-mg dose, bacteriostatic concentrations against susceptible pneumococci are maintained in the serum for at least 5 hr (21). Penicillin V is effective in the treatment of streptococcal pharyngitis, but it must be administered for 10 days to eradicate the organism at an acceptable rate (22).

Penicillin V is also widely employed in the treatment of infections arising from periodontal structures. This oral penicillin may be used as an alternative to parenteral penicillins during dental procedures for the prevention of bacterial endocarditis. A single 2-g dose is administered prior to the procedure; subsequent doses of 500 mg every 6 hr are given for seven doses. This regimen is not currently recommended for patients with prosthetic heart valves (14).

Penicillin V does not provide acceptable cure rates in the treatment of gonorrhea (23) and should not be used for this purpose.

3. Adverse Reactions

The most feared complication of penicillin therapy is anaphylaxis, which occurs in approximately 0.015-0.04% of patients. Fatal anaphylactic reactions occur in about 0.0015-0.002% of patients receiving penicillin (24). Of fatal anaphylactic reactions, the vast majority demonstrate onset of symptoms within 15 min of drug administration (24), so it is prudent to observe patients for 15–30 min following administration of penicillin. It is thought that fatal reactions occur less frequently with oral than with parenteral therapy. If penicillin therapy is clearly indicated in a patient with a history of penicillin allergy, skin testing is warranted (25). Such tests should be performed by individuals skilled in their interpretation and in the treatment of any adverse reaction to the test. The standard intradermal skin test is useful only for predicting immediate hypersensitivity reactions to the penicillins.

A particular reaction has been associated with the intramuscular or accidental intravenous administration of procaine penicillin. Anxiety, dizziness, dyspnea, seizures, and a variety of other symptoms have been reported, as has cardiopulmonary arrest (26,27). Reactions of this type have been attributed to procaine toxicity or to microembolization to the lung of insoluble drug aggregates (27). When procaine penicillin G (or benzathine penicillin) is administered, care must be taken to aspirate with the syringe prior to injection in order to avoid inadvertent intramuscular injection.

Neurotoxicity has been described in patients receiving massive (20 million to 60 million units/day) doses of penicillin. Abnormalities include somnolence, myoclonic jerks, seizures, and coma. Concomitant hyponatremia may increase the likelihood of seizure activity. This reaction appears to be due to direct toxicity of penicillin to neural tissues (28). Although doses of penicillin in excess of 24 million units daily are rarely used today, particular care must be taken to avoid penicillin accumulation to toxic levels in patients with renal insufficiency.

Penicillin therapy has been associated with a variety of adverse hematological reactions, including hemolytic anemia, neutropenia, and thrombocytopenia (29). Phlebitis, rash, gastrointestinal disturbances, and superinfection may result from therapy with any penicillin. Adverse reactions associated primarily with individual agents other than penicillin G are discussed in subsequent sections of this chapter.

B. Penicillinase-Resistant Penicillins

1. General Considerations

The semisynthetic penicillins discussed in this section share the property of resistance to hydrolysis by staphylococcal beta-lactamase. They are used primarily in the treatment of infections due to beta-lactamase-producing *Staphylococcus aureus*. Against strains of *Staph. aureus* which do not produce beta-lactamase, penicillin G is actually more potent than these drugs and is therefore preferred. However, such penicillin-susceptible strains of *Staph. aureus* are distinctly uncommon, accounting for less than 15% of clinical isolates at the present time. None of the penicillinase-resistant penicillins is more active than penicillin G against the streptococci. Enterococci are generally quite resistant, and these agents have no role in the therapy of serious enterococcal infections (30).

Some strains of *Staph. aureus* are resistant to methicillin and the other semi-synthetic penicillins. They constitute a small minority of clinical staphylococcal isolates in the United States, but higher rates of isolation have been noted in Europe and in some American cities (31). Current evidence suggests that methicillin resistance in *Staph. aureus* is due to abnormal penicillin-binding proteins in these strains (32). Despite the fact that combinations of penicillinase-resistant penicillins with gentamicin may be synergistic against such isolates (33), vancomycin remains the preferred antibiotic for serious infections due to methicillin-resistant staphylococci (7).

Methicillin resistance has been noted more frequently in *Staphylococcus epidermidis* isolates, which are a common cause of prosthetic valve endocarditis (34). Populations of such organisms are often heterogeneous, with methicillin-resistant bacteria constituting a small fraction of the total number of organisms present (35). These may not be easily detected under standard conditions of susceptibility testing. Methicillin-resistant *Staph. epidermidis* is also resistant to the other antistaphylococcal penicillins, and infections due to such strains are generally treated with vancomycin alone or in combination with other antibiotics (34).

2. Methicillin

The first of the antistaphylococcal penicillins introduced into clinical practice, methicillin has been shown to be effective in the treatment of infections due to *Staph. aureus* (36). For serious staphylococcal infections parenteral doses of up to 12 g daily may be employed in adults with normal renal function. Although higher doses have been used, these appear to be associated with an increased risk of adverse reactions (37).

The development of acute interstitial nephritis is a well-known complication of methicillin therapy (38). Renal dysfunction accompanying this syndrome may be profound but is usually reversible upon discontinuation of the drug (39). The rate of occurrence of this complication is difficult to assess accurately but has been estimated to be as high as 17% (40). Because this reaction is thought to represent a hypersensitivity phenomenon, it is prudent to avoid re-exposing a patient who has recovered from methicillin-induced nephritis to other penicillins. Rechallenge with another penicillin has resulted in recurrence of renal dysfunction in some patients (41), although such relapse does not appear to be inevitable (39).

3. Oxacillin

Oxacillin has been shown to be effective in the treatment of serious staphylococcal infections (42) and continues to be widely used for this purpose. Parenteral doses of up to 12 g daily are usually adequate to treat serious staphylococcal infections in adults. In contrast to methicillin, no adjustment in dosage is required in the presence of renal dysfunction (43). Less serious infections can be treated with oral oxacillin, which is generally used at doses of 500 mg four to six times daily.

Although acute interstitial nephritis has been reported following the administration of oxacillin (44), this complication appears to be seen less commonly with oxacillin than with methicillin. However, a notable side effect of oxacillin therapy has been the development of hepatitis, which is often asymptomatic. This has occurred in up to 15% of patients receiving doses of 6 g or more daily (45). In some cases the development of fever and eosinophilia suggests that the hepatitis may represent a hypersensitivity phenomenon (45), but in other instances a toxic effect of high doses of the drug seems a more likely explanation (46,47).

4. Nafcillin

Like the other antistaphylococcal penicillins discussed here, nafcillin is effective in the therapy of serious staphylococcal infections such as endocarditis (48). In such cases nafcillin is occasionally used in combination with an aminoglycoside because of the bactericidal synergism which is demonstrated by such combinations in vitro. While such combinations may result in a more rapid clearance of bacteremia in some patients, regimens utilizing nafcillin alone or in combination with an aminoglycoside were found to be equally effective in curing staphylococcal endocarditis in a recently reported study (48). Combinations of nafcillin with gentamicin are synergistic in vitro against enterococci, but the addition of serum negates this synergistic effect (30). Therefore such combinations should not be used in the therapy of enterococcal infections.

In the treatment of serious staphylococcal infections nafcillin is usually administered in doses of 8-12 g daily. No adjustment of dosage is necessary in the presence of renal failure (43).

5. Oral Antistaphylococcal Penicillins

In the United States cloxacillin and dicloxacillin are available for oral administration only. Somewhat higher peak serum levels are obtained with dicloxacillin than with cloxacillin, and both are better absorbed than oral oxacillin (49). Perhaps the most frequent use of these drugs is in the treatment of skin and soft tissue infections from which staphylococci are recovered, or in which there exists a high likelihood that either staphylococci or streptococci are the causative organisms. Although oral cloxacillin is effective in the treatment of streptococcal pharyngitis or pneumococcal pneumonia (50), there is no reason to use any antistaphylococcal penicillin for infections caused by pathogens against which penicillin V is not only more active but also less expensive. Most minor skin and soft tissue infections in adults for which oral therapy can be safely considered respond to cloxacillin or dicloxacillin in daily doses of approximately 1-2 g. The drugs are generally administered every 6 hr. Neither cloxacillin nor dicloxacillin require dose modification in the presence of renal failure (43). In highly selected circumstances oral therapy with larger doses of antistaphylococcal penicillins has been used to treat more serious staphylococcal infections. Such use of these drugs should be undertaken only under close medical supervision by individuals skilled in evaluating therapeutic response.

6. Comments

Both nafcillin and oxacillin provide effective parenteral therapy for serious staphylococcal infections. Despite minor differences in the in vitro activity of these drugs, neither is clearly superior in general clinical use and some hospital formularies include only one or the other of the drugs. Many physicians currently avoid methicillin because of the apparently increased risk of acute interstitial nephritis associated with this agent. In most clinical situations in which an oral antistaphylococcal agent is indicated, either cloxacillin or dicloxacillin can be used effectively.

C. Extended-Spectrum Penicillins

1. Ampicillin

Because ampicillin is active against most strains of *Hemophilus influenzae* as well as streptococci and other respiratory tract pathogens, this drug has been widely used in the treatment of acute otitis media (51), acute sinusitis (52), and tracheobronchitis or pneumonia (53). Ampicillin offers no advantage over penicillin against infections known to be caused by group A streptococci or pneumococci. The drug has been used extensively in pediatrics, where bacteremic infections and meningitis due to *H. influenzae, Listeria monocytogenes,* group B streptococci, and other ampicillin-susceptible organisms are of particular importance (54). The significant prevalence of ampicillin-resistant *H. influenzae* in many areas frequently necessitates the concurrent or alternative use of chloramphenicol or other antibiotics until the susceptibilities of a pathogenic strain can be ascertained. In the treatment of meningitis due to pneumococci or meningococci, ampicillin appears to be as effective as penicillin (55).

Many bacterial isolates causing uncomplicated community-acquired urinary tract infections are susceptible to ampicillin at concentrations achievable in the urine. In such cases ampicillin at doses of 500 mg four times daily (in adults) has been highly effective in eradicating the infection (56). In seriously ill patients with suspected urosepsis, broader coverage against gram-negative bacilli than that provided by achievable serum concentrations of ampicillin is desirable. Once susceptibility of the pathogen to ampicillin is documented, treatment may be continued with parenteral ampicillin. For serious infections in adults with normal renal function, ampicillin is usually administered in doses of 8–12 g daily. Maximum doses are employed in the therapy of central nervous system infections.

Ampicillin is effective in the treatment of enteric fever due to susceptible *Salmonellae* (57,58). However, chloramphenicol appears to be superior to ampicillin in the treatment of enteric fever when oral regimens are compared (59). Both oral ampicillin and parenteral ampicillin have been used successfully in the treatment of shigellosis (60,61).

Single-dose therapy consisting of ampicillin, 3.5 g orally, together with probenecid, may be used for uncomplicated urethritis caused by penicillin-susceptible gonococci and results in cure rates of approximately 90% (13). In 1973 Wiesner et al. (62) found that gonococci which disseminate to produce an arthritis-dermatitis syndrome were generally more susceptible to penicillin than those causing uncomplicated urethritis. Subsequently this group reported successful use of oral ampicillin in the treatment of this syndrome (63). It is important to note, however, that disseminated disease due to a penicillin resistant gonococcus has been described more recently (64), which may limit the usefulness of such oral regimens.

Ampicillin is occasionally useful in the therapy of endocarditis. The drug offers no advantage over penicillin in the treatment of endocarditis due to *viridans* streptococci. Rarely endocarditis may be caused by *Hemophilus* species, against which ampicillin may be more active than penicillin G. Such infections have been satisfactorily treated with high-dose ampicillin alone or in combination with an aminoglycoside (65). Although ampicillin is somewhat more active than penicillin G against enterococci, neither drug is predictably bactericidal against these organisms. Therefore enterococcal endocarditis is treated with ampicillin or penicillin (or vancomycin in penicillin-allergic patients) in combination with an aminoglycoside (7). In most situations there is no clear advantage of ampicillin compared with penicillin in such regimens. Possibly ampicillin may be preferable to penicillin for the treatment of endocarditis due to *Streptococcus faecium*, which is more resistant to penicillin than *Streptococcus faecalis* isolates, or in the treatment of enterococcal infections of the central nervous system. In such cases even a marginal advantage of ampicillin may be critical for successful outcome.

Both ampicillin and penicillin G are active against *L. monocytogenes,* and both drugs have been used successfully in the treatment of meningitis caused by this organism (66). Bactericidal synergism between penicillins and aminoglycosides has been documented in vitro (67), and such combinations are often used in an attempt to maximize killing of the organisms in vivo.

A significant consideration in deciding whether to use ampicillin in preference to penicillin G against pathogens susceptible to both drugs is the fact that ampicillin is more likely to cause drug rash. It has been estimated that approximately 8% of patients receiving ampicillin develop a rash, while only 3% of patients develop a rash with penicillin (68). Nearly all patients with acute infectious mononucleosis due to Epstein-Barr virus will develop a rash if ampicillin is administered, while this occurs in a minority of patients who receive penicillin (69). Patients with mononucleosis due to cytomegalovirus also appear to be at increased risk of ampicillin-related rashes (70).

2. Amoxicillin

Differences between the in vitro susceptibilities of common pathogens to amoxicillin or ampicillin are small; however, amoxicillin is better absorbed following oral administration (71). Although parenteral amoxicillin has been used successfully in the treatment of serious infections (72), it does not appear to provide any major advantage over ampicillin when both drugs are administered parenterally. Only the oral form of the drug is available in the United States.

Pneumococci and *H. influenzae* are the organisms most commonly responsible for acute otitis media (73) and acute maxillary sinusitis (52,74). Amoxicillin, 500 mg three times daily, is as effective as ampicillin, 500 mg four times daily, in therapy of acute maxillary sinusitis in adults (52). For the treatment of otitis media in children, amoxicillin is used in doses of 20–40 mg/kg daily (73). Lower doses of amoxicillin than of ampicillin are required in the treatment of childhood otitis and, in studies comparing the two drugs, diarrhea has been seen less frequently in amoxicillin-treated children (51,75). Neither drug is active against beta-lactamase-producing strains of *H. influenzae* (76). While amoxicillin is effective against group A streptococci, it is more likely than penicillin V to cause rashes in children (77) and therefore should not be used to treat streptococcal pharyngitis.

Amoxicillin is effective in the therapy of urinary tract infections (78). In patients with uncomplicated cystitis a single 3-g dose of amoxicillin has been shown to be as effective as more conventional courses of 250 mg, three of four times daily, administered over 10–14 days (79,80). Rubin et al. (56) reported that in patients with urinary tract infection and negative tests for antibody-coated bacteria, a single 3-g dose of amoxicillin resulted in bacterial eradication rates comparable to those seen with standard 10-day courses of ampicillin or trimethoprim-sulfamethoxazole. Among patients with positive antibody-coated bacteria tests, single-dose amoxicillin therapy was effective in only 33% of patients. However, many of these patients also relapsed following retreatment with conventional therapy. Single-dose amoxicillin therapy is associated with a lower rate of adverse effects (4–6%) than is seen with conventional therapy (12–40%) (56,80).

A single 3-g dose of amoxicillin together with probenecid is effective in uncomplicated urogenital infections due to *N. gonorrhoeae* (18,81). Anorectal gonorrhea in men and pharyngeal gonorrhea in either sex are more difficult to treat, and single-dose oral regimens are not recommended. Infections due to penicillin-resistant strains will not respond to amoxicillin.

Oral amoxicillin at doses of 100 mg/kg daily has been reported to be effective in the treatment of typhoid fever in children (58). High-dose amoxicillin therapy (1 g every 6 hr) appears to be comparable to standard oral chloramphenicol therapy in the treatment of typhoid fever in adults (82). Amoxicillin is less effective than ampicillin in acute shigellosis (83) and should not be used in this disease.

3. Hetacillin

Hetacillin is rapidly hydrolyzed to ampicillin in aqueous solutions as well as upon enteral absorption. Therefore both the in vitro and in vivo activities of this antibiotic are due entirely to the free ampicillin which is generated (84,85). The drug is effective and has been used successfully at doses of 500 mg administered orally or intramuscularly four times daily in the treatment of pneumococcal pneumonia in adults (86).

Since there appears to be no significant advantage of hetacillin over ampicillin or amoxicillin in either antimicrobial activity or pharmacokinetic properties (84,87), there is no reason to choose hetacillin in preference to the other drugs for clinical use.

4. Mecillinam

Mecillinam, or amdinocillin, has recently been approved for clinical use in the United States. The drug is highly active against many gram-negative bacteria but possesses relatively poor activity against gram-positive organisms and *Pseudomonas aeruginosa* (88). Partly in order to broaden the antibacterial spectrum in therapeutic regimens and partly to exploit the possibility of synergistic activity of mecillinam in combination with other beta-lactams (89), several clinical trials have been designed using the drug in combination with other antibiotics. In some of these trials the enterally absorbed pivaloyloxymethyl ester of the drug (pivmecillinam or pivamdinocillin), which is rapidly hydrolyzed to mecillinam, has been used exclusively or after several days of parenteral mecillinam. The worldwide clinical experience with mecillinam has been recently reviewed (90).

In a randomized study of uncomplicated bacterial cystitis in women, pivmecillinam, 400 mg four times daily for 1 week, cleared bacteriuria in 20 of 23 patients, which was comparable to the rate of bacterial eradication seen with trimethoprim-sulfamethoxazole (91). In a multicenter study comparing mecillinam (10 mg/kg four to six times daily) with "standard" therapy, bacteriological cure rates following therapy of urinary tract infections with mecillinam were comparable to those obtained with tobramycin (90). Kosmidis et al. (92) found that combinations of pivmecillinam with pivampicillin were no more effective an pivampicillin alone in the treatment of urinary tract infections due to ampicillin-susceptible organisms. However, the combination was successful in 68% of patients with urinary tract infections due to ampicillin-resistant organisms.

Several studies have investigated the efficacy of mecillinam in the treatment of enteric fever. Mecillinam and/or pivmecillinam used alone have been successful in approximately 90% of patients (93,94). However, some patients have not responded well to such therapy (95). Mecillinam may be less effective in eliminating *Salmonellae* from the stool than trimethoprim–sulfamethoxazole (94). Combinations of mecillinam/pivmecillinam with ampicillin/pivampicillin appear to be highly effective in the treatment of enteric fever (96–98).

In a randomized study of patients with acute purulent exacerbations of chronic bronchitis, pivmecillinam–amoxicillin combinations were superior to amoxicillin alone as judged by both subjective and objective criteria (99). Mecillinam combined with other beta-lactam antibiotics has been used successfully in the treatment of gram-negative septicemia, with cure rates of approximately 80% in a small number of patients (100,101). However, in a comparative trial of mecillinam alone or in combination with cefoxitin or ticarcillin/carbenicillin in febrile cancer patients, most of whom were neutropenic, the overall response rates to all regimens were only 50–60% in documented infections, with less than 40% of septicemic patients responding to such therapy (102).

Mecillinam appears to be relatively well tolerated. Adverse reactions to date have been similar to those seen with other penicillins and have infrequently necessitated discontinuation of therapy (90,101). Unique toxicities have not been reported.

The effectiveness of mecillinam has been best studied in the treatment of urinary tract infections, but whether this drug alone or in combination with another beta-lactam will prove superior to other currently available antibiotics is still unknown. For other serious infections the numbers of patients studied have been small and many of these received concurrent therapy with other antibiotics. Clearly additional comparative studies are needed before the ultimate role of mecillinam in clinical practice can be defined.

D. Antipseudomonal Penicillins

1. Carbenicillin

The development of carbenicillin provided a beta-lactam antibiotic that was active against *P. aeruginosa,* as well as strains of *Enterobacter* and *Serratia* and other gram-negative bacteria that are generally resistant to ampicillin. This expanded spectrum against gram-negative bacilli was accomplished at the expense of diminished potency against gram-positive bacteria (103).

Urinary tract infections due to *P. aeruginosa* have been successfully treated with carbenicillin in doses of 1-6 g daily in adults (104). Eradication of the organism is often influenced by the presence of obstruction, stones, indwelling urethral catheters, or other complicating factors. Minimal inhibitory concentrations of carbenicillin against *P. aeruginosa* are relatively high, and doses in the range of 20 to 40 g daily have been required in the treatment of serious *Pseudomonas* infections in adults with normal renal function. Curreri et al. (105) used carbenicillin alone or in combination with gentamicin to treat *P. aeruginosa* sepsis complicating thermal burns. Although the overall mortality in such patients was high, many patients with *Pseudomonas* pneumonia and septicemia survived. Carbenicillin alone (106) or in combination with gentamicin (107) has been employed in the therapy of infections in cancer patients, many of whom have been neutropenic. While such regimens are often effective, bacteriological cure and patient survival ultimately depend on the severity and course of the underlying disease process.

Chronic disorders of the respiratory tract are often complicated by infections due to *P. aeruginosa*. Carbenicillin has been useful in the treatment of such infections, including chronic otitis and mastoditis (108) and acute exacerbations of pulmonary disease in patients with cystic fibrosis (109,110). Carbenicillin doses of at least 100 mg/kg daily must be used in the treatment of acute pulmonary infections due to *P. aeruginosa* in children with cystic fibrosis (110). While such therapy frequently results in clinical improvement, eradication of the organisms from respiratory tract secretions occurs uncommonly.

From a number of clinical studies it is apparent that when carbenicillin is used to treat chronic or serious *Pseudomonas* infections, strains with increased resistance to the drug may arise (104,109). One rationale for using this agent in combination with an aminoglycoside is to decrease the likelihood that carbenicillin-resistant strains will emerge during therapy (89). However, it is clear that such combinations do not completely prevent the emergence of resistant strains. Carbenicillin–aminoglycoside combinations are also employed in the empiric therapy of febrile episodes in neutropenic or otherwise immunocompromised patients, both to achieve the broadest possible antibacterial spectrum and also because of evidence that the use of two antibiotics that are active against the bacterial pathogen results in improved cure rates in such patients (111).

Hepatitis has been reported in some patients receiving high doses of carbenicillin. Recurrence following rechallenge with lower doses of the drug has been described (112). Acute interstitial nephritis has occurred in association with carbenicillin therapy (113). Neutropenia due to carbenicillin has been reported. This may represent a toxic reaction rather than a hypersensitivity reaction, at least in some cases, since low doses of the drug have been given safely in a patient who had experienced neutropenia during two high-dose courses of the drug (114). Hemostatic abnormalities due to defects in platelet function occur frequently in patients receiving high doses of carbenicillin, although these uncommonly result in hemorrhage (115). The delivery of large quantities of sodium and inorganic anion during therapy with carbenicillin may result in hypokalemia and alkalosis (116).

Carbenicillin and aminoglycosides must not be mixed together in intravenous solutions, since inactivation of the latter can result (117). Inactivation of the aminoglycoside is also possible in vivo, particularly in patients with severe renal impairment in whom excretion of both drugs is reduced and doses are administered at infrequent intervals (118).

2. Indanyl Carbenicillin

Unlike the parent compound, the indanyl ester of carbenicillin resists degradation at an acidic pH and is absorbed following oral administration. The drug is hydrolyzed in the body to yield carbenicillin, with only traces of the original compound detectable in the blood (119). High levels of carbenicillin are achieved in the urine following administration of indanyl carbenicillin, but serum levels are inadequate for the treatment of systemic infections (120). Therefore use of this drug is limited to the treatment of urinary tract infections due to *P. aeruginosa* or other bacteria resistant to achievable concentrations of alternative drugs. Clinical studies have documented the efficacy of this antibiotic in the treatment of urinary tract infections (121,122). Infections caused by *P. aeruginosa* or other relatively resistant pathogens often occur in patients with structural or functional abnormalities of the urinary tract. In this setting bacteriological relapse or reinfection following therapy with any antibiotic is common. The emergence of strains resistant to carbenicillin has been reported following treatment of urinary tract infections with indanyl carbenicillin (122).

Indanyl carbenicillin is available in tablets, each equivalent to 328 mg of carbenicillin. The usual dose in the treatment of *Pseudomonas* urinary tract infections in adults is two tablets, four times daily. In the presence of severe renal impairment attainable urinary levels may be therapeutically inadequate (123) and use of the drug in such circumstances is not recommended.

3. Ticarcillin

The antibacterial spectrum of ticarcillin is similar to that of carbenicillin, but the former is more potent against *P. aeruginosa.* As a result, some strains of this organism which are resistant to carbenicillin will be susceptible to ticarcillin, but, more importantly, lower doses of ticarcillin than of carbenicillin are required for the therapy of *Pseudomonas* infections. The usual dose of ticarcillin in serious *Pseudomonas* infections is 18-24 g daily in adults with normal renal function. The dose must be adjusted in the presence of renal dysfunction. Lower doses can be used in infections limited to the urinary tract.

Parry and Neu (124) reported an overall 81% favorable response rate in patients with serious gram-negative infections treated with ticarcillin. Patients with infections caused by organisms other than *P. aeruginosa* responded significantly better (96% response) than those with *Pseudomonas* infections (74% response). The drug has been used successfully in the therapy of pneumonia caused by a variety of organisms, including *P. aeruginosa* and *H. influenzae* (125). In a prospective randomized trial comparing combinations of ticarcillin plus tobramycin with carbenicillin plus gentamicin in serious infections due to gram-negative bacilli (most of which were *P. aeruginosa*), the ticarcillin–tobramycin combination was shown to be more effective (126). Combinations of ticarcillin with tobramycin or another aminoglycoside have been used as standard empiric therapy of febrile episodes in neutropenic patients at many institutions.

Ticarcillin, like carbenicillin, is active against many anaerobic bacteria. At doses of approximately 20 g daily, both drugs have been used successfully in the treatment of infections due primarily to anaerobes, including pleuropul monary infections, intra-abdominal abscesses, and anaerobic septicemia (127, 128). Combinations of ticarcillin with gentamicin appear to be as effective as chloramphenicol–gentamicin or clindamycin–gentamicin in the treatment of intra-abdominal and female genital tract sepsis (129).

As with carbenicillin, resistant strains may arise during therapy with ticarcillin. Colonization with ticarcillin-resistant organisms, including *Klebsiella* and yeasts, also occurs and may result in superinfection (124,125). The range of adverse reactions to ticarcillin is similar to that seen with carbenicillin. Hepatotoxicity has been observed less frequently with ticarcillin than with carbenicillin (126). Ticarcillin may result in prolongation of the bleeding time by interference with platelet aggregation (130). Although ticarcillin contains more sodium per gram of drug than does carbenicillin (5.2 mEq/g or more versus 4.7 mEq/g), this is offset by the fact that lower doses of ticarcillin are employed. Significant hypokalemia has been reported in as many as 17% of patients treated with ticarcillin (129), but this is readily preventable or treatable if the possibility of this complication is recognized.

E. Acylaminopenicillins

1. Azlocillin

Azlocillin is the latest of the acylaminopenicillins to be approved for clinical use in the United States. It is generally less active than piperacillin or mezlocillin against enteric gram-negative bacilli, but azlocillin and piperacillin are the most active drugs of this class against *P. aeruginosa*.

Most published studies with this agent suffer from the fact that when patients are stratified by site of infection and bacterial pathogen, each group includes only small numbers of treated individuals. Against a variety of infections caused by *P. aeruginosa* and other gram-negative bacteria, favorable response rates of approximately 80-90% have been noted (131,132). However, clinical results depend to a large extent upon the nature and severity of the underlying disease process. Azlocillin in doses of 8 g daily was shown to be comparable to ticarcillin in doses of 12 g daily in the treatment of complicated urinary tract infections, most of which were due to *P. aeruginosa* (133). In a randomized study comparing ticarcillin-tobramycin, azlocillin-tobramycin, and azlocillin alone in the treatment of acute exacerbations of pulmonary disease in patients with cystic fibrosis, similar degrees of clinical improvement were observed for all treatment groups (134). Strains resistant to azlocillin have emerged during therapy with this agent (132,135). Concurrent aminoglycoside therapy may retard the development of such strains but does not prevent their emergence (134).

The recommended dose of azlocillin is 200-300 mg/kg daily, administered intravenously. Doses in excess of 24 g daily are not recommended, and an adjustment in the dose may be required in the presence of impaired renal function. Reported adverse reactions due to azlocillin are similar to those associated with other penicillins. One or more adverse systemic reaction have been noted in 15% of patients treated during clinical trials, but in only 5% of patients was discontinuation of the drug required. In a small number of patients rapid intravenous injection of azlocillin has been associated with the development of chest discomfort, the etiology of which is unclear (136).

2. Mezlocillin

The in vitro activity of mezlocillin against most gram-negative bacteria, including *P. aeruginosa,* is comparable to that of ticarcillin. However, it is more active than ticarcillin against *Klebsiella pneumoniae* and streptococci. In open trials studying the effectiveness of mezlocillin in the treatment of infections of the lung, bone, soft tissues, abdomen, and urinary tract, cure rates of approximately 75-85% have been reported (137,138). Mezlocillin at a dose of 6 g daily was found to be as effective as ticarcillin at 8 g daily in the treatment of urinary tract infections (139). In a randomized study comparing mezlocillin with cefoxitin in the therapy of various infections, similar response rates were observed with the two drugs (140).

Mezlocillin alone has been shown to be inadequate for the empirical therapy of febrile episodes in granulocytopenic patients, with only one-half of such patients responding favorably to therapy (141). However, preliminary reports indicate that mezlocillin in combination with an aminoglycoside appears to be as effective as ticarcillin-aminoglycoside combinations in neutropenic patients (142).

Mezlocillin is administered in doses of 200–300 mg/kg daily in the therapy of serious infections. Doses in excess of 24 g daily are not recommended. Adjustments of drug dosage must be made in patients with renal insufficiency. No unique toxicities have been reported with this antibiotic in comparison with other penicillins. Although abnormalities in platelet aggregation have been noted in volunteers given the drug, mezlocillin appears to be less likely than carbenicillin to cause significant prolongation of the bleeding time (143).

3. Piperacillin

Piperacillin is as active as or perhaps somewhat more active than azlocillin against *P. aeruginosa*, yet it possesses activity comparable to that of mezlocillin against other gram-negative bacteria. Used alone for treatment of various infections, piperacillin has resulted in favorable response rates of approximately 75–95% (144–147). In combination with an aminoglycoside, piperacillin is as effective as carbenicillin or ticarcillin in empiric therapy of febrile episodes in granulocytopenic patients (148,149) and in the treatment of serious gram-negative infections in unselected patients (150). As seen with other broad-spectrum penicillins, organisms resistant to piperacillin have been noted to arise during therapy with this drug (146). A review of over 1000 piperacillin treatment courses revealed that resistant strains emerged in less than 2% of courses, although resistance in *Pseudomonas* isolates developed in approximately 6% of courses (151).

Piperacillin is usually administered in doses of 200–300 mg/kg daily in the treatment of serious infections in adults with normal renal function. Dosage may require adjustment in the presence of diminished renal function. Infections limited to the urinary tract generally require lower doses of the drug. Piperacillin may be administered intravenously or intramuscularly, but the former route is preferred in seriously ill patients or when large doses of the drug are required. Adverse reactions attributed to piperacillin are similar to those seen with other penicillins used in high doses. The sodium content of piperacillin (1.98 mEq/g) is less than one-half that of ticarcillin or carbenicillin. Hypokalemia was seen less often during therapy with piperacillin than during carbenicillin therapy in one study in which the daily dose of piperacillin was approximately one-half that of carbenicillin (148). Piperacillin commonly induces abnormal platelet aggregation responses when administered to healthy volunteers but may be less likely to cause significant prolongation in bleeding time than the older antipseudomonal penicillins (152).

III. SUMMARY

Many of the penicillins discussed in this chapter have been in general clinical use for a number of years and their records of efficacy and safety have been well established. None of these drugs have been shown to be more effective or better tolerated than penicillin G for the treatment of serious infections caused by susceptible bacteria. For the treatment of infections due to beta-lactamase-producing *S. aureus,* nafcillin and oxacillin are equally effective when parenteral therapy is required. Either cloxacillin or dicloxacillin can be used for oral antistaphylococcal therapy. None of the penicillins should be used to treat infections due to methicillin-resistant staphylococci.

The broader activity of ampicillin against gram-negative bacteria in comparison with that of penicillin G permits its use in the therapy of respiratory tract infections due to *H. influenzae*, in urinary tract infections, and in other infections caused by susceptible gram-negative bacteria. However, penicillin G is preferred to ampicillin in the treatment of most streptococcal infections because of the higher incidence of minor adverse reactions seen with the latter drug. Amoxicillin is a useful alternative to oral ampicillin, particularly in children who are less likely to develop diarrhea as a complication of therapy with the better-absorbed antibiotic. The demonstration that single-dose amoxicillin regimens are highly successful in the treatment of uncomplicated bacterial cystitis has been a promising development, since these are often better tolerated than conventional therapy. Mecillinam, now called amdinocillin, provides a broader spectrum of antibacterial activity against gram-negative bacilli than ampicillin. However, the comparative efficacy of mecillinam, used alone or in combination with other antibiotics, relative to other currently available or investigational drugs requires further examination.

Ticarcillin has largely gained acceptance over carbenicillin in the therapy of infections due to *P. aeruginosa* because its increased potency permits the use of lower doses. Based upon studies of in vitro activity, the acylaminopenicillins would appear to provide definite advantages over carbenicillin or ticarcillin. Nevertheless, none is so effective that it can replace standard combination regimens in the empiric therapy of febrile episodes in severely immunocompromised patients. Any major advantage in terms of therapeutic outcome or toxicity of acylaminopenicillin-aminoglycoside combinations compared with ticarcillin-aminoglycoside combinations as empiric therapy in cases of suspected sepsis has yet to be demonstrated.

The broad antibacterial spectrum of the acylaminopenicillins may permit a more parsimonious use of antibiotics in patients with infections due to multiple organisms. In institutions where the prevalence of ticarcillin-resistant organisms is significant, the potential advantages of the acylaminopenicillins are evident. In other circumstances the role of the new penicillins remains unclear. Of particular concern is the fact that against *P. aeruginosa* the acylaminopenicillins are less likely than ticarcillin to be bactericidal at concentrations near the minimal inhibitory concentration. In addition, the in vitro activity of these drugs may be profoundly influenced by the size of the bacterial inoculum used (153). Thus, while current clinical evidence suggests that these new agents are generally both safe and effective, they should be used selectively until comparative studies demonstrate their superiority to other currently available antibiotics.

REFERENCES

1. H. Friedman and G. H. Warren. Enhanced susceptibility of penicillin-resistant staphylococci to phagocytosis after *in vitro* incubation with low doses of nafcillin. *Proc. Soc. Exp. Biol. Med., 146*:707 (1974).
2. I. Ofek, E. H. Beachey, B. I. Eisenstein, M. L. Alkan, and N. Sharon. Suppression of bacterial adherence by subminimal inhibitory concentrations of β-lactam and aminoglycoside antibiotics. *Rev. Infect. Dis., 1*:832 (1979).
3. D. A. Wilson and G. N. Rolinson. The recovery period following exposure of bacteria to penicillins. *Chemotherapy, 25*:14 (1979).
4. M. N. Swartz and P. R. Dodge. Bacterial meningitis – A review of selected aspects. *N. Engl. J. Med., 272*:779 (1965).
5. A. Brewin, L. Arango, W. K. Hadley, and J. F. Murray. High-dose penicillin therapy and pneumococcal pneumonia. *J. Am. Med. Assoc., 230*:409 (1974).
6. J. Ward and H. Koornhof. Antibiotic resistant pneumococci, in *Current Clinical Topics in Infectious Diseases,* Vol. 1 (J. S. Remington and M. N. Swartz, eds.), McGraw-Hill, New York, 1980, p. 265.
7. M. A. Sande and W. M. Scheld. Combination antibiotic therapy of bacterial endocarditis. *Ann. Intern. Med., 92*:390 (1980).
8. A. W. Karchmer, R. C. Moellering, Jr., D. G. Maki, and M. N. Swartz. Single-antibiotic therapy for streptococcal endocarditis. *J. Am. Med. Assoc., 241*:1801 (1979).
9. B. F. Farber, G. M. Eliopoulos, J. I. Ward, K. L. Ruoff, V. Syriopoulou, and R. C. Moellering, Jr. Multiply resistant viridans streptococci: Susceptibility to β-lactam antibiotics and comparison of penicillin-binding protein patterns. *Antimicrob. Agents Chemother., 24*:702 (1983).
10. R. S. Edson, J. E. Rosenblatt, D. T. Lee, and E. A. McVey III. Recent experience with antimicrobial susceptibility of anaerobic bacteria. Increasing resistance to penicillin. *Mayo Clin. Proc., 57*:737 (1982).
11. M. E. Levison, C. T. Mangura, B. Lorber, E. Abrutyn, E. L. Pesanti, R. S. Levy, R. R. MacGregor, and A. R. Schwartz. Clindamycin compared with penicillin for the treatment of anaerobic lung abscess. *Ann. Intern. Med., 98*:466 (1983).
12. W. R. Wilson, R. L. Thompson, C. J. Wilkowske, J. A. Washington II, E. R. Giuliani, and J. E. Geraci. Short-term therapy for streptococcal infective endocarditis. *J. Am. Med. Assoc., 245*:360 (1981).
13. R. E. Kaufman, R. E. Johnson, H. W. Jaffe, C. Thornsberry, G. H. Reynolds, P. J. Wiesner, and the Cooperative Study Group. National gonorrhea therapy monitoring study. Treatment results. *N. Engl. J. Med., 294*:1 (1976).

14. E. L. Kaplan, B. F. Anthony, A. Bisno, D. Durack, H. Houser, H. D. Millard, J. Sanford, S. T. Shulman, M. Stillerman, A. Taranta, and N. Wenger. Prevention of bacterial endocarditis. *Circulation, 56*:139A (1977).
15. G. Peter and A. L. Smith. Group A streptococcal infections of the skin and pharynx. *N. Engl. J. Med., 297*:365 (1977).
16. American Heart Association Committee Report. Prevention of rheumatic fever. *Circulation, 55*:1 (1977).
17. R. R. Babb, J. A. Spittell, Jr., W. J. Martin, and A. Schirger. Prophylaxis of recurrent lymphangitis complicating lymphedema. *J. Am. Med. Assoc., 195*:871 (1966).
18. Treatment of sexually transmitted diseases. *Med. Lett. Drugs Ther., 24*:29 (1982).
19. J. A. Mohr, W. Griffiths, R. Jackson, H. Saadah, P. Bird, and J. Riddle. Neurosyphilis and penicillin levels in cerebrospinal fluid. *J. Am. Med. Assoc., 236*:2208 (1976).
20. B. M. Greene, N. R. Miller, and T. E. Bynum. Failure of penicillin G benzathine in the treatment of neurosyphilis. *Arch. Intern. Med., 140*:1117 (1980).
21. C. G. McCarthy and M. Finland. Absorption and excretion of four penicillins. Penicillin G, penicillin V, phenethicillin and phenylmercaptomethyl penicillin. *N. Engl. J. Med., 263*:315 (1960).
22. R. H. Schwartz, R. L. Wientzen, Jr., F. Pedreira, E. J. Feroli, G. W. Mella, and V. L. Guandolo. Penicillin V for group A streptococcal pharyngotonsillitis. *J. Am. Med. Assoc., 246*:1790 (1981).
23. R. R. Willcox. The newer penicillins in the treatment of gonorrhoea. *Postgrad. Med. J. Suppl., 40*:202 (1964).
24. O. Idsøe, T. Guthe, R. R. Willcox, and A. L. DeWeck. Nature and extent of penicillin side-reactions, with particular reference to fatalities from anaphylactic shock. *Bull. WHO, 38*:159 (1968).
25. A. Saxon. Immediate hypersensitivity reactions to β-lactam antibiotics. *Rev. Infect. Dis. Suppl., 2*:S368 (1983).
26. R. L. Green, J. E. Lewis, S. J. Kraus, and E. L. Frederickson. Elevated plasma procaine concentrations after administration of procaine penicillin G. *N. Engl. J. Med., 291*:223 (1974).
27. J. E. Galpin, A. W. Chow, T. T. Yoshikawa, and L. B. Guze. "Pseudoanaphylactic" reactions from inadvertant infusion of procaine penicillin G. *Ann. Intern. Med., 81*:358 (1974).
28. H. Smith, P. I. Lerner, and L. Weinstein. Neurotoxicity and "massive" intravenous therapy with penicillin. *Arch. Intern. Med., 120*:47 (1967).
29. N. U. Bang and R. B. Kammer. Hematologic complications association with β-lactam antibiotics. *Rev. Infect. Dis. Suppl., 2*:S380 (1983).
30. R. H. Glew and R. C. Moellering, Jr. Effect of protein binding on the activity of penicillins in combination with gentamicin against enterococci. *Antimicrob. Agents Chemother., 15*:87 (1979).
31. L. D. Sabath. Chemical and physical factors influencing methicillin resistance of *Staphylococcus aureus* and *Staphylococcus epidermidis*. *J. Antimicrob. Chemother. Suppl. C, 3*:47 (1977).

32. B. Hartman and A. Tomasz. Altered penicillin-binding proteins in methicillin-resistant strains of *Staphylococcus aureus. Antimicrob. Agents Chemother., 19*:726 (1981).
33. R. J. P. Hemmer, P. Vaudaux, and F. A. Waldvogel. Methicillin potentiates effect of gentamicin on methicillin-resistant *Staphylococcus aureus. Antimicrob. Agents Chemother., 15*:34 (1979).
34. A. W. Karchmer, G. L. Archer, and W. E. Dismukes. *Staphylococcus epidermidis* causing prosthetic valve endocarditis: Microbiologic and clinical observations as guides to therapy. *Ann. Intern. Med., 98*:447 (1983).
35. G. L. Archer. Antimicrobial susceptibility and selection of resistance among *Staphylococcus epidermidis* isolates recovered from patients with infections of indwelling foreign devices. *Antimicrob. Agents Chemother., 14*:353 (1978).
36. J. D. Allen, C. E. Roberts, Jr., and W. M. M. Kirby. Staphylococcal septicemia treated with methicillin. *N. Engl. J. Med., 266*:111 (1962).
37. L. M. Kancir, C. U. Tuazon, T. A. Cardella, and J. N. Sheagren. Adverse reactions to methicillin and nafcillin during treatment of serious *Staphylococcus aureus* infections. *Arch. Intern. Med., 138*:909 (1978).
38. J. Ditlove, P. Weidmann, M. Bernstein, and S. G. Massry. Methicillin nephritis. *Medicine, 56*:483 (1977).
39. J. E. Galpin, J. E. Shinaberger, T. M. Stanley, M. J. Blumenkrantz, A. S. Bayer, G. S. Friedman, J. Z. Montgomerie, L. B. Guze, J. W. Coburn, and R. J. Glassock. Acute interstitial nephritis due to methicillin. *Am. J. Med., 65*:756 (1978).
40. C. M. Nolan and R. S. Abernathy. Nephropathy associated with methicillin therapy. Prevalence and determinants in patients with staphylococcal bacteremia. *Arch. Intern. Med., 137*:997 (1977).
41. D. N. Gilbert, R. Gourley, A. d'Agostino, S. H. Goodnight, Jr., and H. Worthen. Interstitial nephritis due to methicillin, penicillin and ampicillin. *Ann. Allergy, 28*:378 (1970).
42. J. O. Klein, L. D. Sabath, B. W. Steinhauer, and M. Finland. Oxacillin treatment of severe staphylococcal infections. *N. Engl. J. Med., 269*:1215 (1963).
43. W. M. Bennett, R. S. Muther, R. A. Parker, P. Feig, G. Morrison, T. A. Golper, and I. Singer. Drug therapy in renal failure: Dosing guidelines for adults. Part I: Antimicrobial agents, analgesics. *Ann. Intern. Med., 93*:62 (1980).
44. D. B. Tillman, P. A. Oill, and L. B. Guze. Oxacillin nephritis. *Arch. Intern. Med., 140*:1552 (1980).
45. I. M. Onorato and J. L. Axelrod. Hepatitis from intravenous high-dose oxacillin therapy. *Ann. Intern. Med., 89*:497 (1978).
46. A. H. Bruckstein and A. A. Attia. Oxacillin hepatitis. Two patients with liver biopsy, and review of the literature. *Am. J. Med., 64*:519 (1978).
47. A. A. Pollock, S. A. Berger, M. S. Simberkoff, and J. J. Rahal, Jr. Hepatitis associated with high-dose oxacillin therapy. *Arch. Intern. Med., 138*:915 (1978).
48. O. Korzeniowski, M. A. Sande, and the National Collaborative Endocarditis

Study Group. Combination antimicrobial therapy for *Staphylococcus aureus* endocarditis in patients addicted to parenteral drugs and in non-addicts. A prospective study. *Ann. Intern. Med., 97*:496 (1982).

49. C. F. Gravenkemper, J. V. Bennett, J. L. Brodie, and W. M. M. Kirby. Dicloxacillin. In vitro and pharmacologic comparisons with oxacillin and cloxacillin. *Arch. Intern. Med., 116*:340 (1965).
50. M. Turck, A. Ronald, and R. G. Petersdorf. Clinical studies with cloxacillin. *J. Am. Med. Assoc., 192*:961 (1965).
51. V. M. Howie, J. H. Ploussard, and J. Sloyer. Comparison of ampicillin and amoxicillin in the treatment of otitis media in children. *J. Infect. Dis. Suppl., 129*:S181 (1974).
52. B. H. Hamory, M. A. Sande, A. Sydnor, Jr., D. L. Seale, and J. M. Gwaltney, Jr. Etiology and antimicrobial therapy of acute maxillary sinusitis. *J. Infect. Dis., 139*:197 (1979).
53. D. M. Musher, K. R. Kubitschek, J. Crennan, and R. E. Baughn. Pneumonia and acute febrile tracheobronchitis due to *Haemophilus influenzae*. *Ann. Intern. Med., 99*:444 (1983).
54. G. H. McCracken, Jr., and H. F. Eichenwald. Antimicrobial therapy in infants and children. Part II. Therapy of infectious conditions. *J. Pediatr., 93*:357 (1978).
55. A. W. Mathies, Jr., J. M. Leedom, L. D. Thrupp, D. Ivler, B. Portnoy, and P. F. Wehrle. Experience with ampicillin in bacterial meningitis, in *Antimicrobial Agents and Chemotherapy – 1965* (G. L. Hobby, ed.), American Society for Microbiology, Washington, D.C., 1966, p. 610.
56. R. H. Rubin, L. S. T. Fang, S. R. Jones, R. S. Munford, J. M. Slepack, P. A. Varga, L. Onheiber, C. L. Hall, and N. E. Tolkoff-Rubin. Single-dose amoxicillin therapy for urinary tract infection. Multicenter trial using antibody-coated bacteria localization technique. *J. Am. Med. Assoc., 244*:561 (1980).
57. R. A. Sleet, G. Sangster, and J. McC. Murdoch. Comparison of ampicillin and chloramphenicol in the treatment of paratyphoid fever. *Br. Med. Jour., 1*:148 (1964).
58. E. Calderon. Amoxicillin in the treatment of typhoid fever due to chloramphenicol-resistant *Salmonella typhi*. *J. Infect. Dis. Suppl., 129*: S219 (1974).
59. R. P. Robertson, M. F. A. Wahab, and F. O. Raasch. Evaluation of chloramphenicol and ampicillin in *Salmonella* enteric fever. *N. Engl. J. Med., 278*:171 (1968).
60. K. C. Haltalin, J. D. Nelson, H. T. Kusmiesz, and L. V. Hinton. Comparison of intramuscular and oral ampicillin therapy for shigellosis. *J. Pediatr., 73*:617 (1968).
61. K. C. Haltalin, J. D. Nelson, H. T. Kusmiesz, and L. V. Hinton. Optimal dosage of ampicillin for shigellosis. *J. Pediatr., 74*:626 (1969).
62. P. J. Wiesner, H. H. Handsfield, and K. K. Holmes. Low antibiotic resistance of gonococci causing disseminated infection. *N. Engl. J. Med., 288*:1221 (1973).

63. H. H. Handsfield, P. J. Wiesner, and K. K. Holmes. Treatment of the gonococcal arthritis–dermatitis syndrome. *Ann. Intern. Med., 84*:661 (1976).
64. M. I. Leftik, J. W. Miller, and J. D. Brown. Penicillin-resistant gonococcal polyarthritis. *J. Am. Med. Assoc., 239*:134 (1978).
65. J. E. Geraci, C. J. Wilkowske, W. R. Wilson, and J. A. Washington II. *Haemophilus* endocarditis. Report of 14 patients. *Mayo Clin. Proc., 52*:209 (1977).
66. R. E. Nieman and B. Lorber. Listeriosis in adults: A changing pattern. Report of eight cases and review of the literature, 1968–1978. *Rev. Infect. Dis., 2*:207 (1980).
67. R. C. Moellering, Jr., G. Medoff, I. Leech, C. Wennersten, and L. J. Kunz. Antibiotic synergism against *Listeria monocytogenes. Antimicrob. Agents Chemother., 1*:30 (1972).
68. S. Shapiro, D. Slone, V. Siskind, G. P. Lewis, and H. Jick. Drug rash with ampicillin and other penicillins. *Lancet, 2*:969 (1969).
69. H. Pullen, N. Wright, and J. McC. Murdoch. Hypersensitivity reaction to antibacterial drugs in infectious mononucleosis. *Lancet, 2*:1176 (1967).
70. E. Klemola. Hypersensitivity reactions to ampicillin in cytomegalovirus mononucleosis. *Scand. J. Infect. Dis., 2*:29 (1970).
71. H. C. Neu. Antimicrobial activity and human pharmacology of amoxicillin. *J. Infect. Dis. Suppl., 129*:S123 (1974).
72. D. A. Leigh and J. G. Nash. Parenteral amoxycillin treatment for severe infections in hospitalized patients. *J. Antimicrob. Chemother., 5*:109 (1979).
73. C. D. Bluestone. Otitis media in children: To treat or not to treat? *N. Engl. J. Med., 306*:1399 (1982).
74. E. R. Wald, G. J. Milmoe, A'D. Bowen, J. Ledesma-Medina, N. Salamon, and C. D. Bluestone. Acute maxillary sinusitis in children. *N. Engl. J. Med., 304*:749 (1981).
75. H. M. Feder. Comparative tolerability of ampicillin, amoxicillin, and trimethoprim–sulfamethoxazole suspensions in children with otitis media. *Antimicrob. Agents Chemother., 21*:426 (1982).
76. H. C. Neu. Amoxicillin. *Ann. Intern. Med., 90*:356 (1979).
77. M. Stillerman, H. D. Isenberg, and R. R. Facklam. Treatment of pharyngitis associated with group A *Streptococcus*: Comparison of amoxicillin and potassium phenoxymethyl penicillin. *J. Infect. Dis. Suppl., 129*:S169 (1974).
78. D. N. Gilbert. Comparison of amoxicillin and ampicillin in the treatment of urinary tract infections. *J. Infect. Dis. Suppl., 129*:S231 (1974).
79. L. S. T. Fang, N. E. Tolkoff-Rubin, and R. H. Rubin. Efficacy of single-dose and conventional amoxicillin therapy in urinary tract infection localized by the antibody-coated bacteria technic. *N. Engl. J. Med., 298*:413 (1978).
80. M. Savard-Fenton, B. W. Fenton, L. B. Reller, B. A. Laver, and R. L.

Byyny. Single-dose amoxicillin therapy with follow-up urine culture. Effective initial management for acute uncomplicated urinary tract infections. *Am. J. Med., 73*:808 (1982).
81. Centers for Disease Control. Gonorrhea. Centers for Disease Control recommended treatment schedules, 1979. *Ann. Intern. Med., 90*:809 (1979).
82. N. Pillay, E. B. Adams, and D. North-Coombes. Comparative trial of amoxycillin and chloramphenicol in the treatment of typhoid fever in adults. *Lancet, 2*:333 (1975).
83. J. D. Nelson and K. C. Haltalin. Amoxicillin less effective than ampicillin against *Shigella* in vitro and in vivo: Relationship of efficacy to activity in serum. *J. Infect. Dis. Suppl., 129*:S222 (1974).
84. R. Sutherland and O. P. W. Robinson. Laboratory and pharmacological studies in man with hetacillin and ampicillin. *Br. Med. J., 2*:804 (1967).
85. Hetacillin. *Med. Lett. Drugs Ther., 13*:49 (1971).
86. D. B. Louria and M. Schultz. Treatment of pneumonia in adults with hetacillin. *Ann. N.Y. Acad. Sci., 145*:387 (1967).
87. W. M. M. Kirby and A. C. Kind. Clinical pharmacology of ampicillin and hetacillin. *Ann. N.Y. Acad. Sci., 145*:291 (1967).
88. H. C. Neu. Structure–activity relations of new β-lactam compounds and in vitro activity against common bacteria. *Rev. Infect. Dis. Suppl., 2*:S319 (1983).
89. G. M. Eliopoulos and R. C. Moellering, Jr. Antibiotic synergism and antimicrobial combinations in clinical infections. *Rev. Infect. Dis., 4*:282 (1982).
90. C. H. Demos and E. Green. Review of clinical experience with amdinocillin monotherapy and comparative studies. *Am. J. Med., 75*:72 (1983).
91. D. Guttmann. A comparison of pivmecillinam and cotrimoxazole in the treatment of simple cystitis in general practice. *J. Antimicrob. Chemother. Suppl. B, 3*:137 (1977).
92. J. Kosmidis, A. Karagiannis, K. Eliades, C. Dimopoulos, and G. K. Daikos. Miraxid: Therapeutic, pharmacokinetic and in vitro study in urinary tract infections. Proceedings on the 13th International Congress on Chemotherapy, 4.1/1-11, Vienna, Austria, 1983.
93. A. M. Geddes and P. D. Clarke. The treatment of enteric fever with mecillinam. *J. Antimicrob. Chemother. Suppl. B, 3*:101 (1977).
94. A. P. Ball and A. M. Geddes. Management of enteric fever with amdinocillin. *Am. J. Med., 75*:130 (1983).
95. B. K. Mandal, A. G. Ironside, and J. Brennand. Mecillinam in enteric fever. *Br. Med. J., 1*:586 (1979).
96. D. Tanphaichitra, A. Bussayanond, and O. Christensen. The combination of pivmecillinam and pivampicillin in the treatment of acute enteric fever. *J. Antimicrob. Chemother., 8*:23 (1981).
97. B. M. Limson, M. T. Mendoza, E. Liwanag, O. E. Christensen, and P. Menday. Randomized, comparative trial of mecillinam, mecillinam/ampicillin and chloramphenicol in the treatment of enteric fever. *J. Antimicrob. Chemother., 9*:405 (1982).

98. B. M. Limson, M. T. Mendoza, and O. E. Christensen. Myraxid in enteric fever, including drug-resistant salmonellosis. Proceedings of the 13th International Congress on Chemotherapy, 4.1/1-10, Vienna, Austria, 1983.
99. A. Pines, A. R. Nandi, H. Raafat, and M. Rahman. Pivmecillinam and amoxycillin as combined treatment in purulent exacerbation of chronic bronchitis. *J. Antimicrob. Chemother. Suppl. B, 3*:141 (1977).
100. E. Ekwall, A. Scheja, S. Cronberg, K. Ganrot-Norlin, M. Jonsson, I. Juhlin, G. Kahlmetes, A. Thoren, K. E. Thulin, and G. Tunevall. Mecillinam and ampicillin separately or combined in gram-negative septicemia. *Infection, 8*:37 (1980).
101. J. W. King, T. R. Beam, Jr., H. C. Neu, and L. G. Smith. Systemic infections treated with amdinocillin in combination with other beta-lactam antibiotics. *Am. J. Med., 75*:113 (1983).
102. R. D. Lawson, E. H. Estey, and G. P. Bodey. Amdinocillin: Use alone or in combination with cefoxitin or carbenicillin-ticarcillin. *Am. J. Med., 75*: 113 (1983).
103. W. L. Hewitt and R. E. Winters. The current status of parenteral carbenicillin. *J. Infect. Dis. Suppl., 127*:S120 (1973).
104. C. B. Smith, J. N. Wilfert, P. E. Dans, T. A. Kurrus, and M. Finland. In-vitro activity of carbenicillin and results of treatment of infections due to *Pseudomonas* with carbenicillin singly and in combination with gentamicin. *J. Infect. Dis. Suppl., 122*:S14 (1970).
105. P. W. Curreri, R. B. Lindberg, F. C. DiVincenti, and B. A. Pruitt, Jr. Intravenous administration of carbenicillin for septicemia due to *Pseudomonas aeruginosa* following thermal injury. *J. Infect. Dis. Suppl., 122*:S40 (1970).
106. G. P. Bodey, V. Rodriguez, and J. K. Luce. Carbenicillin therapy of gram-negative bacilli infections. *Am. J. Med. Sci., 257*:408 (1969).
107. S. Schimpff, W. Satterlee, V. M. Young, and A. Serpick. Emperic therapy with carbenicillin and gentamicin for febrile patients with cancer and granulocytopenia. *N. Engl. J. Med., 284*:1061 (1971).
108. J. D. Nelson. Carbenicillin therapy of infections due to *Pseudomonas* in children. *J. Infect. Dis. Suppl., 122*:S48 (1970).
109. R. W. Lyons, G. F. Thornton, and V. T. Andriole. Carbenicillin: Clinical and laboratory studies. *J. Infect. Dis. Suppl., 122*:S104 (1970).
110. N. N. Huang, E. J. Hiller, C. M. Macri, M. Capitanio, and K. R. Candy. Carbenicillin in patients with cystic fibrosis. Clinical pharmacology and therapeutic evaluation. *J. Pediatr., 78*:338 (1971).
111. L. S. Young. Combination or single drug therapy for gram-negative sepsis, in *Current Clinical Topics in Infectious Diseases,* Vol. 3 (J. S. Remington and M. N. Swartz, eds.), McGraw-Hill, New York, 1982, p. 177.
112. F. M. Wilson, J. Belamarie, C. B. Lauter, and A. M. Lerner. Anicteric carbenicillin hepatitis. Eight episodes in four patients. *J. Am. Med. Assoc., 232*:818 (1975).
113. G. B. Appel, B. A. Woda, H. C. Neu, M. F. Parry, F. Silva, and C. L. Pirani.

Acute interstitial nephritis associated with carbenicillin therapy. *Arch. Intern. Med., 138*:1265 (1978).
114. M. P. Reyes, M. Palutke, and A. M. Lerner. Granulocytopenia associated with carbenicillin. Five episodes in two patients. *Am. J. Med., 54*:413 (1973).
115. C. H. Brown III, E. A. Natelson, M. W. Bradshaw, T. W. Williams, Jr., and C. P. Alfrey, Jr. The hemostatic defect produced by carbenicillin. *N. Engl. J. Med., 291*:265 (1974).
116. S. V. Cabizuca and K. B. Desser. Carbenicillin-associated hypokalemic alkalosis. *J. Am. Med. Assoc., 236*:956 (1976).
117. L. K. Pickering and P. Gearhart. Effect of time and concentration upon interaction between gentamicin, tobramycin, netilmicin, or amikacin and carbenicillin or ticarcillin. *Antimicrob. Agents Chemother., 15*:592 (1979).
118. L. J. Riff and G. G. Jackson. Laboratory and clinical conditions for gentamicin inactivation by carbenicillin. *Arch. Intern. Med., 130*:887 (1972).
119. K. Butler, A. R. English, B. Briggs, E. Gralla, R. B. Stebbins, and D. C. Hobbs. Indanyl carbenicillin: Chemistry and laboratory studies with a new semisynthetic penicillin. *J. Infect. Dis. Suppl., 127*:S97 (1973).
120. A. K. Knirsch, D. C. Hobbs, and J. J. Korst. Pharmacokinetics, toleration, and safety of indanyl carbenicillin in man. *J. Infect. Dis. Suppl., 127*:S105 (1973).
121. K. M. Ries, C. G. Cobbs, J. Y. Gillenwater, M. E. Levison, G. L. Mandell, M. A. Sande, and D. Kaye. Double-blind comparison of carbenicillin indanyl sodium, ampicillin, and cephalexin in treatment of urinary tract infection. *Antimicrob. Agents Chemother., 4*:593 (1973).
122. M. Turck. The treatment of urinary tract infections with oral carbenicillin. *J. Infect. Dis. Suppl., 127*:S133 (1973).
123. C. E. Cox. Pharmacology of carbenicillin indanyl sodium in renal insufficiency. *J. Infect. Dis. Suppl., 127*:S157 (1973).
124. M. F. Parry and H. C. Neu. Ticarcillin for treatment of serious infections with gram-negative bacteria. *J. Infect. Dis., 134*:476 (1976).
125. F. R. Ervin and W. E. Bullock. Clinical and pharmacological studies of ticarcillin in gram-negative infections. *Antimicrob. Agents Chemother., 9*:94 (1976).
126. M. F. Parry and H. C. Neu. A comparative study of ticarcillin plus tobramycin versus carbenicillin plus gentamicin for the treatment of serious infections due to gram-negative bacilli. *Am. J. Med., 64*:961 (1978).
127. D. Webb, H. Thadepalli, I. Roy, and V. T. Bach. Ticarcillin disodium in anaerobic infections. *Arch. Intern. Med., 138*:1618 (1978).
128. W. Fiedelman and C. D. Webb. Clinical evaluation of carbenicillin in the treatment of infection due to anaerobic bacteria. *Curr. Ther. Res., 18*:441 (1975).
129. G. K. M. Harding, F. J. Buckwold, A. R. Ronald, T. J. Marrie, S. Brunton, J. C. Koss, M. J. Gurwith, and W. L. Albritton. Prospective, randomized comparative study of clindamycin, chloramphenicol, and ticarcillin, each

in combination with gentamicin, in therapy for intraabdominal and female genital tract sepsis. *J. Infect. Dis., 142*:384 (1980).
130. P. Somani, M. R. Smith, A. Gohara, and K. Kapila. The effects of mezlocillin, ticarcillin and placebo on blood coagulation and bleeding time in normal volunteers. *J. Antimicrob. Chemother. Suppl. C, 11*:33 (1983).
131. H. C. Neu, E. L. Francke, C. Ortiz-Neu, and A. S. Prince. The use of azlocillin to treat serious infections. *J. Antimicrob. Chemother. Suppl. B, 11*: 141 (1983).
132. S. Olive, W. J. Mogabgab, B. Holmes, B. Pollock, B. Pauling, and R. Beville. Treatment of serious *Pseudomonas* infections with azlocillin. *J. Antimicrob. Chemother. Suppl. B, 11*:153 (1983).
133. C. E. Cox. A comparison of azlocillin and ticarcillin in the treatment of complicated urinary tract infections. *J. Antimicrob. Chemother. Suppl. B, 11*:183 (1983).
134. F. J. McLaughlin, W. J. Matthews, Jr., D. J. Strieder, B. Sullivan, A. Taneja, P. Murphy, and D. A. Goldmann. Clinical and bacteriological response to three antibiotic regimens for acute exacerbations of cystic fibrosis: Ticarcillin–tobramycin, azlocillin–tobramycin, and azlocillin–placebo. *J. Infect. Dis., 147*:559 (1983).
135. S. J. Eykyn. Azlocillin in the treatment of serious infections with *Pseudomonas aeruginosa. J. Antimicrob. Chemother., 9*:395 (1982).
136. M. F. Parry. The tolerance and safety of azlocillin. *J. Antimicrob. Chemother. Suppl. B, 11*:223 (1983).
137. H. Thadepalli and B. Rao. Clinical evaluation of mezlocillin. *Antimicrob. Agents Chemother., 16*:605 (1979).
138. S. J. Pancoast, J. A. Jahre, and H. C. Neu. Mezlocillin in the therapy of serious infections. *Am. J. Med., 67*:747 (1979).
139. P. O. Madsen and O. S. Nielsen. Comparative study of mezlocillin and ticarcillin in the treatment of urinary tract infections. *Clin. Ther., 3*:311 (1980).
140. J. L. LeFrock, A. Molavi, K. Rolston, B. Smith, R. Schell, P. Chandrasekar, and B. Carr. In-vitro and in-vivo comparison of mezlocillin and cefoxitin. *J. Antimicrob. Chemother. Suppl. C, 11*:83 (1983).
141. B. F. Issell and G. P. Bodey. Mezlocillin for treatment of infections in cancer patients. *Antimicrob. Agents Chemother., 17*:1008 (1980).
142. I. Hann, P. Noone, H. G. Prentice, R. Sage, H. Blacklock, L. Stirling, R. Gray, R. Corringham, F. Boesen, J. Mohiuddin, M. Rubeck, and V. Hoffbrand. The results of a randomized trial of empirical antibiotic treatment in febrile neutropenic patients with four β-lactam/aminoglycoside combinations. *J. Antimicrob. Chemother. Suppl. C, 11*:57 (1983).
143. E. A. Copelan, R. K. Kusumi, L. Miller, and R. J. Fass. A comparison of the effects of mezlocillin and carbenicillin on haemostasis in volunteers. *J. Antimicrob. Chemother. Suppl. C, 11*:43 (1983).
144. S. Pancoast, A. S. Prince, E. L. Francke, and H. C. Neu. Clinical evaluation of piperacillin therapy for infection. *Arch. Intern. Med., 141*:1447 (1981).

145. B. Lutz, W. Mogabgab, B. Holmes, B. Pollock, and R. Beville. Clinical evaluation of the therapeutic efficacy and tolerability of piperacillin. *Antimicrob. Agents Chemother., 22*:10 (1982).
146. G. L. Simon, D. R. Snydman, F. P. Tally, and S. L. Gorbach. Clinical trial of piperacillin and acquisition of resistance by *Pseudomonas* and clinical relapse. *Antimicrob. Agents Chemother., 18*:167 (1980).
147. R. L. Marier, C. V. Sanders, S. Faro, A. Janney, W. W. Williams, F. Derks, and K. E. Aldridge. Piperacillin *v* carbenicillin in the therapy for serious infections. *Arch. Intern. Med., 142*:2000 (1982).
148. D. J. Winston, W. G. Ho, L. S. Young, W. L. Hewitt, and R. P. Gale. Piperacillin plus amikacin therapy *v.* carbenicillin plus amikacin therapy in febrile, granulocytopenic patients. *Arch. Intern. Med., 142*:1663 (1982).
149. J. C. Wade, S. C. Schimpff, K. A. Newman, C. L. Fortner, H. C. Standiford, and P. H. Wiernik. Piperacillin or ticarcillin plus amikacin. A double-blind prospective comparison of empiric antibiotic therapy for febrile granulocytopenic cancer patients. *Am. J. Med., 71*:983 (1981).
150. R. B. Kohler, L. A. Foerster, L. J. Wheat, J. M. Williams, J. Reynolds, and J. Norton. Piperacillin and gentamicin *v.* carbenicillin and gentamicin for treatment of serious gram-negative infections. *Arch. Intern. Med., 142*:1335 (1982).
151. R. L. Marier, A. T. Marinaccio, C. V. Sanders, K. E. Aldridge, and J. W. Mitchell. Susceptibility patterns of bacteria following therapy with piperacillin. *J. Antimicrob. Chemother. Suppl. B, 9*:85 (1982).
152. L. O. Gentry, J. G. Jemsek, and E. A. Natelson. Effects of sodium piperacillin on platelet function in normal volunteers. *Antimicrob. Agents Chemother., 19*:532 (1981).
153. G. M. Eliopoulos and R. C. Moellering, Jr. Azlocillin, mezlocillin and piperacillin: New broad-spectrum penicillins. *Arch. Intern. Med., 97*:755 (1982).

9

Industrial Manufacture of Cephalosporins

CHARLES A. BUNNELL, WAYNE D. LUKE, and
FRED M. PERRY, Jr.
Tippecanoe Laboratories, Eli Lilly and Company, Lafayette, Indiana

I. INTRODUCTION

Cephalosporins are important antibiotics in the arsenal of drugs available to fight infectious disease in humans. A significant portion of worldwide pharmaceutical manufacturing is devoted to the production of cephalosporins. In the United States, as of 1984, the Food and Drug Administration has licensed 18 cephalosporins for clinical use and nearly an equal number are in various stages of clinical trials. In this chapter we shall discuss the general challenges facing large-scale synthesis of cephalosporins in the industrial environment and illustrate solutions to these challenges using specific examples from syntheses of cephalosporins sold in the United States. Cephalosporin antibiotics on the U.S. market and selected cephalosporins nearing approval are listed in Table 1.

II. ECONOMIC ASPECTS

In 1983 worldwide pharmaceutical sales were \$71 billion. Antibiotics accounted for \$9.2 billion of these sales and approximately \$1.2 billion was for cephalosporin antibiotics (1). In 1982, the most recent year for which statistics are available, the total antibiotic market in the United States was \$1.6 billion, with cephalosporins accounting for \$700 million (2). Sales from 10 companies represented 86% of the United States antibiotic market (Table 2; ref. 2).

A total of 75% of antibiotic sales worldwide in 1982 were for oral drugs, but in the United States oral and injectable forms accounted for equal shares of sales. In contrast, cephalosporin antibiotics sales in the United States are 75% for injectable and 25% for oral preparations (Table 1) (3–6, 10–12). American

Table 1 Cephalosporin Antibiotics on U.S. Market or in Final Stages of Clinical Trial

Generic name (generation)	Trade name	Manufacturer	U.S. approval year	Reference
Oral market				
Cefaclor (2)	Ceclor	Lilly	1979	10
Cefadroxil (1)	Ultracef	Bristol	1980	11
Cefadroxil (1)	Duricef	Mead-Johnson	1980	11
Cephalexin (1)	Keflex	Lilly	1970	10
Cephradine (1)	Anspor	Smith Kline and French	1972	
Cephradine (1)	Velosef	Squibb	1972	12
Injectable market				
Cefazolin (1)	Ancef	Smith Kline and French	1973	3
Cefazolin (1)	Kefzol	Lilly	1973	3
Cefamandole (2)	Mandol	Lilly	1978	3
Cefoperazone (3)	Cefobid	Pfizer	1983	
Cefotaxime (3)	Claforan	Hoechst-Roussel	1981	3
Cefoxitin (2)	Mefoxin	Merck	1979	3
Ceftizoxime (3)	Cefizox	Smith Kline and French	1983	
Cefuroxime (2)	Zinacef	Glaxo	1983	
Cephalothin (1)	Keflin	Lilly	1965	3
Cephapirin (1)	Cefadyl	Bristol	1974	3
Cephradine (1)	Velosef	Squibb	1978	3
Moxalactam (3)	Moxam	Lilly	1981	3
Cefonicid (2)	Monocid	Smith Kline and French	1984	
Ceforanide (2)	Precef	Bristol	1984	
Cefmenoxime (3)	Bestcall	Abbott	NA[a]	
Ceftriaxone (3)	Rocephin	Roche	1985	
Ceftazidime (3)	Fortaz	Glaxo	1985	
Ceftazidime (3)	Tazidime	Lilly	1985	

[a]NA = not approved in the United States.

Table 2 The 1982 United States Antibiotic Market Share

Company	Percentage of market
Lilly	38
Pfizer	8
Upjohn	7
Merck	7
Bristol-Myers	6
Lederle	5
Abbott	5
Smith Kline & French	4
Hoechst	3
Squibb	3

Source: Ref. 2.

sales of injectable cephalosporins, which in 1982 amounted to $528 million, were distributed as follows: 30% first-generation, 47% second-generation, and 23% third-generation cephalosporins (3). Cefazolin, developed at Fujisawa and marketed by Lilly and SKF, led the market for first-generation injectable cephalosporins, while cefoxitin and cefmandole split the second generation segment. The oral cephalosporin market is led by the first-generation cephalexin and second-generation cefaclor. All third-generation cephalosporins are injectables. The market for third-generation cephalosporins was led by cefotaxime and moxalactam. Although moxalactam is an oxacephem antibiotic, it resembles the third-generation cephalosporins in many properties and is often listed with these drugs (see the chapter by Jackson et al., this volume).

In 1983, one second-generation injectable cephalosporin, cefuroxime (Glaxo) (4), and two third generation injectable cephalosporins, ceftizoxime (Smith Kline and French) (5), and cefoperazone (Pfizer) (6), were successfully introduced into the United States marketplace.

In 1984, two second-generation and one third-generation injectable cephalosporin antibiotics (7) were approved. The most important approval in 1985 will likely be ceftazidime (Glaxo). Ceftazidime will likely be marketed by both Glaxo and Lilly (3).

The most important determinants of price of cephalosporins are dosage form and generation designation. Oral cephalosporins are less expensive than injectable cephalosporins, and first-generation cephalosporins are less expensive than the second- or third-generation drugs. The price differences among manufacturers are negligible.

The price premium for injectable cephalosporin products can be attributed to several factors. The nucleus and side chains are more expensive to produce. Sterile, particle-free formulations and extra packaging due to the specialized drug administration required for parenteral drugs all add significantly to the cost of producing the marketed product. For injectable drugs the cost to the patient is further increased by the cost of skilled labor to prepare and administer the drug. An often overlooked element in the expense of the antibiotic therapy is the frequency of administration, which can range from two to four doses per day. Cefonicid is being promoted as a once-a-day drug to reduce this element of cost (9). Nevertheless, a self-administered orally absorbed capsule or tablet will cost the patient less.

III. HISTORICAL PERSPECTIVE

Cephalosporin chemistry began with Giuseppi Brotzu's discovery of the antibiotic properties of extracts of *Cephalosporium acremonium*, a fungus isolated from seawater near a sewage outlet at Cagliara, Italy (see Chap. 1, this volume). This discovery eventually led to the isolation and structural elucidation of cephalosporin C [1], which established the unique beta-lactam moiety and con-

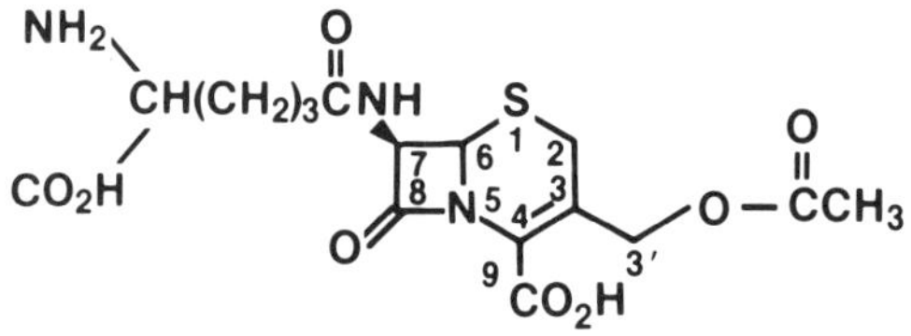

(1)

firmed it to be a structural analogue of penicillin. Early in the development of penicillins the antibiotic activity was shown to be highly dependent on the C-6 acylamido sidechain. The cephalosporin nucleus of cephalosporin C offered similar opportunities for modification at C-7 as well as potential for modifications at C-2, C-3, in the dihydrothiazine ring and at C-3. Structural activity studies have since shown that biological activity is primarily controlled by modifications at C-7, C-3, and C-3′ (13).

Although numerous methods for construction of the beta-lactam ring and the total synthesis of cephalosporins, penicillins, and their nuclear analogs have been reported (14–16), fermentation remains the method of choice for large scale industrial production of penicillins and cephalosporins. Fermentations are routinely scaled up to 25,000 to 100,000 gallon equipment or larger and offer the advantage of rigorous stereochemical control at the two chiral centers in the beta-lactam moiety.

The organisms producing cephalosporins differ in one key aspect from the organism that produces penicillins: *Penicillium chrysogenum, C. acremonium,* and *Nocardia lactamdurans* each possess enzymes that convert inexpensive raw materials to an intracellular beta-lactam, isopenicillin N. An acyltransferase in *P. chrysogenum* allows replacement of the aminoacid side chain of isopenicillin N by exogenously added phenylacetic acid or phenoxyacetic acid to produce penicillin G or V, respectively (18). *Cephalosporium acremonium* and *N. lactamdurans* lack acyltransferase but possess enzymes which convert isopenicillin N to cephalosporin C (*C. acremonium*) or cephamycin C (*N. lactamdurans*). The biosynthesis of these compounds is discussed in Chapters 5 and 13.

Four beta-lactams are commonly fermented in commercial quantities for the manufacture of cephalosporin antibiotics: cephalosporin C, penicillin V, penicillin G, and cephamycin C. Cefoxitin is the only cephalosporin manufactured from cephamycin C and all aspects of this 7-O-methylcephalosporin antibiotic are dealt with in Chapter 13. Cephalosporin C fermentation and isolation are not as efficient as the penicillin fermentations (19). Moreover, oral cephalosporins are not easily derived from cephalosporin C. Thus economic pressure has led to a great deal of research and several economically viable routes for synthesis of the cephalosporin skeleton from penicillins (20–22). The challenges facing industrial synthesis of cephalosporins can be broadly divided into six categories:

1. Selection of the precursor for generating the cephalosporin nucleus: penicillin G or V or cephalosporin C. Penicillin precursors must be rearranged into the cephalosporin skeleton.
2. Cleavage of the acylamide sidechain from the beta-lactam precursor.
3. Acylation of the beta-lactam-7-amino function intermediate with the desired antibiotic C-7 side chain.
4. Alteration of the chemical substituent at the C-3 position.
5. Construction of the C-7 or C-3 side chain.
6. Protection or activation of functional groups during synthetic transformations.

In the industrial setting the selection of materials and the adoption of a synthetic route is governed by cost and not necessarily overall yield. Protecting and activating groups thus may be selected because they impart desirable handling characteristics such as solubility or crystallinity of intermediates, thereby facilitating processing.

IV. STARTING MATERIAL

A. 3′-Heteroatom Cephalosporins

Selection of the starting material (penicillin G or V or cephalosporin C) is heavily influenced by the C-3 substituent desired in the final product. For cephalosporins containing 3-acetoxymethyl, 3-thiomethyl, or 3-aminomethyl substituents, the most direct synthetic route is from cephalosporin C. The mechanism of 3′-acetoxy displacement has been extensively studied and reviewed in the past (23,24). The 3′-acetoxy group can be readily displaced under either aqueous or nonaqueous conditions. Under aqueous conditions mechanistic studies have shown that displacement occurs via an S_N1 process with carboxyl group stabilization of the intermediate carbonium ion. Hence protection of the C-4 carboxyl group is not necessary and, in fact, impedes reaction. Aqueous or mixed-solvent system reactions are typically buffered and conducted at moderately elevated temperatures ranging from 30 to 100°C. Under such conditions lactone formation is not significant.

Two general approaches to improving 3′-acetoxy displacement yields have been reported in the patent literature: These use Lewis or Bronsted acid activation or initial in situ conversion of the acetoxy group to a more facile leaving group.

Boron trifluoride complexes of ethers, alcohols, and acids facilitate displacements under nonaqueous conditions (25). Likewise, protonic acids, particularly methane sulfonic acid, trifluoroacetic acid, and hydrogen iodide, can facilitate 3′-acetoxy displacements (26). Additions of inorganic salts such as potassium iodide and potassium thiocyanate have been reported to enhance displacement yields (27,28). The exact role of the added salts is difficult to assess. Initial acetoxy displacement by the added ions does not appear to occur. Thus the salts may enhance yields by serving as Lewis acids or by altering the ionic strengths of the medium; in some cases where amine displacement leads to betaines the added salts may stabilize the products (28).

Conversion to a more facile, sulfur-based leaving group can be effected by treatment with sodium thiosulfate or salts of a wide variety of thio and dithio acids. Much of this work was reported during the early development of cephaloridine and has been reviewed elsewhere (29). More recently the 3′-acetoxy group has been converted to a bromide by reaction with boron tribromide under anhydrous conditions (30) or to an iodide by reaction with trimethylsilyl iodide (31,32).

B. 3-Methyl Cephalosporins

Penicillins V and G are the preferred starting materials for synthesis of 3-methyl cephalosporin. Although direct reduction of the 3′-acetoxy group of intermediates derived from cephalosporin C has been achieved by catalytic hydrogenation (33,34) and more recently by acid-catalyzed reduction with trialkysilylanes (35), the most economical route to 3-methyl cephalosporins involves acid-catalyzed rearrangement of penicillin sulfoxides. Since Morin first reported rearrangement of penicillin sulfoxides into 3-methyl cephalosporins (36), at least 20 additional U.S. patents have been granted covering specific catalysts, solvents, and substrates and several papers discussing the reaction mechanism have appeared (20,37). Carboxylic acid protection is required and high yields are dependent on judicious choice of protecting groups, acid catalyst, and solvent. The protecting group can be selected so that removal occurs during isolation of the ring-expanded product or the protecting group may be left intact for use during subsequent C-7 side-chain cleavage and reacylation steps. The best of the former conditions involves trimethylsilyl protection of [2] followed by ring expansion with pyridine hydrobromide/bistrimethylsilylurea in toluene followed by hydrolysis of the silyl ester. This process forms [3] in 97% yield (38) (Fig. 1).

The benzhydryl, p-nitrobenzyl, and trichloroethyl esters are more stable protecting groups than trimethylsilyl esters. These more stable esters of penicillin V or G undergo ring expansion best in 1,4-dioxane (39) or 1,1,2-trichloroethane (40) using pyridine salts of phosphonic acids as catalyst, a process developed by Glaxo (41).

The high yield and relatively low cost for preparation of 3-methyl-δ-3-cephalosporins from penicillins has made them attractive as precursors that are potentially economically competitive to cephalosporin C for synthesis of 3-thiomethyl and 3-pyridinium-methyl cephalosporins. Allylic bromination of the methyl group of 3-methyl-δ-3-cephem sulfoxide esters bearing a variety of 7-amino substituents has been reported under photochemical conditions (42–47).

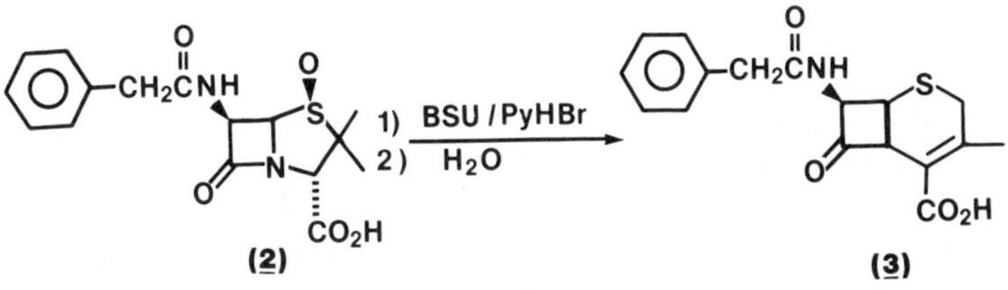

Figure 1

Competing bromination at C-2 is significant and appears to be a function of the 7-amino substituent. For example, the trichloroacetyl side chain completely suppresses C-2 bromination (42). Gist-Brocades has patented the most promising route to 3′-thio cephalosporins by selective reaction at the allylic center (47). By sequential reactions, [4], derived from [3], was photobrominated, leading to a mixture of [5] and [6], which was treated with trimethylphosphite to effect reduction at C-2 followed by thiol displacement at C-3′ to afford [8]. The overall yield from the sulfoxide [4] to isolated [8] was 54% (Fig. 2).

C. 3-Heteroatom Cephalosporins

Synthetically, cephalosporins with direct hydrogen or heteroatom substitution at C-3 require removal of the 3′-carbon atom from the cephalosporin skeleton. Retrosynthesis shows that the 3′-carbon can be excised by ozonolysis of a 3-methylenecepham [9], which could serve as a key intermediate in the synthesis

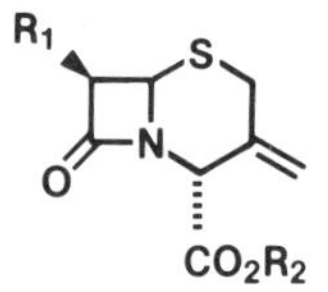

(9)

of all C-3 heteroatom cephalosporins. Several research groups have developed routes to 3-methylenecephams from penicillins and from cephalosporins derived from cephalosporin C.

This chemistry, as well as the conversion of the methylenecephams into cefaclor, has been recently reviewed and will not be discussed here (17,22,48). Economically the most viable routes to 3-methylenecephams are from penicillins; thus industrially penicillins V and G serve as the ultimate precursors for all C-3 heteroatom cephalosporins.

D. 3′-Carbamoyl Cephalosporins

Deacetylcephalosporins serve as starting materials for 3′-carbamoyl cephalosporins. Deacetylcephalosporin C is a minor component in cephalosporin C fermentations (49), and although organisms have been found that produce a preponderance of deacetylcephalosporin C, they have never been commercialized (50).

Hydrolytic deacylation of a cephalosporin acid or ester under basic conditions usually suffers from either double-bond isomerization or beta-lactam

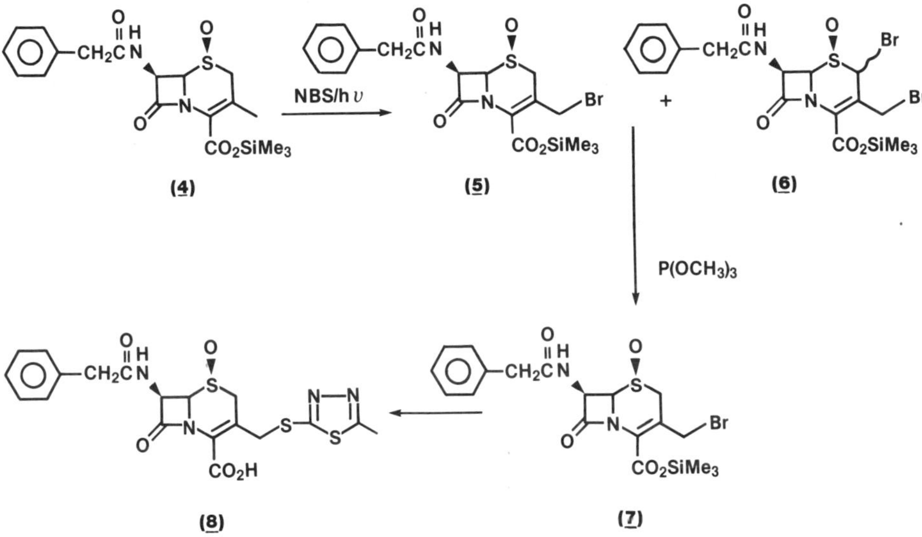

Figure 2

cleavage. Treatment of cephalosporin C under such conditions leads to a low yield of deacetylcephalosporin C and is of little practical utility (51). Deacylation of 7-aminocephalosporanic acid (7-ACA) [10] by treatment with 2 Eq of aqueous NaOH for 0.5 hr at 0°C is reported to afford [11] in 64% yield (52, 53) (Fig. 3). While this is a useful method for generating laboratory quantities of [11], large-scale manufacture by this process is doubtful.

Enzymatic deacylation can be effectively employed with a wide variety of esterases and cephalosporin substrates (51–56,130). The enzymatic cleavage is advantageous because the reaction conditions are mild and the enzyme is potentially

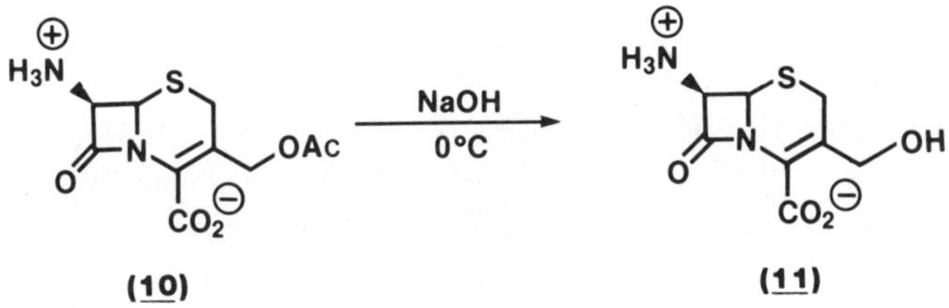

Figure 3

recoverable. The mild conditions minimize beta-lactam cleavage, double-bond isomerization, and lactone formation. Glaxo has reported using an enzymatic process to hydrolyze 7-ACA to [9] in their synthesis of cefuroxime (57).

V. C-7 SIDE-CHAIN CLEAVAGE

The true birth of the industrial production of semisynthetic penicillins and cephalosporins began with the development of successful methods for cleavage of the acylamino side chains of penicillin G, penicillin V, and cephalosporin C. The first efficient method for conversion of cephalosporin C to 7-ACA involved diazotization with nitrosylchloride followed by hydrolysis or alcoholysis to afford 7-ACA in 50% yield (58–60). Diazotization leads to a cyclic imino ether [12]

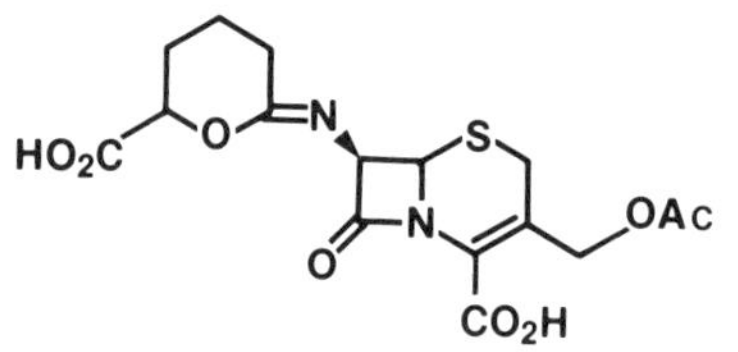

(12)

which hydrolyzes under far milder conditions than those required for direct hydrolysis of the 7-amide bond.

Realizing that other 7-amino intermediates may hydrolyze as easily, Ciba scientists developed a general procedure for penicillin and cephalosporin side-chain cleavage that involves initial conversion of the amide linkage into an imino chloride. This conversion was achieved under anhydrous conditions by reaction with phosphorus trichloride or phosphorus pentachloride, followed by alcoholysis to an imino ether, and subsequent hydrolysis to the free amine (61). More recently Lilly scientists have formed imino chlorides using a complex derived from addition of chlorine to triphenylphosphite (62).

Industrially, phosphorus pentachloride remains the reagent of choice for side-chain cleavage of penicillins and cephalosporins. The mechanisms of imino ether formation and preferred alcohols for effecting this conversion have been recently reviewed (63).

Cephalosporin C side-chain cleavage via the Ciba phosphorus pentachloride process required protection of the free carboxyl and amine groups. Typically these groups were protected by reaction with acetyl chloride in methylene chloride before the cleavage reactions. After this sequence of reactions, the C-4 mixed anhydride was hydrolyzed and 7-ACA was precipitated directly from the reaction mixture by adjusting the pH to its isoelectric point. In a similar manner the desacetoxycephalosporin, protected as its trimethylsilyl ester, had the side chain removed to form 7-aminodesacetoxycephalosporanic acid (7-ADCA).

Technology for enzymatic C-7 side-chain cleavage has been developed in recent years, mainly by Toyo Jozo (64,65). The use of immobilized enzyme systems for industrial productions of 7-ACA and 7-ADCA would seem to have a significant economic advantage over most chemical cleavage methods. Enzymatic cleavage has been reported to give isolated yields of 80-90% of theory. Enzymatic cleavage of cephalosporin C has required protection or removal of the amino group from the aminoadipoyl side chain before enzymatic cleavage of the amide bond (65). This two-step sequence reduces or eliminates the economic advantage over chemical cleavage.

Both 7-ACA and 7-ADCA are chemical items of commerce and are prepared in large scale in the industrial environment (66). As such, 7-ACA and 7-ADCA serve as starting materials for most industrial processes for semisynthetic cephalosporin antibiotics.

VI. 7-AMINO ACYLATION

Virtually all of the known methods for acyl group activation and subsequent N-acylation of amines and amino acids have been reported or patented for N-acylation of cephalosporins. The parallels between peptide chemistry and the acylation of penicillins and cephalosporin are well documented. Industrially, the most common activation involves conversion to an acid chloride or a mixed anhydride. Acid chloride acylations are often effected under Schotten-Bauman conditions, while mixed anhydrides are employed strictly in anhydrous reactions. For example, the C-7 1-(1H)-tetrazolylacetyl side-chain of cefazolin has been introduced by dropwise addition of 1-(1H)-tetrazolylacetyl chloride at 0°C to an aqueous acetone solution of 7-ACA buffered at pH 7.0-8.0 with sodium bicarbonate. The product was isolated by acidification, extraction into ethyl acetate, and subsequent precipitation as its sodium salt (67). Similarly, cefonicid has been prepared by addition of [13] to [14] in aqueous acetone buffered at pH 7.2 with sodium bicarbonate (68).

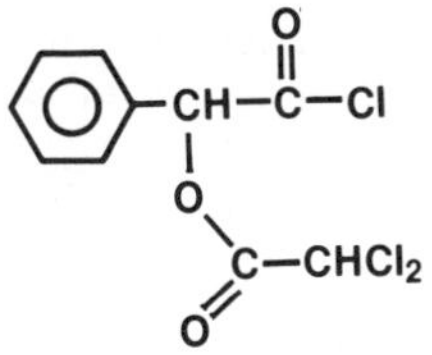

(13)

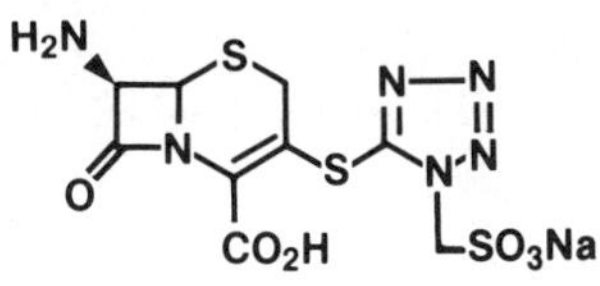

(14)

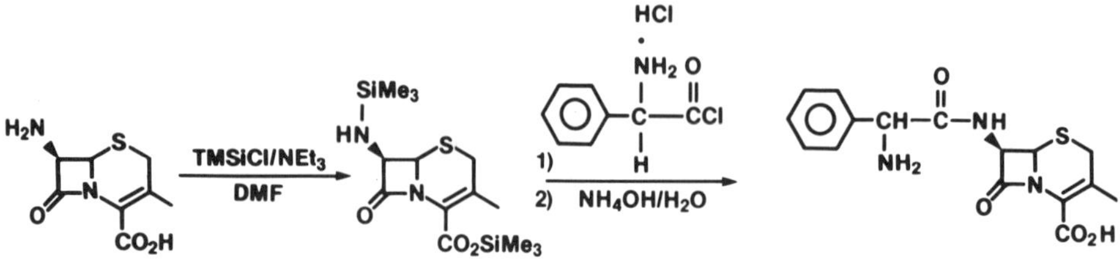

(15) (16) (17)

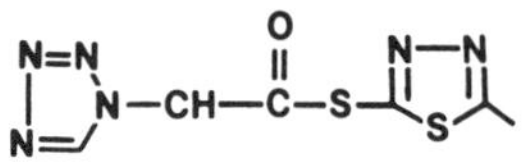

(18)

Figure 4

Acylations of 7-ACA or 7-ADCA under nonaqueous conditions are difficult owing to the very low solubility of these compounds in most organic solvents. Silylation of 7-ACA or 7-ADCA affords readily soluble silyl esters that are easily acylated under anhydrous conditions. Silylation enjoys the advantage that silyl groups are easily introduced at ambient temperature and readily hydrolyzed. The route to cephalexin utilized by Glaxo (Fig. 4) illustrates this method (69). The silylation reaction is effected at ambient temperature and the final product is precipitated from the reaction mixture by pH adjustment with ammonium hydroxide.

A novel type of acyl group activation, unique to cephalosporin chemistry, involves acylation of 7-ACA with a thio ester composed of the C-7 and C-3 side chains of the desired cephalosporin product. As acylation occurs, the thio group is liberated to effect 3′-acetoxy displacement. Asahi has reported that heating an aqueous acetone solution of [18] and 7-ACA at pH 6.4 for 4 hr at 60°C afforded a 90.6% yield of cefazolin (70–72). This route requires that the optimum stoichiometry and reaction conditions in both the acylation and the displacement reactions be identical, which is rarely the case.

VII. SELECTION OF THE SYNTHETIC ROUTE

Three transformations, side-chain cleavage, 7-amino acylation, and 3′-displacement, are required for preparation of most semisynthetic cephalosporins from

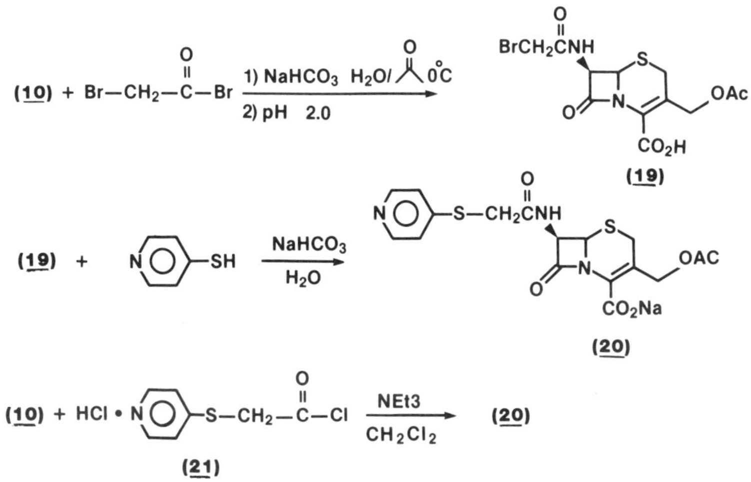

Figure 5

cephalosporin C. The chemical literature describes three possible sequences:

1. 3′-Displacement, side-chain cleavage, 7-amino acylation
2. Side-chain cleavage, 7-amino acylation, 3′-displacement
3. Side-chain cleavage, 3′-displacement, 7-amino acylation

In the industrial environment yield is not the dominant factor in selection of a particular route. More important considerations are cost of raw materials, manufacturing costs, and patent rights—all of which define the final cost of the product. Raw materials costs and step yields require introduction of expensive materials as late as possible in the synthetic sequence. For this reason, the second and third sequences are invariably more cost effective than the first.

Both the C-7 and the C-3 side chains can be introduced as the side chain present in the final antibiotic or as a partial unit further elaborated on the cephalosporin nucleus. An example of the latter is provided in Bristol's two routes to cephapirin [20] (Fig. 5). The first route involves acylation of 7-ACA with bromoacetylbromide to afford [19], which was treated with 4-mercaptopyridine to afford cephapirin [20] (73). In the second route the acid chloride [21] was used to acylate 7-ACA to yield [20] directly (74).

Again cost usually favors complete construction of the side chains before their attachment to the cephalosporin nucleus.

Table 3 Cephalosporins on the U.S. Market or in Final Stages of Clinical Trials

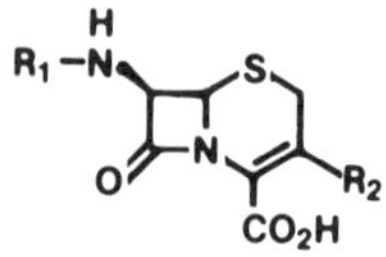

R_1	R_2	Generic Name	References
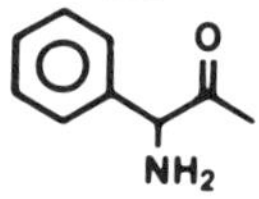	$-CH_3$	Cephalexin	[103-105]
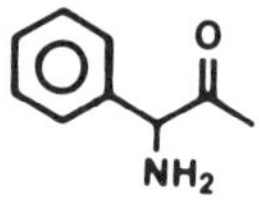	$-Cl$	Cefaclor	[106]
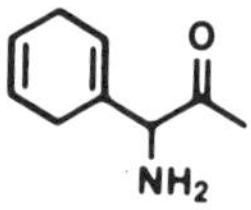	$-CH_3$	Cephradine	[74, 76, 107]
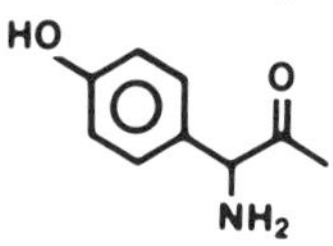	$-CH_3$	Cefadroxil	[108, 109]
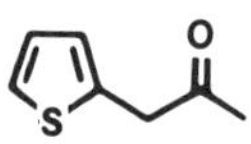	$-CH_2OAC$	Cephalothin	[131]
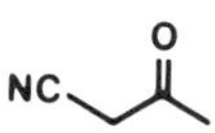	$-CH_2OAC$	Cephacetrile	[110]
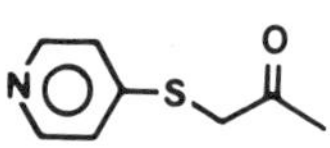	$-CH_2OAC$	Cephapirin	[73, 74, 111]
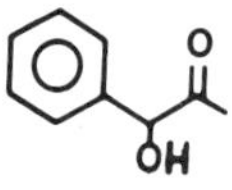	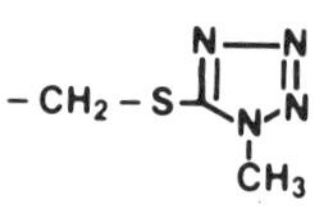	Cefamandole	[83, 112]
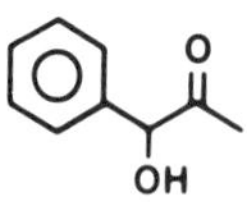	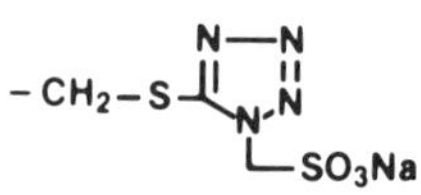	Cefonicid	[128]
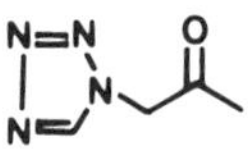	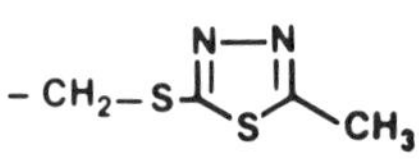	Cefazolin	[77-81]

Table 3 (Continued)

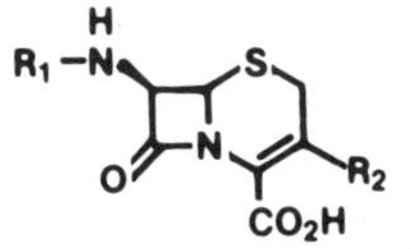

R_1	R_2	Generic Name	References
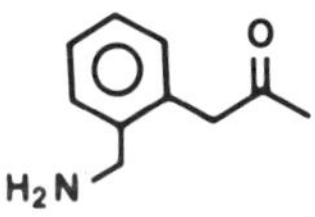	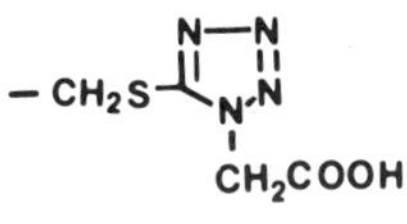	Ceforanide	[113-115]
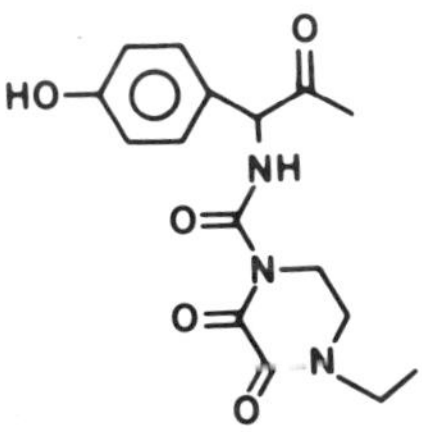	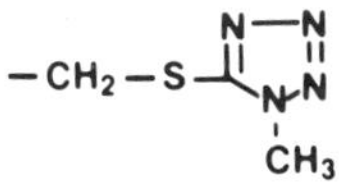	Cefoperazone	[116-118]
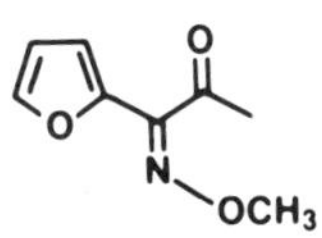	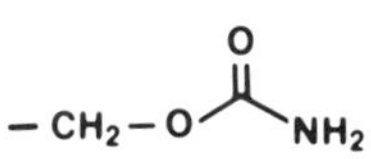	Cefuroxime	[101, 119-122]
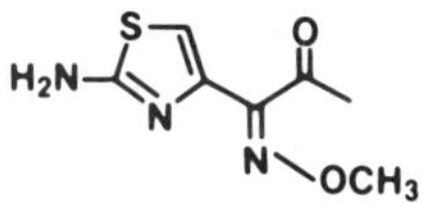	$-CH_2OAC$	Cefotaxime	[123, 124]
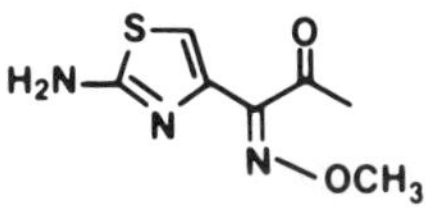	−H	Ceftizoxime	[93, 125]
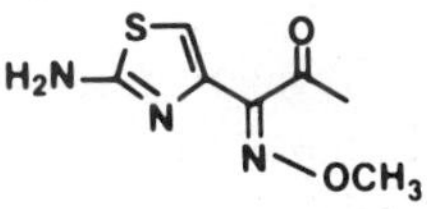	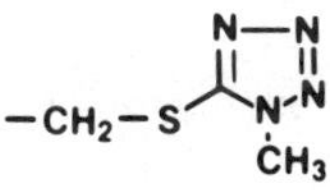	Cefmenoxime	[123, 126]
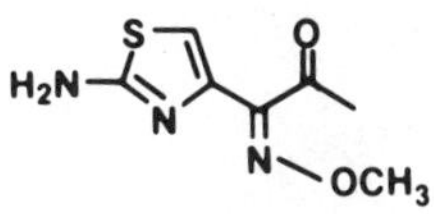	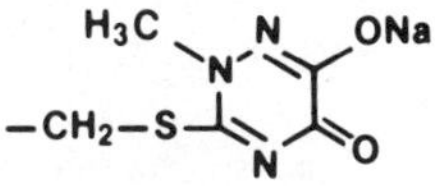	Ceftriaxone	[127]
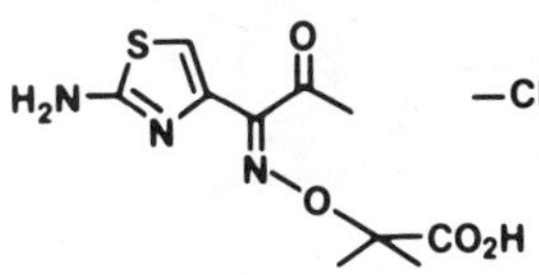	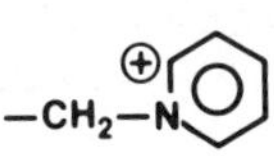	Ceftazidime	[87, 129]

VIII. SIDE-CHAIN SYNTHESIS

A. Introduction

In recent years a significant part of synthesis of new cephalosporin products has been devoted to the synthesis of side chains. There has been a natural evolution from the testing of simpler to more complex chemical structures. Since the synthesis of most cephalosporins from 7-ACA involves only two chemical steps (acylation at C-7 and displacement at C-3′), considerable chemistry may be involved in the synthesis of the side chains, especially for third-generation cephalosporins. Because of the chemical complexity of some side chains, their production adds significantly to the cost of final products. This combination of interesting chemistry and economic importance has led us to include side chain synthesis as a separate section in this chapter.

The side chains specifically discussed here were chosen mainly for their economic importance. Table 3 gives references for the synthesis of the other side chains. Information concerning the exact manufacture of side chains is strictly proprietary; however, synthetic strategies and general methodologies can be obtained from the patent and chemical literature. One should note that the yields from patents generally represent crude yields and no inference can be made concerning the suitability of crude materials in subsequent steps.

B. 2-(1,4-Cyclohexadienyl)glycine

Phenylglycine [22], a rare example of a C-7 side chain that permits good oral absorption, appears in cephalexin and cefaclor. In a modification of this side chain Squibb discovered that 2-(1,4-cyclohexadienyl) glycine, [23] gave ceph-

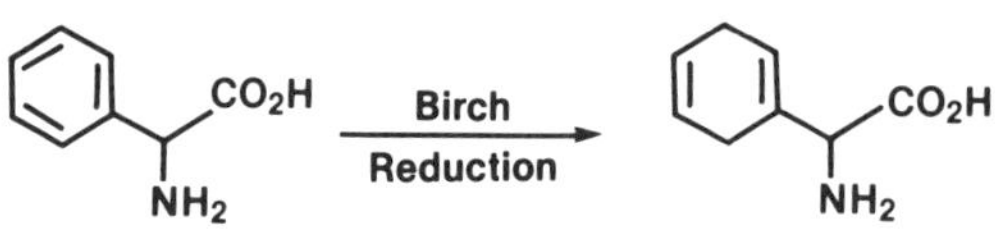

(22) (23)

radine, which is pharmacologically similar to cephalexin. Squibb's original synthesis of [23] involved a Birch reduction using lithium metal, ammonia, and t-butanol (75,76). More recently Nippon Kasei has reported reduction using sodium metal with water as a cosolvent (77).

C. 1H-Tetrazoleacetic Acid and 5-Methyl-1,3,4-Thiadiazole-2-Thiol

Cefazolin, an important injectable antibiotic, contains an interesting and relatively inexpensive side chain at both C-7 and C-3′. Two processes (Fig. 6) for

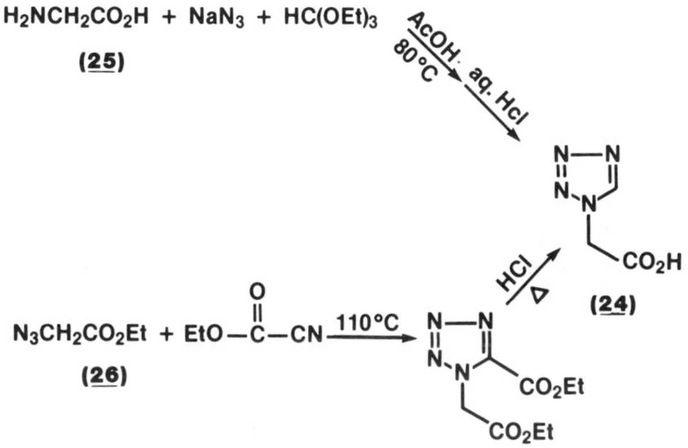

Figure 6

preparing tetrazole acetic acid [24] have been reported. A Fujisawa process (78) starts with glycine [25], while a Lilly process (79) begins with ethyl azidoacetate [26].

The former process has the advantage of using more readily available starting materials. Likewise, both Fujisawa (80) and Lilly (81) have disclosed processes for production of 5-methyl-1,3,4-thiadiazole-2-thiol (Fig. 7).

The processes differ fundamentally only in the order of hydrazine addition to carbon disulfide. The Fujisawa process reacted dithiocarbazic acid [28] derived from hydrazine and carbon disulfide, with several ester synthons, while the Lilly process reacted specifically thioamides [29] first with hydrazine and then with carbon disulfide.

D. 1H-Tetrazole Thiols

Second- and third-generation cephalosporins such as cefamandole, cefoperazone, cefmenoxime, cefonicid, and ceforanide contain the 1H-tetrazole-5-thio group [30]. The paucity of patents on the synthesis of this important side chain may be due to the simple synthesis reported in 1930 from methylisothiocyanate [31] (82).

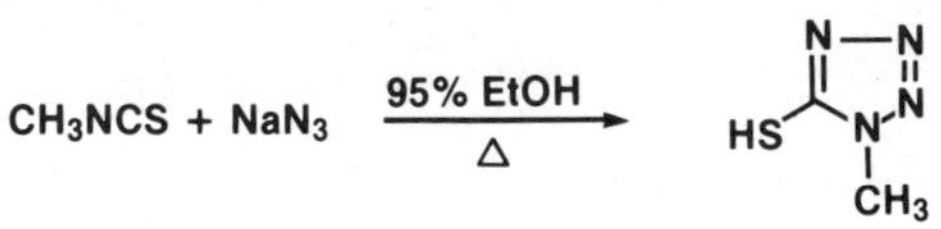

(31) (30)

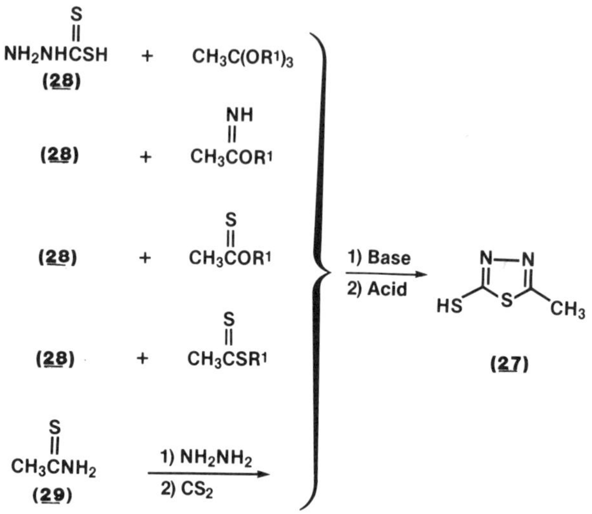

Figure 7

A general synthesis of 1-alkyltetrazole-5-thiols [32] from alkyl thiosemicarbazides [33] has been reported (83); however, industrial production of 1-methyltetrazole-5-thiol by this procedure is doubtful.

An approach via the dithiocarbamates [34] similar to the original route to [30] has been reported for the synthesis of the tetrazole-5-thiol acids [32a] and [32b] (84), which are used in cefonicid and ceforanide, respectively (Fig. 8).

A recently published synthesis of [32b] begins with tetrazoyl-1-acetic acid [24], which is brominated and treated with thiourea, base, and then acid (85).

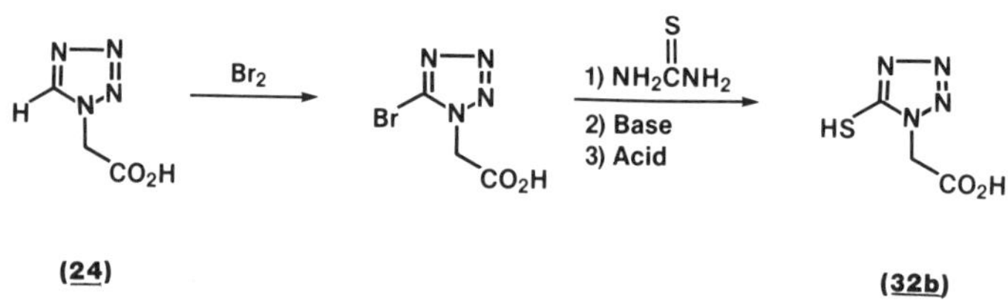

E. 2-(2-Amino-4-Thiazolyl)-2-Oximinoacetic Acid

The potent antibiotic action that is conferred by the 2-(2-amino-4-thiazolyl)-2-oximinoacetic acid [41] side chain has led to proliferation of cephalosporins

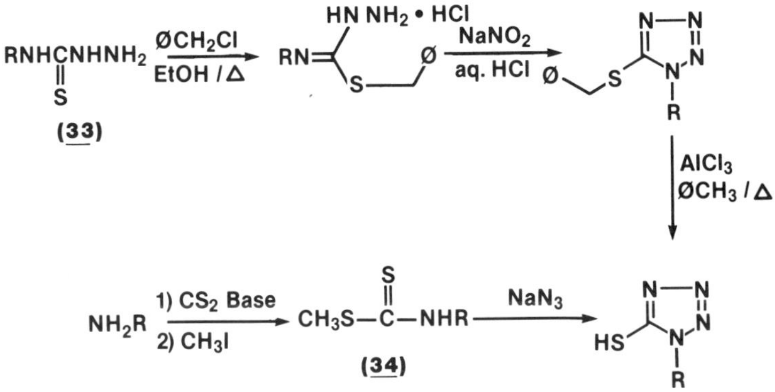

(33)

(34)

(32)

R

a) $-CH_2SO_3H$
b) $-CH_2CO_2H$
c) —alkyl

Figure 8

bearing this moiety. At least five of these compounds have either been approved or are pending approval in the United States. The fierce worldwide competition is exemplified in the patent literature by a morass of overlapping claims and art; consequently, only a fraction of the related patent literature will be mentioned here.

There are a number of synthetic approaches to [41], generally starting from ethyl acetoacetate (Fig. 9), although ethyl acetoglyoxylate [42] (Fig. 10) has also been reported as a starting material. Many paths are available to produce the desired products [40] or [41]. It is not clear from the chemical literature which path is most advantageous. The basic issues for chemical synthesis of this side chain are the sequence for construction of the alkoxime, the method of halogenation, thiazole formation, protection of the thiazole-2-amino group and maintenance of the proper syn geometry of the oxime.

The routes in Figures 9 and 10 are fundamentally different in the order of oximation. The ethyl acetoacetate route (86) establishes the oxime early with a sodium nitrate oxidation to give [35] or [37] (87,88) followed by thiazole ring formation. A comprehensive discussion of the route illustrated in Figure 9 is found in Fujisawa patents (87,89), including an example of the synthesis of pharmaceutically important methoxime compound [51] (Fig. 11). On paper at least, this sequence from [47] to [51] represents the epitomy of a desirable commercial process, that is, the chemistry is simple and the raw materials are inexpensive.

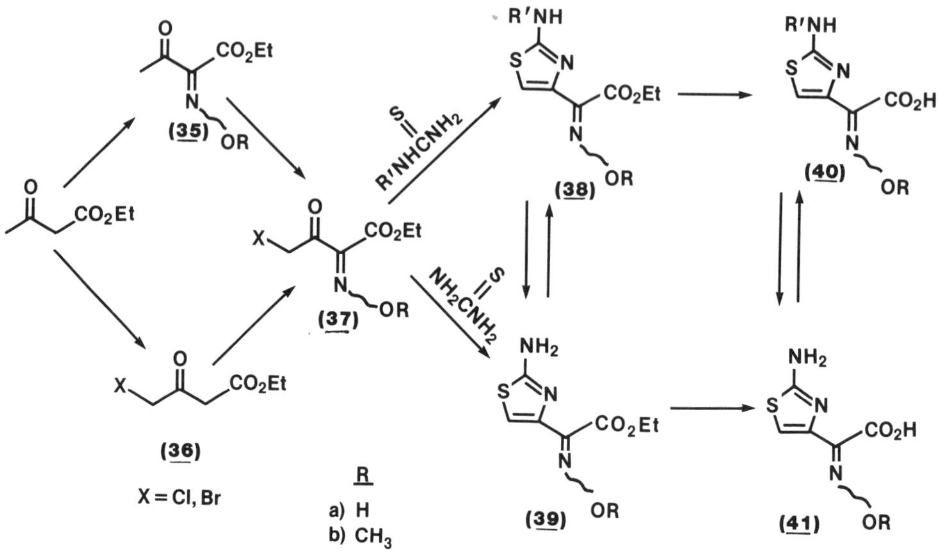

Figure 9

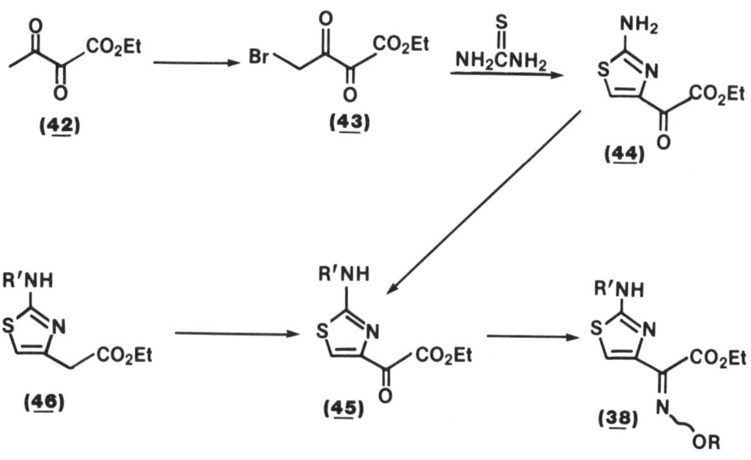

Figure 10

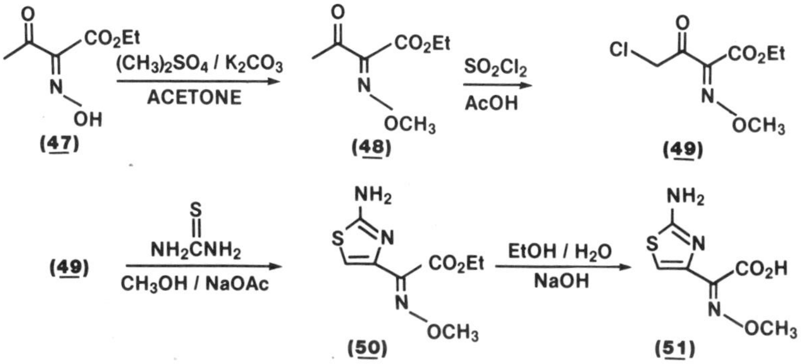

Figure 11

The diketo structures of [42] and [43] (Fig. 10) dictate that construction of the thiazole must occur before oximation. Because of the late entry of the oxime, the use of alkoxyamines more complicated than methoxyamine can occur without loss of the expensive side chain on subsequent steps (90). The keto ester [45] (R′ = mesyl) has also been prepared by selenium dioxide oxidation of [46] (R′ = mesyl) (91).

On the other hand, the timing for halogenation does not seem to be particularly important starting from either ethyl acetoacetate or keto-oxime [35] (Fig. 9). Sulfonyl chloride has been the reagent of choice for chlorination (86, 88,89,92,93), while bromine has typically been used for bromination (92,94). The use of ketals [52] has also been claimed but probably does not represent a commercially viable process (95).

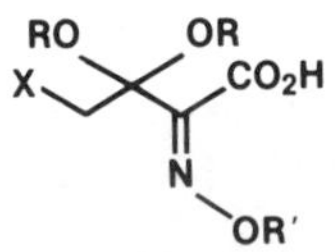

(52)

Thiazole formation is simple conceptually; however, this step is generally the lowest-yielding step (30–70%) in Figure 9. Typical conditions are reaction of keto-oxime [37] with thiourea in an alcohol solvent, either in the presence of a base (88,89,93) or without added base (96,97).

Protection of the thiazole-2-amino group is dependent on the acylation procedure used for attaching the side chain to the cephalosporin nucleus. For example, no protection is needed if the acid function is activated as a thiol ester [53] (98). Using standard activation methods and common protecting groups,

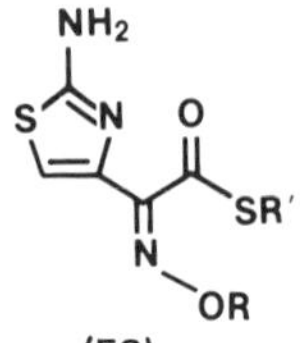

(53)

amine protection has generally been employed. Of these, trityl seems to be one of the more popular, probably because it lends crystallinity to intermediates. Trityl derivatives such as keto-ester [45] (R′ = trityl) (92) and oxime ester [38a] (R′ = trityl) (88) have been prepared by the reaction of [44] and [39a], respectively, with trityl chloride and triethylamine at low temperature (-15 to -30°C) in dimethylformamide (DMF). Direct synthesis of the thiazole [38b] (R′ = CO_2TCE) from the reaction of keto-oxime ester [37b] (X = Br) with trichloroethoxycarbonyl thiourea has been reported by Takeda (97).

It is well-known that the syn isomer [54] is more potent than the anti-isomer [55] (99); therefore preparation and maintenance of the proper oxime stereo-

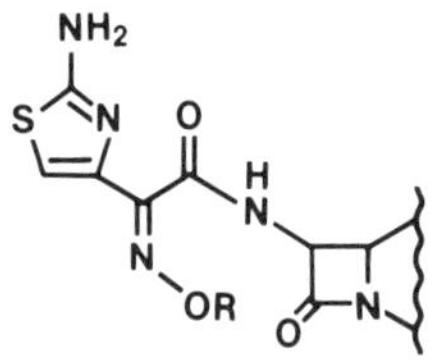

(54)

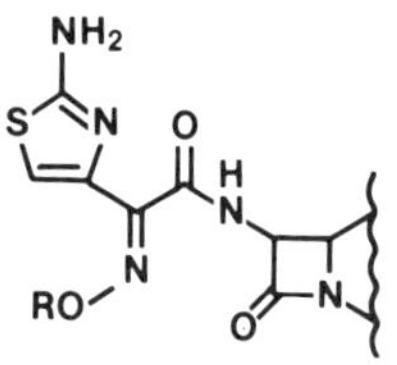

(55)

chemistry is essential. There is little in the patent literature to address the issue. Although it has not been explicitly stated, selective crystallization or stereoselective synthesis must be achieved in the techniques used to produce the syn isomer predominantly. For example, a Fujisawa patent reports preparation of the syn isomer of [50] by selective crystallization of the anti-isomer as its hydrobromide salt from a reaction mixture (100).

Glaxo has patented a procedure to enrich a mixture of aryloxime esters [56] and [57] in favor of the syn isomer [57] by selective hydrolysis of the anti-isomer [56] to the anti-acid [58] (99). The acid [58] was recycled by esterification and reequilibration to a syn/anti-mixture under acidic conditions.

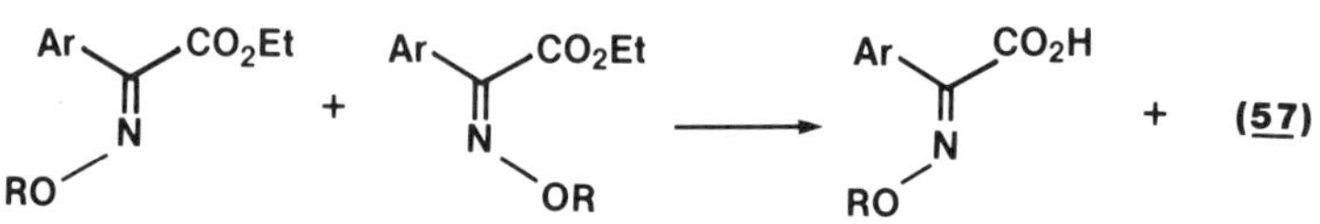

(56) (57) (58)

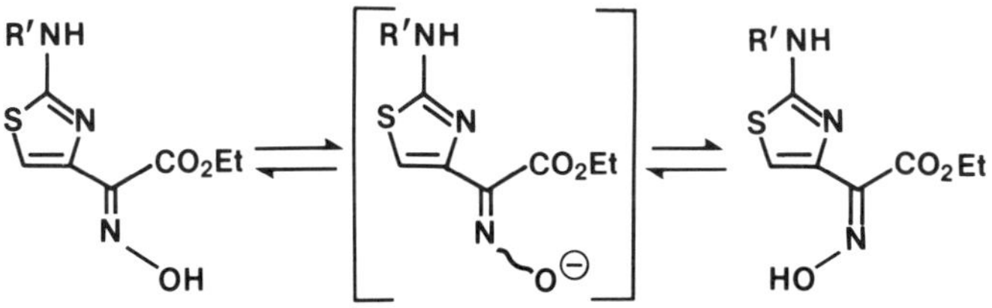

(59) (60) (61)

Figure 12

Fujisawa reports the direct synthesis of the syn oxime [51] from the corresponding keto acid and methoxyamine hydrochloride (91).

Despite the sensitivity of the oxime to isomerization, the proper syn stereochemistry can be maintained in the sequence from keto-oxime [35] to either [40] or [41] (89).

Isomerization of the parent oxime [59] to [61] can occur under basic conditions via the anion [60] (Fig. 12). In the synthesis of the ceftazidime side-chain precursor [63], conditions have been found that allow O-alkylation of the oxime [62] in good yield (101) (Fig. 13) with little syn/anti-isomerization.

Finally, there are several methods using standard procedures that allow preparation of the acid chloride [65] from the acid [64a] without substantial isomerization of the oxime (91,96,102) (Fig. 14). Glaxo particularly cites the use of the sodium salt [64b] with oxalyl chloride in the presence of DMF as a method for making [65] without oxime isomerization (96) (Fig. 14).

Although there are patents claiming processes and compounds for attaching part of the side chain to the cephalosporin nucleus before finishing construction of the oximinothiazole group, these routes have not been discussed because they are economically unfeasible. In particular, formation of the aminothiazole of a cephalosporin derivative is unreasonable, since thiazole formation is such a low-yielding step.

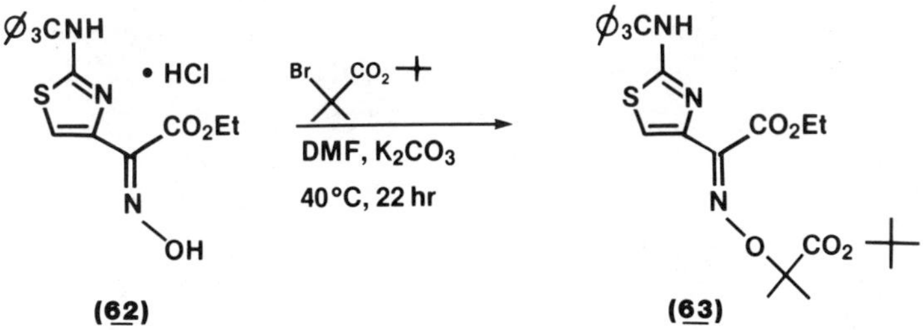

(62) (63)

Figure 13

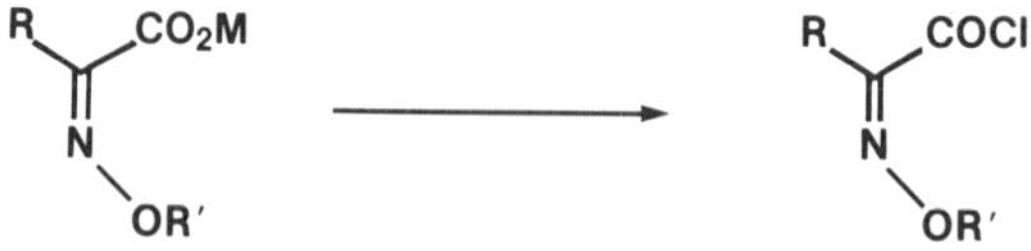

(64)

M
a) H
b) Na

Figure 14

IX. FUTURE PROSPECTS

The pharmaceutical use of cephalosporins has not reached its zenith, judging from the number of cephalosporins in various stages of clinical trials in the United States and elsewhere. The introduction of new cephalosporin antibiotics coupled with the fact that several of the early cephalosporins in the U.S. market are reaching the end of their patent life will have a major impact on future cephalosporin production. Both factors will lead to a more competitive market and hence the continued development and optimization of cost-effective routes to cephalosporins. All of the current cephalosporins (excluding cefoxitin; see Chap. 13), as well as those presently in clinical trials, are prepared semisynthetically from penicillin V or G or cephalosporin C. Thus the optimization of penicillin and cephalosporin C fermentation, coupled with isolation and conversion of these primary fermentation products into the common precursors 7-ACA and 7-ADCA, will remain an important challenge to the commercial cephalosporin industry.

Industrial use of enzymatic processes for amide side-chain cleavage in penicillin production has been discussed in Chapter 6. Enzymatic hydrolysis has the advantages of high yield, recyclable reagents, and operation at moderate temperature, in addition to the avoidance of expensive solvents, toxic reagents, and hazardous by-products which have a poor environmental impact. Consideration of these advantages suggests that development of an efficient enzymatic process for aminoadipoyl side-chain cleavage in cephalosporin C, without amine protection, would be highly desirable and will certainly see greater work in the future.

REFERENCES

1. World pharmaceutical market forecast by French analyst. *IMS Pharm. Market Lett.*, Feb. 20, p. 11 (1984).
2. R. B. Sykes and J. P. Valles. Business outlook: Antibiotics market still peaking. *High Technol.*, Dec. p. 66 (1983).

3. Injectable cephalosporin market analyzed. *Scrip-World Pharm. News,* April 11, p. 11 (1983).
4. C. Clark. Glaxo Co. Update. *Scrimgeour, Kemp-Gee and Co.,* Report No. 400440, p. 7 (1984).
5. R. Victor. Smith Kline Beckman Corporation Up-date. *Drexel Burnham Lambert Inc.,* Report No. 306038, p. 5 (1983).
6. A. H. Snider and M. N. Kampf. Pfizer, Inc. Company Follow-Up, *Kidder, Peabody and Co. Inc.,* Report No. 304260, p. 14 (1983).
7. News U.S. drug approval predictions. *Scrip-World Pharm. News,* Feb. 8, p. 14 (1984).
8. *1984 Redbook – Drug Topics Annual Pharmacists' Reference,* 88th ed., Medical Economics, Oradell, New Jersey, 1984.
9. Smith Klines drug sales + 9.7% in '82. *Scrip-World Pharm. News,* April 13, p. 7 (1983).
10. D. L. Smith and J. D. France. Eli Lilly and Co. A basic study. *Smith Barney, Harris Upham and Co. Inc.,* Report No. 200061, p. 39 (1982).
11. K. Blair. Bristol-Meyers – Action Recommendation. *Donaldson Lufkin and Jenrett, Inc.,* Report No. 303415, p. 3 (1982).
12. D. L. Smith. Squibb Corp – An Update. *Smith Barney, Harris Upham and Co. Inc.,* Report 200108, p. 18 (1982).
13. M. Gorman and C. W. Ryan. Structure–activity relationships of β-lactam antibiotics, in *Cephalosporins and Penicillins Chemistry and Biology* (E. H. Flynn, ed.), Academic, New York, 1972, p. 532.
14. K. Heusler. Total synthesis of penicillins and cephalosporins, in *Cephalosporins and Penicillins Chemistry and Biology* (E. H. Flynn, ed.), Academic, New York, 1972, p. 255.
15. K. G. Holden. Total synthesis of penicillins, cephalosporins and their nuclear analogs, in *Chemistry and Biology of β-Lactam Antibiotics,* Vol. 2 (R. B. Morin and M. Gorman, eds.), Academic, New York, 1982, p. 99.
16. B. G. Christensen and T. N. Salzmann. Strategy in the total synthesis of β-lactam antibiotics, in *Antibiotics Containing the β-Lactam Structure* (A. L. Demain and N. A. Solomon, eds.), Springer-Verlag, New York, 1983, p. 329.
17. F. A. Jung, W. R. Pilgrim, J. P. Poysen, and P. J. Siret. The chemistry and antimicrobial activity of new synthetic β-lactam antibiotics, in *Topics in Antibiotic Chemistry,* Vol. 4 (P. G. Sammes, ed.), Wiley, New York, 1980.
18. A. L. Demain. Biosynthesis of β-lactam antibiotics, in *Antibiotics Containing the Beta-Lactam Structure* (A. L. Demain and N. A. Solomon, eds.), Springer-Verlag, New York, 1983, p. 189.
19. R. Burcourt. Synthetic or semisynthetic pathways? An open question for the routes to cephalosporin of the new generation, in *Recent Advances in the Chemistry of β-Lactam Antibiotics* (G. I. Gregory, ed.), Royal Society of Chemistry, London, 1980, p. 1.
20. R. D. G. Cooper and D. O. Spry. Rearrangements of cephalosporins and penicillins, in *Cephalosporins and Penicillins Chemistry and Biology* (E. H. Flynn, ed.), Academic, New York, 1972, p. 183.

21. R. Scartazzini and H. Bickel. New orally active cephalosporins. *Heterocycles, 7*:1165 (1977).
22. M. Gorman, R. R. Chauvette, and S. Kukolja. Cefaclor, in *Chronicles of Drug Discovery,* Vol. 2 (J. S. Bindra and D. Lednicer, eds.), Wiley, New York, 1983, p. 49.
23. A. B. Taylor. Cephalosporin acids. Part III. Reactions with pyridine: kinetics and mechanism. *J. Chem. Soc., 1965*:7020 (1965).
24. L. D. Hatfield, J. W. Fischer, J. M. Dunigan, R. W. Burchfield, J. M. Greene, J. A. Webber, R. T. Vasileff, and M. D. Kinnich. Cephalosporin acids; a new look at reactions at the C-3′ position. *Philos. Trans. R. Soc. London, B289*: 173 (1980).
25. U.S. patent 4,317,907 (1982).
26. U.S. patent 4,014,874 (1977).
27. U.S. patent 3,270,012 (1966).
28. J. L. Spencer, F. Y. Siu, B. G. Jackson, H. M. Higgens, and E. H. Flynn. Chemistry of cephalosporin antibiotics. IX. Synthesis of cephaloridine. *J. Org. Chem., 32*:500 (1967).
29. C. F. Murphy and J. A. Webber. Alteration of the dihydrothiazine ring moiety, in *Cephalosporins and Penicillins Chemistry and Biology* (E. H. Flynn, ed.), Academic, New York, 1972, p. 134.
30. H. Yazawa, H. Nakamura, K. Tanaka, and K. Kariyone. Direct displacement of the acetoxy group by halogen using boron trihalide in the cephalosporin series. *Tetrahedr. Lett.,* 3991 (1974).
31. R. Bonjouklian and M. L. Phillips. Reactions of TMSI with cephalosporin esters. *Tetrahedr. Lett.,* 3915 (1981).
32. U.S. patent 4,266,049 (1981).
33. U.S. patent 3,124,576 (1964).
34. R. J. Stedman, K. Swered, and J. R. E. Hoover. 7-Aminodesacetoxycephalosporanic acid and its derivatives. *J. Med. Chem., 7*:117 (1964).
35. U.S. patent 4,346,219 (1982).
36. U.S. patent 3,275,626 (1966).
37. R. D. G. Cooper, L. D. Hatfield, and D. O. Spry. Chemical interconversion of the β-lactam antibiotics. *Accounts, 6*:32 (1973).
38. U.S. patent 4,003,894 (1977).
39. U.S. patent 3,725,399 (1973).
40. U.S. patent 3,953,440 (1976).
41. U.S. patent 3,879,379 (1975).
42. I. Miskolczi, F. Sztariczkai, and R. Bognar. New selective synthesis of 3-bromomethyl-3-cephem esters. *Org. Prep. Proc. Int., 13*:315 (1981).
43. Japanese patent 82005791 (1982).
44. U.S. patent 4,182,870 (1979).
45. U.S. patent 4,107,431 (1978).
46. U.S. patent 4,112,591 (1978).
47. European patent appl. 34,394 (1981).
48. R. D. G. Cooper and G. A. Koppel. The chemistry of penicillin sulfoxide, in

Chemistry and Biology of β-Lactam Antibiotics, Vol. 1 (R. B. Morin and M. Gorman, eds.), Academic, New York, 1982, p. 1.
49. F. M. Huber, R. H. Baltz, and P. G. Caltrider. Formation of desacetylcephalosporin C in cephalosporin C fermentation. *Appl. Microbiol., 16*:1011 (1968).
50. R. P. Elander. Strain improvement and preservation of β-lactam producing microorganisms, in *Antibiotics Containing the β-Lactam Structure* (A. L. Demain and N. A. Solomon, eds.), Springer-Verlag, New York, 1983, p. 97.
51. J. D. Jeffrey, E. P. Abraham, and G. G. F. Newton. Desacetylcephalosporin C. *Biochem. J., 81*:591 (1961).
52. N. Nomura, T. Fugono, T. Hitake, I. Minami, T. Azuma, S. Morimoto, and T. Masuda. Semisynthetic β-lactam antibiotics. 6. Sulfocephalosporins and their antipseudomonal activities. *J. Med. Chem., 17*:1312 (1974).
53. T. Takaya, H. Takasugi, T. Murakawa, and H. Nakano. Studies on β-lactam antibiotics. III. Synthesis and enzymatic stability of 3-acyloxymethyl-7-β-[(z)-2-(2-amino-4-thiazoyl)-2-(methoxyimino)acetamido]-3-cephem-4-carboxylic acids. *J. Antibiot., 34*:1300 (1981).
54. U.S. patent 3,239,394 (1966).
55. U.S. patent 3,436,310 (1969).
56. U.S. patent 3,304,236 (1967).
57. E. M. Wilson. A tale of two cephalosporins. *Chem. Ind. London, 6*:217 (1984).
58. R. B. Morin, B. G. Jackson, E. H. Flynn, and R. W. Roeske. Chemistry of cephalosporin antibiotics I. 7-Aminocephalospoanic acid from cephalosporin C. *J. Am. Chem. Soc., 84*:3400 (1962).
59. U.S. patent 3,367,933 (1968).
60. R. B. Morin, B. G. Jackson, E. H. Flynn, R. W. Roeske, and S. L. Andrew. Chemistry of cephalosporin antibiotics. XIV. The reaction of cephalosporin C with nitrosyl chloride. *J. Am. Chem. Soc., 91*:1396 (1969).
61. B. Fechtig, H. Peter, and E. Vischer. Modifikationen von Antibiotika. *Helv. Chim. Acta, 51*:1108 (1968).
62. U.S. patent 4,211,702 (1980).
63. L. D. Hatfield, W. H. W. Lunn, B. G. Jackson, L. R. Peters, L. C. Blaszczak, J. W. Fischer, J. P. Gardner, and J. M. Dunigan. Application of phosphorous–halogen compounds in cleavage of the 7-amide group of cephalosporins, in *Recent Advances in the Chemistry of β-Lactam Antibiotics* (G. I. Gregory, ed.), Royal Society of Chemistry, London, 1980, p. 109.
64. U.S. patent 3,960,662 (1976).
65. Y. Shibuya, K. Matsumoto, and T. Fujii. Isolation and properties of 7β-(4-carboxylbutanamido) cephalosporanic acid acylase-producing bacteria. *Agric. Biol. Chem., 45*:1561 (1981).
66. *Script-World Pharm. News,* Jan. 12, p. 13 (1983).
67. K. Kariyone, H. Harada, M. Kurita, and T. Takano. Cefazolin. A new semisynthetic cephalosporin antibiotic. I. Synthesis and chemical properties of cefazolin. *J. Antibiot., 13*:131 (1970).

68. U.S. patent 4,093,723 (1978).
69. U.S. patent 2,957,773 (1960).
70. U.S. patent 4,314,059 (1982).
71. U.S. patent 4,258,195 (1981).
72. European patent appl. 4,570 (1979).
73. U.S. patent 3,422,100 (1969).
74. U.S. patent 3,503,967 (1970).
75. U.S. patent 3,485,819 (1969).
76. J. E. Dolfini, H. E. Applegate, G. Bach, H. Basch, J. Bernstein, J. Schwartz, and F. L. Weisenborn. New class of semisynthetic penicillin and cephalosporins derived from D-2-(1,4-cyclohexadienyl)glycine. *J. Med. Chem., 14*: 117 (1971).
77. U.S. patent 4,338,461 (1982).
78. U.S. patent 3,767,667 (1973).
79. U.S. patent 3,962,272 (1976).
80. U.S. patent 3,798,229 (1974).
81. U.S. patent 3,824,246 (1974).
82. R. Stolle and F. Henke-Stark. Uber Tetrazolabkömmlinge. *J. Prakt. Chem., 124*:261 (1930).
83. U.S. patent 4,110,338 (1978).
84. D. A. Berges, G. W. Chan, T. J. Polansky, J. J. Taggart, and G. L. Dunn. 4,5-Dihydro-5-thioxo-1H-tetrazole-1-alkanoic and alkanesulfonic acids and their amide derivatives. *J. Heterocycl. Chem., 15*:981 (1978).
85. U.S. patent 4,374,994 (1983).
86. M. Hatanaka and T. Ishimaru. Synthetic penicillins, heterocyclic analogs of ampicillin structure-activity relationships. *J. Med. Chem., 16*:978 (1973).
87. U.S. patent 4,331,664 (1982).
88. U.S. patent 4,258,041 (1981).
89. Great Britain patent 2,025,933 (1980).
90. European patent appl. 88,454 (1983).
91. U.S. patent 4,316,019 (1982).
92. U.S. patent 4,201,779 (1980).
93. H. Tankasugi, H. Kochi, T. Masugi, H. Nakano, and T. Takaya. Studies on β-lactam antibiotics. VII. *J. Antibiot., 37*:846 (1983).
94. M. Ochiai, A. Morimoto, T. Okada, Y. Matsushita, H. Yamamoto, O. Aki, and M. Kidi. Synthesis and structure-activity relationships of 7β-(2-aminothiazol-4-yl)acetamido)-cephalosporin derivatives. *J. Antibiot., 33*:1022 (1980).
95. U.S. patent 4,298,529 (1981).
96. U.S. patent 4,152,432 (1979).
97. U.S. patent 4,205,180 (1980).
98. European patent appl. 37,380 (1981).
99. U.S. patent 3,903,113 (1975).
100. U.S. patent 4,331,669 (1982).
101. European patent appl. 88,183 (1983).

102. U.S. patent 4,017,515 (1977).
103. U.S. patent 3,507,861 (1970).
104. U.S. patent 3,946,002 (1976).
105. U.S. patent 3,957,773 (1976).
106. U.S. patent 3,925,372 (1975).
107. U.S. patent 3,912,726 (1975).
108. U.S. patent 3,489,752 (1970).
109. U.S. patent 3,985,741 (1976).
110. U.S. patent 3,483,197 (1969).
111. U.S. patent 3,578,661 (1971).
112. U.S. patent 3,641,021 (1972).
113. U.S. patent 3,796,716 (1974).
114. U.S. patent 4,100,346 (1978).
115. U.S. patent 4,374,994 (1983).
116. U.S. patent 4,110,327 (1978).
117. U.S. patent 4,304,909 (1981).
118. T-1551. *Drugs Future, 4*:675 (1979).
119. U.S. patent 4,013,680 (1977).
120. U.S. patent 4,093,803 (1978).
121. Cefuroxime. *Drugs Future, 3*:267 (1978).
122. U.S. patent 3,974,153 (1976).
123. U.S. patent 4,098,888 (1978).
124. HR-756. *Drugs Future, 3*:749 (1978).
125. U.S. patent 4,166,115 (1979).
126. SCE-1365. *Drugs Future, 5*:146 (1980).
127. U.S. patent 4,349,672 (1982).
128. U.S. patent 4,159,373 (1979).
129. Ceftazidime. *Drugs Future, 6*:612 (1981).
130. R. P. Chauvette, E. H. Flynn, B. G. Jackson, E. R. Lavagnino, R. B. Morin, R. A. Meuller, R. P. Pioch, R. W. Roeske, J. L. Spencer, and E. VanHeyningen. Chemistry of cephalosporin antibiotics II. Preparation of a new class of antibiotics and the relation of structure to activity. *J. Am. Chem. Soc., 84*:3401 (1962).
131. R. R. Chauvette, E. H. Flynn, B. G. Jackson, E. R. Lavagnino, R. B. Morin, R. A. Mueller, R. P. Pioch, R. W. Roeske, C. W. Ryan, J. L. Spencer, and E. VanHeyningen. Structure–activity relationships among 7-acylamidocephalosporanic acids. *Antimicrob. Agents Chemother.* -1962, 687 (1962).

10

Pharmacology of the Cephalosporins

KAREN I. PLAISANCE
Hartford Hospital and School of Pharmacy, University of Connecticut, Hartford, Connecticut

CHARLES H. NIGHTINGALE and
RICHARD QUINTILIANI
Hartford Hospital, Hartford, Connecticut

I. INTRODUCTION

Modifications of the substituents on the cephem nucleus (see Appendix 1) have resulted in rapidly increasing numbers of cephalosporin antibiotics over the past decadt. These compounds have been traditionally grouped on the basis of their antimicrobial spectra into first, second, and third generations, but pharmacokinetic properties differ within each generation. The purpose of this chapter is to review the basic pharmacokinetics of each of these agents, with particular emphasis on protein binding and its influence on tissue distribution, elimination pathways, and antimicrobial activity. Following a brief introduction to these concepts, the individual agents will be discussed.

II. GENERAL CONCEPTS

A. Protein Binding and Tissue Distribution

Since cephalosporins are distributed within total body water, protein binding may affect the penetration into various body compartments. A linear relationship exists between the unbound fraction of drug in the plasma and the volume of distribution at steady state (VD_{SS}; see Fig. 1). Furthermore, as protein binding increases, the concentration of unbound cephalosporin in the plasma available for diffusion into extravascular sites decreases (1,2).

*Current affiliation: Clinical Pharmacy Department, School of Pharmacy, University of Maryland, Baltimore, Maryland

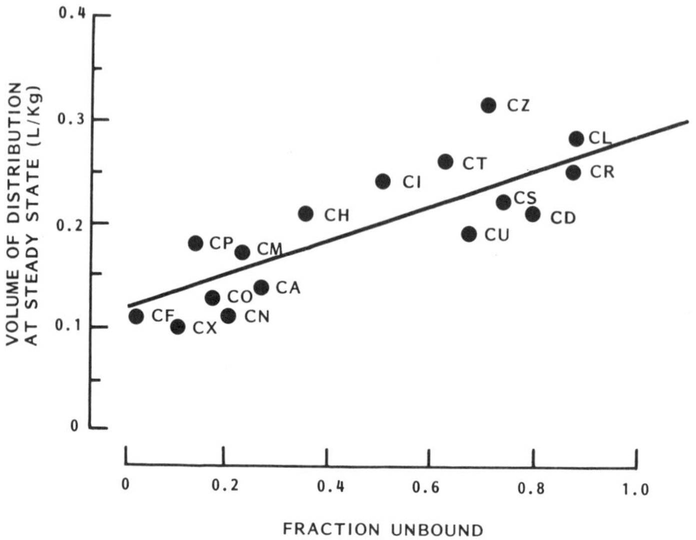

Figure 1 Relationship between fraction of unbound drug in plasma and steady state volume of distribution for 16 cephalosporins. The regression equation is: VD_{SS} = 0.181 (fraction unbound) + 0.113. The correlation coefficient, r = 0.827. Abbreviations: CF = cefonicid; CX = ceftriaxone; CP = cefoperazone; CO = ceforanide; CN = cefazolin; CM = cefmenoxime; CA = cefamandole; CH = cephalothin; CI = cephapirin; CZ = ceftizoxime; CS = cefsulodin; CD = ceftazidime; CR = cephradine; CL = cephalexin; CT = cefotaxime; CU = cefuroxime.

A major concern for the clinician is the concentration of antibiotic at the site of infection. Passage of antibiotic into tissue depends, in part, on the physiochemcial properties of the antibiotic (e.g., lipid solubility) and the amount of drug not bound to plasma proteins (3-7). The antibiotic content of tissues is the sum of the concentrations in at least three distinct compartments: interstitial fluid, the vascular system, and the cellular mass of the tissue. Because tissue cells are not well penetrated by beta-lactams, measurement of concentrations of antibiotics in extracellular fluid, where most infections are thought to occur, may be more appropriate than measurements in whole tissue (6). Workers have inferred a uniform distribution of drug throughout the entire tissue from conventional assays on tissue homogenates (8). The error in this assumption was recently illustrated when ceftazidime concentrations in excised muscle were shown to be approximately 10-fold lower than concurrent extracellular fluid concentrations (9).

A second problem with conventional tissue assays results from local degradation of the antibiotic, by either enzymes present in the tissue or bacteria in infected tissues. For example, our laboratory has demonstrated rapid degradation of cephalothin to deacetylcephalothin during processing of bone specimens. Cephalothin recovery was increased from 10.8 ± 4.2 to 68.9 ± 9.1% using a quick-frozen-crush technique to process the bone samples (10).

While whole tissue concentrations may seriously underestimate actual beta-lactam concentrations at the site of infection (extracellular fluid), these concentrations may be useful for comparisons between agents of the same class.

B. Protein Binding and Elimination

Renal excretion is the major route of elimination for most cephalosporins. Renal excretion is the net result of three processes: filtration, secretion, and reabsorption. Glomerular filtration and tubular secretion act to eliminate the drug. Reabsorption from the renal tubule returns a portion of the drug to the bloodstream and diminishes excretion. Both tubular secretion and reabsorption appear to be independent of protein binding (1,4,5,7,11). The rate of filtration is diminished by protein binding because only unbound drug is filtered by the glomeruli. Diseases that decrease protein binding of the drugs may increase the amount of drug filtered by the glomerulus (12).

Some cephalosporins are readily secreted and have renal clearances essentially independent of protein binding. Other cephalosporins are eliminated predominantly by filtration and exhibit renal clearance that is highly dependent on free drug concentration.

Hepatic clearance of cephalosporins occurs by either metabolism, as in the case of cephalothin, cephapirin, and cefotaxime, or biliary excretion (e.g., cefoperazone and ceftriaxone). The metabolism of currently available cephalosporins consists of deacetylation to metabolites that have less antimicrobial activity than the parent compound. Metabolism occurs via esterases that are present in the liver as well as other tissues (13).

In general, hepatic clearance (Cl_H) may be described by $Cl_H = (Qf_u Cl_i)/(Q + f_u Cl_i)$, where Q is blood flow to the liver, f_u is the fraction of unbound drug, and Cl_i is the intrinsic clearance, an indicator of hepatocyte activity. With cephalosporin antibiotics, the intrinsic clearance is significantly less than hepatic blood flow, and hepatic clearance is directly proportional to the degree of protein binding: $Cl_H = f_u Cl_i$.

The pharmacokinetic and molecular basis of biliary excretion remains poorly understood. The ability of a drug to bind to intracellular proteins such as ligandin has been suggested to influence the uptake and transport of antibiotics in the liver (13). The hepatic tissue protein binding of beta-lactams is directly correlated with the degree of biliary excretion (14). The extent of biliary excretion of cephalosporins in rats is directly proportional to the molecular weight above 450 (15). In humans cefoperazone, which has the highest molecular weight of the currently available cephalosporins, exhibits the highest degree of biliary excretion (13). Biliary secretion appears to be an active transport system which can be inhibited by concomitant administration of probenecid, similar to the active transport system involved in renal tubular secretion (16,17). Since active transport processes are thought to be independent of plasma protein binding, biliary secretion of cephalosporins is likely to be independent of plasma protein binding.

C. Protein Binding and Antimicrobial Activity

It is well established in vitro that antibiotics which are highly bound to plasma proteins show diminished microbiological activity in the presence of plasma (4, 5). We recently demonstrated an increase in the MIC_{50} and MIC_{90} of *Staphylococcus aureus* to cefonicid (98% protein bound) from 4 to 32 μg/ml and from 4 to 64 μg/ml, respectively, in Mueller–Hinton broth supplemented with human serum (18). For penicillins a direct correlation was observed between the in vivo activity against experimental *S. aureus* infections and the extent of protein binding of the antimicrobial (3). With other factors being equal, therapeutic activity in vivo should be diminished as a result of high plasma protein binding.

A high degree of plasma protein binding may have significant effects on both the pharmacokinetics and pharmacodynamics of cephalosporins. The longer elimination half-life observed with highly protein-bound cephalosporins as a consequence of reduced renal or metabolic clearance may allow less frequent dosing. Less frequent dosing may be possible if the pathogen is highly susceptible to the antibiotic, so that the concentration of unbound active cephalosporin at the site of infection is not reduced by protein binding below the concentration required for therapeutic benefit.

III. PHARMACOKINETICS OF THE ORAL CEPHALOSPORINS

The oral agents that will be reviewed in this section are cephalexin, cephradine, cefadroxil, and cefaclor. Pharmacokinetic parameters for these drugs are presented in Table 1 and serum concentration profiles are illustrated in Figure 2.

A. Cephalexin and Cephradine

Cephalexin and cephradine differ in structure by a single double bond in a six-membered ring within the side chain. The drugs have essentially identical pharmacokinetic parameters and microbiological activity. These agents are quite active against gram-positive cocci, with the exception of enterococci and methicillin-resistant staphylococci, and have good activity against gram-positive rods, excluding *Listeria monocytogenes.* Among the gram-negative enteric bacilli, *Escherichia coli, Klebsiella pneumoniae,* and *Proteus mirabilis* are regularly susceptible to these antibiotics. Both agents are less than 20% bound to plasma proteins (19,20).

Table 1 Pharmacokinetic Parameters of Oral Cephalosporins[a]

Parameter	Cephalexin	Cephradine	Cefadroxil	Cefaclor
α (hr^{-1})	4.35 ± 0.32	–	–	–
β (hr^{-1})	0.85 ± 0.17	0.86 ± 0.16	0.49 ± 0.06	1.02 ± 0.18
K_a (hr^{-1})	2.38 ± 1.15	2.12 ± 1.03	2.16 ± 0.76	2.73 ± 0.66
K_{12} (hr^{-1})	1.15 ± 0.02	–	–	–
K_{21} (hr^{-1})	2.45 ± 0.30	–	–	–
K_{10} (hr^{-1})	1.62 ± 0.02	–	–	–
Lag time (hr)	0.34 ± 0.09	0.32 ± 0.09	0.36 ± 0.01	0.20
$t_{1/2,\alpha}$	0.16 ± 0.01	–	–	–
$t_{1/2,\beta}$	0.89 ± 0.18	0.83 ± 0.13	1.45 ± 0.18	0.73 ± 0.12
V_C (liters)	10.95 ± 2.04	–	–	–
VD_{SS} (liters)	25.60 ± 8.63	–	–	–
VD_{β} (liters)	20.51 ± 5.38	–	–	16.7 ± 0.69
VD_{ext} (liters)	24.29 ± 5.47	20.27 ± 1.96	20.65	–
Percent protein bound	10–15	6	20	25
Clearance (ml/min)	327.6 ± 68.4	327.4 ± 54.4	172.0 ± 7.45	329.3 ± 97.9

[a]Values given are the mean ± SD.
Source: Ref. 31.

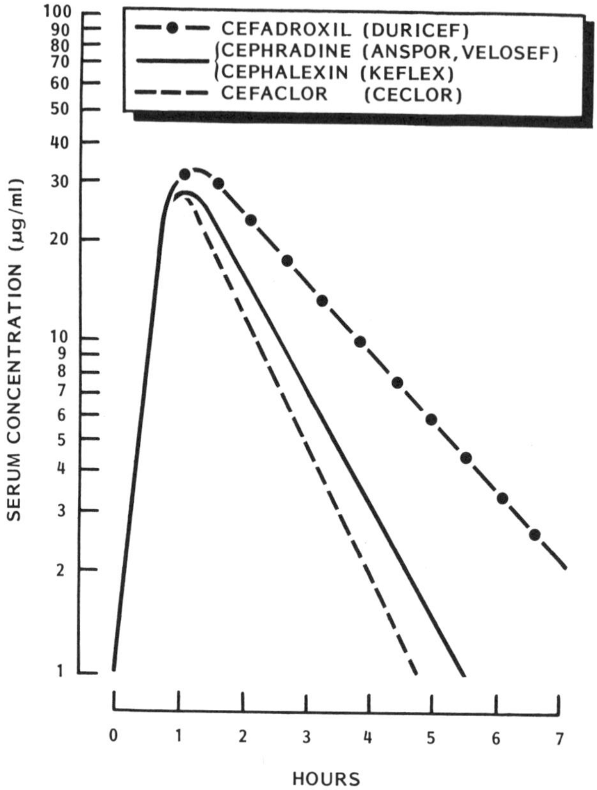

Figure 2 Serum concentrations of oral cephalosporins after a 1-g dose.

1. Absorption

The absorption, distribution, metabolism, and excretion of cephalexin (two 500-mg capsules, one 1-gram tablet) and cephradine (two 500-mg capsules) were described in nine healthy volunteers in a randomized three-way crossover study (21). No significant pharmacokinetic differences exist between cephalexin and cephradine in absorption, elimination half-life, area under the serum concentration curve (AUC), peak serum concentration, time of peak, or lag time for absorption. Absorption of both agents was very good, with high urinary recovery. Administration of either agent with food resulted in a delay in the time to peak concentrations and a reduction in the peak concentration; however, no effect on extent of absorption as determined by either AUC or elimination half-life was observed. When administered with food, cephradine is absorbed by infants and children in a manner similar to that observed in adults (22). For cephalexin, however, the AUC was reduced, suggesting decreased absorption with food in this age group (23). No clinical significance is associated with these observations.

2. Distribution and Tissue Penetration

Peak serum concentrations of approximately 30 μg/ml occurred 1 hr after an oral dose of 1 g of either cephalexin or cephradine (20,24). In two studies concentrations of cephalexin achieved after two 500-mg doses or a single 1-g dose were high enough to be clinically useful for deep-seated *S. aureus* infections (25,26). Synovial concentrations of 3.8–15.5 μg/ml were measured 3–4 hr after a 1-g dose (25), while mandibular bone concentrations ranged from 0 to 9.3 μg/ml 1 hr after a 500-mg dose (26). Skin exudate concentrations of cephalexin were approximately 75% of serum concentrations 1 hr after administration (27).

Concentrations of these two agents in other tissues are low. Neither agent appears to penetrate into the cerebrospinal fluid in the absence of meningeal inflammation (28,29). Aqueous humor concentrations were below 2 μg/ml after a 2-g dose of cephalexin (28). In bile, concentrations were 0.3-32 μg/ml after an oral dose of 0.5 or 1 g of cephalexin (28), and 2.2-41 μg/ml 3-7.5 hr after 500 mg of cephradine (28). The penetration of cephalexin and cephradine into other tissues has been reviewed elsewhere (28–31).

3. Elimination

Both cephalexin and cephradine are excreted unchanged by the kidneys, with renal clearance approximating total body clearance. Excretion involves both glomerular filtration and tubular secretion (28,29). The elimination half-lives of cephalexin and cephradine are 0.8–0.9 hr (28–32). Probenecid enhances both the peak serum concentrations of cephalexin and cephradine, as well as the duration of activity (28,29). The elimination half-lives of these antibiotics are prolonged in patients with creatinine clearances below 20 ml/min, and dosage adjustments have been recommended (28,29). A delay in the peak serum concentrations of cephradine and cephalexin has also been observed in patients with significant renal impairment (28,29).

Because of their almost identical pharmacokinetics and microbiological activity, cephalexin and cephradine are considered by many clinicians to be therapeutic alternatives and are used interchangeably. These drugs have replaced the older, poorly absorbed cephaloglycine.

B. Cefadroxil

The antimicrobial spectrum of cefadroxil is similar to that of cephalexin and cephradine. Its pharmacokinetic properties, however, are quite different and may reflect the substantial difference in chemical properties conferred by replacing a simple aromatic ring in cephalexin and cephradine with the acidic phenolic ring in cefadroxil. Higher and more prolonged serum and urinary concentrations result after the administration of cefadroxil than with equal doses of cephalexin and cephradine.

1. Absorption

Like cephalexin, cefadroxil is completely absorbed when given orally with peak concentrations and AUC values being dose related. Ingestion of cefadroxil with food does not appear to significantly affect the extent of absorption in either adults or children (34-37).

2. Distribution and Tissue Penetration

Cefadroxil is approximately 20% protein bound, with a volume of distribution smaller than that of cephalexin (see Table 1) (31,33-35,37-41). The penetration of cefadroxil into various tissues has recently been reviewed (42). Cefadroxil achieves better concentrations in lung and tonsils than cephalexin (42). Satisfactory concentrations of cefadroxil are also obtained in bone, muscle, synovial fluid, prostate gland, liver, gallbladder, and bile duct after a 1-g oral dose (42).

3. Elimination

Cefadroxil is eliminated predominantly by the kidney, with urinary recoveries being about 90% (33,34,36,39,40). During the first 3 hr after administration of 0.5 g, mean urine concentrations of cefadroxil were 1200 μg/ml compared to 2000 μg/ml for cephalexin (33). The maximum rate of tubular secretion of cefadroxil appears to be one-half that of cephalexin (33). This difference may be the primary reason for the longer half-life of cefadroxil, 1.5 versus 0.8 hr for cephalexin. The longer half-life of cefadroxil permits the accumulation of serum concentrations upon multiple dosing and allows for longer dosage intervals.

As for other oral cephalosporins, the clearance of cefadroxil is decreased in the presence of renal insufficiency (39,43). Total body clearance is reduced to 18 ml/min in anephric individuals (see Table 1). This change results in an increase in elimination half-life to 10-18 hr in anuric patients (39). Dosage adjustment is usually not necessary until creatinine clearance falls below 25 ml/min.

C. Cefaclor

Cefaclor differs from cephalexin by the substitution of a chlorine at the 3-position. This change confers greater in vitro activity against gram-negative bacteria, especially *Hemophilus influenzae.*

1. Absorption

From a pharmacokinetic viewpoint, only relatively minor differences exist between cefaclor and cephalexin. Cefaclor is rapidly and completely absorbed (34, 40,44,45). As with cephalexin, food appears to decrease the peak plasma concentrations, delay the time to peak, and prolong the duration of antibiotic levels in plasma (46). In children food had less of an effect on the pharmacokinetics of cefaclor than for cephalexin (47).

2. Distribution and Tissue Penetration

Plasma protein binding of cefaclor is 20%, similar to the other oral cephalosporins (31). Penetration into tissues is also good with cefaclor. Cefaclor concentrations in middle ear fluid were 3.8 ± 2.8 μg/ml during the first 30 min after a 15-mg/kg dose and remained above 1 μg/ml 90–120 min after dose administration (48). Adequate concentrations in prostatic tissue are maintained for up to 8 hr with 250- or 500-mg doses (49). Concentrations of cefaclor are also adequate in aqueous humor and sputum (50,51). In none of these studies were comparisons made between cefaclor and other cephalosporins.

3. Elimination

Cefaclor is eliminated by the renal route, but its half-life is slightly shorter than that of cephalexin (see Table 1). The urinary recovery of cefaclor is 50–70%, lower than that of cephalexin, probably because cefaclor is chemically unstable in normal acidic urine (52). Probenecid decreased urinary concentrations and recovery, suggesting some inhibition of tubular secretion (46). Dosage reduction may be necessary in renally impaired patients, but anephric patients exhibit only a moderate prolongation of elimination half-life (46,53). Cefaclor is removed by hemodialysis, resulting in a dialysis half-life of approximately 2 hr (53).

Based upon the moderate increase in serum half-life in the presence of severe renal failure, chemical degradation or biotransformation of cefaclor has been suggested (46). Less than 1% of the drug is excreted via the biliary tract (37).

D. Summary of the Oral Cephalosporins

Pharmacokinetically, the oral cephalosporins are remarkably similar, with the exception of cefadroxil (which has a longer half-life). The agents are all poorly bound to human albumin (below 20%). Similarities in serum pharmacokinetics are reflected in tissue distribution, and no advantage in distribution can be assigned to any one of these drugs. The predominant clearance mechanism for the oral cephalosporins is via renal pathways.

IV. PHARMACOKINETICS OF THE PARENTERAL CEPHALOSPORINS

The parenteral agents that will be discussed here are listed in Table 2. The pharmacokinetic parameters are presented in Tables 3-5. After bolus intravenous administration these antibiotics exhibit pharmacokinetics that are best described

Table 2 Parenteral Cephalosporins

First generation	Second generation	Third generation
Cephradine	Cefamandole	Cefotaxime[a]
Cefazolin	Cefonicid	Ceftizoxime
Cephalothin[a]	Ceforanide	Ceftazidime
Cephapirin[a]	Cefotiam	Cefmenoxime
	Cefuroxime	Cefsulodin
		Cefoperazone
		Ceftriaxone

[a]Metabolized cephalosporins.

by a two-compartment model. Within each generation of cephalosporins marked differences exist in protein binding and drug elimination. These differences will be compared within each generation and summarized at the end of each section.

A. Pharmacokinetics of the First-Generation Cephalosporins

Of the first-generation cephalosporins, cephradine and cefazolin are excreted unchanged by the kidney, while cephalothin and cephapirin undergo biotransformation as well as renal elimination. The pharmacokinetic parameters for these agents are described in Table 3 and their serum concentration profiles are illustrated in Figure 3.

1. Cephradine

The pharmacokinetics and tissue distribution of cephradine after oral administration were discussed in the section on oral cephalosporins.

Absorption. Intramuscular administration of 1 g of cephradine results in peak serum concentrations of 10.4 μg/ml after 2 hr (54). While the peak concentration of cephradine was lower when given by the intramuscular route as compared to orally, the areas under the curves for the two routes were identical, indicating similar extents of absorption (54). Urinary recoveries also suggest nearly complete bioavailability (54).

After intramuscular administration of 500 mg, concentrations of cephradine in lung tissue were approximately 40% of simultaneous serum concentrations. One hour after administration mean lung tissue concentrations of 2.6 μg/ml were observed (55).

Elimination. Intravenous administration of 1 g of cephradine produces serum concentrations of 86.3 μg/ml at 5 min, with essentially no drug detectable

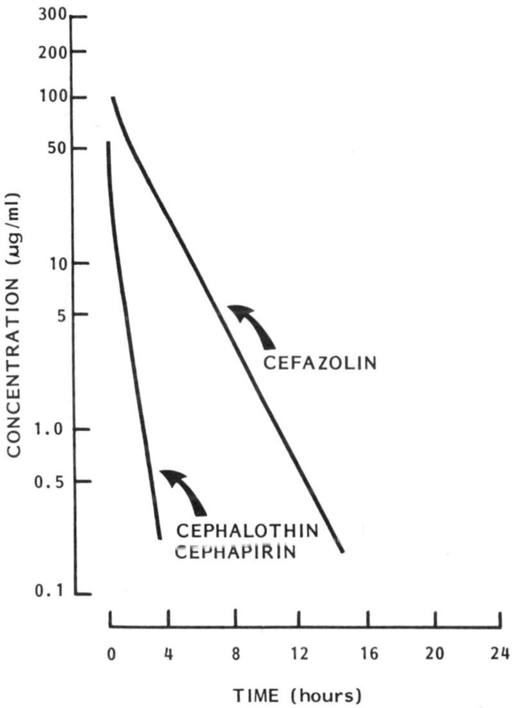

Figure 3 Serum concentrations of first-generation parenteral cephalosporins after a 1-g dose.

in the serum after 6 hr (56). A two-compartment open model best describes the pharmacokinetics of cephradine. Its elimination half-life is 0.7–0.85 hr when given intravenously and 1.5 hr after intramuscular administration (28,29,56). Renal impairment results in accumulation of cephradine and a prolongation of serum elimination half-life. Dosage adjustments are recommended for patients with creatinine clearances below 20 ml/min (29).

2. Cefazolin

Absorption. After intramuscular administration peak concentrations occur in 1–2 hr and reach approximately 70 μg/ml after a 1-g dose. Urinary recovery is approximately 80% after 24 hr (29,57–61).

Distribution and Tissue Penetration. Cefazolin is more highly protein bound (about 85%) and has a smaller apparent volume of distribution than the other first-generation cephalosporins (see Table 2) (19,28,60,61). This high degree of protein binding may affect antimicrobial activity; in one study the presence of

Table 3 Pharmacokinetic Parameters of the First-Generation Cephalosporins[a]

	Cephradine	Cefazolin			
	Refs. 31 and 60	Ref. 28	Ref. 63	Refs. 31 and 60	Ref. 28
α (hr^{-1})	6.39 ± 1.39	3.97	3.07	4.30 ± 2.56	7.28
β (hr^{-1})	0.99 ± 0.38	0.40	0.46	0.42 ± 0.08	1.56
K_{12} (hr^{-1})	2.26 ± 0.13	1.73	0.93	1.72 ± 1.31	2.01
K_{21} (hr^{-1})	2.81 ± 1.54	1.67	1.83	2.00 ± 1.28	2.73
K_{10} (hr^{-1})	2.32 ± 0.10	0.97	0.77	1.00 ± 0.32	4.09
$t_{1/2,\alpha}$ (hr)	0.11 ± 0.03	0.24	0.23	0.23 ± 0.14	0.10
$t_{1/2,\beta}$ (hr)	0.76 ± 0.30	1.80	1.51	1.74 ± 0.36	0.56
V_C (liters)	9.23 ± 1.88	4.44	4.74	4.10 ± 1.68	7.76
VD_{SS} (liters)	16.04 ± 2.22	8.48	7.15	8.32 ± 1.92	14.29
VD_{β} (liters)	21.20 ± 3.03	10.27	7.93	12.38 ± 4.43	22.20
Percent protein bound	6–20	75–85	–	–	65
Clearance (ml/min)	435	62	–	–	472

[a]References from which the data are taken are given at the head of each column. Means ± SD were calculated by averaging data cited in review articles.

human serum decreased the antimicrobial activity by 41–48% (62). However, the AUC for unbound drug (AUC_f) was 54.2 for cefazolin but 49.0 for cephalothin (63), casting doubt on the clinical relevance of the difference in protein binding between the two drugs.

Peak serum concentrations are approximately 200 μg/ml after intravenous injection of 1 g and decline to 75 μg/ml at 1 hr (29,63). In a study comparing heart tissue and pericardial fluid concentrations of cefazolin (85% protein binding) with cephradine (less than 20% protein binding), unbound concentrations of drug in pericardial fluid were higher for cephradine than for cefazolin, although both were in the therapeutic range (64). This result may be explained by the albumin content of pericardial fluid (about 50%) to which cefazolin can bind. Atrial appendage homogenate concentrations of cefazolin were higher than for cephradine, suggesting that cefazolin may bind to tissue proteins as well. Higher total cefazolin concentrations were also observed in synovial fluid, knee, and hip and occurred even though the free serum concentrations of cefazolin were lower than those of cephradine (10,65,66). High tissue concentrations of cefazolin also have been reported in aqueous humor, tonsils, peritoneal fluid, skeletal muscle, and pleural fluid (28,29,67,68). Concentrations in bile averaged

Cephalothin			Cephapirin				
Ref. 89	Ref. 63	Refs. 31 and 60	Ref. 28	Ref. 89	Ref. 63	Ref. 109	Refs. 31 and 60
6.0	7.15	6.95 ± 1.93	5.32	5.7	4.69	5.52	5.31 ± 0.44
1.3	1.42	1.50 ± 0.48	1.00	1.2	0.91	1.91	1.05 ± 0.12
1.5	1.77	1.82 ± 0.83	0.99	1.4	1.07	1.14	1.15 ± 0.18
2.1	2.21	2.52 ± 0.88	1.37	1.9	1.34	1.52	1.53 ± 0.26
3.7	4.59	4.12 ± 0.87	3.96	3.6	3.19	3.94	3.67 ± 0.36
0.12	0.10	0.11 ± 0.03	0.13	0.12	0.15	0.13	0.13 ± 0.01
0.53	0.49	0.53 ± 0.28	0.71	0.58	0.76	0.64	0.67 ± 0.08
10.15	7.28	8.08 ± 2.68	9.27	9.88	8.84	10.31	9.58 ± 0.65
17.40	13.11	14.61 ± 5.59	15.87	17.60	15.90	18.04	16.85 ± 1.13
28.88	23.53	23.54 ± 8.48	34.94	29.64	30.99	37.28	33.21 ± 3.52
–	–	–	44–50	–	–	54	–
626.2	–	–	–	580.2	–	–	–

67 μg/ml for the first 3 hr following an intravenous dose of 1.5 g, but in patients with obstructed cystic ducts the concentrations in the common bile duct were below serum levels (69–73). Poor penetration into prostate, milk, and spinal fluid were also observed (29,74–76).

Elimination. Cefazolin is eliminated from the body primarily through renal mechanisms. Urinary recovery in 24 hr is 80–100% following intravenous dosage, with total body and renal clearance values being identical (77,78).

The elimination half-life in patients with normal renal function is approximately 1.5 hr (28,29,59). Decreased clearance and prolonged half-lives are seen in patients with renal dysfunction (61,78–80). Patients with normal kidney function excreted 55% of a dose within the first 6 hr and 81.5% within 24 hr. Moderate renal impairment (creatinine clearance of 47–69 ml/min) reduced excretion to 36% within the first 6 hr and to 68% within 24 hr. Severe renal impairment (creatinine clearance of 5–21 ml/min) reduced excretion to 5.9% in 6 hr and to 22% in 24 hr. In patients with creatinine clearances below 5 ml/min the half-life is 35.3 ± 9.6 hr (31,81,82). Hemodialysis decreases the serum half-life during dialysis to about 5 hr (31,81–84). Peritoneal dialysis has little effect on elimination half-life (32 hr in these patients), although 19% of the dose may be recovered in the dialysate (81).

3. Cephalothin

Absorption. Cephalothin is not absorbed after oral administration and is therefore marketed only in parenteral form. Intramuscular administration may be quite painful and is not often used, but bioavailability following intramuscular administration is approximately 100% (87,89). Peak serum concentration of 15-20 μg/ml were achieved 0.5-1 hr after a 1-g intramuscular dose (77,86-89). Intraperitoneal administration yields serum concentrations of 4.4 μg/ml in 1 hr (90).

Distribution and Tissue Penetration. Cephalothin is moderately (60-65%) bound to human serum proteins (19,77,88). After intravenous administration of 1 g of cephalothin, serum concentrations were 65-102 μg/ml at 5 min after dosing but fell to 5.2-6.2 μg/ml at 1 hr (29,63,89,91). Intravenous injection of 2 g of cephalothin to patients with meningitis yielded concentrations in spinal fluid approaching 0.31 μg/ml within 1 hr; in patients without meningitis, spinal fluid concentrations were below the limit of the assay (92). Aqueous humor concentrations of 0.5 μg/ml were measured 0.5 hr after a 1-g intravenous dose (93). Atrial appendage concentrations were < 5μg/g after a 2-g intravenous dose (94,95). Synovial fluid concentrations of 12.6 μg/ml were measured 20 min after a 1-g intravenous injection (29,96), and peak bone concentrations of 2.8 μg/g were achieved by 25-45 min (10). Peak concentrations in the bile 1-3 hr following a 1-g intravenous dose ranged from 0.4 to 42 μg/ml and were less than 1 μg/ml in the gallbladder bile of patients with obstructed cystic ducts (28,97, 98). Cephalothin concentrations in uterine myometrium were 15.5 μg/g 20 min after a 2-g intravenous dose (99). Concentrations of 30.2 and 12.5 μg/ml were found in the mother and fetus, respectively, after an intravenous injection of 1 g (28,29,100). The concentration of cephalothin in mother's milk is low (28).

Elimination. Cephalothin is rapidly metabolized in the body to deacetylcephalothin, a compound with approximately 20% of the activity of the parent compound against organisms used in microbiological assays (29). The metabolism of cephalothin by esterases occurs in most tissues, with minor metabolism in the serum (101). The metabolite and parent compound are eliminated from the body via the kidneys, with active tubular secretion accounting for the majority of metabolite excretion (102,103). Approximately 44% of the total amount of drug recovered in the urine is present as the metabolite (102-105). Probenecid administration approximately doubles serum elimination half-life and enhances serum concentrations of cephalothin (91). Renal clearance accounts for 58% of total body clearance (77). In patients with normal renal function the elimination half-life of cephalothin is 0.5 hr (63,77,102,103). No desacetyl metabolite was detectable in serum by high-pressure liquid chromatography (HPLC) methods after 6 hr. In this same study the elimination half-life of cephalothin in patients with creatinine clearances of less than 10 ml/min was 3.5 hr, and no apparent decline in metabolite concentration was evident in 14 hr (103). Because of alternate elimination pathways, severe renal dysfunction only moderately prolongs the elimination half-life of the parent compound. Hemodialysis has little effect on the clearance of cephalothin (28,81). Serum concentrations were reduced by as much as 50% with peritoneal dialysis, although the elimination half-life was not significantly affected (106).

4. Cephapirin

Absorption. The absorption of cephapirin by the oral route is negligible; administration is solely by the intramuscular and intravenous routes. Cephapirin is well absorbed after intramuscular administration, with peak serum concentrations of about 20 μg/ml achieved 0.5-1 hr after injection of a 1-g dose (89,107).

Distribution and Tissue Penetration Cephapirin is moderately bound (50-60%) to serum proteins (28,29,31,108). After intravenous administration of a 1-g dose, peak concentrations of 64-73 μg/ml have been reported; concentrations decline rapidly to 3-6 μg/ml 1 hr after administration (89,107,109). Few studies compare the tissue penetration of cephalothin and cephapirin, but the penetration of cephapirin into atrial appendage in adults and children has been compared with that of cephalothin (95,110). Adults had higher concentrations of cephapirin (5-10 μg/g of atrial appendage 1 hr after dosing) than of cephalothin; in children the concentrations were similar (below 5 μg/g at 1 hr). Like other first-generation cephalosporins, cephalothin and cephapirin penetrate poorly into inflamed and noninflamed meninges and are not recommended for treatment of central nervous system infection.

More recent work has reported cephalosporin distribution into prostate and seminal vesicles, bone, female reproductive tissues, amniotic fluid, and cord serum (111-115). Tissue concentration comparisons between metabolized and nonmetabolized cephalosporins are difficult to assess in these studies because of design and methodological differences. However, it appears that metabolized drugs (cephalothin and cephapirin) exhibit lower tissue concentrations than the nonmetabolized agents (31). This difference may be explained in part by the lower serum concentrations observed with metabolized agents, as well as by the direct contribution of tissue metabolism, both in vivo and in vitro. The above studies are therefore likely to have underestimated tissue concentrations of the metabolized drugs.

Elimination. The elimination half-life of cephapirin after intravenous administration is short, 0.5-0.7 hr (29,31,60). Like cephalothin, cephapirin is sub-

Table 4 Pharmacokinetic Parameters of Second-Generation Parenteral Cephalosporins[a]

	Cefamandole					Cefuroxime		
	Ref. 139	Ref. 123[b]	Ref. 122	Ref. 119	Refs. 31 and 60	Ref. 171	Ref. 166	Ref. 167
α (hr^{-1})	2.66	3.13	3.13	3.74	3.21 ± 0.45	2.36	2.83	4.31
β (hr^{-1})	0.74	0.72	0.80	0.97	0.81 ± 0.11	0.49	0.62	0.56
K_{12} (hr^{-1})	–	0.73	0.82	0.72	0.76 ± 0.06	0.70	0.77	1.76
K_{21} (hr^{-1})	–	1.14	1.39	1.40	1.31 ± 0.15	0.99	1.55	1.60
K_{10} (hr^{-1})	–	1.98	1.90	2.58	2.15 ± 0.37	1.18	1.12	1.50
$t_{1/2,\alpha}$ (hr)	0.26	0.22	0.20	0.19	0.22 ± 0.03	0.29	0.25	0.16
$t_{1/2,\beta}$ (hr)	0.94	0.96	0.87	0.71	0.87 ± 0.11	1.41	1.12	0.62
V_C (liters)	–	5.01	9.41	4.17	6.20 ± 2.81	8.09	9.80	5.47
VD_{SS} (liters)	–	8.22	14.90	6.30	9.81 ± 4.51	13.78	14.64	11.46
VD_{β} (liters)	–	13.78	21.95	11.09	15.62 ± 5.68	19.39	17.83	14.86
Percent protein bound	–	–	–	–	74	–	–	–
Clearance (ml/min)	232.8	198.4	293.6	–	–	162.9	158.9	–

[a]References from which the data are taken are given at the head of each column. Means ± SD were calculated by averaging data cited in review articles.
[b]Data reanalyzed using a two-compartment model.

ject to deacetylation in various tissues, with subsequent excretion of the parent compound and metabolite by the kidneys (109,116). The desacetyl metabolite of cephapirin accounts for approximately 48% of the total amount of drug recovered in the urine (109,116). Severe renal dysfunction (creatinine clearance of 12 ml/min or less) decreases the renal clearance of cephapirin, with only 19% of a dose recovered in the urine (117). Saturable renal reabsorption may occur with cephapirin (108). Less than 1% of administered cephapirin is excreted via the bile (29).

B. Summary of the First-Generation Cephalosporins

Of the first-generation agents, cefazolin is clearly the most highly protein bound. Although in vitro evidence suggests that cefazolin is less active in the presence of human serum, the bulk of clinical and scientific data suggest that cefazolin is efficacious in the therapy of serious staphylococcal infections.

The pharmacokinetic parameters of first-generation cephalosorins shown in Table 3 as well as the tissue concentrations of metabolized cephalosporins are uncertain because they were derived from studies where drug concentrations were determined by microbiological analysis. Activity of metabolites could not be separated from the activity of the parent compound by these methods. The curves actually represent the decline of microbiological activity (produced by a

	Cefonicid		Ceforanide				Cefotiam	
Refs. 31 and 60	Refs. 141 and 145	Refs. 142 and 145	Ref. 152	Ref. 153	Ref. 157	Refs. 151 and 37	Ref. 160	Ref. 37
3.17 ± 1.02	4.5	–	–	–	–	2.39	–	–
0.56 ± 0.06	0.2	–	0.257	0.266	0.232	0.259	0.866	–
1.08 ± 0.59	1.9	–	–	–	–	–	–	–
1.38 ± 0.34	2.5	–	–	–	–	–	–	–
1.27 ± 0.20	0.4	–	–	–	–	–	–	–
0.23 ± 0.07	0.15	–	–	–	–	0.29	–	–
1.05 ± 0.40	3.5	4.4	2.7	2.6	3.0	2.67	0.8	–
7.79 ± 2.18	3.9	–	–	–	–	–	–	–
13.29 ± 1.64	6.6	9.3	–	–	–	–	–	–
17.30 ± 2.40	–	–	11.6	10.6	8.9	8.6	–	–
33	–	–	81	–	–	85	–	40
–	23.3	27.1	49.5	46.9	34.4	37.1	378.6	–

mixture of unknown proportions of parent drug and metabolite) as a function of time, but the pharmacokinetic parameters are expressed only in terms of the parent drug.

The clearance mechanism for all the first-generation cephalosporins is predominantly renal, with a contribution of glomerular filtration of free drug and active tubular secretion of total drug. Evidence suggests that tubular secretion is in excess of glomerular filtration for all of these agents, with the exception of cefazolin. Cefazolin has the longest elimination half-life and is usually given at 8-hr intervals, while cephapirin, cephalothin, and cephradine are given every 4–6 hr. Renal dysfunction will decrease the clearance of these drugs and prolong their elimination half-lives. Cephalothin and cephapirin are eliminated by both renal and metabolic mechanisms, and therefore renal dysfunction prolongs the elimination half-lives of these two drugs to a lesser extent than for cefazolin and cephradine.

Dosage adjustments are not necessary for these agents until creatinine clearance falls to 20–30 ml/min. The first-generation cephalosporins are not concentrated in bile, with cefazolin having the highest bile levels (28 μg/ml, or 0.13% of dose). There is no evidence for differences in therapeutic efficacy, however, between cephalosporins that are highly concentrated in the bile and those which are not.

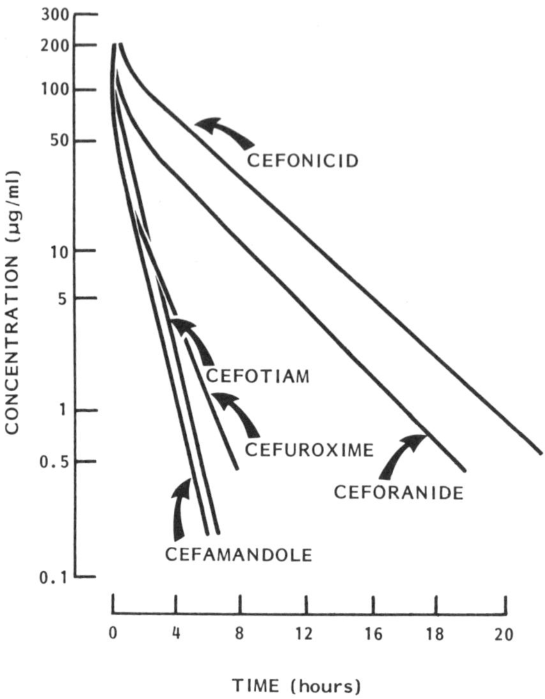

Figure 4 Serum concentrations of second-generation parenteral cephalosporins after a 1-g dose.

C. Pharmacokinetics of the Second-Generation Cephalosporins

The pharmacokinetic parameters for the second-generation cephalosporins are described in Table 4, and serum concentration profiles are illustrated in Figure 4.

1. Cefamandole

Cefamandole exhibits greater microbiological activity than first-generation cephalosporins against indole-positive *Proteus, Enterobacter, Citrobacter, Providencia, H. influenzae,* and *E. coli.*

Administered as cefamandole nafate, the drug undergoes rapid hydrolysis (half-life, 13 min) to cefamandole in the body, with hydrolysis complete within 2 hr (29).

Absorption. Following intramuscular administration, absorption is rapid, with serum peaks of 20-35 μg/ml occurring 0.5-1 hr after administration; 80-

100% of the dose can be recovered within 24 hr, suggesting nearly complete absorption (118-124).

Distribution and Tissue Penetration. Cefamandole is 70-80% bound to serum proteins (29,31,119,120). Serum concentrations 15 min after a 1-g intravenous dose are approximately 90-100 μg/ml (29,119,121). Cefamandole distributes poorly into aqueous humor and inflamed or noninflamed meninges but does penetrate heart tissue well, with atrial appendage concentrations as high as 50 μg/g observed 40 min after a 2-g intravenous dose (125-130). Synovial fluid concentrations of 40.8 ± 6.3 μg/ml were reported approximately 30 min after a 2-g dose (131). In patients undergoing total hip replacement, cancellous bone concentrations ranged from 2.4 to 38.5 μg/g 20-70 min after a 1-g intravenous injection (132). Biliary concentrations of 352 μg/ml have been reported after a 1-g dose of cefamandole (133-135). Cefamandole concentrations in the bile of patients with hepatobiliary disease ranged from 1.6 to 1400 μg/ml 0.5-2.5 hr after an intravenous dose of 1 g. Only with complete aseptic cystic duct obstruction was cefamandole undetectable in gallbladder bile (135).

Elimination. The 50-min elimination half-life of cefamandole is shorter than that of cefazolin, despite its similar degree of protein binding (29,31,120,122, 123,136,137). Most renal elimination occurs by active tubular secretion; concomitant administration with probenecid decreases renal clearance by 70% (124, 136,137). The elimination half-life is prolonged to 11.5 hr (range, 6.3-19.2 hr) in functionally anephric individuals (138-140). Nonrenal mechanisms, such as biliary excretion, may play a minor role in the elimination of cefamandole in patients with normal renal function, but may assume a proportionately larger role in patients with severe renal disease (140). Cefamandole does not appear to undergo metabolic degradation.

2. Cefonicid

Cefonicid is a tetrazolethiomethyl cephalosporin that resembles cefamandole in both structure and in vitro antimicrobial activity. Cefonicid is less active against *S. aureus* than other currently available first- and second-generation cephalosporins.

Distribution and Tissue Penetration. Cefonicid is highly bound to serum proteins. At concentrations of cefonicid between 50 and 200 μg/ml in human serum, cefonicid is 98% bound and the apparent volume of distribution is small (1). Peak plasma concentrations immediately following an intravenous bolus of 1 g exceed 200 μg/ml and, as with other cephalosporins, the pharmacokinetics best fit a two-compartment model (141,142). Peak concentrations in most tissues are achieved rapidly. We have measured interstitial fluid concentrations obtained by suction-blister and paper disk techniques in volunteers. After a

30-mg/kg intravenous dose, disk concentrations declined in parallel with serum concentrations, with peak concentrations of 55 ± 15 μg/ml observed 30 min after the dose. Peak concentrations in blister fluid were similar but delayed, suggesting that the blister fluid tends to act as a reservoir for the accumulation of highly protein-bound drugs (143).

Sputum concentrations of cefonicid in patients with pneumonia were 2–4 μg/ml, approximately twice those observed for cefamandole (144). Pleural fluid concentrations of cefonicid approximately 1 hr following a 1-g dose ranged from trace levels to 42.9 μg/ml (145).

Cefonicid concentrations in surgical wound fluid, subcutaneous fat, and pus 1 hr after an intramuscular dose ranged from 0.4 to 70.2 μg/ml (145). Bile and gallbladder wall concentrations were 0–20 and 15–40 μg/ml, respectively, 2–3 hr after a 1-g intravenous dose, higher than those observed after the same dose of cefoxitin (145). Cefonicid concentrations in breast milk are low (less than 0.3 μg/ml) (145). Prostate concentrations approximately 1 hr after a 1-g intramuscular dose averaged 13 μg/g of tissue (145). Bone concentrations obtained approximately 1 hr after a 30-mg/kg intravenous dose were 30 μg/g of tissue and were approximately twice as high as those observed following a 30-mg/kg dose of cefazolin (146). Peak uterine tissue concentrations following administration of 30 or 15 mg/kg intravenously were approximately 30 μg/g of tissue, approximately twice those achieved by the same dose of cefoxitin (146). Atrial appendage concentrations ranged between 30 and 130 μg/g of tissue, approximately twice as high as cefazolin concentrations in tissue obtained at the same time following a 30-μg/kg intravenous dose (146). Atrial appendage concentrations 2 hr after a 2-g intramuscular dose were lower, 10.2 ± 7.4 μg/g (147). The decline in cefonicid concentrations in bone, uterine tissue, and atrial appendage occurred at the same rate as the decline observed in serum (146). Cerebrospinal fluid penetration, although not studied, would be expected to be low owing to high plasma protein binding.

Elimination. The major route of elimination for cefonicid is renal excretion, with approximately 90% of the renal clearance of cefonicid due to tubular secretion (141). Renal clearance of cefonicid is approximately 24% of creatinine clearance (145). The slow renal clearance results in the notably long elimination half-life of 4 hr (141,142).

Serum concentrations following a single 7.5-mg/kg dose ranged from 6 to 12 μg/ml at 12 hr and were still detectable 24 hr after dosing (142). Probenecid markedly decreases the tubular secretion of cefonicid and results in a prolongation of the elimination half-life to 7.5 hr (141). Severe renal dysfunction significantly prolongs the half-life to 40–60 hr (148,149). Removal by hemodialysis is low and supplementary doses postdialysis are not necessary (148,149).

3. Ceforanide

Ceforanide, like cefonicid, is closely related to cefamandole in both structure and antimicrobial spectrum. Ceforanide is less active, however, than cefamandole against gram-positive cocci and has slightly greater activity against the Enterobacteriaceae.

Absorption. Following intramuscular administration of 1 g of ceforanide, serum peak concentrations of 67 μg/ml were obtained in 1 hr (150,151). Approximately 90% of the dose may be recovered in the urine within 12 hr (150, 151). Bioavailability of ceforanide from the intramuscular route is 100% (151).

Distribution and Tissue Penetration. Ceforanide is highly bound to serum proteins (about 85%), and this binding appears to be concentration dependent, decreasing to 65% at serum concentrations of 400 μg/ml (37,152). Peak concentrations following intravenous administration of 1- and 2-g doses of ceforanide are approximately 135 and 250 μg/ml, respectively (151-153). A nonlinear increase in the AUC was observed with a dosage increase from 2 to 4 g because renal clearance increased as protein binding fell at higher drug concentrations (152).

Limited information exists on tissue penetration of ceforanide in humans. The tissue penetration of ceforanide and cefamandole in patients undergoing open heart surgery has been studied at our institution (154). Three hours after an intravenous dose of 30 mg/kg, samples of pericardial fluid, atrial appendage, sternal bone, and intercostal muscle contained 68 μg/ml and 28, 17, and 13 μg/g of ceforanide, respectively. These concentrations were higher and more sustained than those observed for cefamandole (154). Gallbladder bile concentrations 2 hr after a 1-g intravenous dose in patients without billiary disease and in patients with obstructed cystic ducts were 131 ± 61 and 14 ± 7 μg/ml, respectively (155).

Elimination. The main advantage of ceforanide over cefamandole is the prolonged elimination half-life of 2.6-3.0 hr which may allow less frequent dosing (151-153,156,157). Ceforanide is not metabolized and 85-90% of a dose may be recovered in the urine unchanged (151-153). Approximately 50% of the clearance is via glomerular filtration, with the remainder via tubular secretion (152,153). Probenecid does not appear to alter the plasma pharmacokinetics or urinary excretion of ceforanide (150). The elimination half-life is prolonged in patients with renal dysfunction, with reported half-lives as long as 20-40 hr in patients with severe renal disease (157,158). Hemodialysis removes approximately 20-50% of a dose, with a dialysis half-life of 5.5 hr (157,158). The elimination half-life of ceforanide in children 1-2 years old is significantly shorter (1.5 ± 0.5 hr) than in either neonates (2.2 ± 0.2 hr) or children over 10 years old (2.3 ± 0.5 hr). This phenomena may be caused by age-related differences in glomerular filtration rate or protein binding (159).

4. Cefotiam

Cefotiam has antibacterial activity similar to that of other second-generation cephalosporins; although it is more sensitive to beta-lactamase, cefotiam penetrates the outer cell membrane of pathogenic bacteria to a greater extent than other second-generation drugs (37).

Distribution and Tissue Penetration. Cefotiam is moderately (40%) bound to human serum proteins (37). Peak concentrations observed after a 30-min infusion of 1 g were 52 μg/ml (160). Tissue penetration data are limited in humans. The penetration of cefotiam into heart valves, muscle, and subcutaneous tissue produced concentrations of 22.0, 6.5, and 9.1 μg/g, respectively, 30–60 min after a 2-g intravenous dose (161). Peak concentrations of cefotiam in umbilical cord blood were 13.0–23.9 μg/ml 15–30 min after a 1-g intravenous dose. Amniotic fluid concentrations of 19.6–23.5 μg/ml were attained approximately 2.5 hr after dosing (162).

Elimination. The pharmacokinetics of cefotiam have been described in 16 volunteers (160). Peak plasma concentrations and AUC more than doubled as the dose was increased from 1 to 2 g, suggesting dose-dependent pharmacokinetics. Decreasing values for clearance were also observed at the higher doses, suggesting that saturation of tubular secretion may occur. The elimination half-life for the 1-g dose was 0.6–0.7 hr, but for the 2-g dose it was 1.0–1.1 hr (160). Biliary excretion plays a role in elimination of cefotiam in animal species, but its role in human elimination has yet to be determined (137).

5. Cefuroxime

Cefuroxime has a broad spectrum of antimicrobial activity similar to that of other second-generation cephalosporins.

Absorption. Cefuroxime is poorly absorbed after oral administration, with 1% of the dose recovered in the urine (29). Recently cefuroxime 1-acetoxyethyl ester has been developed as a prodrug for oral administration (163–165). The pharmacokinetics of cefuroxime axetil was studied in 52 volunteers (163). Intact cefuroxime axetil was absorbed from the gastrointestinal tract and rapidly cleaved by esterases such that the ester was not detected in systemic circulation. Bioavailability as measured by urinary recovery was 40–50% if taken after food and 30% if taken after an overnight fast. Peak serum concentrations were 6.3 ± 0.4 μg/ml approximately 2 hr after a 250-mg dose (163). The pharmacokinetics did not change after repeated administration (164). After intramuscular administration, peak serum concentrations reached 32.2–39.1 μg/ml 1 hr after a 1-g dose (166,167). Approximately 100% of the intramuscular dose may be recovered in the urine 24 hr after dosing (166).

Distribution and Tissue Penetration. The human serum protein binding of cefuroxime is 33% (60,166). Like other cephalosporins, cefuroxime is largely distributed into the extravascular compartment. After intravenous administration of cefuroxime, peak concentrations of 72 μg/ml were reported, but concentrations declined rapidly to 25 μg/ml 1 hr after dosing (168,171).

Cerebrospinal fluid contained 4.3 ± 3.0 μg/ml of cefuroxime after doses of 75 mg/kg in 19 specimens collected from children with bacterial meningitis (169). Aqueous humor concentrations of 1.6 μg/ml were measured after a single 1.5-g dose (170). Sputum concentrations obtained from the lower main-stem bronchus in 49 adults requiring bronchoscopy were 0.95 μg/ml after 7 doses of 750 mg of cefuroxime and 1.78 μg/ml after a single dose of 1.5 g (172). Another study reported lower sputum concentrations following single doses (173). Peak concentrations in bone rose with increasing dose up to 1.5 g but did not appear to differ between 1.5 and 3.0 g, although there was a prolongation of the high concentrations observed in bone at the higher dosage level (174,175). In patients with severely ischemic limbs prior to amputation, cefuroxime concentrations were in excess of 4 μg/ml in 38 of 40 wound exudates (176). Biliary tract concentrations measured approximately 25 min following a 1.5-g intravenous dose were 39.2 μg/ml in common bile duct bile, 5.4 μg/ml in gallbladder bile, and 42.8 μg/g in gallbladder wall (177,178). Prostatic tissue concentrations after a 1.5-g intravenous dose were 29.2 μg/g (179). Peak amniotic fluid concentrations of 0–43.4 μg/ml were measured 3–5 hr after a 1.5-g dose. Cefuroxime was detectable in the newborn for up to 6 hr after delivery (180).

Elimination. Cefuroxime is eliminated by renal mechanisms, with over 90% of a dose being excreted in the urine unchanged; most is excreted within the first 6 hr (166–168). The elimination half-life is approximately 80 min in normal adults (166,167,171). Probenecid decreased the renal clearance and prolonged the elimination half-life. Tubular secretion accounts for 43–54% of renal elimination of cefuroxime (166). Patients with creatinine clearances below 20 ml/min per 1.73 m^2 excreted only 35% of the dose within 24 hr and had a mean elimination half-life of 17.6 hr (168,181). Hemodialysis decreases serum concentrations to one-quarter of predialysis concentrations, and supplemental doses are recommended after dialysis (179).

D. Summary of the Second-Generation Cephalosporins

The second-generation parenteral cephalosporins are a pharmacokinetically diverse group of agents. Of these antibiotics, cefonicid is the most highly protein bound (98%), ceforanide and cefamandole are moderately bound, and cefotiam and cefuroxime exhibit low protein binding (below 50%). The microbiological consequence of the high degree of protein binding is diminished antibacterial activity in the presence of human serum. Because only a small amount of antibiotic may be available for diffusion into tissues, a highly protein-bound antibiotic may not reach free concentrations in tissue in excess of the MIC of pathogenic organisms. At the present time the marketing trend is to develop antibiotics with long serum half-lives so that infrequent dosing is possible. While infrequent dosing is a desirable feature, caution is urged with highly protein-bound agents in situations where the pathogens are only moderately susceptible.

Of the available second-generation cephalosporins, cefamandole is notable because it reaches high concentrations in the bile. The therapeutic consequences of high bile concentrations, however, are controversial. There is no evidence of the therapeutic superiority of any cephalosporin, regardless of its biliary excretion, in the treatment of biliary tract infection.

E. Pharmacokinetics of the Third-Generation Cephalosporins

Pharmacokinetic properties of the third-generation cephalosporins are compared in Table 5. Serum concentration profiles are illustrated in Figure 5. These agents

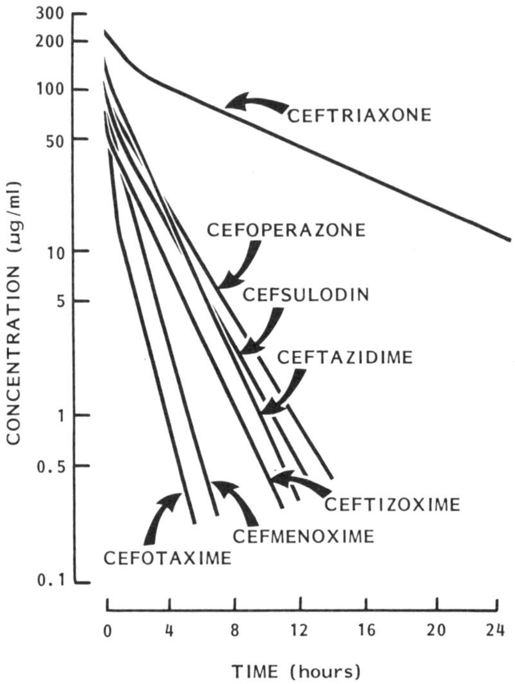

Figure 5 Serum concentrations of third-generation cephalosporins after 1-g dose.

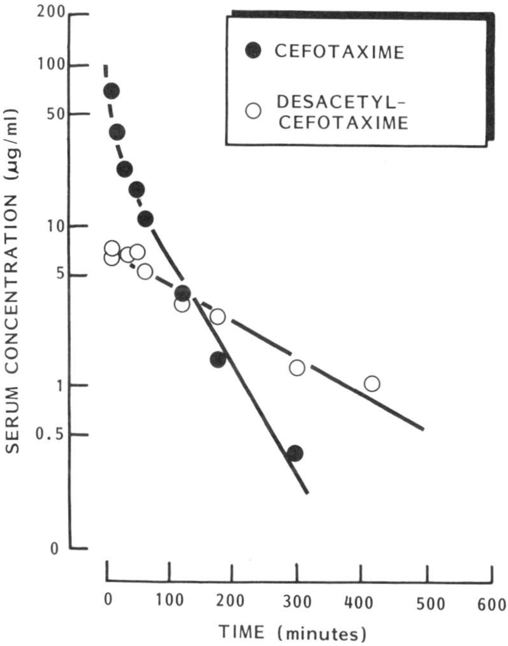

Figure 6 Serum concentrations of cefotaxime and desacetylcefotaxime after a 15-mg/kg dose of cefotaxime.

are active against more gram-negative organisms and less active against gram-positive pathogens than the second-generation drugs. The first of these agents to be released on the American market was cefotaxime.

1. Cefotaxime

The aminothiazole ring in cefotaxime confers a high affinity for bacterial wall transpeptidase. Together with the cis configuration of the methoximino group, which enhances beta-lactamase stability, these structural modifications give rise to exceptionally high activity against gram-negative organisms (37). Like all cephalosporins with a 3-acetoxymethyl group (cephalothin, cephapirin), cefotaxime is deactylated. Desacetylcefotaxime appears rapidly after an intravenous dose of cefotaxime (Fig. 6); the apparent half-life is longer than that of the parent compound and the antimicrobial activity is lower (182). Microbiological assays do not permit independent measurement of unchanged cefotaxime in the presence of its metabolite. For this reason the studies reviewed in the following section primarily utilize specific bioassay or HPLC assays.

Table 5 Pharmacokinetic Parameters of Third-Generation Parenteral Cephalosporins

	Cefotaxime[a]	Ceftizoxime[b]	Ceftazidime[c]
α (hr^{-1})	3.2 ± 0.70	4.05	1.38 ± 0.37
β (hr^{-1})	0.59 ± 0.10	0.42 ± 0.05	0.37 ± 0.05
K_{12} (hr^{-1})	1.05 ± 0.23	4.2	–
K_{21} (hr^{-1})	1.29 ± 0.47	1.56	–
K_{10} (hr^{-1})	1.60 ± 0.21	1.8	–
$t_{1/2,\alpha}$ (hr)	0.23 ± 0.04	–	0.52 ± 0.14
$t_{1/2,\beta}$ (hr)	1.16 ± 0.23	1.66 ± 0.20	1.94 ± 0.38
V_C (liters)	10.8 ± 1.7	15.9	8.94 ± 0.82
VD_{SS} (liters)	18.0 ± 4.5	24.6 ± 2.16	14.8 ± 1.14
VD_{β} (liters)	30.8 ± 8.1	28.7 ± 2.35	17.7 ± 1.30
Percent protein bound	37–38	30–31	16–26
Clearance (ml/min)	358 ± 37.9	162.2 ± 31.1	111.2 ± 16.4

[a]From Refs. 31, 37, 182, 184, 185, 187, and 189–191.
[b]From Refs. 37, 216, 217, 225, and 227–229.
[c]From Refs. 37, 232, 234, 235, 237, 239, 247, 250, and 251.
[d]From Refs. 37, 258, 259, 263, and 264.
[e]From Refs. 37, 265, 268, and 269.
[f]From Refs. 37, 182, 237, 270, 273, 275, 293, 294, 298, and 299.
[g]From Refs. 37, 304, 305, 307, 309, 321, and 326.

Absorption. Cefotaxime is rapidly absorbed when administered by the intramuscular route, with peak concentrations of 20–25 μg/ml 30 min after a 1-g dose; bioavailability is 90–100% (183–185).

Distribution and Tissue Penetration. Cefotaxime is only 38% bound to human serum proteins at therapeutic concentrations, as measured by ultrafiltration or dialysis (183,186–188). Peak concentrations after an intravenous bolus dose of 1 g of cefotaxime are 80–100 μg/ml (37,182,187,189–191), but peak concentrations attained after a 30-min infusion of 1 g are 41 μg/ml (184).

Cefotaxime concentrations 2–4 hr after an intravenous dose of 1 g were 0.22–0.70 μg/ml in sputum and 7.2 μg/ml in pleural fluid (193). Bronchial tissue concentrations 1 hr after injection were 1.6 μg/g (194). Cefotaxime concentrations in the cerebrospinal fluid (CSF) of patients without meningitis were generally below 1 μg/ml, but in patients with meningitis 1.1–7.1 μg/ml was measured in

Cefmenoxime[d]	Cefsulodin[e]	Cefoperazone[f]	Ceftriaxone[g]
1.97 ± 0.65	1.51	1.89 ± 1.04	2.28 ± 2.72
0.55 ± 0.20	0.39 ± 0.03	0.39 ± 0.06	0.11 ± 0.02
0.58 ± 0.30	2.35	0.15	0.12
0.94 ± 0.52	1.78	0.36	0.27
1.50 ± 0.41	1.32	0.56	0.18
0.37 ± 0.13	0.46	0.44 ± 0.18	1.03 ± 1.22
1.40 ± 0.58	1.79 ± 0.17	1.82 ± 0.32	6.60 ± 1.06
9.64 ± 2.13	10.15 ± 1.91	14.8	5.2 ± 2.3
28.1	15.7 ± 1.13	12.7 ± 7.6	7.2 ± 0.08
26.1 ± 9.4	20.2 ± 0.57	12.2 ± 3.0	9.6 ± 1.51
77	15–37	85–90	83–96
222.0 ± 35.0	130.6 ± 13.3	80.0 ± 10.3	17.4 ± 3.4

CSF 1–4 hr after a 2-g dose (187,188,195–197). Concentrations in the CSF as high as 30 μg/ml have been reported (187,198). Mean CSF concentrations of 5.2 μg/ml cefotaxime and 5.9 μg/ml desacetylcefotaxime were observed 1 hr after multiple dosages of cefotaxime. These concentrations represented 10 and 55% of the average serum concentrations, respectively (199).

Interstitial fluid concentrations vary according to the study methodology. Mean blister concentrations of 25 μg/ml measured by microbiological assays were observed after a 1-g intramuscular dose (200). A total of 2 and 4 hr after a 1-g intravenous dose, concentrations of cefotaxime and desacetylcefotaxime were 4 and 1.6 μg/ml, respectively, as measured by HPLC (201).

In 10 patients undergoing cataract extraction, cefotaxime concentrations in the anterior chamber of the eye ranged from 0 to 2.3 μg/ml after an intravenous injection of 2 g (202). In children with acute otitis media treated with 50 mg/kg cefotaxime, effusion concentrations of 2.1-3.3 and 1.2 μg/ml were measured 1 hr after intravenous and intramuscular injection, respectively (203).

Bone concentrations of cefotaxime have been studied in patients with hip fractures after multiple intramuscular dosages of either 1 g four times daily or 2 g three times daily; 2-6 hr after the last dose, concentrations in bone ranged from 0.5 to 15.4 μg/g (181); 0.5-3 hr after a 2-g intravenous bolus, concentrations in bone were 2.1-7.6 μg/g (182).

Cefotaxime and desacetylcefotaxime concentrations have been measured in both common duct and gallbladder bile. In patients receiving multiple 1-g doses, common duct bile concentrations of cefotaxime and desactylcefotaxime were 36 and 243 μg/ml, respectively, 1.3 hr after injection (187). Gallbladder bile concentrations after multiple 1-g intravenous doses were 33.7-82.4 μg/ml cefotaxime while gallbladder wall concentrations were approximately 1 μg/g by bioassay (204). In 10 subjects 2-g intravenous doses produced average bile concentrations of 87.6 μg/ml and gallbladder wall concentrations of 15.8 μg/g (187). The biliary penetration of cefotaxime and that of its metabolites were compared in patients undergoing endoscopic retrograde choliopancreaography (ERCP) and patients with indwelling T-tubes at our institution. In ERCP patients peak bile cefotaxime concentrations of 25 μg/ml were reached 40-60 min after a 15-mg/kg dose. Metabolite concentrations in bile were 100 μg/ml. Cefotaxime concentrations of 26.1 μg/ml were reached 30 min after dosing in patients with T-tubes. The desacetyl metabolite showed a delayed peak in bile of 29.6 μg/ml 90 min after a dose (205).

In noninfected ascitic fluid cefotaxime concentrations varied from 3.8 to 17.6 μg/ml in six patients 2 hr after 1-g intramuscular doses (206). Breast milk concentrations in postpartum women were low, averaging below 1 μg/ml (207). The range of concentrations of cefotaxime reported in the ovary, oviduct, endometrium, myometrium, and fallopian tubes 0.3–4 hr after a 2-g intravenous dose was 0.26-6.4 μg/g (187).

Cefotaxime concentrations measured in prostatic tissue following a 1-g intramuscular dose were 2.6 μg/g in deep tissue and 3.9 μg/g in superficial tissue (208). The same dose produced renal tissue concentrations of 1.9-7.0 (inner cortex), 1.9-10.8 (outer medulla), and 2.3-14 μg/g (inner medulla) (208).

Concentrations in the pericardium and myocardium 15 min after a 50-mg/kg intravenous dose were 32 and 22 μg/g, respectively. The average myocardial concentration 2 hr following the dose was 3.8 μg/g (187). Because the MIC values of many gram-negative organisms are less than 1 μg/ml, this drug appears to achieve tissue concentrations high enough to eradicate infection.

Elimination. Approximately 50-60% of an intravenous dose of either 1 or 2 g is excreted as unchanged cefotaxime (37,182,183,187,189,190). Cefotaxime is also transformed in the liver, and possibly other tissues, to desacetylcefotaxime, with peak serum concentrations of the metabolite appearing within 5 min of dosing. The extent of this metabolism ranges from 35 to 56% (37,187,209, 210). A total of 24% of a dose can be recovered in the urine as desacetylcefotaxime within 24 hr (37,182,183,187,189,190,210). The metabolite possesses appreciable microbiological activity and will accumulate in patients with renal dysfunction. In addition, two inactive metabolites, isomers of desacetylcefotaxime lactone in which the beta-lactam ring has been opened, are generally detectable only in the urine of healthy individuals, but may be detectable in the serum of patients with renal insufficiency (37,185,187,191,209-211).

Total plasma clearance is greater than renal clearance, reflecting the contribution of metabolism (37,182,185,187,189). Renal clearance is significantly decreased with an increase in AUC after the concomitant administration of probenecid (183,189). The elimination half-life is 0.9-1.1 hr for cefotaxime and 1.3-1.6 hr for desacetylcefotaxime following intravenous administration of cefotaxime in healthy subjects (182,183,185,187,189).

The pharmacokinetics of both cefotaxime and its major metabolite have been studied in patients with renal dysfunction (185,191,213-215). Only studies using specific assays are discussed in this section. In patients with severe renal impairment (creatinine clearances below 10 ml/min) total plasma clearance, renal clearance, and urinary recovery of unchanged cefotaxime are all significantly decreased. The mean elimination half-life of cefotaxime is prolonged to only 2-2.6 hr, which reflects the alternate excretion routes for cefotaxime (185, 213). The apparent elimination half-life of the desacetyl metabolite is altered to a greater extent, increasing to 10-15 hr (185,213). Total urinary recovery of cefotaxime and desacetylcefotaxime decreases with renal impairment, but the ratio of the urinary recovery of desacetylcefotaxime to that of cefotaxime increases with declining renal function. Hence the percentage of the dose recovered in the urine as metabolite exceeds the percentage excreted unchanged in patients with severe renal dysfunction (187). Hemodialysis improves the clearance of cefotaxime, with the mean half-life decreasing from 3.4 to 1.6 hr (185). Desacetylcefotaxime is also removed by hemodialysis, with the apparent half-life decreasing from 14 to 3 hr (185). Peritoneal dialysis appears to be of little value in increasing the clearance of cefotaxime (213).

Six patients with acute drug-related hepatocellular damage, five of whom had creatinine clearance above 40 ml/min, had cefotaxime half-life values within the normal range. However, the amount of desacetylcefotaxime formed by these patients, as reflected by peak concentrations, was reduced (213).

2. Ceftizoxime

Ceftizoxime bears the same side chain as cefotaxime but lacks the acetoxymethyl group at the 3-position on the ring. This molecular modification does not greatly alter microbiological activity. Since ceftizoxime lacks the substituent at the 3-position, it is not subject to deacetylation.

Absorption. Serum concentrations of ceftizoxime peak 1 hr after a 1-g intramuscular dose at 40.9 μg/ml, and at 14–16 μg/ml after a 500-mg dose, with 75.6% of the dose recovered in the urine within 6 hr (216–218). Approximately 78% of a ceftizoxime dose is absorbed from peritoneal dialysis fluid containing ceftizoxime during a 6-hr dwell time (219).

Distribution and Tissue Penetration. Ceftizoxime is 31% plasma protein bound in humans (220). Peak serum concentrations following a 1-g intravenous dose were 84 μg/ml (217). In normal individuals with uninflamed meninges undergoing myelography we observed that concentrations above 1 μg/ml were not obtainable following a single 30-mg/kg dose (221,222). Single doses of 30 mg/kg were also administered on days 1, 3, 7, 10, and 14 to 12 patients with bacterial meningitis. Two hours following administration, CSF concentrations ranged from undetectable to 17 μg/ml (mean of 41 samples, 4.9 μg/ml). Higher CSF concentrations were observed in patients with high protein concentrations or high leukocyte counts during earlier days of therapy and in samples obtained more than 120 min following drug administration (215). In 24 patients receiving multiple doses of 29 mg/kg intravenously in the presence of meningitis, the average CSF concentration 1.5 hr after administration was 3.8 ± 2.9 μg/ml. In 23 of 27 specimens CSF concentrations were below 1 μg/ml (224). In a small group of patients treated with ceftizoxime (200 mg/kg daily) for pneumococcal, meningicoccal, and *Hemophilus* meningitis, CSF concentrations ranged from below 0.5 to 29 μg/ml. All patients had sterile CSF concentrations at 24 and 36 hr after initiation of therapy (223). Aqueous humor concentrations in three patients about 1.5 hr after a 1-g dose were low, 1.5 ± 0.7 μg/ml (200).

Extravascular tissue penetration in humans has recently been reviewed (224, 225). Concentrations of ceftizoxime in pleural fluid and sputum remained below 10 μg/ml in patients receiving intravenous doses (224). Concentrations measured in gallbladder bile or common duct bile were above 40 μg/ml and gallbladder tissue concentrations approached 70 μg/g (224,226). Prostatic tissue and uterine wall concentrations above 10 μg/g may be achieved (224). Atrial appendage concentrations were 7.9 ± 3.5 μg/g 1–2 hr after a 1.3-g dose in 14 patients (224). Bone concentrations of 6.3 ± 4.6 μg/g were observed 1 hr after a 1-g dose of ceftizoxime in five patients (224). Amniotic fluid concentrations measured in 76 women were 14.0 ± 8.9 μg/ml 127–210 min after a 1-g dose (224). Breast milk contained below 1 μg/ml ceftizoxime (224).

Elimination. The elimination half-life of ceftizoxime is approximately 1.5 hr in individuals with normal renal function; urinary recovery of ceftizoxime accounts for approximately 90% of the dose (216,217,227,229). Concurrent administration of probenecid results in higher serum concentrations of ceftizoxime, with an increase in elimination half-life to 2.3 hr and a decrease in renal clearance (138 ± 13 to 85 ± 3), indicating that this drug is eliminated by tubular secretion (216). Other authors, however, suggest that tubular secretion plays only a minor role in ceftizoxime elimination (229). Patients with severe renal disease (creatinine clearance below 10 ml/min) exhibit a prolongation of the mean elimination half-life to 19.3 ± 7.5 hr, in contrast to the moderate prolongation in half-life seen with cefotaxime (218,227,229). Reduction in the frequency of administration is necessary in patients with severe renal dysfunction (227). Peritoneal dialysis with a 6-hr dwell time removes only 4–5% of the dose (219). Hemodialysis clearance has been calculated as 44.8 ± 21.5 ml/min at an average blood flow rate of 205 ± 11.7 ml/min. Supplemental dosage of ceftizoxime after dialysis is not necessary (229).

3. Ceftazidime

Ceftazidime shows low protein binding, a relatively long half-life, and minimal tubular secretion. Ceftazidime and cephaloridine have the same substituent at the 3-position and are similar in their pharmacokinetic properties. Animal studies have failed to reveal nephrotoxicity from ceftazidime, although a slight but significant decrease in glomerular filtration rate measured by [^{51}Cr] EDTA clearance was demonstrated. Proximal tubular function measured by urinary β_2-microglobulin excretion was not affected (230,231).

Absorption. Mean peak ceftazidime concentrations of 37.2 μg/ml appear approximately 1 hr after a 1-g intramuscular dose (232). The 24-hr urinary recovery of ceftazidime after intramuscular administration was 80-90%. The bioavailability after intramuscular administration was approximately 100% (232, 233).

Intraperitoneal administration of ceftazidime produced serum peak concentrations adequate to treat infection caused by common pathogens. Two hours after a 1-g intraperitoneal dose, serum concentrations were 40 ± 13 μg/ml, and after 12 hr of peritoneal dialysis with dialysate containing 200 mg of ceftazidime, serum concentrations were 25.3 ± 3.1 μg/ml (236).

Distribution and Tissue Penetration. Plasma protein binding is low, approximately 16–26% (232–235). Intravenous bolus injections of 1 g of ceftazidime produced initial serum concentrations of 121 μg/ml, while 1-hr infusions of 1 g produced peak concentrations of 69.5 μg/ml (232).

The extracellular fluid penetration of ceftazidime has been evaluated utilizing both skin blister (238,239) and subcutaneous thread techniques (238,240,241). Although results vary somewhat with the method used, all studies suggest high penetration into extravascular fluid, with peak concentrations ranging from 20 to 64 μg/ml 1–2 hr after a 1-g intravenous dose (238–241). Lymphatic concentrations and pharmacokinetics appeared similar to those of blister fluid (242). Concentrations of ceftazidime in the CSF of patients with noninflamed meninges following a 2-g bolus dose were below 1 μg/ml (242); however, in five patients with meningitis concentrations ranged from 0.8 to 18 μg/ml 0.5 and 1 hr after a 2-g intravenous bolus dose, in spite of apparently similar degrees of meningeal inflammation (242). Upon multiple intravenous doses of 2 g CSF concentrations ranged from 2 to 30 μg/ml in 11 patients with meningitis (243).

Mean ceftazidime concentrations in aqueous humor 1–3 hr after a 2-g intravenous bolus dose were 11 ± 4 μg/ml, whereas mean pleural fluid concentrations were 28 ± 2 μg/ml 4 hr after dosing (242). Sputum concentrations in patients with cystic fibrosis ranged from 0.7 to 9.8 μg/ml 1 hr after 50-mg/kg doses administered intravenously every 8 hr for 5–6 days (244). Breast milk concentrations of ceftazidime in 11 women receiving 2 g of ceftazidime every 8 hr for 2–4 days remained above 3.8 ± 2 μg/ml throughout therapy (245). A total of 31 patients undergoing abdominal or vaginal hysterectomy received 2 g of ceftazidime 1–6 hr before the procedure; peak tissue concentrations not corrected for contamination with blood, attained within 1–2 hr after the dose, were 18–19 μg/ml in the myometrium, endometrium, and salpinges (246).

Ceftazidime concentrations in blood-free femoral bone averaged 31.1 ± 1.7 μg/g approximately 30 min after a 2-g intravenous injection and 24.5 ± 1.3 μg/g 2 hr after injection in 12 patients, with similar levels in periprothetic fluid (247). In 39 patients receiving 2 g of ceftazidime intravenously as much as 5 hr prior to cardiac surgery, mean tissue concentrations corrected for blood contamination were 6.6, 9.4, 9.2, 20.0, and 12.7 μg/g of skin, skeletal muscle, fat, bone, and heart muscle, respectively (249). These concentrations are sufficient to prevent infection by common pathogens.

Ceftazidime concentrations in bile after a 2-g intravenous dose were 30–40 μg/ml 1 hr after dosing and remained above 6 μg/ml for over 8 hr (247,248). Peak biliary concentrations in another study were not attained until 4 hr after a 1-g dose (247). Concentrations of ceftazidime in gallbladder tissue after a 1-g dose were maintained above 8 μg/g for over 4 hr (237). Concentrations in peritoneal fluid after a 2-g intravenous dose of ceftazidime peaked at 27.6 ± 1.2 μg/ml 1 hr following the dose (247).

Elimination. A total of 70–90% of a dose of ceftazidime is recovered unchanged in the urine within 24 hr. The elimination half-life is about 1.8 hr (232–235,237,243,244,250). No active metabolites were detected in the urine by bioautography, and renal clearance (93 ml/min) approximated total body clearance (116 ml/min) (37,232–234,237,250). Probenecid has no effect on elimination half-life, AUC, or clearance (233,237,250). Hence ceftazidime appears to be removed from the body primarily by glomerular filtration.

Urinary recovery is decreased in patients with renal impairment. In patients with creatinine clearances of less than 10 ml/min, 15.6% of the dose was recovered in the urine within 24 hr (237). In a study of 19 patients and 5 volunteers with various degrees of renal function, the elimination half-life increased from 1.5 ± 0.2 hr in normals to 3.6 ± 0.7, 9.0 ± 1.0, and 16.1 ± 4.0 hr in patients with creatinine clearances of 30–80, 13–29, and 2–12 ml/min per 1.73 m^2, respectively. The mean elimination half-life of ceftazidime was 25.5 ± 4.6 hr between dialyses and 2.8 ± 0.2 hr during dialysis, indicating good removal of ceftazidime by hemodialysis (252). Recommendations to reduce ceftazidime dosage in renal insufficiency have been made based on correlations between creatinine clearance or serum creatinine concentrations and ceftazidime elimination (252, 253). Peritoneal dialysis effectively lowers serum concentrations and shortens elimination half-life (236).

The pharmacokinetics of ceftazidime varies with age. After single intravenous doses of 30 mg/kg, the elimination half-life for infants less than 2 months old was 4.2 ± 1.6 hr and for those 2–12 months it was 2.0 ± 0.6 hr (254). Neonates also appear to have a larger distribution volume than older children (254,256). Children with cystic fibrosis appear to eliminate ceftazidime more rapidly after single doses of 50 mg/kg than normal adults (256). The elimination half-life was about 1 hr in seven neonates with cystic fibrosis, compared with 4.7 hr in normal neonates, and the total body clearance was 6.0 ± 3.1 versus 2.0 ± 0.5 ml/min per kilogram, respectively (256). Older patients with cystic fibrosis (8–30 years old), however, had elimination half-lives similar to those of normal controls (257). Elderly patients (63–83 years old) with serum creatinines of 0.7–1.5 mg/dl, demonstrated an increase in serum elimination half-life (2.9 hr, as compared to 1.7 hr in normals) and a reduction in 12-hr urinary excretion from 86% in controls to 69% in the elderly (251). This result probably reflects an age-related reduction in renal function.

4. Cefmenoxime

Cefmenoxime is characterized by an intermediate degree of protein binding. Elimination, primarily renal with no important metabolic route of clearance, with a half-life of 1 hr is similar to that of many cephalosporins.

Absorption. Peak plasma concentrations of cefmenoxime attained 40 min after intramuscular administration of 250, 500, and 1000 mg were about 9, 15, and 27 μg/ml, respectively (258). Following intramuscular administration 24-hr urinary recoveries were 72% and were comparable to those following intravenous bolus dosing (75%). The bioavailability of the intramuscular route (determined by comparisons of AUC) was nearly 100% (258).

Distribution and Tissue Penetration. Serum concentrations of cefmenoxime over time are best described by a two-compartment pharmacokinetic model, as for other cephalosporins (258). After intravenous injections of 0.5-, 1-, and 2-g doses, peak concentrations in serum were 64, 101, and 198 μg/ml, respectively (258,259). The plasma protein binding reported in normal volunteers for cefmenoxime was 77%, but protein binding was considerably lower and more variable (43.5 ± 13%) in critically ill patients with mild to moderate renal impairment (258,260).

In five patients with either pneumonia or chronic respiratory infections, sputum concentrations after a 1-g dose infused over 1 hr peaked at 0.32–1.97 μg/ml, representing 0.8–2.6% of serum peak concentrations (259). Aqueous humor concentrations in 11 patients undergoing cataract extraction after receiving 1 g of cefmenoxime intravenously ranged from 0.3 to 1.1 μg/ml 20–60 min after injection (261). Concentrations of 0.15–1.4 μg/ml were measured in the CSF of 12 normal volunteers undergoing myelograms after receiving three doses of 30 mg/kg every 6 hr (262).

Elimination. The elimination half-life of cefmenoxime after intravenous administration is 0.8–1.1 hr, with approximately 70% of a dose recovered in the urine within 24 hr (258,259,263). In addition, about 11% of a dose of radiolabeled cefmenoxime underwent biliary secretion (263).

Serum concentrations observed 30 min after a 0.5-hr infusion of 1 g of cefmenoxime with probenecid were 84.2 μg/ml, compared with 73.5 μg/ml without probenecid, and the elimination half-lives were 1.8 and 1.1 hr, respectively (263). Hence tubular secretion appears to play a significant role in the elimination of cefmenoxime. In 20 patients with renal disease who received 2 g intravenously, the AUC increased when renal function was impaired. Correlations between the AUC and the plasma creatinine or glomerular filtration rate allow establishment of dosage guidelines for patients with renal dysfunction (264).

5. Cefsulodin

Cefsulodin is characterized by low protein binding. Elimination, primarily renal with no important metabolic route of clearance, with a half-life of 1.5–2 hr is similar to that of many cephalosporins.

Absorption. In 28 volunteers peak serum concentrations of cefsulodin were 5.5, 11.8, and 19.4 μg/ml approximately 1.4 hr after a 250-, 500-, and 1000-mg doses, respectively (265). No statistically significant differences exist in 24-hr urinary recoveries with intramuscular (52.1 ± 9.3%) and intravenous (55.6 ± 11.0%) administration. Simultaneous regression analysis showed that the AUC with intramuscular dosing was 82% of that obtained with intravenous infusion, the small reduction perhaps explained by degradation. Preliminary experiments have suggested that at 37°C the in vitro cefsulodin half-life in human plasma is approximately 6 hr (265).

Distribution and Tissue Penetration. The protein binding of cefsulodin is low, ranging between 25 and 37%. Mean peak concentrations in heart valves, muscle, and subcutaneous tissue were 8, 19, and 8.3 μg/g, respectively, with a simultaneous serum concentration of 147 μg/ml (266). Extravascular penetration of cefsulodin is significant; blister fluid concentrations 2 hr after dosing averaged 15.4 μg/ml and dermabrasion fluid concentrations were 8.3 μg/ml, with corresponding serum concentrations of 20.6 μg/ml (267).

Elimination. The elimination half-life of cefsulodin is 1.5-2.0 hr in normal individuals (265,267-269). A total of 60-90% of a dose is recovered unchanged in the urine. In pateints with normal renal function plasma clearance and renal clearance of cefsulodin are 136 and 84 ml/min, respectively (268). The observation that renal clearance was less than creatinine clearance suggested that cefsulodin undergoes tubular reabsorption, in contrast to other cephalosporins (268).

Two groups have found linear relationships between renal function (glomerular filtration rate and creatinine clearance) and the total plasma clearance of cefsulodin (268,269). The elimination half-life was prolonged to 10.1 hr in patients with creatinine clearances below 10 ml/min and to 13 hr in anuric patients (268,269). During hemodialysis plasma drug concentration was reduced by 60% and the elimination half-life fell to 2.1 hr (269).

6. Cefoperazone

Cefoperazone is characterized by high protein binding. The drug penetrates into the CSF but achieves variable concentrations. Elimination is primarily biliary, with a 2-hr half-life.

Absorption. The intramuscular absorption of cefoperazone following the administration of 0.25-, 0.5-, and 1-g doses gave peak blood concentrations of 21.8, 33.4, and 73.9 μg/ml, respectively, 1 hr after administration (270). The AUC was the same with 15-min intravenous infusion as with intramuscular administration, indicating nearly complete bioavailability (12). Bioavailability following intraperitoneal administration of cefoperazone in dialysate was about 95% (271).

Distribution and Tissue Penetration. Peak serum concentrations following intravenous administration of 2 g of cefoperazone infused over 15-30 min averaged about 250 μg/ml (272-276). These high concentrations reflect in part the small volume of distribution and the high degree of protein binding of cefoperazone (12,270,273,277,278). The binding sites for cefoperazone appear to be the same as for cefazolin (277). The protein binding of cefoperazone is 94, 89, and 43% at serum concentrations of 25, 250, and 5000 μg/ml, respectively (278). Cefoperazone did not displace bilirubin from serum albumin, but bilirubin easily displaced cefoperazone from albumin (270).

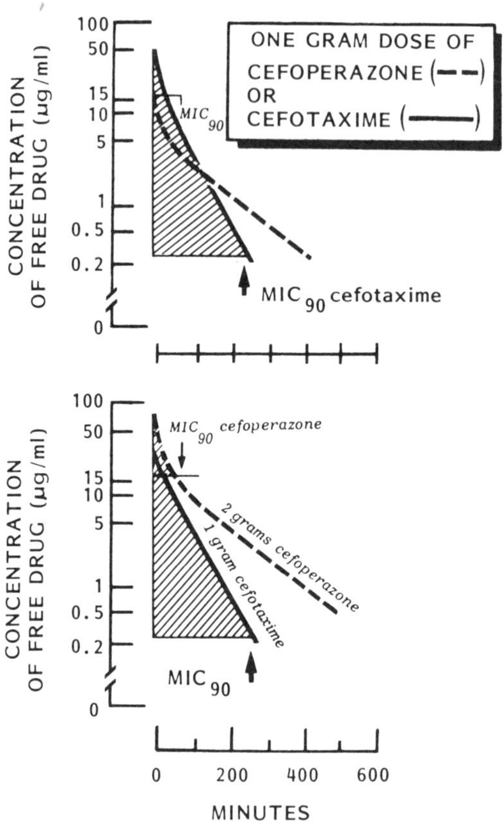

Figure 7 Time during which the concentration of unbound cefotaxime and cefoperaone are above the MIC_{90} for *E. coli* and *Klebsiella.*

High protein binding may limit the amount of free drug available to penetrate into tissue and exert microbiological activity. Cefoperazone in the unbound form is only available for approximately 5 min at or above the MIC_{90} for *E. coli* and *K. pneumoniae* after a single 1-g intravenous dose (Fig. 7). Cefotaxime, a less highly bound drug, is available for approximately 4.5 hr longer at the same dose. Increasing the cefoperazone dose to 2 g does little to increase the duration of the free drug concentration.

In pateints receiving cefoperazone for the treatment of respiratory infections, peak sputum concentrations of 0.08–6.1 μg/ml occur after intravenous doses of 0.5–3 g (270,274). After a 0.5- and a 1-g dose, concentrations in tonsillar tissue and maxillary sinus were 4–8 μg/ml, while middle ear fluid concentrations were 3 μg/ml after a 2-g dose (270).

Extravascular fluid concentrations peak at approximately 8 μg/ml within 1 hr after a 2-g intravenous dose (279). The area under the concentration–time curve for extravascular fluid was 7.3% of the area under the serum concentration–time curve, as expected with the high degree of protein binding of cefoperazone (279). However, concentrations were above the MIC of susceptible organisms. Concentrations in ascitic fluid can approach 65 μg/ml during therapy (270,274).

Cefoperazone penetrates into cerebrospinal fluid (CSF). In 11 children (1 month to 8 years old) CSF concentrations ranging from 0.44 to 7.3 μg/ml were observed 2.5–4 hr after infusion (280). In a patient treated for *K. pneumoniae* meningitis, the CSF concentration was 9 μg/ml on day 4 of therapy, about 6 hr after a 2-g dose (281). In 15 patients with bacterial meningitis given a single 50-mg/kg dose, a single 100-mg/kg dose, or three doses of 100 mg/kg at 8 hr intervals, CSF concentrations ranged from below 1 to 5.2, below 1 to 8.2, and below 1 to 11.5 μg/ml, respectively (282). At our institution the penetration of cefoperazone into the CSF was studied in 10 volunteers undergoing lumbar myelography 9–141 min after receiving 30 mg/kg intravenously; CSF concentrations were below 1 μg/ml in these volunteers with noninflamed meninges (283).

Patients pretreated with 2–4 g of cefoperazone before undergoing cataract extraction had aqueous humor concentrations ranging from 0.9 to 3.4 μg/ml 1–6 hr after administration (284).

Concentrations of cefoperazone in breast milk are below 1 μg/ml after a 1-g intravenous dose. Placental transfer of drug is approximately 33% of the administered dose (285). Amniotic fluid concentrations of 2.8–4.8 μg/ml appear after 1- and 2-g doses (270). Peak pelvic tissue concentrations were 24.6 ± 9.9, 21.0 ± 7.1, and 25.6 ± 9.4 μg/g in fundal myometrium, lower uterine segment, and fallopian tube, respectively, 2–3 hr after a 2-g intramuscular dose (286).

Peak bile concentrations were 81.5 and 292.5 μg/ml in patients with pancreatic cancer and cholelithiasis, respectively (287). Other studies have indicated that therapeutic cefoperazone concentrations are achieved in lung tissue, bone, prostatic tissue, renal tissue, appendix, muscle, fat, and ureter (288–290).

Elimination. Two hydrolysis products of cefoperazone, representing less than 1% of the total drug recovered, have been detected in human urine and bile by high-performance liquid chromatography (12,270,291). The elimination half-life of cefoperazone ranges from 1.6 to 2.4 hr, depending in part upon drug dose (12,270,273,274).

Renal clearance of cefoperazone is approximately 25% of total body clearance and 15–36% of a dose is recovered in the urine within 6 hr (12,270–274). The ratio of renal clearance to creatinine clearance was 13%, which is similar to the unbound fraction of cefoperazone circulating in the serum (12,271–274). This fact suggests that the primary mechanism for renal excretion is glomerular filtration. Probenecid only slightly increased the serum elimination half-life (109 versus 92 min) and had no observable effect on the fraction of the dose recovered in the urine from 0 to 6 hr (270). Hence tubular secretion probably plays only a minor role in the renal excretion of cefoperazone.

The major route of elimination of cefoperazone is via biliary excretion. Patients with T-tubes and without apparent hepatic insufficiency demonstrated peak biliary concentrations of cefoperazone of 675–6113 μg/ml (270). This type of patient also demonstrated a longer elimination half-life (mean 4.1 hr, versus 1.6 hr in controls) and lower total clearance (31.3 ml/min, versus 77.7 ml/min in controls) (292). Total urinary excretion reached 40–59%, approximately twice that in normals (23.6%).

In the presence of biliary obstruction, renal elimination becomes the major route of excretion of cefoperazone. The elimination of cefoperazone was studied in 13 patients after a single 1-g dose and compared with normal subjects (12). In three patients with a high degree of biliary tract obstruction, 90% of the administered dose was recovered in the urine within 24 hr. These three pateints also demonstrated greater renal clearance (21 versus 14 ml/min), with a doubling of the ratio of renal clearance of cefoperazone to creatinine clearance. The authors postulate that this is due to the marked reduction in protein binding (from 90 to 65%) observed in these pateints, perhaps caused by displacement by bilirubin (12). Urinary recovery of cefoperazone in five cirrhotic patients appeared directly related to the extent of hyperbilirubinemia. The elimination half-life in these 13 patients ranged from 2.8 to 7.0 hr, with a mean of 5 hr (12). Similar results were obtained independently in six patients with cirrhosis (293).

In another study hepatic injury (viral hepatitis, alcoholic fatty liver, cirrhosis) prolonged the elimination half-life and significantly lowered total and extrarenal clearance; renal clearance was unchanged (294,295). These authors could not relate the pharmacokinetic changes they observed to the nature of hepatic disease.

Peak bile concentrations of cefoperazone in five postcholecystectomy patients with T-tube drainage ranged from 2.8 to 1100 μg/ml and were correlated (r = 0.986) with serum bilirubin concentration (296).

The elimination half-life of cefoperazone in patients with liver impairment is still shorter than the common dosage interval of 12 hr and therefore in patients with good renal function relatively little accumulation should take place. This hypothesis was verified in five patients after five 1-g doses of cefoperazone given every 12 hr; mean serum concentrations on day 3 were 3–22% higher than those on day 1.

The renal clearance in the presence of normal hepatic function only accounts for 25% of the total body clearance of cefoperazone; hence one would not expect a large increase in the elimination half-life in patients with poor renal function. Studies on patients with severe chronic renal failure receiving 1 g as a bolus showed a prolongation of elimination half-life (5.0 to 15.1 hr) in 6 of the 10 patients studied (297). None of these patients had a history of hepatobiliary disease, nor were any taking medications that might affect the pharmacokinetics of cefoperazone. Further studies with multiple doses of 1 or 2 g every 12 hr for 5-14 days in eight patients with severe chronic renal failure showed no drug accumulation. Another group, studying functionally anephric dialysis subjects while off dialysis, observed similar elimination half-lives for cefoperazone (2.07 hr in normals; 2.03 hr in dialysis subjects) and similar total body clearance (96.2 ml/min for normals; 92.9 ml/min for dialysis subjects) (298). Similar findings were reported by others (12,278). On the basis of these reports, the pharmacokinetics of cefoperazone does not appear to be substantially altered in patients with renal insufficiency uncomplicated by hepatobiliary disease. Dosage reduction is recommended for patients with creatinine clearances below 20 ml/min (299).

Our institution has reported an increase in the elimination half-life in four critically ill patients with concomitant renal and hepatic dysfunction (283). The longest estimated half-life was 28.1 hr in a patient with severe renal impairment and jaundice. Based on these and other case reports, it may be prudent to adjust cefoperazone dosage in the presence of concomitant renal and hepatobiliary disease, although more information is needed on the pharmacokinetics in this group of patients (12,278).

The elimination half-life was 5.6 hr and the total body clearance was 36 ml/hr per kilogram in 15 preterm infants (gestional age from 32 to 36 weeks; postnatal age from 1 to 6 days) receiving either 50 or 250 mg/kg by intravenous infusion (300). The elimination rate constant (r = 0.57) and clearance (r = 0.67) were correlated with gestational age. In 28 full-term and premature neonates with sepsis, the elimination half-life of cefoperazone was 7-9 hr, but when 14 of these infants were restudied on days 5-7, the mean serum half-lives were 5-7 hr (301).

The pharmacokinetics of cefoperazone in 34 patients with neoplastic disease but normal hepatic and renal function was similar to results obtained from normal volunteers (302).

7. Ceftriaxone

The antimicrobial properties of ceftriaxone are similar to those of other third-generation cephalosporins. Pharmacokinetically ceftriaxone is notable for its high degree of protein binding (95%), and its unusually long serum elimination half-life of about 8 hr.

Absorption. Peak serum concentrations of 42 and 45 μg/ml were attained 2.5-3 hr after a 0.5-g intramuscular dose of ceftriaxone. Peak concentrations of 95.2 ± 53.0 μg/ml were seen 3 hr after a 1-g intramuscular dose (303,304). Coadministration of lidocaine has no effect on the already high bioavailability of intramuscular doses (303,304). A total of 25% of the administered dose was collected in urine within 24 hr following intramuscular dosing, compared with 37% following intravenous dosing (304).

Distribution and Tissue Penetration. Intravenous doses of 1 g administered every 12 hr result in peak concentrations of 145 ± 11 μg/ml on day 1 and 168 ± 25 μg/ml on day 4 of therapy (305). Following intravenous administration of 150, 500, and 1500 mg to healthy volunteers, total (bound plus unbound) ceftriaxone concentrations and AUC do not increase in proportion to the increase in dose, resulting in dose-dependent increases in total body clearance from 9.7 ml/min at 150 mg to 13 ml/min at 1500 mg (306,307). These dose-related changes in pharmacokinetic parameters can be explained, at least in part, by concentration-dependent plasma protein binding. The free fraction of ceftriaxone in human plasma increase from 0.04 (96% bound) at plasma concentrations of 0.5 μg/ml to 0.17 (83% bound) at plasma concentrations of 300 μg/ml and 0.2–0.5 at concentrations of 500–1000 μg/ml (306–308). The high protein binding is also reflected in a relatively small volume of distribution, 9.1 liters (309, 310).

Since only free drug is available for distribution into various tissues, it may be assumed that little drug would be available for extravascular penetration. However, high protein binding notwithstanding, ceftriaxone appears to readily penetrate blister fluid, albeit slowly. Peak blister fluid concentrations averaged 32.7 ± 7 μg/ml in six subjects about 6.5 hr after a 0.5-g intravenous dose (311).

The ability of ceftrixone to penetrate into the CSF has been studied in pediatric patients with bacterial meningitis (312–315). The CSF concentrations averaged 5.16 ± 2.1 μg/ml 6 hr after an average dose of 46 mg/kg administered intramuscularly (312). After a single 50-mg/kg dose of ceftriaxone, CSF concentrations peaked at 6 hr and averaged 4.2 ± 2.1 μg/ml in 19 patients, and in 30 pediatric patients receiving single doses of either 50 or 75 mg/kg, mean concentrations in the CSF 1–6 hr after infusion were 5.4 and 6.4 μg/ml, respectively (313,314). The CSF concentrations averaged 5–10% of concomitant plasma concentrations. These CSF concentrations exceed the MIC for common pathogens by at least 10-fold and are typically accompanied by rapid sterilization of the CSF.

Ceftriaxone concentrations were studied in 15 patients undergoing cardiopulmonary bypass surgery who received a 1-g intravenous dose approximately 2 hr before surgery. Concentrations were 4.7 ± 2.1 μg/g in sternal bone and 7.7 ± 1.8 μg/g in atrial appendage (316).

The penetration of ceftriaxone into reproductive tissues has been studied in 31 women after a 2-g intravenous infusion of ceftriaxone at various times before abdominal or vaginal hysterectomy (317). Tissue concentrations peaked approximately 2 hr after administration and were 37.8 ± 5.2, 31.8 ± 8.4, and 53.1 ± 5.5 μg/g in myometrium, endometrium, and salpinges, respectively. Tissue concentrations in excess of 20 μg/g could be maintained in all tissues sampled for at least 5 hr. Unfortunately, blood was simply swabbed from the outside of the tissues; therefore the likelihood of these concentrations being influenced by blood contamination is great (317). The penetration of ceftriaxone into the fetus at parturition was studied in 17 women after a 2-g intravenous bolus injection over 2-5 min (318). Mean umbilical cord serum concentrations peaked 4 hr after ceftriaxone administration and ranged from 23.0 to 28.9 μg/ml. Amniotic fluid and placental concentrations averaged 17.0 and 15.5 μg/ml 6 and 2 hr after the dose, respectively. Ceftriaxone concentrations in newborn urine was variable and ranged from 17.0 to 92.0 μg/ml 1-12 hr after ceftriaxone administration to the mother (318). Breast milk concentrations after a 1-g intravenous or intramuscular dose were also studied in 20 patients 3 days postpartum. Peak milk concentrations were approximately 0.7 and 0.5 μg/ml 5 hr following intravenous and intramuscular administration, respectively (318).

Elimination. Ceftriaxone has an elimination half-life of 6-8 hr, with both renal and nonrenal clearance mechanisms (306-308). After 48 hr approximately 65% of a 1.5-g dose can be recovered as ceftriazone in the urine. Dosage appears to influence the percentage of dose excreted in the urine during early intervals, with 12.8% of a 150-mg dose excreted during the first 2 hr and 21.9% of a 1500-mg dose excreted in the same interval (306,307). Neither dose nor time had any influence on the renal clearance of unbound drug. The mean renal clearance of free ceftriaxone was 173 ml/min, somewhat higher than the average glomerular filtration rate, implying a minor role for tubular secretion in the renal elimination of ceftriaxone (307).

A substantial portion of a dose of ceftriaxone is eliminated by nonrenal mechanisms. In two subjects 56% of a 150-mg intravenous dose of ^{14}C-labeled ceftriaxone was recovered in the urine while 44% of the dose was recovered as microbiologically inactive products in the feces after 100 hr (309). The concentration of ceftriaxone in bile-rich duodenal fluid in four male volunteers after intravenous administration of 500 mg peaked at 150-200 μg/ml 60-120 min after injection (319). Ceftriaxone concentrations have also been measured in the bile and gallbladder wall of 13 patients undergoing cholecystectomy after receiving a 15-mg/kg intravenous dose of ceftriaxone at various times before the removal of tissue. Concentrations in bile ranged from 25.6 to 4633 μg/ml, while gallbladder wall concentrations ranged from 12.5 to 387.5 μg/g of tissue (320).

Since ceftriaxone clearance is approximately two-thirds renal and one-third nonrenal (presumably biliary), the need for dosage modification in patients with mild to moderate impairment is probably minimal. Nine patients with renal insufficiency requiring hemodialysis or peritoneal dialysis but with normal liver function were studied after a 7-mg/kg dose (322). In these patients the mean elimination half-life was prolonged to 13.4 hr and the mean total body clearance was reduced to 6.9 ml/kg per hour (normal, 13.5 ml/kg per hour) (322). In 10 of 12 patients with end-stage renal failure but intact nonrenal elimination pathways, ceftriaxone's elimination half-life increased to 12 hr (normal, 8 hr). Two patients with normal liver function tests, however, exhibited marked prolongation of the elimination half-life (20 and 34 hr). With impairment of both routes of elimination, a decrease in dosage may be recommended (322).

The pharmacokinetics of ceftriaxone has also been studied in eight subjects requiring hemodialysis (323). Variability in the elimination half-lives was reported in these patients, with an interdialysis half-life range of 7.7–38.5 hr (mean, 13.9 hr); during dialysis the elimination half-lives ranged from 11.7 to 33.4 hr (mean, 16.1 hr). Statistical analysis detected no differences in half-life, plasma clearance, and volume of distribution during dialysis and interdialysis intervals (323). Three patients undergoing peritoneal dialysis did not have detectable ceftriaxone concentrations in the dialysate after receiving a 7-mg/kg dose (321). Hence it does not appear that ceftriaxone is removed by peritoneal dialysis.

Ceftriaxone concentrations have been studied in newborns 1–45 days old (324), infants 7–15 months old (325), and children 24–70 months (325). In newborns peak serum concentrations after a 15-min infusion of 50 mg/kg were 136–173 μg/ml and the mean elimination half-life ranged from 5.2 to 7.4 hr in infants weighing more than 1500 g and from 7.7 to 8.4 hr in infants weighing less than 1500 g (324). Infants and children receiving a 50-mg/kg intravenous dose over 5 min exhibited similar pharmacokinetic parameters, with an average elimination half-life of 6.5 hr, a total body clearance of 0.71 ml/min per kilogram, and VD_β of 0.394 liter/kg (325).

Ceftriaxone pharmacokinetics was studied in eight subjects 65–78 years old. A 24% reduction in renal clearance corresponding to a 19% reduction in creatinine clearance occurred. However, no statistically significant alterations in either total body clearance or elimination half-life was observed, suggesting that dosage adjustment in elderly patients is not necessary (326).

In patients with various neoplastic disorders but normal renal and hepatic function who received 2 g of ceftriaxone every 8 hr as a continuous infusion, the mean concentrations in the serum were maintained at 135 μg/ml during the infusion period (327). Patients receiving either 1- or 2-g intravenous single doses demonstrated similar pharmacokinetic parameters as in other studies. The intramuscular administration of 500 mg, however, produced peak serum concentrations of only 32.9 μg/ml 2 hr after administration, lower than the 42–45 μg/ml concentrations reported by other workers. The reasons for the lower peak concentrations following intramuscular administration in this study may relate to absorption changes caused by muscle wasting in these patients or to variations in assay techniques (327).

F. Summary of the Third-Generation Cephalosporins

The third-generation cephalosporins are pharmacokinetically diverse. Of these antibiotics, cefotaxime is the only agent that is metabolized to a significant extent (35–56%) to an active metabolite. Nonrenal clearance plays a significant role in the elimination of both cefoperazone and ceftriaxone, with biliary excretion accounting for the majority of the clearance of cefoperazone and one-third of the clearance of ceftriaxone. Of the third-generation agents, ceftriaxone has the longest elimination half-life (6–8 hr), which may allow for once-daily dosing. Ceftriaxone and cefoperazone are the most highly protein bound of this group at 95 and 90%, respectively. Cefmenoxime is moderately bound and the other third-generation cephalosporins discussed in this chapter all have low protein binding. The relationship of protein binding to therapeutic efficacy is not clear-cut; with higher protein binding lower concentrations are theoretically available for diffusion into tissues. This expectation is not always borne out by the data, as illustrated by several studies reviewed in this chapter.

V. CONCLUSIONS

Any new antibiotic must be compared with older agents with respect to therapeutic efficacy, protection against infection, toxicity, cost, and pharmacokinetic properties. For a new drug to be considered an "advance," it should achieve some definite advantage in one or more of these areas. With expanded microbiological activity and greatly increased potency, a number of new beta-lactam antibiotics have become very useful agents in the therapy of difficult infections, particularly those occurring in patients with generalized immunodeficiencies or those in body sites of localized immunodeficiency (e.g., bone, CSF). Of additional clinical relevance has been the ability of some of these new drugs to replace the necessity of combination antibiotic therapy, reducing the chances for adverse reactions.

To use the new beta-lactam antibiotics properly, one must know much more than whether an organism is merely resistant or sensitive to the drug. One must know how sensitive and how resistant the bacterium is to the drug and for how long serum and tissue levels remain above inhibitory or bactercidal concentrations of the drug for the suspected or proven pathogen. Of course, we cannot forget the cost of the drug and its potential for adverse reactions. The newer cephalosporins offer new tools to the clinician and demand attention to the pharmacokinetic principles in applying these drugs effectively.

REFERENCES

1. M. N. Dudley and C. H. Nightingale. Effects of protein binding on the pharmacology of cephalosporins, in *New Beta-Lactam Antibiotics: A Review From Chemistry to Clinical Efficacy of the New Cephalosporins,* Proceedings of the Cephalosporin Symposium of the American College of Clinical Pharmacology, College of Physicians of Philadelphia, Philadelphia, 1982, pp. 227–239.

2. R. Wise, A. P. Gillett, B. Cadge, et al. The influence of protein binding upon tissue fluid levels of six β-lactam antibiotics. *J. Infect. Dis., 142*:77–82 (1980).
3. D. J. Merrikin, J. Briant, and G. N. Rolinson. Effect of protein binding on antibiotic activity *in vivo. J. Antimicrob. Chemother., 11*:233–238 (1983).
4. W. A. Craig and B. Suh. Theory and practical impact of binding of antimicrobials to serum proteins and tissue. *Scand. J. Infect. Dis. Suppl. 14, 10* 92–99 (1978).
5. S. M. Singhvi, A. F. Heald, and E. C. Schreiber. Pharmacokinetics of cephalosporin antibiotics: Protein binding considerations. *Chemotherapy, 24*: 121–133 (1978).
6. M. Barza. Principles of tissue penetration of antibiotics. *J. Antimicrob. Chemother. Suppl. C, 8*:7–28 (1981).
7. D. M. Ryan and O. Cars. Antibiotic assays in muscle: Are conventional tissue levels misleading as indicator of the antibacterial activity? *Scand. J. Infect. Dis., 12*:307–309 (1980).
8. W. A. Craig and P. G. Welling. Protein binding of antimicrobials: Clinical pharmacokinetic and therapeutic implications. *Clin. Pharmacokinet., 2*: 252–268 (1977).
9. D. M. Ryan and O. Cars. A problem in interpretation of β-lactam antibiotic levels in tissues. *J. Antimicrob. Chemother., 12*:281–284 (1983).
10. B. A. Cunha, H. R. Gossling, H. S. Pasternak, et al. The penetration characteristics of cefazolin, cephalothin, and cephradine into bone in patients undergoing total hip replacement. *J. Bone Joint Surg., 59A*:857–859 (1977).
11. H. C. Standiford, M. C. Jordan, and W. M. M. Kirby. Clinical pharmacology of carbenicillin compared with other penicillins. *J. Infect. Dis. Suppl., 122*: 9–13 (1970).
12. R. A. Greenfield, A. U. Gerber, and W. A. Craig. Pharmacokinetics of cefoperazone in patients with normal and impaired hepatic and renal function. *Rev. Infect. Dis. Suppl., 5*:127–136 (1983).
13. J. D. Turnidge and W. A. Craig. Beta-lactam pharmacology in liver disease. *J. Antimicrob. Chemother., 11*:499–501 (1983).
14. T. Komatsu, H. Nishiya, K. Iwata, et al. Binding of antibiotics to human liver ligandin, in *Current Chemotherapy and Immunotherapy*, American Society for Microbiology, Washington, D.C., 1982, pp. 150–151.
15. W. E. Wright and V. D. Line. Biliary excretion of cephalosporins in rats: Influence of molecular weight. *Antimicrob. Agents Chemother., 17*:842–846 (1980).
16. R. E. Kates and T. N. Tozer. Biliary secretion of methotrexate in rats and its inhibition be probenecid. *J. Pharm. Sci., 65*:1348–1352 (1976).
17. N. Baber, L. Halliday, R. Sibeon, et al. The interaction between indomethacin and probenecid. *Clin. Pharmacol. Ther., 24*:298–307 (1978).
18. M. N. Dudley, C. H. Nightingale, R. Quintiliani, and R. C. Tilton. *In vitro* activity of cefonicid, ceforanide and cefazolin against *Staphylococcus aureus* and *Staphylococcus epidermidis* and the effect of human serum. *J. Infect. Dis., 148*:78 (1983).

19. S. M. Singhvi, A. F. Heald, H. H. Gadebasch, et al. Human serum protein binding of cephalosporin antibiotics *in vitro*. *J. Lab. Clin. Med., 89*:414-420 (1977).
20. G. Renzini, G. Ravagnan, B. Oliva, and E. Salvetti. Cephradine microbiological activity *in vitro* and *in vivo*. Serum and tissue levels. *Med. Act. Drugs Today Suppl., 10*:75-83 (1974).
21. E. Finkelstein, R. Quintiliani, R. Lee, et al. Pharmacokinetics of oral cephalosporins: Cephradine and cephalexin. *J. Pharm. Sci., 67*:1447-1450 (1978).
22. C. M. Ginsburg and G. H. McCracken, Jr. Pharmacokinetics of cephradine suspension in infants and children. *Antimicrob. Agents Chemother., 16*:74-76 (1979).
23. G. H. McCracken, Jr., C. M. Ginsburg, J. C. Clahsen, and M. L. Thomas. Pharmacologic evaluation of orally administered antibiotics in infants and children: Effect of feeding on bioavailability. *Pediatrics, 62*:738-743 (1978).
24. M. Chow, R. Quintiliani, B. A. Cunha, et al. Pharmacokinetics of high dose oral cephalosporins. *J. Clin. Pharmacol., 19*:185-194 (1979).
25. S. Jalava, H. Saarimma, and R. Elfving. Cephalexin levels in serum, synovial fluid and joint tissues after oral administration. *Scand. J. Rheumatol., 6*:250-252 (1977).
26. G. M. Shuford. Concentrations of cephalexin in manibular alveolar bone, blood, and oral fluids. *J. Am. Dent. Assoc., 99*:47-50 (1979).
27. A. P. Gillett and R. Wise. Penetration of four cephalosporins into tissue fluid in man. *Lancet, 1*:962-964 (1978).
28. C. H. Nightingale, D. C. Greene, and R. Quintiliani. Pharmacokinetics and clinical use of cephalosporin antibiotics. *J. Pharm. Sci., 64*:1899-1927 (1975).
29. J. M. Brogard, G. Comte, and M. Pinget. Pharmacokinetics of cephalosporin antibiotics. *Antibiot. Chemother., 25*:123-162 (1978).
30. R. Quintiliani and C. H. Nightingale. The oral cephalosporins: Cephalexin, cephradine, cefaclor and cefadroxil, in *Infectious Disease Reviews* (W. J. Holloway, ed.), Futura, Mt. Kisco, New York, 1981, pp. 125-142.
31. C. H. Nightingale, M. A. French, and R. Quintiliani. Cephalosporin pharmacokinetics, in *Beta-Lactam Antibiotics* (S. Mitsuhashi, ed.), Japan Scientific Societies, Tokyo, 1981, pp. 259-295.
32. D. S. Greene, D. R. Flanagan, R. Quintiliani, and C. H. Nightingale. Pharmacokinetics of cephalexin: An evaluation of one and two-compartment model pharmacokinetics. *J. Clin. Pharmacol., 16*:257-264 (1976).
33. M. Pfeffer, A. Jackson, J. Ximens, and J. Perde-De Menezes. Comparative human oral clinical pharmacology of cefadroxil, cephalexin and cephradine. *Antimicrob. Agents Chemother., 11*:331-338 (1977).
34. H. Lode, R. Stahlmann, and P. Koeppe. Comparative pharmacokinetics of cephalexin, cefaclor, cefadroxil and CGP9000. *Antimicrob. Agents Chemother., 16*:1-6 (1979).
35. E. R. Jolly, D. M. Henness, and D. Richards, Jr. Human safety, tolerance and pharmacokinetic studies of cefadroxil: A new cephalosporin antibiotic

for oral administration. *Curr. Ther. Res., 22*:727–736 (1977).
36. D. M. Henness, D. Richards, P. J. Santella, and J. Rubinfeld. Oral bioavailability of cefadroxil, a new semisynthetic cephalosporin. *Clin. Ther., 1*: 263–273 (1978).
37. J. M. Brogard and F. Comte. Pharmacokinetics of the new cephalosporins. *Antibiot. Chemother., 31*:145–210 (1982).
38. R. E. Buck and K. E. Price. Cefadroxil, a new broad-spectrum cephalosporin. *Antimicrob. Agents Chemother., 11*:324–330 (1977).
39. G. Humbert, A. Leroy, J. P. Fillastre, and M. Godin. Pharmacokinetics of cefadroxil in normal subjects and in patients with renal insufficiency. *Chemotherapy, 25*:189–195 (1979).
40. B. Hampel, H. Lode, J. Wagner, and P. Koeppe. Pharmacokinetics of cefadroxil and cefaclor during an eight-day dosage period. *Antimicrob. Agents Chemother., 22*:1061–1063 (1982).
41. F. LaRosa, S. Ripa, M. Prenna, et al. Pharmacokinetics of cefadroxil after oral administration in humans. *Antimicrob. Agents Chemother., 21*:320–322 (1982).
42. R. Quintiliani. A review of the penetration of cefadroxil into human tissue. *J. Antimicrob. Chemother. Suppl. B, 10*:33–38 (1982).
43. R. E. Cutler, A. D. Blair, and M. R. Kelly. Cefadroxil kinetics in patients with renal insufficiency. *Clin. Pharmacol. Ther., 25*:514–521 (1979).
44. G. R. Hodges, C. Liu, D. R. Hinthorn, et al. Pharmacological evaluation of cefaclor in volunteers. *Antimicrob. Agents Chemother., 14*:454–456 (1978).
45. O. M. Korzeniowski, W. M. Scheld, and M. A. Sande. Comparative pharmacology of cefaclor and cephalexin. *Antimicrob. Agents Chemother., 12*: 157–160 (1977).
46. J. Santoro, B. N. Agarwal, R. Martinelli, et al. Pharmacology of cefaclor in normal volunteers and patients with renal failure. *Antimicrob. Agents Chemother., 13*:951–954 (1978).
47. G. H. McCracken, Jr., C. M. Ginsburg, J. C. Clahsen, and M. L. Thomas. Pharmacokinetics of cefaclor in infants and children. *J. Antimicrob. Chemother., 4*:515–521 (1978).
48. P. J. Krause, N. J. Owens, C. H. Nightingale, et al. Penetration of amoxicillin, cefaclor, erythromycin–sulfisoxazole, and trimethoprim–sulfamethoxazole into the middle ear fluid of patients with chronic serous otitis media. *J. Infect. Dis., 145*:815–821 (1982).
49. R. P. Smith, G. P. Schmid, A. L. Baltch, et al. Concentration of cefaclor in human prostatic tissue. *Am. J. Med. Sci., 281*:19–24 (1981).
50. J. L. Axelrod and R. S. Kochman. Cefaclor levels in human aqueous humor. *Arch. Ophthalmol., 98*:740–742 (1980).
51. C. Simon and U. Gutzemeier. Serum and sputum levels of cefaclor. *Postgrad. Med. J. Suppl. 4, 55*:30–34 (1979).
52. M. A. Foglesong, J. W. Lamb, and J. V. Dietz. Stability and blood level determinations of cefaclor, a new oral cephalosporin antibiotic. *Antimicrob. Agents Chemother., 13*:49–52 (1978).
53. G. Gartenberg, B. R. Meyers, S. Z. Hirschman, and E. Srulevitch. Pharma-

cokinetics of cefaclor in patients with stable renal impairment and patients undergoing hemodialysis. *J. Antimicrob. Chemother.*, *5*:465–470 (1979).
54. E. S. Neiss. Cephradine: A summary of preclinical studies and clinical pharmacology. *J. Irish Med. Assoc. Suppl.*, *66*:1–12 (1973).
55. I. J. Kiss, E. Farago, and J. Pinter. Serum and lung tissue levels of cephradine in thoracic surgery. *Br. J. Clin. Pharmacol.*, *3*:891–895 (1976).
56. E. S. Rattie, P. D. Bernardo, and L. J. Ravin. Pharmacokinetic interpretation of cephradine levels in serum after intravenous and extravascular administration in humans. *Antimicrob. Agents Chemother.*, *10*:283–287 (1976).
57. M. M. Cahn, E. J. Levy, P. Actor, and J. F. Pauls. Comparative serum levels and urinary recovery of cefazolin, cephaloridine and cephalothin in man. *J. Clin. Pharmacol.*, *14*:61–66 (1974).
58. S. H. Landesman and S. L. Gorbach. Cefazolin: Pharmacology and clinical usefulness, in *Cefazolin Sodium in Clinical Use,* Excerpta Medica, Amsterdam, 1978.
59. R. Quintiliani and C. H. Nightingale. Cefazolin. *Ann. Intern. Med.*, *89*: 650–656 (1978).
60. K. E. Andersson. On the pharmacokinetics of cephalosporin antibiotics. *Scand. J. Infect. Dis. Suppl. 13*, *10*:37–46 (1978).
61. P. G. Welling, W. A. Craig, G. L. Amidon, and C. M. Kunin. Pharmacokinetics of cefazolin in normal and uremic subjects. *Clin. Pharmacol. Ther.*, *15*: 344–353 (1974).
62. W. E. Wick and D. A. Preston. Biological properties of three 3-heterocyclic-thiomethyl cephalosporin antibiotics. *Antimicrob. Agents Chemother.*, *1*:221–234 (1972).
63. T. Bergan. Comparative pharmacokinetics of cefazolin, cephalothin, cephacetril and cephradine after intravenous administration. *Chemotherapy, 23*: 389–404 (1977).
64. C. H. Nightingale, J. J. Klimek, and R. Quintiliani. Effect of protein binding on the penetration of non-metabolized cephalosporins into atrial appendage and pericardial fluids in open-heart surgical patients. *Antimicrob. Agents Chemother.*, *17*:595–598 (1980).
65. B. A. Cunha, R. Quintiliani, and C. H. Nightingale. Unpublished data.
66. D. J. Schurman, H. P. Hirshman, G. Kajiyama, et al. Cefazolin concentrations in bone and synovial fluid. *J. Bone Joint Surg.*, *60A*:359–362 (1978).
67. E. Sinagowitz, K. Pelz, A. Burgert, et al. Tissue concentrations of cefazolin in man, in *Ninth International Congress of Chemotherapy,* London, 1975.
68. D. R. Cole and J. Pung. Penetration of cefazolin into pleural fluid. *Antimicrob. Agents Chemother.*, *11*:1033–1035 (1977).
69. J. P. Thys, B. Vanderkelen, and J. Klastersky. Pharmacological study of cefazolin during intermittent and continuous infusion: A crossover investigation in humans. *Antimicrob. Agents Chemother.*, *10*:395–398 (1976).
70. A. R. McLeish, C. J. L. Strachan, S. J. A. Powis, et al. The influence of biliary disease on the excretion of cefazolin in human bile. *Surgery, 81*:426–430 (1977).

71. M. D. Ram and S. Watanatittan. Biliary excretion and concentration of cefazolin. *Am. J. Gastroenterol., 66*:540–545 (1976).
72. K. Shibata and M. Fujii. Clinical studies of cefazolin in the surgical field. *Antimicrob. Agents Chemother., 10*:467–472 (1970).
73. M. D. Ram and S. Watanatittan. Levels of cefazolin in human bile. *J. Infect. Dis. Suppl., 128*:361–363 (1973).
74. A. S. Litvak, C. D. Franks, S. K. Vaught, and J. W. McRoberts. Cefazolin and cephalexin levels in prostatic tissue and sera. *Urology, 7*:497–498 (1976).
75. H. Yoshioka, K. Cho, T. Masatoshi, et al. Transfer of cefazolin into human milk. *J. Pediatr., 94*:151–152 (1979).
76. H. P. Bassaris, R. Quintiliani, E. Maderazo, et al. Pharmacokinetics and penetration characteristics of cefazolin into human spinal fluid. *Curr. Ther. Res., 19*:110–120 (1976).
77. W. M. M. Kirby and C. Regamey. Pharmacokinetics of cefazolin compared with 4 other cephalosporins. *J. Infect. Dis. Suppl., 128*:341–353 (1973).
78. M. F. Rein, F. B. Westervelt, and M. A. Sande. Pharmacodynamics of cefazolin in the presence of normal and impaired renal function. *Antimicrob. Agents Chemother., 4*:366–371 (1973).
79. T. Bergan, E. K. Brodwall, and O. Orjavik. Pharmacokinetics of cefazolin in patients with normal and impaired renal function. *J. Antimicrob. Chemother., 3*:435–443 (1977).
80. A. W. Czerwinski, J. A. Pederson, and J. P. Barry. Cefazolin plasma concentrations and urinary excretion in patients with renal impairment. *J. Clin. Pharmacol., 14*:560–566 (1974).
81. V. T. Andriole. Pharmacokinetics of cephalosporins in patients with normal or reduced renal function. *J. Infect. Dis. Suppl., 137*:88–97 (1978).
82. J. M. Brogard, M. Pinget, C. Brandt, and J. Lavillaureix. Pharmacokinetics of cefazolin in patients with renal failure: Special reference to hemodialysis. *J. Clin. Pharmacol., 17*:225–230 (1977).
83. T. Madhavan, K. Yaremchuk, N. Levin, et al. Effects of renal failure and dialysis on cefazolin pharmacokinetics. *Antimicrob. Agents Chemother., 8*:63–66 (1975).
84. C. P. Craig and S. I. Rifkin. Pharmacokinetics and hemodialyzability of cefazolin in uremic patients. *Clin. Pharmacol. Ther., 19*:825–829 (1976).
85. C. M. Bunke, G. R. Aronoff, M. E. Brier, et al. Cefazolin and cephalexin kinetics in continuous ambulatory peritoneal dialysis. *Clin. Pharmacol. Ther., 33*:66–72 (1983).
86. J. O. Klein, T. C. Eichkoff, J. G. Tilles, and M. Finland. Cephalothin: Activity *in vitro,* absorption and excretion in normal subjects and clinical observation in 40 patients. *Am. J. Med. Sci., 248*:640–656 (1964).
87. E. S. Rattie and L. J. Ravin. Pharmacokinetic interpretation of blood levels and urinary excretion data for cefazolin and cephalothin after intravenous and intramuscular administration in humans. *Antimicrob. Agents Chemother., 7*:606–613 (1975).
88. C. Regamey, R. C. Gordon, and W. Kirby. Cefazolin versus cephalothin and

cephaloridine: A comparison of their clinical pharmacology. *Arch. Intern. Med., 133*:407–410 (1974).

89. A. Z. Lane, G. M. Chudzik, and S. B. Siskin. Comparative pharmacokinetic studies on cephapirin and cephalothin following intravenous and intramuscular administration. *Curr. Ther. Res., 21*:117–127 (1977).
90. D. E. Wilson, T. C. Chalmers, and M. A. Madoff. The passage of cephalothin into and out of ascitic fluid. *Am. J. Med. Assoc., 253*:449–452 (1967).
91. C. S. Goodwin, E. B. Raftery, A. D. Goldberg, et al. Effects of rate of infusion and probenecid on serum levels, renal excretion and tolerance of intravenous doses of cefoxitin in humans: Comparison with cephalothin. *Antimicrob. Agents Chemother., 6*:338–346 (1974).
92. N. J. Vianna and D. Kaye. Penetration of cephalothin into the spinal fluid. *Am. J. Med. Sci., 254*:216–220 (1967).
93. R. E. Records. Intraocular penetration of cephalothin. *Am. J. Ophthalmol., 66*:441–443 (1968).
94. P. Eigel, A. Tschirkov, P. Satter, and H. Knothe. Assays of cephalosporin antibiotics administered prophylactically in open heart surgery. *Infection, 6*:23–28 (1978).
95. R. Quintiliani, J. Klimek, and C. H. Nightingale. Penetration of cephapirin and cephalothin into the right appendage and pericardial fluid of patients undergoing open heart surgery. *J. Infect. Dis., 139*:348–352 (1979).
96. D. W. Gump and R. L. Lipson. The penetration of cephalothin into synovial fluid and other body fluids. *Curr. Ther. Res., 10*:583–591 (1968).
97. K. R. Ratzan, C. Ruiz, and G. L. Irvin, III. Biliary tract excretion of cefazolin, cephalothin and cephaloridine in the presence of biliary tract disease. *Antimicrob. Agents Chemother., 6*:426–431 (1974).
98. N. J. Mendelson, J. Portnoy, H. Sigman, and V. Dick. Pharmacology of cephalothin in the biliary tract of humans. *Antimicrob. Agents Chemother., 6*:659–665 (1974).
99. N. Yamada, K. Kido, H. Uchida, et al. Application of cephalosporins to obstetrics and gynecology: Transfer of cefazolin and cephalothin to uterine tissue. *Am. J. Obstet. Gynecol., 136*:1036–1040 (1980).
100. M. A. MacAulay and D. Charles. Placental transfer of cephalothin. *Am. J. Obstet. Gynecol., 100*:940–946 (1968).
101. C. C. Lee, E. B. Herr, and R. C. Anderson. Pharmacological and toxicological studies on cephalothin. *Clin. Med., 70*:1123–1138 (1963).
102. K. W. Miller, K. K. H. Chan, H. G. McKoy, et al. Cephalothin kinetics: Before, during and after cardiopulmonary bypass surgery. *Clin. Pharmacol. Ther., 26*:54–62 (1979).
103. I. Nilsson-Ehle and P. Nilsson-Ehle. Pharmacokinetics of cephalothin: Accumulation of its desacetylated metabolite in uremic patients. *J. Infect. Dis., 139*:712–716 (1979).
104. W. M. M. Kirby, J. B. DeMaine, and W. S. Serrill. Pharmacokinetics of the cephalosporins in healthy volunteers and uremic patients. *Postgrad. Med. J. Suppl., 47*:41–46 (1971).

105. T. F. Rolewicz, B. L. Mirkin, M. J. Cooper, and M. W. Anders. Metabolic disposition of cephalothin in desacetylcephalothin in children and adults: Comparison of a high performance liquid chromatographic and microbial assay procedures. *Clin. Pharmacol. Ther., 22*:928-935 (1977).
106. R. L. Perkins, E. J. Smith, and S. Saslaw. Cephalothin and cephaloridine: Comparative pharmacodynamics in chronic uremia. *Am. J. Med. Sci., 257*: 116-124 (1969).
107. J. Axelrod, B. R. Meyers, and S. Z. Hirschman. Cephapirin: Pharmacology in normal volunteers. *J. Clin. Pharmacol., 12*:84-88 (1972).
108. A. Arvidsson, O. Borga, and G. Alvan. Renal excretion of cephapirin and cephaloridine: Evidence for saturable tubular reabsorption. *Clin. Pharmacol. Ther., 25*:870-876 (1979).
109. B. E. Cabana, D. R. Van Harken, and G. H. Hottendorf. Comparative pharmacokinetics and metabolism of cephapirin in laboratory animals and humans. *Antimicrob. Agents Chemother., 10*:307-317 (1976).
110. E. R. Green, S. Subramanian, H. Faden, et al. A comparison of the penetration characteristics of cephapirin and cephalothin into right atrial appendage, muscle, fat and pericardial fluid of pediatric patients undergoing open heart operation. *Ann. Thorac. Surg., 31*:155-160 (1981).
111. R. Rubi and H. M. Galan. Cephapirin concentrations in prostatic and seminal vesicle tissues. *Int. J. Clin. Pharmacol. Biopharm., 17*:87-89 (1979).
112. D. J. Schurman, D. S. Burton, G. Kajiyama, et al. Sodium cephapirin disposition and distribution into human bone. *Curr. Ther. Res., 20*:194-203 (1976).
113. W. Fry, J. Ximenes, and S. B. Sisken. Concentrations of cephapirin sodium in plasma and gynecologic tissue after a single preoperative case. *Int. J. Clin. Pharmacol. Ther. Toxicol., 18*:92-96 (1980).
114. G. Creatsas, M. Pavlatos, D. Lolis, and D. Kaskarelis. A study of the kinetics of cephapirin and cephalexin in pregnancy. *Curr. Med. Res. Opin., 7*: 43-46 (1980).
115. I. Archer and T. C. Forster. Materno-fetal cephradine transfer in pregnancy. *Antimicrob. Agents Chemother., 14*:924-926 (1978).
116. B. E. Cabana, D. R. Van Harken, and G. H. Hottendorf. The role of the kidney in the elimination of cephapirin in man. *J. Pharmacokinet. Biopharm., 3*:419-438 (1975).
117. R. V. McCloskey, E. E. Terry, A. W. McCracken, et al. Effect of hemodialysis and renal failure on serum and urine concentrations of cephapirin sodium. *Antimicrob. Agents Chemother., 1*:90-93 (1972).
118. N. K. Shemonsky, J. Carrizosa, and M. E. Levinson. *In vitro* activity and pharmacokinetics in patients of cefamandole, a new cephalosporin antibiotic. *Antimicrob. Agents Chemother., 8*:679-683 (1975).
119. R. S. Griffith, H. R. Black, G. L. Brier, and J. D. Wolny. Cefamandole: *In vitro* and clinical pharmacokinetics. *Antimicrob. Agents Chemother., 10*:814-823 (1976).
120. M. Barza, S. Melethil, S. Berger, and E. C. Ernst. Comparative pharmacokinetics of cefamandole, cephapirin and cephalothin in healthy subjects

and effect of repeat dosing. *Antimicrob. Agents Chemother., 10*:421–425 (1976).

121. B. R. Meyers, B. Ribner, S. Yancovitz, and S. Z. Hirschman. Pharmacological studies with cefamandole in human volunteers. *Antimicrob. Agents Chemother., 9*:140–144 (1976).
122. R. E. Polk, G. L. Archer, and R. Lower. Cefamandole kinetics during cardiopulmonary bypass. *Clin. Pharmacol. Ther., 23*:473–480 (1978).
123. N. S. Aziz, J. G. Gambertoglio, E. T. Lin, et al. Pharmacokinetics of cefamandole using a HPLC assay. *J. Pharmacokinet. Biopharm., 6*:153–164 (1978).
124. R. S. Griffith, H. R. Black, G. L. Brier, and J. D. Wolny. Effect of probenecid on the blood levels and urinary excretion of cefamandole. *Antimicrob. Agents Chemother., 11*:809–812 (1977).
125. J. L. Axelrod and R. Kochman. Cefamandole levels in primary aqueous humor in man. *Am. J. Ophthalmol., 85*:342–348 (1978).
126. E. A. Steinberg, G. D. Overturf, L. J. Baraff, and J. Wilkins. Penetration of cefamandole into spinal fluid. *Antimicrob. Agents Chemother., 11*:933–935 (1977).
127. C. Liu, D. R. Hinthorn, G. R. Hodges, et al. Penetration of cefoxitin into human cerebrospinal fluid: Comparison with cefamandole, ampicillin and penicillin. *Rev. Infect. Dis., 1*:127–131 (1979).
128. N. Olson, C. H. Nightingale, and R. Quintiliani. Penetration characteristics of cefamandole into right atrial appendage and pericardial fluid in patients undergoing open-heart surgery. *Ann. Thorac. Surg., 29*:104–108 (1980).
129. G. L. Archer, R. E. Polk, R. J. Duma, and R. Lower. Comparison of cephalothin and cefamandole prophylaxis during insertion of prostethic heart valves. *Antimicrob. Agents Chemother., 13*:924–929 (1978).
130. C. S. Bryan, C. W. Smith, and J. P. Sutton. Comparison of cefamandole and cefazolin during cardiopulmonary bypass. *J. Thorac. Cardiovasc. Surg., 86*:222–225 (1983).
131. D. J. Schurman, H. P. Hirshman, and D. S. Burton. Cephalothin and cefamandole penetration into bone, synovial fluid, and wound drainage fluid. *J. Bone Joint Surg., 62A*:981–985 (1980).
132. D. A. Leigh, J. Marriner, D. Nisbet, et al. Bone concentrations of cefuroxime and cefamandole in the femoral head in 96 patients undergoing total hip replacement surgery. *J. Antimicrob. Chemother., 9*:303–311 (1982).
133. K. R. Ratzan, H. B. Baker, and I. Lauredo. Excretion of cefamandole, cefazolin and cephalothin into T-tube bile. *Antimicrob. Agents Chemother., 13*:985–987 (1978).
134. J. U. Levi, A. S. Livingstone, O. V. Martinez, et al. Biliary concentrations of cefamandole and its use in biliary tract surgery. *Scand. J. Infect. Dis. Suppl. 25, 12*:55–57 (1980).
135. M. Uwaydan, H. Kantarjian, M. Osseiran, and F. Bal'A. Cefamandole bile levels in patients with hepatobiliary disease. *Antimicrob. Agents Chemother., 22*:1087–1089 (1982).

136. H. C. Neu. Comparison of the pharmacokinetics of cefamandole and other cephalosporin compounds. *J. Infect. Dis. Suppl., 137*:80–87 (1978).
137. D. S. Greene, R. Quintiliani, M. Thompson, and C. H. Nightingale. Effect of probenecid on the renal clearance of cefamandole. *Curr. Ther. Res., 22*: 737–740 (1977).
138. M. J. Ahern, F. O. Finkelstein, and V. T. Andriole. Pharmacokinetics of cefamandole in patients undergoing hemodialysis and peritoneal dialysis. *Antimicrob. Agents Chemother., 10*:457–461 (1976).
139. J. M. Brogard, J. Kopferschmitt, M. O. Spach, et al. Cefamandole pharmacokinetics and dosage adjustments in relation to renal function, *J. Clin. Pharmacol., 19*:366–377 (1979).
140. A. W. Czerwinski and J. A. Pederson. The pharmacology of cefamandole in patients with reduced renal function. *Scand. J. Infect. Dis. Suppl. 25, 12*:45–48 (1980).
141. D. Pitkin, J. Dubb, P. Actor, et al. Kinetics and renal handling of cefonicid. *Clin. Pharmacol. Ther., 30*:587–593 (1981).
142. S. L. Barrier, G. J. Hatheway, J. G. Gambertoglio, et al. Pharmacokinetics of cefonicid, a new broad spectrum cephalosporin. *Antimicrob. Agents Chemother., 21*:935–938 (1982).
143. W. C. Shyu and C. H. Nightingale. Unpublished data.
144. R. J. Wallace, S. L. Niefield, S. Waters, et al. Comparative trial of cefonicid and cefamandole in the therapy of community acquired pneumonia. *Antimicrob. Agents Chemother., 21*:231–235 (1982).
145. M. N. Dudley, R. Quintiliani, and C. H. Nightingale. Review of cefonicid, a long acting cephalosporin. *Clin Pharm., 3*:23–32 (1984).
146. C. H. Nightingale, R. Quintiliani, M. N. Dudley, et al. Tissue penetration and half-life of cefonicid. *Rev. Infect. Dis.* (in press).
147. R. P. Sterling, D. J. Connor, J. C. Norman, and D. A. Cooley. Cefonicid concentrations in serum and atrial tissue during open heart surgery. *Antimicrob. Agents Chemother., 23*:790–792 (1983).
148. D. P. Alexander, S. L. Barriere, J. C. Gambertoglio, and J. E. Conte, Jr. Pharmacokinetics of cefonicid in patients undergoing chronic hemodialysis. Paper presented at the 22nd Interscience Conference on Antimicrobial Agents and Chemotherapy, Miami, Florida, 1982, Abstract 786.
149. A. D. Blair, S. C. Forland, and R. E. Cutler. Cefonicid pharmacokinetics in renal insufficiency. Paper presented at the 22nd Interscience Conference on Antimicrobial Agents and Chemotherpy, Miami, Florida, 1982, Abstract 787.
150. J. F. Jovanovich, L. D. Saravolatz, K. Burch, and D. J. Pohlod. Failure of probenecid to alter the pharmacokinetics of ceforanide. *Antimicrob. Agents Chemother., 20*:530–532 (1981).
151. S. Ripa, F. LaRosa, A. Ghezzi, et al. Pharmacokinetics of ceforanide. *Antimicrob. Agents Chemother., 21*:323–326 (1982).
152. R. D. Smyth, M. Pfeffer, A. Glick, et al. Clinical pharmacokinetics and safety of high doses of ceforanide (BL-S786R) and cefazolin. *Antimicrob. Agents Chemother., 16*:615–621 (1979).

153. F. H. Lee, M. Pfeffer, D. R. Van Harken, et al. Comparative pharmacokinetics of ceforanide (BL-S786R) and cefazolin in laboratory animals and humans. *Antimicrob. Agents Chemother.*, *17*:188–192 (1980).
154. L. D. Mullany, M. A. French, C. H. Nightingale, et al. Penetration of ceforanide and cefamandole into right atrial appendage, pericardial fluid, sternum, and intercostal muscle of patients undergoing open heart surgery. *Antimicrob. Agents Chemother.*, *21*:416–420 (1982).
155. D. E. Kenady and M. D. Ram. Biliary levels of ceforanide. *Antimicrob. Agents Chemother.*, *23*:706–709 (1983).
156. E. H. Estey, S. S. Weaver, B. M. LeBlane, et al. Ceforanide kinetics. *Clin. Pharmacol. Ther.*, *30*:398–403 (1981).
157. S. S. Hawkins, R. H. Alford, W. J. Stone, et al. Ceforanide kinetics in renal insufficiency. *Clin. Pharmacol. Ther.*, *30*:468–474 (1981).
158. J. R. Hess, S. J. Berman, W. H. Boughton, et al. Pharmacokinetics of ceforanide in patients with end-stage renal disease on hemodialysis. *Antimicrob. Agents Chemother.*, *17*:251–253 (1980).
159. A. S. Dajani, M. C. Thirumoorthi, R. E. Bawdon, et al. Pharmacokinetics of intramuscular ceforanide in infants, children and adolescents. *Antimicrob. Agents Chemother.*, *21*:282–287 (1982).
160. F. D. Daschner, K. A. Hemmer, P. Offermann, and J. Slanicka. Pharmacokinetics of cefotiam in normal humans. *Antimicrob. Agents Chemother.*, *22*:958–960 (1982).
161. H. M. Von Just, V. Schlosser, G. Spillner, et al. Konzentrationen von Cefotiam in Serum, Herzklappen, Muskel und Fettgewel wahrend herzchirurgischer Eingriffe. *Arzneim. Forsch.*, *33*:578–579 (1983).
162. I. Miyakawa, H. Inoue, T. Kuroki, et al. Placental transfer of cefotiam dihydrochloride. *Antimicrob. Agents Chemother.*, *25*:147–148 (1984).
163. S. M. Harding, P. E. O. Williams, and J. Ayrton. Pharmacology of cefuroxime as the 1-acetoxyethylester in volunteers. *Antimicrob. Agents Chemother.*, *25*:78–82 (1984).
164. D. K. Sommers, M. Van Wyk, P. E. O. Williams, and S. M. Harding. Pharmacokinetics and tolerance of cefuroxime axetil in volunteers during repeated dosing. *Antimicrob. Agents Chemother.*, *25*:344–347 (1984).
165. P. E. O. Williams and S. M. Harding. The absolute bioavailability of oral cefuroxime axetil in male and female volunteers after fasting and after food. *J. Antimicrob. Chemother.*, *13*:191–196 (1984).
166. R. D. Foord. Cefuroxime: Human pharmacokinetics. *Antimicrob. Agents Chemother.*, *9*:741–747 (1976).
167. G. K. Daikos, J. C. Kosmidis, C. H. Stathakis, and H. Giamarellou. Cefuroxime: Antimicrobial activity, human pharmacokinetics and therapeutic efficacy. *J. Antimicrob. Chemother.*, *3*:555–562 (1977).
168. R. W. Bundtzen, R. D. Toothaker, O. S. Nielson, et al. Pharmacokinetics of cefuroxime in normal and impaired renal function: Comparison of high-pressure liquid chromatography and microbiological assays. *Antimicrob. Agents Chemother.*, *19*:443–449 (1981).
169. M. DelRio, D. F. Chrane, S. Shelton, et al. Pharmacokinetics of cefurox-

ime in infants and children with bacterial meningitis. *Antimicrob. Agents Chemother.*, *22*:990–994 (1982).

170. A. B. Richards, A. J. Bron, B. McLendon, et al. The intraocular penetration of cefuroxime after parenteral administration. *Br. J. Ophthalmol.*, *63*:687–689 (1979).
171. P. E. Gower and C. H. Dash. The pharmacokinetics of cefuroxime after intravenous injection. *Eur. J. Clin. Pharmacol.*, *12*:221–227 (1977).
172. T. H. Peirce, R. A. Kenny, A. F. Dawson, and P. M. Hobbs. Levels of cefuroxime in bronchial secretion. *Curr. Med. Res. Opin.*, *6*:649–652 (1980).
173. C. W. H. Havard, R. P. Bax, T. C. Samanta, et al. Sputum and blood concentrations of cefuroxime in lower respiratory tract infections. *Thorax*, *35*:379–383 (1980).
174. K. Dornbusch, H. Hugo, and A. Lidstrom. Antibacterial activity of cefuroxime in human bone. *Scand. J. Infect. Dis.*, *12*:49–53 (1980).
175. H. H. Jung and T. Mischkowsky. Measurements of cefuroxime concentration in bone in dogs and man. *Arch. Orthop. Trauma Surg.*, *94*:25–28 (1979).
176. B. R. Bullen, C. H. Ramsden, and R. C. Kester. Cefuroxime levels attained in tissues and wound exudates from severely ischaemic limbs. *J. Antimicrob. Chemother.*, *7*:163–169 (1981).
177. M. H. Thomas, C. H. Dash, K. G. Burnand, and A. B. Woodyer. The excretion of cefuroxime in human bile. *Br. J. Surg.*, *68*:290–291 (1981).
178. M. Thomas, A. K. Browning, and R. J. McFarland. Excretion of cefuroxime in biliary disease. *Surg. Gynecol. Obstet.*, *158*:272-274 (1984).
179. B. Gold and W. J. Rodriguez. Cefuroxime: Mechanism of action, antimicrobial activity, pharmacokinetics, clinical applications, adverse effects and therapeutic indications. *Pharmacotherapy*, *3*:82–100 (1983).
180. P. Bousfield, A. K. Browning, B. M. Mullinger, and M. Elstein. Cefuroxime: Potential use in pregnant women at term. *Br. J. Obstet. Gynecol.*, *88*:146–149 (1981).
181. B. Trollfors, M. Suurkula, J. D. Price, and R. Norrby. Renal function during cefuroxime treatment in patients with pre-existing renal impairment. *J. Antimicrob. Chemother.*, *6*:665–670 (1980).
182. B. Kemmerich, H. Lode, G. Belmega, et al. Comparative pharmacokinetics of cefoperazone, cefotaxime and moxalactam. *Antimicrob. Agents Chemother.*, *23*:429–434 (1983).
183. F. Esmieu, J. Guibert, H. C. Rosenkilde, et al. Pharmacokinetics of cefotaxime in normal human volunteers. *J. Antimicrob. Chemother. Suppl. A*, *6*:83–92 (1980).
184. K. P. Fu, P. Aswapokee, I. Ho, et al. Pharmacokinetics of cefotaxime. *Antimicrob. Agents Chemother.*, *16*:592–597 (1979).
185. R. M. J. Ings, J. P. Fillastre, M. Godin, et al. The pharmacokinetics of cefotaxime and its metabolite in subjects with normal and impaired renal function. *Rev. Infect. Dis. Suppl.*, *4*:379–391 (1982).
186. H. C. Neu, N. Aswapokee, P. Aswapokee, and K. P. Fu. HR 756, a new cephalosporin active against gram-positive and gram-negative aerobic and

anaerobic bacteria. *Antimicrob. Agents Chemother., 15*:273–281 (1979).

187. A. A. Carmine, R. N. Brogden, R. C. Heel, et al. Cefotaxime: A review of its antibacterial activity pharmacological properties and therapeutic use. *Drugs, 25*:223–289 (1983).
188. M. N. Dudley and S. L. Barriere. Cefotaxime: Microbiology, pharmacology and clinical use. *Clin. Pharm., 1*:114–124 (1982).
189. R. Luthy, J. Blase, A. Bonetti, et al. Comparative multiple-dose pharmacokinetics of cefotaxime, moxalactam and ceftazidime. *Antimicrob. Agents Chemother., 20*:567–575 (1981).
190. H. C. Neu, P. Aswapokee, K. P. Fu, et al. Cefotaxime kinetics after intravenous and intramuscular injection of single and multiple doses. *Clin. Pharmacol. Ther., 27*:677–685 (1980).
191. J. T. Doluisio. Clinical pharmacokinetics of cefotaxime in patients with normal and reduced renal function. *Rev. Infect. Dis. Suppl., 4*:333–345 (1982).
192. C. Morel, N. Monrocq, and Y. Besnard. Concentrations of cefotaxime in bronchial secretions. *J. Antimicrob. Chemother. Suppl. A, 6*:123–124 (1980).
193. H. Lode, B. Kemmerich, G. Gruhlke, et al. Cefotaxime in bronchopulmonary infections – A clinical and pharmacological study. *J. Antimicrob. Chemother. Suppl. A, 6*:193–198 (1980).
194. R. Blind, A. Bikfalvi, K. Seeger, et al. Cefotaxime in human lung tissue. *Arzneim. Forsch., 32*:1319–1321 (1982).
195. A. Karimi, K. Seeger, D. Stolke, and H. Knothe. Cefotaxime concentration in cerebrospinal fluid. *J. Antimicrob. Chemother. Suppl. A, 6*:119–120 (1980).
196. W. J. Novick. Levels of cefotaxime in body fluids and tissues: A review. *Rev. Infect. Dis. Suppl., 4*:346–353 (1982).
197. O. Bruckner, H. Collmann, and H. G. Hoffmann. Cefotaxime in treatment of meningitis and ventriculitis? Evaluation of drug concentrations in cerebrospinal fluid. *Intens. Care Med., 8*:33–38 (1982).
198. B. M. Belohradsky, D. Geiss, W. Marget, et al. Intravenous cefotaxime in children with bacterial meningitis. *Lancet, 1*:61–63 (1980).
199. C. E. Cherubin, M. L. Corrado, S. R. Nair, et al. Treatment of gram-negative bacillary meningitis: Role of the new cephalosporin antibiotics. *Rev. Infect. Dis. Suppl., 4*:453–464 (1982).
200. R. F. Frongillo, L. Galuppo, and A. Moretti. Suction skin blister, skin window and skin chamber techniques to determine extravascular passage of cefotaxime in humans. *Antimicrob. Agents Chemother., 19*:22–28 (1981).
201. T. Bergan, T. Kalager, K. B. Hellum, and C. O. Solberg. Penetration of cefotaxime and desacetylcefotaxime into skin blister fluid. *J. Antimicrob. Chemother., 10*:193–196 (1982).
202. H. Busse, K. Seeger, and P. Wreesman. Concentrations of cefotaxime in the anterior chamber of the eye in rabbits and humans. *J. Antimicrob. Chemother. Suppl. A, 6*:143–145 (1980).

203. J. Danon. Cefotaxime concentrations in otitis media effusions. *J. Antimicrob. Chemother. Suppl. A, 6*:131–132 (1980).
204. C. J. Soussy, L. P. Deforges, J. LeVan Thoi, et al. Cefotaxime concentration in the bile and wall of the gall bladder. *J. Antimicrob. Chemother. Suppl. A, 6*:125–130 (1980).
205. W. C. Shyu, C. H. Nightingale, R. Quintiliani, et al. Biliary excretion of cefotaxime. *Curr. Ther. Res., 35*:727–734 (1984).
206. L. Moreau, H. Durand, and P. Biclet. Cefotaxime concentrations in ascites. *J. Antimicrob. Chemother. Suppl. A, 6*:121–122 (1980).
207. D. A. Kafetzis, C. V. Lazarides, C. A. Siafas, et al. Transfer of cefotaxime in human milk and from mother to foetus. *J. Antimicrob. Chemother. Suppl. A, 6*:135–141 (1980).
208. M. Grabe, K. E. Andersson, A. Forsgren, and S. Hellsten. Concentrations of cefotaxime in serum, urine and tissues of urological patients. *Infection, 9*:154–158 (1981).
209. J. Chamberlain, J. D. Coombes, D. Dell, et al. Metabolism of cefotaxime in animals and man. *J. Antimicrob. Chemother. Suppl. A, 6*:69–78 (1980).
210. D. S. Reeves, L. O. White, H. A. Holt, et al. Human metabolism of cefotaxime. *J. Antimicrob. Chemother. Suppl. A, 6*:93–101 (1980).
211. J. D. Coombes. Metabolism of cefotaxime in animals and humans. *Rev. Infect. Dis. Suppl., 4*:325–332 (1982).
212. R. Luthy, J. Blaser, A. Bonetti, et al. Human pharmacokinetics of ceftazidime in comparison to moxalactam and cefotaxime. *J. Antimicrob. Chemother. Suppl. B, 8*:273–276 (1981).
213. R. Wise, N. Wright, and P. J. Wills. Pharmacology of cefotaxime and its desacetyl metabolite in renal and hepatic disease. *Antimicrob. Agents Chemother., 19*:526–531 (1981).
214. J. Chodos, E. L. Franke, M. Saltzman, and H. C. Neu. Pharmacokinetics of intravenous cefotaxime in patients undergoing chronic hemodialysis. *Ther. Drug Monitor, 3*:71–74 (1981).
215. W. M. Glockner, U. Hoffler, J. Kindler, et al. Elimination kinetics of cefotaxime in patients with renal insufficiency requiring hemodialysis. *J. Antimicrob. Chemother. Suppl. A, 6*:219–223 (1980).
216. J. Dubb, P. Actor, D. Pitkin, et al. Ceftizoxime kinetics and renal handling. *Clin. Pharmacol. Ther., 31*:516–521 (1982).
217. H. C. Neu and S. Srinivasan. Pharmacology of ceftizoxime compared with that of cefamandole. *Antimicrob. Agents Chemother., 20*:366–369 (1981).
218. M. Ohkawa, A. Okasho, T. Sugata, and K. Kuroda. Elimination kinetics of ceftizoxime in humans with and without renal insufficiency. *Antimicrob. Agents Chemother., 22*:308–311 (1982).
219. M. L. Gross, P. Somani, B. S. Ribner, et al. Ceftizoxime elimination kinetics in continuous ambulatory peritoneal dialysis. *Clin. Pharmacol. Ther., 34*:673–680 (1983).
220. T. Murakawa, H. Sakamota, S. Fukada, et al. Pharmacokinetics of cefti-

zoxime in animals after parenteral dosing. *Antimicrob. Agents Chemother., 17*:157–164 (1980).
221. R. Quintiliani and C. H. Nightingale. Comparative pharmacokinetics of ceftizoxime and other third-generation cephalosporins in humans. *J. Antimicrob. Chemother. Suppl. C, 10*:99–104 (1982).
222. R. A. Hamilton, N. J. Owens, C. H. Nightingale, et al. Pharmacokinetics and cerebrospinal fluid penetration of ceftizoxime in patients undergoing myelography. (In preparation.)
223. D. Cable, G. Edralin, and G. D. Overturf. Human cerebrospinal fluid pharmacokinetics and treatment of bacterial meningitis with ceftizoxime. *J. Antimicrob. Chemother. Suppl. C, 10*:121–127 (1982).
224. D. N. Gerding and L. R. Peterson. Comparative tissue and extra-vascular fluid concentrations of ceftizoxime. *J. Antimicrob. Chemother. Suppl. C, 10*:105–116 (1982).
225. H. C. Neu. Ceftizoxime: A beta-lactamase stable, broad-spectrum cephalosporin. *Pharmacotherapy, 4*:47–58 (1984).
226. B. A. Cunha, A. M. Ristuccia, M. Jonas, et al. Tissue penetration characteristics of ceftizoxime and cefazolin in human bile and gallbladder wall. *J. Antimicrob. Chemother. Suppl. C, 10*:117–120 (1982).
227. S. F. Kowalsky, R. M. Echols, A. R. Venezia, et al. Pharmacokinetics of ceftizoxime in subjects with various degrees of renal function. *Antimicrob. Agents Chemother., 24*:151–155 (1983).
228. W. C. Shyu, N. S. Jordan, R. Quintiliani, and C. H. Nightingale. Comparative pharmacokinetics of ceftizoxime and cefotaxime. Paper presented at the 13th International Congress of Chemotherapy, Vienna, 1983.
229. R. E. Cutler, A. D. Blair, E. D. Burgess, and D. Parks. Pharmacokinetics of ceftizoxime. *J. Antimicrob. Chemother. Suppl. C, 10*:91–97 (1982).
230. S. R. Norrby, L. A. Burman, H. Linderholm, and B. Trollfors. Ceftazidime: Pharmacokinetics in patients and effects on the renal function. *J. Antimicrob. Chemother., 10*:199–206 (1982).
231. K. Alestig, B. Trollfors, R. Andersson, et al. Ceftazidime and renal function. *J. Antimicrob. Chemother., 13*:177–181 (1984).
232. S. M. Harding, A. J. Monro, J. E. Thomton, et al. The comparative pharmacrokinetics of ceftazidime and cefotaxime in healthy volunteers. *J. Antimicrob. Chemother. Suppl. B, 8*:263–272 (1981).
233. C. H. O'Callaghan, P. Acred, P. B. Harper, et al. GR20263; A new broad spectrum cephalosporin with anti-pseudomonal activity. *Antimicrob. Agents Chemother., 17*:876–883 (1980).
234. B. Kemmerich, H. Warns, H. Lode, et al. Multiple-dose pharmacokinetics of ceftazidime and its influence on fecal flora. *Antimicrob. Agents Chemother., 24*:333–338 (1983).
235. H. Warns, H. Lode, C. M. Harnoss, et al. Multiple dose pharmacokinetics and therapeutic results with ceftazidime. *J. Antimicrob. Chemother. Suppl. A, 12*:235–240 (1983).
236. A. Tourkantonis and P. Nicolaidis. Pharmacokinetics of ceftazidime in

patients undergoing peritoneal dialysis. *J. Antimicrob. Chemother. Suppl. A, 12*:263–267 (1983).

237. A. Saito. Studies on absorption, distribution, metabolism and excretion of ceftazidime in Japan. *J. Antimicrob. Chemother. Suppl. A, 12*:255–262 (1983).
238. D. M. Ryan, B. Hodges, G. R. Spencer, and S. M. Harding. Simultaneous comparison of three methods for assessing ceftazidime penetration into extravascular fluid. *Antimicrob. Agents Chemother., 22*:995–998 (1982).
239. G. C. Armstrong, R. Wise, R. M. Brown, and J. Hancox. Comparison of ceftazidime and cefamandole pharmacokinetics and blister fluid concentrations. *Antimicrob. Agents Chemother., 20*:356–358 (1981).
240. B. Hoffstedt and M. Walder. Penetration of ceftazidime into extracellular fluid in patients. *J. Antimicrob. Chemother. Suppl. B, 8*:289–292 (1981).
241. D. M. Ryan, U. Mason, and S. M. Harding. The penetration of ceftazidime into extravascular fluid. *J. Antimicrob. Chemother. Suppl. B, 8*:283–288 (1981).
242. R. A. Walstad, K. B. Hellum, S. Blinka, et al. Pharmacokinetics and tissue penetration of ceftazidime: Studies on lymph, aqueous humor, skin blister, cerebrospinal and pleural fluid. *J. Antimicrob. Chemother. Suppl. A, 12*:275–282 (1983).
243. J. Modal, D. Vittecoq, J. M. Decazes, et al. Penetration of ceftazidime into cerebrospinal fluid of patients with bacterial meningitis. *Antimicrob. Agents Chemother., 24*:126–128 (1983).
244. B. Strandvik, A. Malmborg, H. Alfredson, and A. Ericsson. Clinical results and pharmacokinetics of ceftazidime treatment in patients with cystic fibrosis. *J. Antimicrob. Chemother. Suppl. A, 12*:283–287 (1983).
245. J. D. Blanco, J. H. Jorgensen, Y. S. Castaneda, et al. Ceftazidime levels in human breast milk. *Antimicrob. Agents Chemother., 23*:479–480 (1983).
246. F. D. Daschner, E. E. Petersen, H. M. Just, and H. G. Hillemanns. Penetration of ceftazidime into serum, myometrium, endometrium, salpinges and subcutaneous tissue. *J. Antimicrob. Chemother. Suppl. A, 12*:247–249 (1983).
247. D. H. Wittmann, H. H. Schassan, F. Kohler, and W. Siebert. Pharmacokinetic studies of ceftazidime in serum, bone, bile, tissue fluid and peritoneal fluid. *J. Antimicrob. Chemother. Suppl. B, 8*:293–297 (1981).
248. E. Bouza, T. Hellin, M. Rodriguez Creixems, et al. Comparison of ceftazidime concentrations in bile and serum. *Antimicrob. Agents Chemother., 24*:104–106 (1983).
249. D. Adam, B. Reichart, and K. J. Williams. Penetration of ceftazidime into human tissue in patients undergoing cardiac surgery. *J. Antimicrob. Chemother. Suppl. A, 12*:269–273 (1983).
250. R. Luthy, J. Blaser, A. Bonetti, et al. Human pharmacokinetics of ceftazidime in comparison to moxalactam and cefotaxime. *J. Antimicrob. Chemother. Suppl. B, 8*:273–276 (1981).

251. K. G. Naber, F. Kees, and H. Grobecker. Ceftazidime: Pharmacokinetics in young volunteers versus elderly patients and therapeutic efficacy with complicated urinary tract infections. *J. Antimicrob. Chemother. Suppl. A, 12*:41–45 (1983).
252. J. P. Fillastre, G. Humbert, B. Olier, et al. Pharmacokinetics of ceftazidime in renal failure. *J. Antimicrob. Chemother., 11*:487–488 (1983).
253. D. Hoffler, P. Koeppe, and K. J. Williams. The pharmacokinetics of ceftazidime in normal and impaired renal function. *J. Antimicrob. Chemother. Suppl. A, 12*:241–245 (1983).
254. J. G. Prinsloo, S. D. Delport, J. Moncrieff, and A. M. Paton. A preliminary pharmacokinetic study of ceftazidime in premature, newborn and small infants. *J. Antimicrob. Chemother. Suppl. A, 12*:361–364 (1983).
255. A. Boccazzi, M. Rizzo, M. L. Caccamo, and B. M. Assael. Comparison of the concentrations of ceftazidime in the serum of newborn infants after intravenous and intramuscular administration. *Antimicrob. Agents Chemother., 24*:955–956 (1983).
256. B. M. Assael, A. Boccazzi, M. L. Caccamo, et al. Clinical pharmacology of ceftazidime in pediatrics. *J. Antimicrob. Chemother. Suppl. A, 12*:341–346 (1983).
257. C. M. Kercsmar, R. C. Stern, M. D. Reed, et al. Ceftazidime in cystic fibrosis: Pharmacokinetics and therapeutic response. *J. Antimicrob. Chemother. Suppl. A, 12*:289–295 (1983).
258. G. R. Granneman, L. T. Sennello, F. J. Steinberg, and R. C. Sonders. Intramuscular and intravenous pharmacokinetics of cefmenoxime, a new broad-spectrum cephalosporin, in healthy subjects. *Antimicrob. Agents Chemother., 21*:141–145 (1982).
259. K. Matsumoto, T. Nagatake, Y. Uzuka, et al. Laboratory evaluation of cefmenoxime: A new cephalosporin. *Chemotherapy, 29*:80–88 (1983).
260. D. P. Reitberg, T. J. Cumbo, I. L. Smith, and J. J. Schentag. Effect of protein binding on cefmenoxime steady-state kinetics in critical patients. *Clin. Pharmacol. Ther., 35*:64–73 (1984).
261. N. Takahashi, K. Takahashi, and M. Takagi. Intraocular penetration of cefmenoxime (SCE-1365), a new cephalosporin, in humans. *Nippon Ganka Gakkai Zasshi, 86*:337–340 (1982).
262. K. V. I. Rolston, P. H. Chandraskekar, B. R. Smith, and J. L. LeFrock. The penetration of cefmenoxime into cerebrospinal fluid across non-inflammed meninges. *J. Antimicrob. Chemother., 12*:519–521 (1983).
263. L. T. Sennello, D. Quinn, D. E. Rollins, et al. Effect of probenecid on the pharmacokinetics of cefmenoxime. *Antimicrob. Agents Chemother., 23*:803–807 (1983).
264. D. Hoffler and P. Koeppe. Pharmacokinetics of cefmenoxime in normal and impaired renal function. *Arzneim. Forsch., 33*:269–272 (1983).
265. G. R. Granneman, L. T. Sennello, R. C. Sonders, et al. Cefsulodin kinetics in healthy subjects after intramuscular and intravenous injection. *Clin. Pharmacol. Ther., 31*:95–103 (1982).

266. F. D. Daschner, B. Metz, G. Spillner, et al. Concentrations of cefamandole and cefsulodin in serum, heart valves, subcutaneous tissue, and muscle of patients undergoing open-heart surgery. *J. Infect. Dis.*, *142*:290 (1980).
267. S. R. Durham and R. Wise. Human pharmacology and tissue levels of CGP 7174/E: A new antipseudomonal cephalosporin. *J. Antimicrob. Chemother.*, *6*:743–747 (1980).
268. G. R. Matzke and W. F. Keane. Cefsulodin pharmacokinetics in patients with various degrees of renal function. *Antimicrob. Agents Chemother.*, *23*:369–373 (1983).
269. T. P. Gibson, G. R. Granneman, J. E. Kallal, and L. T. Sennello. Cefsulodin kinetics in renal impairment. *Clin. Pharmacol. Ther.*, *31*:602–608 (1982).
270. K. Shimizu. Cefoperazone: Absorption, excretion, distribution and metabolism. *Clin. Ther.*, *3*:60–79 (1980).
271. E. Keller, A. Jansen, K. Pelz, et al. Intraperitoneal and intravenous cefoperazone kinetics during continuous ambulatory peritoneal dialysis. *Clin. Pharmacol. Ther.*, *35*:208–213 (1984).
272. C. M. Warns, H. Lode, G. Belmega, and T. Jendroschek. Pharmacokinetic profile of cefoperazone in healthy volunteers. *Infection Suppl. 1*, *9*:13–16 (1981).
273. W. A. Craig. Single dose pharmacokinetics of cefoperazone following intravenous administration. *Clin. Ther.*, *3*:46–49 (1980).
274. W. A. Craig and A. U. Gerber. Pharmacokinetics of cefoperazone: A review. *Drugs Suppl. 1*, *22*:35–45 (1980).
275. S. Srinivasan, E. L. Francke, and H. C. Neu. Comparative pharmacokinetics of cefoperazone and cefamandole. *Antimicrob. Agents Chemother.*, *19*:298–301 (1981).
276. H. Lode, B. Kemmerich, P. Koeppe, et al. Comparative pharmacokinetics of cefoperazone and cefotaxime. *Clin. Ther.*, *3*:80–88 (1980).
277. Y. Watanabe, T. Hayashi, R. Takada, et al. Studies on protein binding of antibiotics: Effect of cefazolin on protein binding and pharmacokinetics of cefoperazone. *J. Antibiot.*, *33*:625–635 (1980).
278. L. Balant, P. Dayer, M. Rudhardt, et al. Cefoperazone: Pharmacokinetics in humans with normal and impaired renal function and pharmacokinetics in rats. *Clin. Ther.*, *3*:50–59 (1980).
279. B. Hoffstedt and M. Walder. Influence of serum protein binding and mode of administration on penetration of five cephalosporins into subcutaneous tissue fluid in humans. *Antimicrob. Agents Chemother.*, *20*:783–786 (1981).
280. R. Ellis-Pegler. Symposium on cefoperazone sodium. Chairman, panel discussion; Section II. *Drugs Suppl.*, *22*:65–68 (1981).
281. R. Ellis-Pegler and S. Lang. Cefoperazone in *Klebsiella* meningitis: A case report. *Drugs Suppl.*, *22*:69–71 (1981).
282. D. Cable, G. Overturf, and G. Edralin. Concentrations of cefoperazone in cerebrospinal fluid during bacterial meningitis. *Antimicrob. Agents Chemother.*, *23*:688–691 (1983).

283. N. J. Owens, M. A. French, C. H. Nightingale, et al. Penetration of cefoperazone into cerebrospinal fluid in patients undergoing myelography and its pharmacokinetics in critically ill patients. *Curr. Ther. Res., 33*:513–523 (1983).
284. J. L. Axelrod and R. S. Kochman. Cefoperazone concentrations in human aqueous humor after intravenous administration. *Am. J. Ophthalmol., 94*: 103–105 (1982).
285. J. A. Lyon. Ceforperazone. *Drug Intell. Clin. Pharm., 17*:7–11 (1983).
286. R. E. Bawdon, D. L. Hemsell, and S. P. Guss. Comparison of cefoperazone and cefoxitin concentrations in serum and pelvic tissue of abdominal hysterectomy patients. *Antimicrob. Agents Chemother., 22*:999–1003 (1982).
287. T. Hirayama and K. Kikuchi. Clinical studies on cefoperazone treatment for bile duct infections. *Jpn. J. Antibiot., 34*:934–938 (1981).
288. J. Ayarra, M. C. Garcia-Iglesias, J. Loscertales, et al. Lung tissue concentrations of cefoperazone, in *Abstracts of the Twelfth International Congress of Chemotherapy,* Florence, 1981, abstract 766.
289. D. H. Wittmann, H. H. Schassan, and H. Seidel. Bone concentrations of six new beta-lactam antibiotics, in *Abstracts of the Twelfth International Congress of Chemotherapy,* Florence, 1981, abstract 410.
290. K. Schalkhauser and D. Adam. Concentrations of cefoperazone in various tissues of the urogenital system, in *Abstracts of the Twelfth International Congress of Chemotherapy,* Florence, 1981, abstract 409.
291. L. A. Wheeler, N. Kaplowitz, and S. M. Finegold. Pharmacokinetic study of cefoperazone and metabolites in patients with liver disease, in *Program and Abstract of the 21st Interscience Conference on Antimicrobial Agents and Chemotherapy,* American Society for Microbiology, Washington, D.C., 1981, abstract 755.
292. M. C. Marti, C. Farquet, J. Fabre, and M. Rundhardt. Pharmacokinetics and biliary excretion of cefoperazone in patients with bile duct drainage. *Infection Suppl. 1, 9*:34–36 (1981).
293. J. A. Boscia, O. M. Korzeniowski, R. Snepar, et al. Cefoperazone pharmacokinetics in normal subjects and patients with cirrhosis. *Antimicrob. Agents Chemother., 23*:385–389 (1983).
294. B. Cochet, J. Belaieff, A. F. Allaz, et al. Decreased extra-renal clearance of cefoperazone in hepatocellular disease. *Br. J. Clin. Pharmacol., 11*:389–390 (1981).
295. B. Cochet, J. Belaieff, A. F. Allaz, et al. Serum levels and urinary excretion of cefoperazone in patients with hepatic insufficiency. *Infection Suppl. 1, 9*: 37–39 (1981).
296. M. B. Rosenfeld and K. R. Ratzan. A comparison of the biliary tract excretion of cefoperazone and cefamandole. Unpublished data on file, Pfizer Pharmaceuticals, New York, 1981.
297. R. R. Bailey, B. Peddie, and E. Blake. Serum and urine concentrations of cefoperazone in severe chronic renal failure. *Drugs Suppl. 1, 22*:46–51 (1981).

298. W. K. Bolton, W. M. Scheld, D. A. Spyker, and M. A. Sande. Pharmacokinetics of cefoperazone in normal volunteers and subjects with renal insufficiency. *Antimicrob. Agents Chemother., 19*:821–825 (1981).
299. D. Hoffler, P. Koeppe, and C. Piper. The pharmacokinetics of cefoperazone in normal and impaired renal function. *Infection Suppl. 1, 9*:24–29 (1981).
300. J. A. Bosso, G. M. Chan, and J. M. Masten. Cefoperazone pharmacokinetics in preterm infants. *Antimicrob. Agents Chemother., 23*:413–415 (1983).
301. W. N. Rosenfeld, H. E. Evans, R. Batheja, et al. Pharmacokinetics of cefoperazone in full-term and premature neonates. *Antimicrob. Agents Chemother., 23*:866–869 (1983).
302. A. W. Maksymiuk, B. M. LeBlanc, N. S. Brown, et al. Pharmacokinetics of cefoperazone in patients with neoplastic disease. *Antimicrob. Agents Chemother., 19*:1037–1041 (1981).
303. I. H. Patel, R. E. Weinfeld, J. Konikoff, and M. Parsonnet. Pharmacokinetics and tolerance of ceftriaxone in humans after single-dose intramuscular administration in water and lidocaine diluents. *Antimicrob. Agents Chemother., 21*:957–962 (1982).
304. B. R. Meyers, E. S. Srulevitch, J. Jacobson, and S. Z. Hirschman. Crossover study of the pharmacokinetics of ceftriaxone administered intravenously or intramuscularly to healthy volunteers. *Antimicrob. Agents Chemother., 24*:812–814 (1983).
305. A. A. Pollock, P. E. Tee, I. H. Patel, et al. Pharmacokinetic characteristics of intravenous ceftriaxone in normal adults. *Antimicrob. Agents Chemother., 22*:816–823 (1982).
306. K. Stoeckel. Pharmacokinetics of Rocephin[R], a highly active new cephalosporin with an exceptionally long biological half-life. *Chemotherapy Suppl. 1, 27*:42–46 (1981).
307. K. Stoeckel, P. J. McNamara, R. Brandt, et al. Effect of concentration-dependent plasma protein binding on ceftriaxone kinetics. *Clin. Pharmacol. Ther., 29*:650–657 (1981).
308. P. J. McNamara, K. Stoeckel, and W. H. Ziegler. Pharmacokinetics of ceftriaxone following intravenous administration of a 3 gram dose. *Eur. J. Clin. Pharmacol., 22*:71–75 (1982).
309. I. H. Patel, S. Chen, M. Parsonnet, et al. Pharmacokinetics of ceftriaxone in humans. *Antimicrob. Agents Chemother., 20*:634–641 (1981).
310. I. H. Patel, K. Miller, R. Weinfeld, and J. Spicehandler. Multiple intravenous dose pharmacokinetics of ceftriaxone in man. *Chemotherapy Suppl. 1, 27*:47–56 (1981).
311. M. Seddon, R. Wise, A. P. Gillett, and R. Livingston. Pharmacokinetics of RO 13-9905, a broad-spectrum cephalosporin. *Antimicrob. Agents Chemother., 18*:240–242 (1980).
312. M. Cadoz, F. Denis, H. Felix, and I. DiopMar. Treatment of purulent meningitis with a new cephalosporin – Rocephin[R] (RO 13-9904). *Chemotherapy Suppl. 1, 27*:57–61 (1981).

313. M. DelRio, G. H. McCracken, Jr., J. D. Nelson, et al. Pharmacokinetics and cerebrospinal fluid bactericidal activity of ceftriaxone in the treatment of pediatric patients with bacterial meningitis. *Antimicrob. Agents Chemother., 22*:622–627 (1982).
314. R. W. Steele, L. B. Eyre, R. W. Bradsher, et al. Pharmacokinetics of ceftriaxone in pediatric patients with meningitis. *Antimicrob. Agents Chemother., 23*:191–194 (1983).
315. M. D. Reed, H. L. Rekate, S. C. Aronoff, et al. Single-dose plasma and cerebrospinal fluid pharmacokinetics of ceftriaxone in infants and children. *Clin. Pharm., 2*:558–563 (1983).
316. C. S. Bryan, S. L. Morgan, A. B. Jordan, et al. Ceftriaxone levels in blood and tissue during cardiopulmonary bypass surgery. *Antimicrob. Agents Chemother., 25*:37–39 (1984).
317. F. D. Daschner, E. E. Petersen, J. Brandle, and H. G. Hillemanns. Concentrations of ceftriaxone in serum and gynecological tissues. *Chemotherapy, 29*:153–155 (1983).
318. D. A. Kafetzis, D. C. Brater, J. E. Fanourgakis, et al. Ceftriaxone distribution between maternal blood and fetal blood and tissues at parturition and between blood and milk postpartum. *Antimicrob. Agents Chemother., 23*:870–873 (1983).
319. D. P. Maudgal, J. D. Maxwell, L. J. Lees, and R. N. Wild. Biliary excretion of amoxycillin and ceftriaxone after intravenous administration in man. *Br. J. Clin. Pharmacol., 14*:213–217 (1982).
320. N. Owens, R. Quintiliani, and C. H. Nightingale. Penetration of ceftriaxone into gallbladder and bile of patients undergoing cholecystectomies for chronic cholecystitis. (In preparation)
321. T. Ti, L. Fortin, J. H. Kreeft, et al. Kinetic disposition of intravenous ceftriaxone in normal subjects and patients with renal failure on hemodialysis or peritoneal dialysis. *Antimicrob. Agents Chemother., 25*:83–87 (1984).
322. K. Stoeckel, P. J. McNamara, G. Hoppe-Seyler, et al. Single dose ceftriaxone kinetics in functionally anephric patients. *Clin. Pharmacol. Ther., 33*:633–641 (1983).
323. D. Cohen, G. B. Appel, B. Scully, and H. C. Neu. Pharmacokinetics of ceftriaxone in patients with renal failure and in those undergoing hemodialysis. *Antimicrob. Agents Chemother., 24*:529–532 (1983).
324. G. H. McCracken, Jr., J. D. Siegel, N. Threlkeld, and M. Thomas. Ceftriaxone pharmacokinetics in newborn infants. *Antimicrob. Agents Chemother., 23*:341–343 (1983).
325. U. B. Schaad and K. Stoeckel. Single-dose pharmacokinetics of ceftriaxone in infants and young children. *Antimicrob. Agents Chemother., 21*:248–253 (1982).
326. J. R. Luderer, I. H. Patel, J. Durkin, and D. W. Schneck. Age and ceftriaxone kinetics. *Clin. Pharmacol. Ther., 35*:19–25 (1984).
327. P. Salvador, R. G. Smith, R. E. Weinfeld, et al. Clinical pharmacology of ceftriaxone in patients with neoplastic disease. *Antimicrob. Agents Chemother., 23*:583–588 (1983).

PART 3
CEPHALOSPORINS

11
Clinical Use of Cephalosporins

RICHARD B. KOHLER, LAWRENCE JOSEPH WHEAT, and ARTHUR C. WHITE
Indiana University School of Medicine, Indianapolis, Indiana

I. INTRODUCTION

Since the introduction of cephalothin over two decades ago, cephalosporins have been widely used in the treatment of a variety of infections. At one time they accounted for over one-half of the total expenditures of hospital pharmacies for injectable antibiotics. Cephalosporins have been classified as first-, second-, or third-generation cephalosporins. The first-generation has activity similar to that of cephalothin, the second generation (e.g., cefamandole) demonstrated increased in vitro activity against certain organisms, and the third generation (e.g., cefotaxime and cefoperazone) had in vitro activity against organisms resistant to first- or second-generation cephalosporins. If one believes that one generation follows another in time, the sequence of introduction of cephalosporins in the United States does not follow logically; cefuroxime, a second-generation cephalosporin, was introduced after both cefotaxime and cefaperazone, third-generation cephalosporins.

The number of newer cephalosporins and related compounds such as monobactams, penems, and oxycephem has increased rapidly and is likely to continue to increase in the next few years. There are very few clinical data on the relative efficacy of these compounds as compared with either each other or previous therapies such as clindamycin and aminoglycoside for mixed aerobic-anaerobic infections or aminoglycoside and ticarcillin for fever in granulocytopenic fever. Several years will be required before good clinical trials will answer these questions.

This chapter will review in vitro data of the various cephalosporins, current recommendations for their use in treatment and prophylaxis, and advantages and disadvantages known at this time.

II. SPECIFIC DRUGS

A. First-Generation Cephalosporins

When cephalothin was first introduced for clinical use, its major in vitro activity was against most gram-positive organisms, including *Streptococcus pneumoniae* (pneumococcus), *Streptococcus pyrogenes,* other streptococci, and *Staphylococcus aureus,* both penicillinase and nonpenicillinase producers, but cephalothin had limited activity against enterococcal streptococci (1-3). Against gram-negative bacteria, cephalothin was active against most *Escherichia coli, Proteus mirabilis,* and *Klebsiella,* but was largely inactive against most other aerobic gram-negative bacteria. For treatment of other gram-negative aerobic organisms such as *Pseudomonas aeruginosa,* the aminoglycosides were the drugs of choice, often combined with a semisynthetic penicillin such as carbenicillin or ticarcillin. For most gram-positive infections, penicillin G or semisynthetic penicillins such as nafcillin or ampicillin were listed as the drugs of choice, and for most of the gram-negative infections ampicillin was as effective as cephalothin. Only for *Klebsiella* infections were first-generation cephalosporins indicated as the initial drug of choice. Despite these limitations, first-generation cephalosporins were extensively used for inpatient and outpatient infections to cover many of the possibilities when the infecting organism was not known and in patients who had mild allergic reactions to penicillins when penicillin would have been otherwise the drug of choice.

B. Second-Generation Cephalosporins

In many hospitals there have been changes in both the types of organisms seen in seriously ill patients and their antimicrobial susceptibility. Many *E. coli, Klebsiella,* and *Prot. mirabilis* have developed resistance to the first generation of cephalosporins. In addition, many organisms have developed resistance against the aminoglycosides tobramycin and gentamicin. Table 1 shows the frequencies of aerobic gram-negative blood isolates, excluding *Hemophilus influenzae,* during 1 year at Indiana University Hospital and their susceptibilities to the first-generation cephalosporin cephalothin, the second-generation cephalosporin cefamandole and the related drug cefoxitin, and tobramycin. Although *E. coli* has remained the single most common aerobic gram-negative bacteria isolated, a wide variety of organisms is isolated from patients with bacteremia; many such *Enterobacter aerogenes, Ps. aeruginosa,* and *Serratia* are rarely susceptible to the first-generation cephalosporins. In contrast, 74% of the *E. coli* and 90% of the *Klebsiella pneumoniae* were susceptible to the first-generation cephalosporin cephalothin. Overall, 49% of the organisms isolated from patients with aerobic gram-negative bacteremia were susceptible to cephalothin. Many organisms were also resistant to the aminoglycoside tobramycin, so that 9% of aerobic gram-nega-

Table 1 Aerobic Gram-Negative Blood Culture Isolates (Percentage of Strains Susceptible to Each Antibiotic) From University Hospital, Indiana

	Cephalothin	Cefoxitin	Cefamandole	Tobramycin
Acinetobacter (9)[a]	0	11	11	89
Enterobacter aerogenes (12)	12	0	42	83
Enterobacter cloacae (12)	0	0	67	100
Escherichia coli (65)	74	98	91	88
Klebsiella oxytoca (4)	100	100	100	100
Klebsiella pneumoniae (29)	90	90	86	100
Proteus (6)	86	100	86	100
Pseudomonas (41)	0	0	0	93
Serratia (14)	0	29	0	64
Total	49	61	64	89

[a]The numbers of isolates tested are given in parentheses.

Table 2 Comparative In Vitro Activity of New Cephalosporin Agents Against Major Pathogens

Organism	Cefotaxime MIC (μg/ml)	Ceftizoxime MIC (μg/ml)
Streptococcus pyrogenes (group A)	< 0.01 - 0.1	< 0.01 - 0.1
Strep. agalactiae (group B)	< 0.01 - 0.1	< 0.01 - 0.1
Strep. faecalis	4 ->128	8 ->128
Strep. pneumoniae	≤ 0.01 - 0.25	≤ 0.01 - 0.25
Streptococci (alpha, nonhemolytic, not group D)[a]	0.01 - 32	0.01 - 32
Staphylococcus aureus[b]	< 0.5 ->125	< 0.5 ->128
Staph. epidermidis[c]	0.5 ->128	0.5 ->128
Hemophilus influenzae	≤ 0.01 - 0.03	≤ 0.01 - 0.03
Neisseria gonorrhoeae	< 0.01 - 0.3	< 0.01 - 0.3
Neisseria meningitidis	< 0.01 - 0.025	< 0.01 - 0.25
Listeria monocytogenes	>128	>128
Escherichia coli	< 0.1 - 8	< 0.1 - 8
Klebsiella pneumoniae	< 0.1 - 2	< 0.1 - 2
Enterobacter aerogenes	< 0.01 - 4	< 0.01 - 4
Enterobacter cloacae	< 0.1 ->128	< 0.1 ->128
Citrobacter freundii	0.02 - 1.6	0.02 - 1.6
Citrobacter diversus	< 0.1 - 16	< 0.01 - 16
Serratia marcescens	0.2 ->128	0.2 ->128
Proteus mirabilis	< 0.001 - 0.05	< 0.001- 0.5
Morganella morganii	0.2 - 4	0.2 - 4
Providencia rettgeri and *stuartii*	< 0.1 - 4	< 0.1 - 4
Salmonella sp.	0.1 - 0.5	0.1 - 0.5
Shigella sp.	< 0.1 - 0.5	< 0.1 - 0.5
Pseudomonas aeruginosa[d]	2 ->128	2 ->128
Pseudomonas (*Ps. maltophilia, Ps. cepacia, Ps. fluorescens, Ps. putida*)	2 ->128	2 ->128
Acinetobacter	2 ->128	2 ->128
Bacteroides fragilis[e]	1 ->128	1 ->128

[a]Cephalothin: range, 0.1–32 μg/ml; MIC, 0.25 μg/ml.
[b]Cephalothin: range, 0.01->128 μg/ml; MIC, 0.5 μg/ml.
[c]Cephalothin: range, 0.1->128 μg/ml; MIC, 1 μg/ml.
[d]Ticarcillin: range, 1->128 μg/ml; MIC, 64 μg/ml. Gentamicin: range, 0.1->16 μg/ml; MIC, >16 μg/ml.
[e]Cefoxitin: range, 1–128 μg/ml; MIC, 16 μg/ml.

Ceftazidime MIC (μg/ml)	Cefoperazone MIC (μg/ml)	Moxalactam MIC (μg/ml)	Cefazolin MIC (μg/ml)
0.06 - 0.5	0.01 - 0.25	< 0.5 - 8	< 0.01- 0.1
0.06 - 0.5	0.01 - 0.25	0.1 - 8	0.01- 0.1
32 ->128	4 ->128	32 ->128	>128
0.06 - 0.25	0.06 - 0.25	0.5 - 4	0.01- 1
0.03 -> 64	0.1 - 32	1 -> 32	–
2 ->128	< 0.1 ->128	1 ->128	–
0.5 ->128	0.1 ->128	1 ->128	–
≤ 0.01 - 0.5	≤ 0.01 - 0.5	≤ 0.03 - 0.25	2 - 32
< 0.01 - 0.25	< 0.01 - 0.25	< 0.01 - 1	1 - 16
< 0.01 - 0.025	< 0.01 - 0.1	< 0.01 - 0.1	> 0.01- 0.25
>128	>128	>128	>128
< 0.1 - 8	< 0.1 ->128	< 0.1 - 8	2 ->128
< 0.1 - 2	< 0.1 - 128	< 0.1 - 4	0.5 ->128
< 0.01 - 4	0.1 - 16	0.006- 3.1	6 ->128
< 0.1 ->128	< 0.1 ->128	< 0.1 ->128	>128
0.02 - 1.6	0.02 ->128	0.02 - 16	>128
< 0.1 - 16	< 0.1 - 16	< 0.1 - 16	–
0.2 ->128	0.2 ->128	0.2 ->128	>128
< 0.001- 0.5	< 0.001- 0.5	< 0.001- 0.05	1 - 32
0.2 - 4	0.2 ->128	0.1 - 0.5	16 ->128
< 0.1 - 4	< 0.1 - 32	< 0.1- 4	16
0.1 - 0.5	< 0.1 - 128	< 0.1 - 0.5	4 ->128
< 0.1 - 0.5	< 0.1 - 64	< 0.1 - 0.5	1 ->128
0.5 - 32	0.25 ->128	1 ->128	–
2 ->128	2 ->128	2 ->128	–
2 ->128	2 ->128	4 ->128	>128
1 ->128	1 ->128	1 ->128	–

Table 3 Comparative In Vitro Activity of New Cephalosporin Agents Against Major Pathogens

Organism	Cefotaxime MIC_{90} (μg/ml)	Ceftizoxime MIC_{90} (μg/ml)	Ceftazidime MIC_{90} (μg/ml)	Cefoperazone MIC_{90} (μg/ml)	Moxalactam MIC_{90} (μg/ml)	Cefazolin MIC_{90} (μg/ml)
Streptococcus pyrogenes (group A)	0.12	0.03	0.25	0.12	4	0.05
Strep. agalactiae (group B)	0.1	0.1	0.25	0.25	4	–
Strep. faecalis	>128	>128	>128	>128	>128	128
Strep. pneumoniae	0.12	0.12	0.25	0.25	2	0.1
Streptococci (alpha, nonhemolytic, not group D)[a]	0.25	0.25	4	1	32	–
Staphylococcus aureus[b]	2	2	8	4	16	–
Staph. epidermidis[c]	8	8	8	8	32	–
Hemophilus influenzae	0.03	0.03	0.12	0.12	0.06	32
Neisseria gonorrhoeae	0.015	0.015	0.12	0.06	0.06	8
Neisseria meningitidis	< 0.01	< 0.01	< 0.01	0.05	0.05	0.01
Listeria monocytogenes	>128	>128	>128	>128	>128	>128
Escherichia coli	0.25	0.25	0.5	16	0.25	>128
Klebsiella pneumoniae	0.25	0.25	0.25	16	0.25	>128
Enterobacter aerogenes	0.2	0.2	0.2	2	0.2	>128

Enterobacter cloacae	8	8	8	32	4	>128
Citrobacter freundii	8	8	8	16	8	>128
Citrobacter diversus	0.5	0.25	0.5	1	0.5	–
Serratia marcescens	4	2	2	16	4	>128
Proteus mirabilis	0.1	0.1	0.2	1	0.2	16
Morganella morganii	2	0.5	2	4	0.5	>128
Providencia rettgeri and *Prov. stuartii*	2	2	1	16	2	> 12
Salmonella sp.	0.25	0.25	0.25	1	0.25	32
Shigella sp.	0.25	0.25	0.25	1	0.25	8
Pseudomonas aeruginosa[d]	64	64	8	32	32	–
Pseudomonas (*Ps. maltophilia, Ps. cepacia, Ps. fluorescens, Ps. putida*	>128	>128	> 64	>128	128	–
Acinetobacter	> 64	>128	> 32	>128	>128	>128
Bacteroides fragilis[e]	64	32	128	64	16	–

[a]Cephalothin: range, 0.1–32 μg/ml; MIC, 0.25 μg/ml.
[b]Cephalothin: range, 0.01–>128 μg/ml; MIC, 0.5 μg/ml.
[c]Cephalothin: range, 0.1–>128 μg/ml; MIC, 1 μg/ml.
[d]Ticarcillin: range, 1–>128 μg/ml; MIC, 64 μg/ml. Gentamicin: range, 0.1–>16 μg/ml; MIC, >16 μg/ml.
[e]Cefoxitin: range, 1–128 μg/ml; MIC, 16 μg/ml.
Source: Data from Ref. 5.

tive organisms isolated from patients with bacteremia were resistant to tobramycin.

The second generation of cephalosporins had increased activity against some but not all aerobic gram-negative organisms. Cephamandole was active in vitro against *Enterobacter* strains; cefoxitin, a cephamycin similar in many ways to second-generation cephalosporins, had increased activity against some *Serratia*. In addition, both were active against more strains of *E. coli* than the first-generation drug cephalothin.

Cefuroxime, a more recently introduced second-generation cephalosporin, is active against the major pathogens in pediatrics, including *H. influenzae, Strep. pneumoniae, Strep. pyrogenes,* and *Staph. aureus* (4). In addition, it is active against some but not all *Klebsiella, E. coli,* and *Enterobacter* resistant to first-generation cephalosporins.

C. Third-Generation Cephalosporins

The major advantage of the third-generation cephalosporins is their increased activity against aerobic gram-negative bacteria. Tables 2 and 3 show minimal inhibitory concentration (MIC) and MIC_{90} values, respectively, as published by Neu (5), of five beta-lactams currently on the U.S. market, cefotaxime, cefoperazone, ceftizoxime, and moxalactam, as well as ceftazidime, which is the latest to be introduced, and the first-generation cephalosporin cefazolin. Against gram-positive organisms, these drugs have no advantage; in fact, as a group they are less active against streptococci and staphylococci than the first-generation cephalosporins. Moxalactam, an oxycephem resembling the third-generation cephalosporins, is the least active against *Strep. pneumoniae* and *Staph. aureus*; all are inactive against enterococci. In comparison with first-generation cephalosporins, the third-generation drugs are more active against *H. influenzae* (both beta-lactamase producers and non-beta-lactamase producers), against *E. coli, Klebsiella,* and *Prot. mirabilis* resistant to first-generation cephalosporins, and against *Ent. aerogenes* and *Serratia,* which have never been susceptible to the first-generation cephalosporins. Among organisms susceptible to both first- and third-generation cephalosporins, the third-generation cephalosporins are generally much more active on a weight basis, with concentrations as low as 0.01 μg/ml inhibiting *Prot. mirabilis* and some *Enterobacter* and *E. coli.* Over 90% of the *E. coli, Klebsiella,* and *Ent. aerogenes* are inhibited by 0.25 μg/ml or less. Of the third-generation cephalosporins, more *E. coli* and *Klebsiella* are resistant to cefoperazone than to the other third-generation cephalosporins. The ranges of concentrations required to inhibit *Ps. aeruginosa, Acinetobacter,* and *Bacteroides fragilis* are considerably greater, with many isolates being resistant to achievable concentrations of most of the third-generation cephalosporins. Cefoperazone and ceftazidime are the most active third-generation cephalosporins against *Ps. aeruginosa.*

Table 4 Resistance of *B. fragilis* to Nine Antibiotics

Antimicrobial agent	Percent resistant
Cefoperazone	51(32)[a]
Cefotaxime	45(32)
Cefoxitin	6(32)
Chloramphenicol	0(16)
Clindamycin	7(8)
Metronidazole	0(8)
Moxalactam	19(32)
Piperacillin	8(128)
Tetracycline	60(4)

[a]The antibiotic concentration that defines "resistance" is given in parentheses for each antibiotic and is expressed in micrograms per milliliter.

Against anaerobic organisms other than *B. fragilis,* cephalosporins are active in vitro, although penicillin G has been the drug of choice for most of these organisms. However, *Bacteroides melaninogenicus* is more resistant to penicillin G. Against *B. fragilis,* the in vitro activity of the third-generation cephalosporins is less predictable, as shown in Table 4 (6). Cefoxitin has the greatest in vitro activity of this group of antibiotics, followed by moxalactam and, with considerably less activity, cefoperazone and cefotaxime. Ceftazidime is not active in vitro against most *B. fragilis.* With increasing resistance of *B. fragilis* to clindamycin, the proportion of *B. fragilis* susceptible to cefoxitin and to a lesser degree moxalactam is similar to that susceptible to clindamycin. Only chloramphenicol and metronidazole were consistently active in vitro.

III. CLINICAL INDICATIONS

First-generation cephalosporins have been widely used antibiotics. In a variety of studies they have been shown to be effective in respiratory, skin, and soft tissue infections, urinary tract infections, a variety of bacteremias, and infections of bones and joints due to susceptible organisms. However, in most infections other drugs were considered the drugs of choice; only rarely were cephalosporins indicated as the preferred drug. For the pneumococcus and group A streptococci, penicillin G is the drug of choice; for *H. influenzae,* ampicillin; for staphylococci, the semisynthetic penicillins; and for *E. coli* and *Prot. mirabilis,* ampicillin or the sulfonamides are usually listed as drugs of choice (3).

A. Upper Respiratory Infections

Most pharyngitis is due to viral agents which are not treatable with antibiotics. Group A streptococci and *Mycoplasma pneumoniae* are the major infections effectively treated with antibiotics. For group A streptococcal infections penicillin G has remained the drug of choice, with erythromycin preferred in patients allergic to penicillin. However, oral cephalexin and other oral cephalosporins have been effective in treating patients with mild, non-life-threatening allergic reactions to penicillin G (3).

B. Otitis Media

Otitis media is a common infection in the pediatric population. The major aerobic organisms isolated from most patients are *Strep. pneumoniae, H. influenzae,* and group A streptococci (7). Ampicillin has been the most widely used drug in the treatment of otitis media because of its activity against all of these pathogens. However, between 5 and 15% of *H. influenzae* are beta-lactamase producers and therefore resistant to ampicillin. The oral cephalosporin cefaclor, the parenteral cephalosporins cefamandole and cefuroxime, and most third-generation cephalosporins are active against most strains of *H. influenzae* resistant to ampicillin. As ampicillin resistance becomes more widespread, the use of these drugs or the combination trimethoprim–sulfamethoxazole may become more frequently indicated.

C. Lower Respiratory Infections

Pneumonias acquired in the community may be due to a wide variety of agents, including *Strep. pneumoniae, H. influenzae, Staph. aureus,* mixed aerobic and anaerobic bacteria, *M. pneumoniae,* and *K. pneumoniae.* Cephalosporins are the drugs of choice only for *K. pneumoniae,* semisynthetic penicillins (nafcillin or oxacillin) for *Staph. aureus,* penicillin or clindamycin for anaerobic infections, erythromycin for *M. pneumoniae* or *Legionella* infections, and ampicillin for *H. influenzae* strains which are not beta-lactamase producers. In the severely ill patient with community-acquired pneumonia, cephalosporins have frequently been used as initial drugs, since they are active against *Strep. pneumoniae, Staph. aureus,* and *Klebsiella.* In the pediatric population, in which *H. influenzae* is so frequent, cefuroxime would cover all these possibilities and as well as both beta-lactamase-positive and beta-lactamase-negative *H. influenzae* (8). Nelson (9) has predicted that cefuroxime may be the drug of choice in the pediatric population for community-acquired pneumonias in the future. Aspiration pneumonia acquired while outside the hospital is usually due to anaerobic organisms. Although penicillin G has been recommended as the drug of choice, there is considerable evidence now that an increasing number of respiratory anaerobes, including *B. melaninogenicus,* are beta-lactamase producers and are resistant to penicillin G. In one study it was suggested that clindamycin was more effective in treating anaerobic lung abscesses than penicillin G (10). The cephalosporins might be used as alternative drugs in patients who are allergic to penicillin G.

Hospital-acquired pneumonias are rarely due to pneumococci or *H. influenzae* and are likely to be due to either anaerobic organisms in approximately half of the patients or a wide variety of multiple-drug-resistant aerobic organisms, including *Ps. aeruginosa, Staph. aureus, E. coli, Proteus,* and *Serratia.* Previous therapy for these infections has usually included an aminoglycoside and a penicillin, such as ticarcillin or carbenicillin. Except for *Ps. aeruginosa* infections, third-generation cephalosporins would be active against most of these pathogens and allow single-drug therapy instead of combined therapy with two drugs and at the same time avoid the ototoxicities and nephrotoxicities of aminoglycoside. In the case of *Ps. aeruginosa* the range of MIC values is quite wide for the third-generation cephalosporins, and *Pseudomonas* has become resistant to the third generation cephalosporins during the course of therapy. Therefore most experts recommend treating pneumonia due to *Pseudomonas* with ticarcillin and an aminoglycoside or, in patients with mild penicillin allergies, with a third-generation cephalosporin plus an aminoglycoside. Cefoperazone is less resistant to degradation by some of the beta-lactamases than the other third-generation cephalosporins, and more *E. coli* and *Klebsiella* would be resistant to cefoperazone than to the other third-generation cephalosporins, including cefotaxime and moxalactam. On the other hand, cefoperazone and ceftazidime are the most active of the currently available third-generation cephalosporins against *Pseudomonas.*

D. Endocarditis

The major causes of endocarditis include group D organisms, both enterococcal and nonenterococcal, *Staph. aureus,* and streptococci of the *Streptococcus viridans* group, particularly *Streptococcus mutans* and *Streptococcus sanguis.* For these infections penicillin G with or without an aminoglycoside has been the drug of choice for *Strep. viridans* and group D infections, enterococcal or nonenterococcal. The semisynthetic penicillins nafcillin and oxacillin have been the primary drug to use for *Staph. aureus* strains, which are usually penicillinase producers and therefore resistant to penicillin G. Occasionally *Staph. aureus* is methicillin resistant and cross-resistant to the other semisynthetic penicillins, nafcillin and oxacillin, as well as to all cephalosporins. For therapy of methicillin-resistant *Staph. aureus* vancomycin is the drug of choice. In patients with a history of mild allergic reactions to penicillin G, the first-generation cephalosporins have been used in the treatment of endocarditis due to methicillin-sensitive *Staph. aureus, Strep. viridans,* and to group D nonenterococcal streptococci (3). Against enterococci the cephalosporins are essentially inactive and vancomycin has been the drug of choice. In patients with severe life-threatening penicillin reactions, vancomycin has been the drug of choice for all gram-positive organisms. For endocarditis occurring after the insertion of prosthetic valves, the most common organisms are *Staphylococcus epidermidis* and *Staph. aureus.* Most *Staph. aureus* are still susceptible to nafcillin and oxacillin, and these are drugs of choice except in patients with penicillin allergy, as cited above. *Staphylococcus epidermidis* is frequently resistant to penicillins of all types, including methicillin, nafcillin, and oxacillin; some of these strains are susceptible in vitro to the first-generation cephalosporins, but most investigators would prefer to use vancomycin for *Staph. epidermidis* resistant to methicillin, nafcillin, and oxacillin. For the infrequent gram-negative organisms causing prosthetic valve endocarditis, the third-generation cephalosporins may be effective; with *Ps. aeruginosa,* as mentioned above, most investigators would include aminoglycosides.

E. Skin and Soft Tissue Infections

Most skin and soft tissue infections, including furuncules, impetigo, and cellulitis, as well as infections following minor injuries, are due to either group A streptococci or coagulase-positive staphylococci. For group A streptococcal infections penicillin G is the drug of choice, with erythromycin as an alternative in the penicillin-allergic patient. Since most staphylococci are resistant to penicillin G, oral semisynthetic penicillin, dicloxacillin, or cloxacillin is preferred for staphylococcal infections. Oral cephalosporins, including cephradine and cephalexin, would be effective against both staphylococci and group A streptococci and have been used extensively in penicillin-allergic patients. In children cellulitis is frequently caused by *H. influenzae* and, if severe, should be treated with ampicillin, to cover most *H. influenzae,* or chloramphenicol initially, to cover ampicillin-resistant *H. influenzae.* Cefuroxime would be an alternative drug to cover both ampicillin-sensitive and ampicillin-resistant *H. influenzae* and could be used in patients with mild allergic reactions to penicillin G.

Decubitus ulcers are usually infected with mixed aerobic and anaerobic bacteria, including *B. fragilis.* In patients with severe sepsis from decubitus ulcers, drugs of choice have included clindamycin or metronidazole with an aminoglycoside. Cefoxitin is effective against 90% of the *B. fragilis* and would be an alternative drug, avoiding the toxicity of the aminoglycosides. Of the currently available cephalosporins, only moxalactam has activity against *B. fragilis* similar to that of cefoxitin. Diabetic foot ulcers are also frequently infected with aerobic and anaerobic bacteria, as is the osteomyelitis in diabetics associated with foot ulcers. Cefoxitin would cover most of these possibilities but would not be active against *Ps. aeruginosa* or enterococci, which also are frequent isolates in these patients.

F. Urinary Tract Infections

Initial urinary tract infections acquired outside of hospitals are usually due to sensitive *E. coli* and can be treated with a number of oral and parenteral drugs which include sulfonamides, ampicillin, and first-generation cephalosporins (3).

Recurrent urinary tract infections, particularly in the presence of stones or urinary tract obstructions, are more frequently due to organisms resistant to the first-generation cephalosporins, ampicillin, tetracycline, and sulfonamides. In addition, hospital-acquired urinary tract infections are frequently due to multiple-drug-resistant organisms, including a high frequency of organisms resistant to the aminoglycosides in many hospitals. The third-generation cephalosporins are particularly effective in severe forms of hospital-acquired urinary tract infections caused by multiple-resistant organisms.

G. Bacteremias

Most bacteremias are secondary to documented infections of the urinary tract, intra-abdominal sepsis, and pneumonias. The treatment for these bacteremias is similar to that for primary underlying disease. In patients who are severely leukopenic because of underlying disease or treatment, the source of bacteremia may not be evident and organisms frequently cannot be identified by blood cultures, but patients' fever respond to broad-spectrum antimicrobial agents. In this group bacteremias due to *Ps. aeruginosa* are particularly frequent, but also resistant *Klebsiella, E. coli,* and staphylococci are commonly isolated organisms. In these circumstances most authorities have administered initial therapy with a semisynthetic penicillin active against *Pseudomonas,* such as ticarcillin or carbenicillin in combination with aminoglycosides (3). In hospitals where *Pseudomonas* is infrequent, therapy with the third-generations cephalosporins has been as effective as treatment with ticarcillin and aminoglycosides.

H. Abdominal Pelvic Infections

Most infections within abdominal abscesses or peritonitis are secondary to diverticulitis, appendicitis, intra-abdominal injuries, or surgery. Mixed aerobic–anaerobic infections, including the *B. fragilis* group, are frequently isolated. Standard therapy for these infections has been the combination of clindamycin for anaerobes, including *B. fragilis,* and aminoglycosides to cover the aerobic gram-negative flora. In severe infections some have recommended that ampicillin be also added to cover enterococci, which are a frequent isolate. Other studies suggest that enterococci need to be treated infrequently. If the disease is acquired outside the hospital, *Ps. aeroginosa* seems to be an uncommon occurrence and therefore a cephalosporin active against both anaerobes, including *B. fragilis*, and most of the aerobic organisms might replace combined therapy with gentamicin and clindamycin, resulting in less ototoxicity and nephrotoxicity from the aminoglycosides. Cefoxitin can be effective in these circumstances (11) and other third-generation cephalosporins have also been demonstrated to be effective (12). However, many clinicians still prefer the combination of aminoglycosides and clindamycin (3).

I. Sexually Transmitted Disease

Of the sexually transmitted diseases, only the gonococcus can be treated with cephalosporins. Cefoxitin, 2 g, plus probenecid or 1 g of cefotaxime alone has been effective in treating both penicillinase-producing and non-penicillinase-producing gonococci (13,14). Such therapies can replace spectinomycin with penicillinase-producing gonococci and are an effective alternative in patients with mild penicillin allergies.

J. Meningitis

Three organisms, *Strep. pneumoniae, H. influenzae,* and *Neisseria meningitides,* are the major bacterial causes of meningitis; in the newborn group B streptococci and *E. coli* are the most frequent isolates. First-generation cephalosporins are ineffective in treating any of these causes of meningitis (3). In the pediatric population the standard therapy in a patient with an unknown meningitis has been ampicillin, which is effective against *N. meningitides, Strep. pneumoniae,* and most *H. influenzae.* Chloramphenicol is usually added as an initial treatment of suspected beta-lactamase-producing ampicillin-resistant *H. influenzae,* with discontinuation of the chloramphenicol if organisms should be ampicillin-susceptible *H. influenzae* or the discontinuation of the ampicillin if the isolates should be ampicillin resistant. Cefotaxime, moxalactam, and cefuroxime are all highly active in vitro against beta-lactamase-positive ampicillin-resistant *H. influenzae* and may replace the other regimens for meningitis in the pediatrics group or serve as alternative drugs in patients allergic to penicillin (15–18). Since moxalactam has poor activity against gram-positive cocci, it should never be used alone in patients with meningitis of unknown type but should be combined with drugs active against *Strep. pneumoniae.* None of the cephalosporins currently available should be used to treat meningitis due to *Ps. aeruginosa,* enterococci, or *Listeria.* Gram-negative meningitis due to *E. coli* or *Klebsiella* can now be treated effectively with third-generation cephalosporins such as cefotaxime or the oxycephem moxalactam (19–24). Such therapy is possible both because these drugs penetrate well in the cerebrospinal fluid space and therefore levels of 4–5 μg/ml can be obtained, but more important is the increased activity at low concentrations of these drugs against *E. coli* and *Klebsiella,* with spinal fluid levels 8-16 times the bactericidal concentrations. Therefore concentrations are obtained in the cerebrospinal fluid that are much higher than the sensitivity of *E. coli* or *Klebsiella. Pseudomonas* is more resistant to the third-generation cephalosporins, so that 4-8 μg/ml may be required to inhibit sensitive organisms. In addition, a significant number of strains are highly resistant. The drugs of choice for treatment of *Pseudomonas* meningitis still include the aminoglycosides plus a semisynthetic penicillin such as ticarcillin or carbenicillin. Most authorities recommend also that the aminoglycoside be given intrathecally in adults with *Pseudomonas* meningitis (3).

K. Bone and Joint Infections

First-generation cephalosporins have been useful in the treatment of staphylococcal osteomyelitis or arthritis in patients with mild penicillin allergies. Osteomyelitis or septic arthritis caused by susceptible gram-negative bacilli could be treated with newer cephalosporins. They are less toxic than the aminoglycosides for prolonged use. However, with current information, no cephalosporin should be used alone for the treatment of osteomyelitis due to *Pseudomonas,* but an aminoglycoside plus a cephalosporin active against *Pseudomonas,* including cefotaxime, moxalactam, cefoperazone, and ceftazidime is appropriate.

L. Surgical Prophylaxis

Cephalosporins have been widely used in surgical prophylaxis for several reasons. They have a broad range of activity, including penicillin G-susceptible and penicillin G-resistant *Staph. aureus,* as well as *Staph. epidermidis,* including some methicillin-resistant strains. They are also active against most *E. coli* and *Klebsiella.* Side effects are minimal, including allergic reactions. There are no control studies demonstrating that the newer cephalosporins are more effective for prophylaxis. Since the first-generation cephalosporins are more active against *Staph. aureus* and are cheaper, they are generally preferred for surgical prophylaxis. Of the first-generation cephalosporins, cefazolin has the added advantage of a longer half-life. Because of the increased cost, decreased antistaphylococcal activity, and the probability of developing resistance if used extensively, it is not recommended that third-generation cephalosporins be used for prophylaxis (3).

1. Biliary Tract Surgery

Infection rates of 2-20%, including bacteremia and wound infections, have been reported. Infections occur more frequently in patients with infected bile, including patients with positive bile cultures or smears. It is recommended that prophylaxis be used in high-risk groups, including patients who are over 70 years of age, patients with obstructions, jaundiced patients with acute cholecystitis or cholangitis, and patients with common duct stones. Prophylactic cephalosporins administered to this group reduced infections from 24 to 5% (25).

2. Gynecological Surgery

The use of prophylaxis with the first generation of cephalosporins has been effective with vaginal hysterectomy, abdominal hysterectomy, and cesarean sections carried out under emergency conditions (26,27).

3. Orthopedic Surgery

In clean cases prophylaxis is not indicated unless a prosthesis is inserted. Prophylaxis is indicated for prosthetic devices because of the serious consequence of infections. Organisms likely to be involved are *Staph. aureus* and *Staph. epidermidis.* Cefazolin and cefamandole are most frequently used as prophylactic agents. In open fractures the wounds are already contaminated and the use of antimicrobial agents is early treatment of an infected wound rather than prophylaxis. Treatment should be more prolonged than the 24 hr usually administered for required prophylaxis.

4. Intestinal Surgery

Upper gastrointestinal surgery has a low rate of infection and usually does not require prophylaxis in patients with normal gastric acidity and normal gastrointestinal motility. However, upper gastrointestinal surgery does have a high risk of infections, and prophylaxis is justified in patients with abnormal gastric motility or acidity secondary to obstructing duodenal ulcer, gastric ulcer, gastric malignancy, or long-term therapy with cimetidine or other agents that decrease acidity. A first-generation cephalosporin is most frequently used (27). In colon or rectal surgery prophylaxis with oral neomycin and erythromycin plus mechanical preparations is the accepted practice. In comparative studies oral neomycin prophylaxis plus mechanical bowel preparation resulted in fewer postoperative complications than mechanical preparation plus a parenteral first-generation cephalosporin (26–30). In emergency surgery such as intestinal obstruction, one cannot use oral antibiotics plus mechanical preparations; therefore a parenteral agents is indicated. Cefoxitin may be the most effective beta-lactam because of its activity against gram-negative bacteria and *B. fragilis.* If there is bowel perforation at operation, patients should be treated for peritonitis with a full course of antibiotics.

5. Urological Procedures

Antimicrobial prophylaxis is not recommended for patients with negative urine cultures undergoing most urological procedures. Patients with positive urine cultures should be treated appropriately, usually with a cephalosporin preoperatively and paraoperatively to avoid postoperative complications.

6. Miscellaneous Procedures

Prophylaxis may be useful in head and neck surgery with a first-generation cephalosporin. There are no well-controlled studies on the prophylaxis with cephalosporins or other agents in neurosurgery procedures. Prophylactic antibiotics with cephalosporins or cefamandole have been used extensively in open heart procedures. There are good data supporting the use of prophylactic antibiotics with cefazolin for vascular grafts involving the abdominal aorta and lower extremities (27).

IV. ADVERSE REACTIONS

Cephalosporins are usually safe antibiotics and adverse reactions are uncommon and usually reversible, including sensitivity reactions, which can be due to cross-reactivity to penicillins, thrombophlebitis, diarrhea, and transient liver chemistry abnormalities and positive Coombs' tests. Concurrent use of cephalothin with an aminoglycoside has been documented to increase nephrotoxicity of the aminoglycoside (31). Second- and third-generation cephalosporins have not been demonstrated to increase nephrotoxicity of aminoglycoside. Patients treated with cefamandole, moxalactam, and cefoperazone have had serious bleeding due to prothrombin deficiencies or platelet dysfunction most frequently reported in patients receiving moxalactam (5,32–43). Most authorities would recommend that vitamin K therapy be given to patients receiving large doses of these drugs, particularly when therapy must be prolonged or the patient was previously malnourished.

The increased cost of the newer cephalosporins suggests that the earlier compounds be used when organisms are susceptible, reserving the newer compounds for organisms resistant to the early cephalosporins or for meningitis, which can be treated only with the newer cephalosporins. The *Medical Letter* estimates that the cost of 10 days of treatment based on the usual maximum adult dosage to the pharmacist ranges from $385.41 for cefazolin, to $785.76 and $981.74 for cefamandole and cefoxitin, respectively, to $1199.40 to $1464.58 to $1353.60 for the third-generation cephalosporins cefotaxime, moxalactam, and cefoperazone, respectively (3).

V. SUMMARY

The number of new and older cephalosporins now available or likely to be available in the next few years poses problems for the clinician in selecting appropriate antibiotics. It also creates difficulty for the laboratory in deciding how much time and money should be spent in determining antimicrobial susceptibilities for these compounds and other antibiotics such as the newer penicillins, penems, and monobactams.

The newer cephalosporins offer few advantages in the treatment of gram-positive aerobic infections. They clearly allow treatment of meningitis due to gram-negative bacteria, which was difficult to treat previously. One potential advantage of the newer cephalosporins is to allow therapy with single cephalosporins, avoiding both the cost of combined therapy and the nephrotoxicities and ototoxicities of aminoglycosides which are usually included in combined therapy. There are insufficient data to determine whether therapy with a single cephalosporin is as effective as present combined therapy for many infections. For known or suspected *Pseudomonas* infections current recommendations are to include an aminoglycoside with either a new cephalosporin active against *Pseudomonas* or a penicillin such as ticarcillin, azlocillin, or piperacillin. For prophylaxis only first-generation cephalosporins are recommended as drugs of choice.

REFERENCES

1. G. L. Mandell. Cephalosporins, in *Principles and Practice of Infectious Diseases* (G. L. Mandell, R. G. Douglas, and J. E. Bennett, eds.), Wiley, New York, 1979, p. 115.
2. D. J. Winston and L. S. Young. Cephalosporins, in *Antimicrobial Therapy*, 3rd ed. (B. J. Kagan, ed.), Saunders, Philadelphia, 1980.
3. *Medical Letter.* Choice of cephalosporins. *Med. Lett. Drugs Ther., 25*:57 (1983).
4. B. R. Smith and J. L. LeFrock. Cefuroxime: Antimicrobial activity, pharmacology, and clinical efficacy. *Ther. Drug Monitor., 5*:149 (1983).
5. H. C. Neu. The new beta-lactamase-stable cephalosporins. *Ann. Intern. Med., 97*:408 (1983).
6. G. Cuchural, N. Jacobus, S. L. Gorbach, and S. P. Tally. A survey of *Bacteroides* susceptibility in the United States. *J. Antimicrob. Chemother., 8*: S27 (1981).
7. *Medical Letter.* Chemoprophylaxis for recurrent acute otitis media. *Med. Lett. Drugs Ther., 25*:102 (1983).
8. J. D. Nelson, H. Kusmiesz, and S. Shelton. Cefuroxime therapy for pneumonia in infants and children. *Pediatr. Infect. Dis., 1*:159 (1982).
9. J. D. Nelson. Cefuroxime: A cephalosporin with unique applicability to a pediatric practice. *Pediatr. Infect. Dis., 2*:394 (1983).
10. M. E. Levison, C. T. Mangura, B. Lorber, E. Abrutyn, E. L. Pesanti, R. S. Levy, R. R. Macgregor, and A. R. Schwartz. Clindamycin compared with penicillin for the treatment of anaerobic lung abscesses. *Ann. Intern. Med., 98*:466 (1983).
11. F. P. Talley, K. McGowan, J. M. Kellum, S. L. Gorbach, and T. F. O'Donnell. A randomized comparison of cefoxitin with or without amikacin and clindamycin plus amikacin in surgical sepsis. *Ann. Surg., 193*:318 (1981).
12. H. H. Stone, P. R. Strom, T. C. Fabian, and W. E. Dunlop. Third-generation

cephalosporins for polymicrobial surgical sepsis. *Arch. Surg., 118*:193 (1983).

13. S. W. Berg, M. E. Kilpatrick, W. O. Harrison, and J. A. McCutchan. Cefoxitin as a single-dose treatment for urethritis caused by a penicillinase-producing *Neisseria gonorrhoeae. N. Engl. J. Med., 301*:509 (1979).
14. H. H. Handsfield. Treatment of uncomplicated gonorrhea with cefotaxime. *Rev. Infect. Dis., 4*:S448 (1982).
15. R. Norrby. Cefuroxime versus ampicillin and chloramphenicol for the treatment of bacterial meningitis. *Lancet, 1*:795 (1982).
16. D. A. Kafetzis, D. C. Brater, and A. N. Kapiki. Treatment of severe neonatal infections with cefotaxime: Efficacy and pharmacokinetics. *J. Pediatr., 100*:443 (1982).
17. D. T. Mullaney and J. F. John. Cefotaxime therapy of serious bacterial infections in adults. *Antimicrob. Agents Chemother., 21*:421 (1982).
18. D. A. Kafetzix, J. Mathioudakis, and A. N. Kapiki. Cefotaxime, a new antibacterial agent for treating bacterial meningitis in pediatrics. *Drug Ther., S9*: 14 (1981).
19. D. T. Mullaney and J. F. John. Cefotaxime therapy. *Arch. Intern. Med., 143*:1705 (1983).
20. J. J. Rahal and M. S. Simberkoff. Host defense and antimicrobial therapy in adult gram-negative bacillary meningitis. *Ann. Intern. Med., 96*:468 (1982).
21. S. H. Landesman, M. L. Corrado, P. M. Shah, M. Armengaud, M. Barza, and C. E. Cherubin. Past and current roles for cephalosporin antibiotics in treatment of meningitis. Emphasis on use of gram-negative bacillary meningitis. *Am. J. Med., 71*:693 (1981).
22. M. L. Corrado, M. E. Gombert, and C. E. Cherubin. Designing appropriate therapy in the treatment of gram-negative bacillary meningitis. *J. Am. Med. Assoc., 248* (1982).
23. J. J. Rahal. Moxalactam therapy for gram-negative bacillary meningitis. *Rev. Infect. Dis., 4*:5606 (1982).
24. D. A. Olson, P. D. Hoeprich, S. M. Nolan, and E. Goldstein. Successful treatment of gram-negative bacillary meningitis with moxalactam. *Ann. Intern. Med., 95*:302 (1981).
25. D. W. Elliott. Biliary tract surgery. *South. Med. J., 70*:31 (1977).
26. *Medical Letter.* Antimicrobial prophylaxis for surgery. *Med. Lett. Drugs Ther., 21*:73 (1979).
27. J. V. Hirchman and T. S. Inui. Antimicrobial prophylaxis: A critque of recent trials. *Rev. Infect. Dis., 2*:1 (1980).
28. J. E. Clarke, R. E. Condon, J. G. Bartlett, S. L. Gorbach, R. L. Nichols, and S. Ochi. Preoperative oral antibiotics reduce septic complications of colon operations. *Ann. Surg., 186*:251 (1977).
29. D. M. Matheson, R. D. Meyer, J. M. Thompson, and S. M. Finegold. Clinical evaluation of moxalactam. *Br. J. Surg., 65*:597 (1978).
30. R. L. Nichols. Use of prophylactic antibiotics in surgical practice. *Am. J. Med., 70*:686 (1981).

31. J. C. Wade, B. G. Petty, G. Conrad, C. R. Smith, J. J. Lipsky, J. Ellner, and P. S. Lietman. Cephalothin plus an aminoglycoside is more nephrotoxic than methicillin plus an aminoglycoside. *Lancet, 2*:604 (1978).
32. R. L. Pakter, T. R. Russell, C. H. Mielke, and D. West. Coagulopathy with the use of moxalactam. *J. Am. Med. Assoc., 248*:1100 (1982).
33. M. R. Weitekamp and R. C. Aber. Prolonged bleeding times and bleeding diathesis associated with moxalactam administration. *J. Am. Med. Assoc., 249*:69 (1983).
34. N. U. Bang, S. S. Tessler, S. S. Heidenreich, R. O. Marks, and L. E. Mattler. Effects of moxalactam on blood coagulation and platelet formation. *Rev. Infect. Dis., 4*:S546 (1982).
35. Editorial. Bleeding in patients with infections: Are antibiotics helping or hurting? *Arch. Intern. Med., 142*:1440 (1982).
36. C. A. Hooper, B. B. Haney, and H. H. Stone. Gastrointestinal bleeding due to vitamin K deficiency in patients on parenteral cefamandole. *Lancet, 1*: 39 (1980).
37. J. Reddy and R. R. Bailey. Vitamin K deficiency developing in patients with renal failure treated with cephalosporin antibiotics. *N. Z. Med. J., 92*:378 (1980).
38. K. Bruch. Hypoprothrombinaemia and cephalosporins. *Lancet, 1*:535 (1983).
39. Editorial. Antimicrobials and haemostasis. *Lancet, 1*:510 (1983).
40. R. Quintiliani. Bleeding disorders associated with newer cephalosporins. *Clin. Pharm., 2*:360 (1983).
41. A. Panwalker and J. Rosenfeld. Hemorrhage, diarrhea, and superinfection associated with the use of moxalactam. *J. Infect. Dis., 147*:171 (1983).
42. S. J. Childs. Bleeding problems. *Arch. Intern. Med., 143*:183 (1983).
43. G. E. Mathisen, R. D. Meyer, J. M. Thompson, and S. M. Finegold. Clinical evaluation of moxalactam. *Antimicrob. Agents Chemother., 21*:780 (1982).

12

Moxalactam (Latamoxef)

BILL G. JACKSON and ROBERT B. KAMMER
Eli Lilly and Company, Indianapolis, Indiana

MITSURU YOSHIOKA and HIDEO YAMADA
Shionogi and Company, Osaka, Japan

I. INTRODUCTION

Moxalactam (latamoxef)* is the first and only clinically available beta-lactam antibiotic whose nucleus is not naturally occurring. It is characterized by an oxygen atom substituted for the sulfur atom in the cephalosporin (cephamycin) nucleus, as shown in Figure 1.

This oxygen substitution was responsible for a several-fold increase in the intrinsic antibacterial activity as compared with that of its 1-thia congener (1), but it introduces the difficult problem of producing the novel ring system, the 1-oxacephem nucleus, on an industrial scale. A 7α-methoxy group and an α-carboxy group at the 7β-amide side chain are common in cephamycins (see Chap. 13) and carbenicillin (also ticarcillin; see Chap. 6), respectively. These two groups complementarily provide enhanced resistance to both beta-lactamases, that is, penicillinase and cephalosporinase (2). A 3-(1-methyl-1H-tetrazol-5-yl)thiomethyl group (together with the α-carboxy group) is important in enhancing gram-negative activity and has been selected as a preferable 3-substituent in many second- and third-generation antibiotics (see Chaps. 9 and 11). A para-hydroxy group on the benzene ring (as in amoxicillin) is effective in increasing the blood level and prolonging the half-life.

Like carbenicillin, moxalactam exists as two interconvertible epimers. The 7β-para-hydroxyphenylmalonamido grouping is either R or S. The R form is

---

*Moxalactam is the generic name approved in the United States (U.S. Adopted Name) and latamoxef is the internationally approved one (International Nonproprietary Name). This antibiotic has been referred to as 6059-S, LY-127935, and lamoxactam in earlier papers.

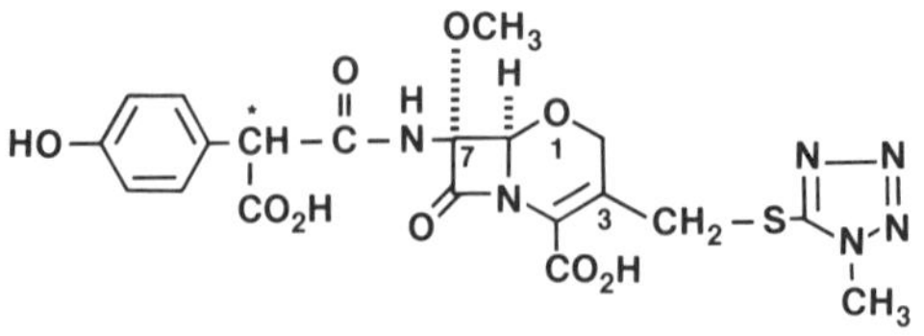

Figure 1 Structure of moxalactam showing the numbering for key atoms.

about twice as active as the S form against most bacteria in vitro. Production of a preparation containing only the more active R form was found impractical owing to rapid interconversion between the two epimers in acid solutions (3) and insufficient stability of a crystalline R-epimer sodium salt prepared by a tedious process (4).

Since being marketed in 1981–1982, moxalactam has been employed widely in the world as a representative, life-saving, third-generation cephalosporin-like antibiotic. In the first section of this chapter chemical syntheses of this antibiotic are reviewed, with an emphasis on industrial production of its unnatural nucleus. The second section summarizes the clinical applications of moxalactam. The last section describes the pharmacokinetic properties of moxalactam, including time courses of the R and S epimers in plasma after administration of this drug.

II. CHEMICAL SYNTHESES OF MOXALACTAM

Potential starting materials for producing the moxalactam (1-oxacephem) nucleus in the optically active form are naturally occurring, inexpensive penicillins and cephalosporins which share such essential parts as the beta-lactam (azetidinone) ring as well as the amino substituent and the carboxymethyl moiety on the ring. Synthetic routes to 1-oxacephems from these natural sources have been studied extensively and comprehensive reviews published (5,6). The key is stereocontrolled introduction of an oxygen function to become the future 1-position. Cephalosporins, though more similar to the 1-oxacephem nucleus than penicillins, have not been found to be as good as penicillins for starting materials.

This section treats only the chemical syntheses of moxalactam from penicillins which were actually employed at Shionogi during development of this antibiotic: First, the key reactions in earlier synthetic routes are described and then the current industrial route is presented, followed by probable future improve-

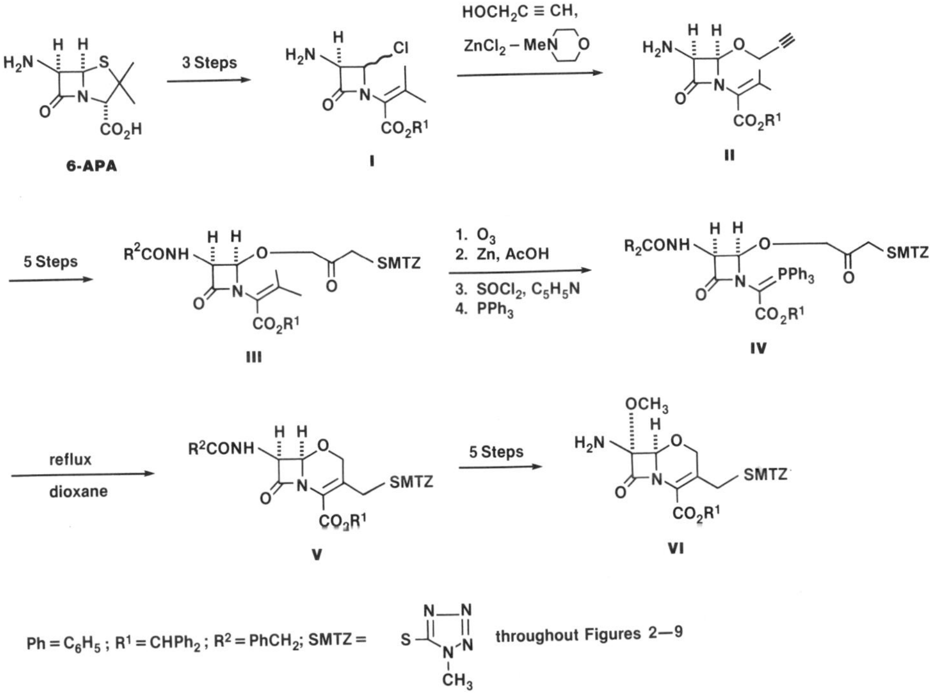

Figure 2 First route to the 1-oxacephem nucleus.

ments in the route. Readers are advised to refer to earlier reviews (7,8) and the literature cited therein for more details.

A. Earlier Synthetic Routes

In the first route shown in Figure 2 (9,10), 4-chloro-azetidinone I, easily prepared from 6-aminopenicillanic acid (6-APA), is converted on zinc chloride-catalyzed substitution with 2-propyn-1-ol into cis-ether II with an overall yield of about 5% after chromatographic separation from the corresponding trans epimer. Ketone III, derived by conventional procedures in 60% overall yield, is smoothly converted into phosphorane IV, whose Wittig condensation gives a 1-oxacephem derivative V in 48% overall yield. The 7β-amino-7α-methoxy nucleus VI is prepared in 74% yield by known methods. Transformation of nucleus VI to moxalactam is described later.

The multistep, low-yield synthesis of the nucleus VI by the above route is moderately improved in the second route (Fig. 3) (11), where only the desired

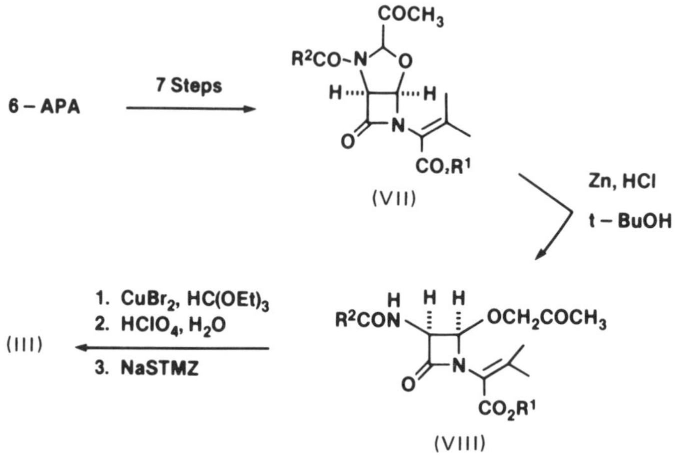

Figure 3 Second route to the 1-oxacephem nucleus.

cis derivative VIII is obtained in 40–50% yield by novel reduction cleavage of oxazolidino compound VII, prepared from 6-APA in about 30% overall yield. Regioselective bromination of methyl ketone VIII followed by facile nucleophilic substitution gives intermediate III in 53% yield.

Though vital for preparing various 1-oxacephem compounds for primary screening and further biological evaluation, these first and second routes involving several chromatographic separation steps were not suitable for the production of moxalactam on a large scale. A kilogram-scale production was realized first by the third route (Fig. 4), using α-oxazolino derivative IX for stereocontrolled β-face introduction of an oxygen function (12). Intermediate IX can be produced from penicillin G in 36% overall yield on a large scale. Acid-catalyzed cleavage of the α-oxazoline ring in IX with allyl alcohol occurs predominantly from the less-hindered β-face, giving 4β-allyloxyazetidinone X in a greater than 80% yield. The 4β-allyloxy group now guides the α-side introduction of the methoxy group at the 3-position in X to give a 3β-amido-3α-methoxy compound XI in 80% yield. Derivative XII is obtained in 34% overall yield by conventional procedures, and its side-chain cleavage affords the desired nucleus VI in 54% yield. In this cleavage an undesired epimer (XIII) is formed in a negligible amount, in contrast to predominant formation of the corresponding 7α-amino-7β-methoxy epimer in the cleavage of conventional cephamycin (1-thia) derivatives. The favorable thermodynamic stability of the 7β-amino-7α-methoxy isomer VI under cleavage conditions is essential to the success of this as well as the fourth route described later.

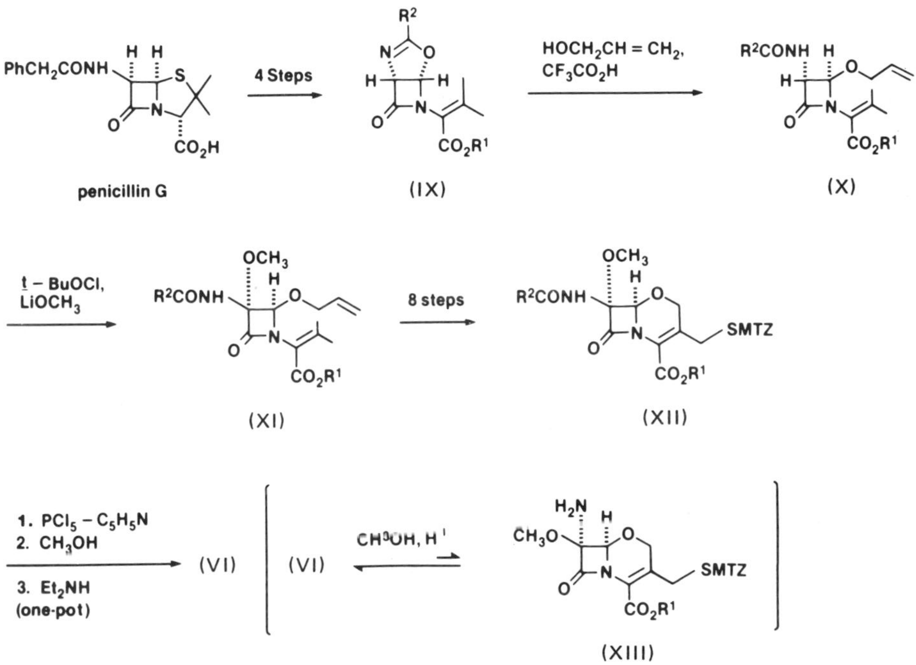

Figure 4 Third route to the 1-oxacephem nucleus.

Although the third route (4.2% overall yield in 15 steps) is much superior to the first or second route (1.1 or 2.8% overall yield in 19 or 21 steps), chromatographic separations in two or three steps hindered further scale-up of this route and encouraged exploration of novel sophisticated synthetic methodologies.

B. Current Industrial Route (Fourth Route)

Current production of moxalactam is based on the fourth route (13), which retains all the carbon atoms in the starting penicillin nucleus as shown in Figure 5. Three novel, key reactions have been explored in this route. The first key reaction is conversion of epipenicillin sulfoxide XIV, produced easily by known procedures in 80% overall yield from 6-APA, into α-oxazolinoazetidinone XV (by treatment with triphenylphosphine). The bicyclic beta-lactam XV, obtained in 80% yield, possesses an unconjugated pentenoate grouping at the beta-lactam nitrogen. The second key reaction, exclusive allylic chlorination, was unexpectedly achieved with chlorine as the chlorinating agent to give allylic chloride XVI

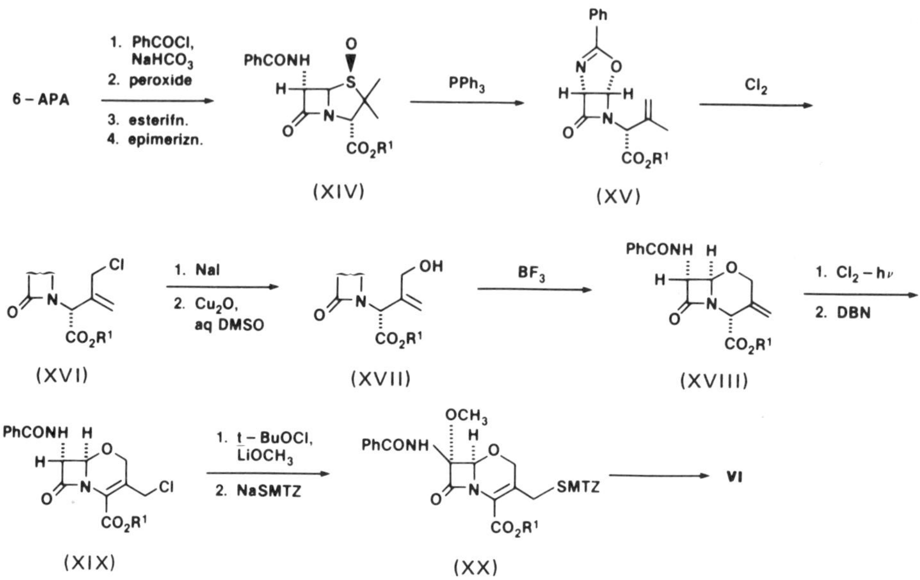

DMSO = $(CH_3)_2SO$; DBN = 1, 5 – diazabicyclo [3.4.0] nonene – 5

Figure 5 Fourth route to the 1-oxacephem nucleus.

in 75% yield with little formation of a chlorine addition product. Conversion of the chloro into the hydroxy group without double-bond migration, the third key reaction, is effected by transformation to a more reactive iodide followed by mild hydrolysis with cuprous oxide in aqueous dimethyl sulfoxide, giving allylic alcohol XVII in 90% yield. Intramolecular etherification of XVII proceeds exclusively from the less-hindered β-side to afford exomethylene derivative XVIII in 90% yield. The desired 7α-methoxy compound XX is obtained in 76% overall yield via a 3-chloromethyl derivative XIX using procedures well known in cephalosporin chemistry. The use of phenyl rather than benzyl for the amide side chain is crucial not only for compatibility in the two chlorination steps but also for improving the yield during side-chain cleavage. Amide XX is cleaved by the one-pot procedure shown in Figure 4 to give nucleus VI in 90% yield (compared with the 54% yield from XII in the third route). In this fourth route the overall yield of 1-oxacephem nucleus VI from 6-APA is improved to 26% and the number of steps reduced to 13.

Moxalactam can be produced from nucleus VI in high yield by acylation with a protected acid chloride XXI to afford diester XXII followed by a new deprotection procedure (14) that employs aluminum chloride as shown in Figure 6.

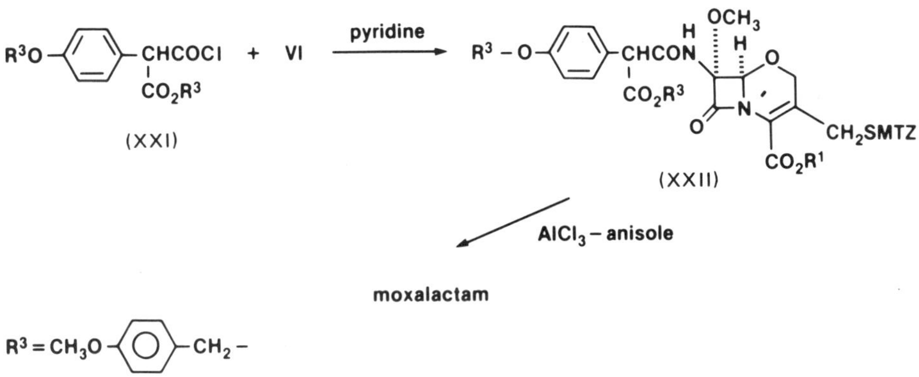

Figure 6 Synthesis of moxalactam from the 1-oxacephem nucleus.

With some modifications and extensive process improvements, industrial production of moxalactam has been carried out without the use of tedious chromatographic separation.

C. Probable Future Improvements

Since publication of the above industrial route, only a few papers relating to moxalactam synthesis have appeared. Apparently less practical is preparation of allylic alcohol XVII from the relatively inaccessible 7-epicepham-1-oxide XXIII (15) (Fig. 7).

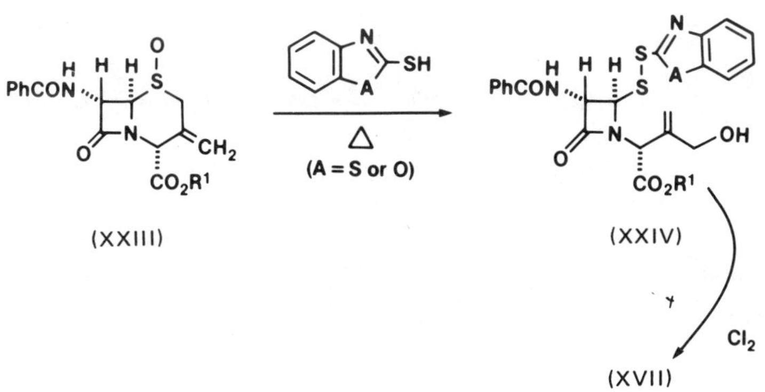

Figure 7 Synthesis of 1-oxacephem from 7-epiexomethylene cepham sulfoxide.

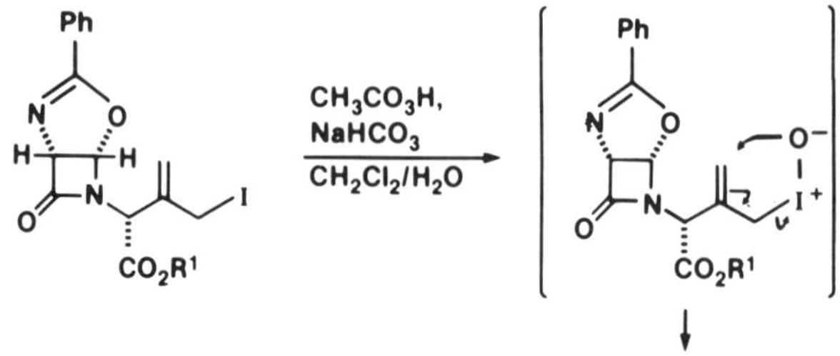

(XVI) (XVII)

Figure 8 Alternate synthesis of allylic alcohol precursor to 1-oxacephem nucleus.

Oxidative hydrolysis of allylic iodide XVI' (16) involving a new [2,3]-sigmatropic rearrangement (Fig. 8) will be industrially applicable, because the reagents are inexpensive and the yield of alcohol XVII is high (93%).

An alternative route to moxalactam from the exomethylene intermediate XVIII (Fig. 9) is characterized by performing necessary chemical manipulations

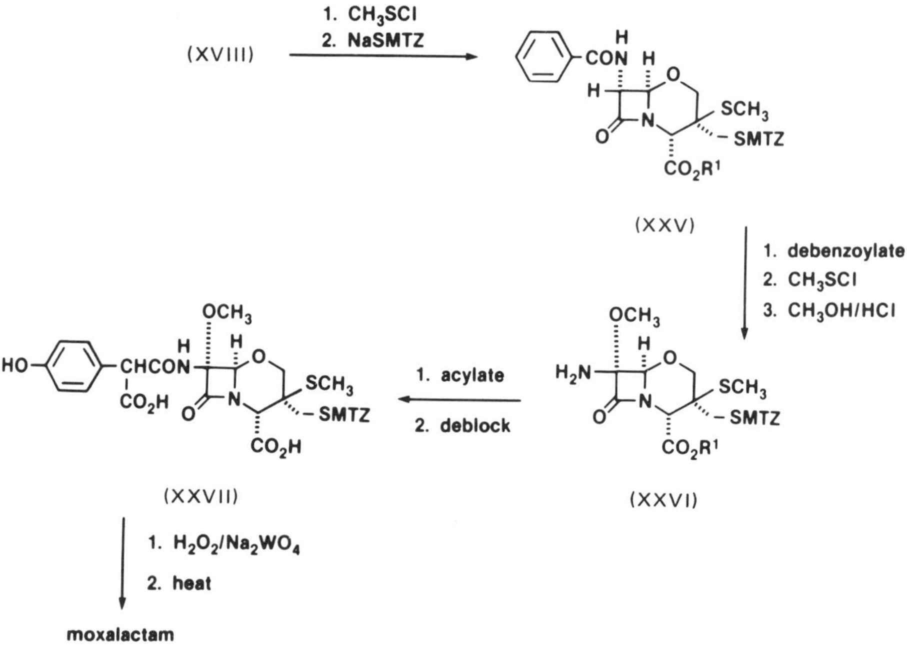

Figure 9 Alternate synthesis of moxalactam from exomethylene 1-oxacepham.

in high yield on novel 3β-methylthio-1-oxacepham derivatives XXV–XXVII, which, without the susceptible 3,4-double bond, are more compatible to otherwise detrimental reagents (8,17). Industrial application of this new route would be highly promising if further improvements could lead to process simplification and a better overall yield of moxalactam.

III. CLINICAL EFFICACY AND SAFETY OF MOXALACTAM

A. Evaluation Criteria

Moxalactam was evaluated for effectiveness and safety in the treatment of bacterial infections of the lower respiratory and urinary tracts, abdomen, pelvis, skin and skin structures, bones and joints, and central nervous system.

The effectiveness of moxalactam therapy was assessed utilizing strict clinical and bacteriological criteria. Clinical diagnosis was established by a medical history and physical examination. Following antibiotic therapy, a repeat clinical evaluation as well as a bacteriological and radiological assessment was required. In all cases evaluable for efficacy, appropriate bacterial pathogens were isolated from clinical specimens and tested for susceptibility to moxalactam. Follow-up bacteriological examination was performed in all patients in whom clinical specimens were available at the end of antimicrobial therapy. Appropriate susceptibility testing was performed on all of these isolates.

Moxalactam therapy was evaluated on the basis of clinical and bacteriological responses unless otherwise specified. Satisfactory bacteriological response was defined as eradication of causative pathogen or reduction of causative pathogen to insignificant numbers. Symptomatic clinical responses were satisfactory if the patient's signs and symptoms due to the primary infection disappeared or significantly improved during drug therapy. A satisfactory response with recurrence was defined similarly, with signs and symptoms recurring after the completion of antimicrobial therapy. No improvement in the patient's signs and symptoms was defined as an unsatisfactory clinical response. Bacteriological responses were based solely on the eradication or significant reduction of causative pathogens during moxalactam therapy.

Safety evaluation was conducted in all patients. The following tests were required before and after treatment with moxalactam: hemoglobin or hematocrit, white blood cell count and differential, platelet count, Coombs' test, blood urea nitrogen, urinalysis, serum creatinine, serum bilirubin, serum glutamic oxaloacetic transaminase (SGOT) or serum glutamic pyruvic transaminase (SGPT), and alkaline phosphatase.

Table 1 Overall Efficacy (Bacteriological Response) of Moxalactam Therapy for Bacterial Infections in 2234 Patients

Type of infection	Usual dosage[a]	Duration of treatment	Number of satisfactory responses per number of patients treated (%)[b]
Urinary tract	250–500 mg every 8 or 12 hr	10–14 days	455/572 (80)
Intra-abdominal	1–2 g every 8 hr	5–14 days	125/137 (91)
Obstetric and gynecological	1–2 g every 8 hr	5–14 days	227/250 (91)
Lower respiratory tract	1–2 g every 8 hr	5–14 days	382/417 (92)
Skin and skin structure	0.5–2 g every 8 or 12 hr	5–10 days	428/464 (92)
Bone and joint	1–2 g every 8 hr	4–6 weeks	110/122 (90)
Bacteremia	1–2 g every 8 hr	2–4 weeks	227/241 (94)
Central nervous system	4 g every 8 hr	2–3 weeks	29/31 (94)
Total			1983/2234 (89)

[a]Dosage for pediatric patients was 75–200 mg/kg per day, given every 8 or 12 hr. In severe infections or in those due to less susceptible organisms, doses of up to 12 g per day in adults and 300 mg/kg per day in children were administered.
[b]Satisfactory bacteriological response is defined as eradication of the causative pathogen or reduction to insignificant numbers.

B. Efficacy Results

1. Overall Efficacy

Overall efficacy based on bacteriological response to moxalactam for 2234 patients is summarized in Table 1. The usual dosage, duration of antibiotic therapy, and outcome are listed separately in this table. The data cited in this and all subsequent tables comes from work at the Lilly Laboratory for Clinical Research and is on file with Eli Lilly and Company (Indianapolis, Indiana).

A listing of causative pathogens isolated during the clinical trials of moxalactam is presented in Table 2. Rate of clinical cure ranged from 69% for infections caused by *Pseudomonas aeruginosa* to 92% for infections caused by species of *Bacteroides, Peptococcus, Peptostreptococcus,* and *Proteus.*

Table 2 Clinical Response to Moxalactam Therapy by Causative Pathogens[a]

Organism (number isolated)	Number of clinical cures (%)
Escherichia coli (279)	255 (91)
Klebsiella species (66)	60 (91)
Proteus species (48)	44 (92)
Enterobacter species (36)	32 (89)
Serratia species (48)	42 (88)
Pseudomonas aeruginosa (134)	93 (69)
Staphylococcus aureus (72)	65 (90)
Bacteroides fragilis (57)	51 (89)
Bacteroides species (118)	109 (92)
Peptococcus and *Peptostreptococcus* species (159)	146 (92)

[a]Satisfactory clinical response was defined as disappearance or decrease of the patient's signs and symptoms during therapy.

2. Urinary Tract Infections

Moxalactam was utilized to treat urinary tract infections in 572 patients, and satisfactory results were obtained in 455 cases (80%). A total of 387 (68%) patients had some anatomical abnormalities of the urinary tract demonstrated. Most patients received 500 mg to 1 g of antibiotic per day. Of these 572 patients, 185 were defined as pyelonephritis. A total of 153 (83%) had a satisfactory response, 23 had a satisfactory response with a subsequent recurrence, and 9 failed therapy. The most frequent bacteria isolated from these cases were *Escherichia coli* and *Proteus* and *Klebsiella* species. Twenty patients had pyelonephritis due to *P. aeruginosa.* Eleven of these patients failed therapy, probably because these infections are both complicated and the dosage of moxalactam was too low to treat organisms somewhat less susceptible to the drug than the *Enterobacteriaceae.*

3. Intra-Abdominal Infections

Clinical response to moxalactam by diagnosis and patient type with intra-abdominal infections is presented in Table 3. The most frequent diagnosis was

Table 3 Clinical Response, by Diagnosis, of Patients with Intra-Abdominal Infections to Moxalactam Therapy

Diagnosis	Number of satisfactory responses per number of patients treated (%)[a]
Peritonitis	80/87 (92)
Intra-abdominal abscess	23/25 (92)
Cholecystitis/cholangitis	11/12 (92)
Ruptured appendix	7/7 (100)
Miscellaneous	4/6 (67)
Total	125/137 (91)

[a]Satisfactory clinical response was defined as disappearance or decrease of patient's signs and symptoms of infection during therapy.

peritonitis followed by intra-abdominal abscess. In all patients treated appropriate surgical drainage and/or other procedures accompanied antibiotic therapy. Pathogens isolated from this group of patients with intra-abdominal infections are listed in Table 4. Bacteriological failures occurred in three patients with

Table 4 Rate of Failure of Moxalactam Treatment, by Pathogen, in 137 Cases of Intra-Abdominal Infection

Organism (number isolated)	Number of therapeutic failures (%)[a]
Escherichia coli (70)	5 (7)
Peptococcus and *Peptostreptococcus* species (33)	1 (3)
Bacteroides fragilis (31)	2 (6)
Other *Bacteroides* species (22)	1 (5)
Pseudomonas species (26)	3 (2)
Klebsiella species (23)	3 (13)
Enterobacter species (13)	2 (15)
Proteus species (12)	1 (8)

[a]There were 12 cases of therapeutic failure. Therapeutic failure was defined as an unsatisfactory symptomatic or bacteriological response.

Table 5 Response, by Diagnosis, of Patients with Obstetric and Gynecological Infections to Moxalactam Therapy

Diagnosis	Number of satisfactory responses per number of patients treated (%)[a]
Endometritis	127/142 (89)
Pelvic inflammatory disease	42/43 (98)
Pelvic cellulitis	40/43 (93)
Salpingitis/oophoritis	12/15 (80)
Pelvic abscess	6/7 (86)
Total	227/250 (91)

[a]Satisfactory response was defined as the disappearance or reduction of patient's signs and symptoms of infection during therapy.

Psedomonas and *Klebsiella* infections and in two patients infected with *Enterobacter* species. Excellent clinical results were obtained in patients with *E. coli* infections and those due to *Bacteroides fragilis.* Many patients in this group were infected with multiple organisms, both aerobes and anaerobes.

4. Obstetric and Gynecological Infections

Moxalactam was used in conjunction with appropriate surgical therapy to treat obstetric and gynecological infections in 250 women. Postpartum or postcesarean endometritis was the most frequent diagnosis, followed by pelvic inflammatory disease and pelvic cellulitis. The results of these treatments are presented in Table 5. Overall clinical response in these women was 91%, ranging from 80% for salpingitis to 98% for pelvic inflammatory disease. Clinically significant microorganisms isolated from this group of 250 patients are listed in Table 6. Therapeutic failures associated with these organisms are also presented. Many patients were infected with multiple organisms in this group as well. Species of *Clostridium* were associated with the highest rate of therapeutic failure, while strains of *Neisseria gonorrhoeae* were eradicated in 95% of treated patients. *Bacteroides* species accounted for 120 clinical isolates in these patients.

5. Lower Respiratory Tract Infections

Moxalactam was studied in 417 patients with infections of the lower respiratory tract. Most were male (75%), over 45 years of age, and half were in serious or critical condition on admission to the hospital. Most patients received 3-6 g of moxalactam daily for the treatment of their infections. A total of 289 patients had pneumonia. Bronchopneumonia was the diagnosis in 92, empyema in

Table 6 Rate of Failure of Moxalactam Treatment of Obstetric and Gynecological Infections Due to Frequently Isolated Organisms

Organism (number isolated)	Number of therapeutic failures (%)[a]
Bacteroides fragilis (23)	4 (17)
Other *Bacteroides* species (97)	8 (8)
Peptostreptococcus species (74)	10 (14)
Peptococcus species (51)	2 (4)
Clostridium species (21)	8 (38)
Fusobacterium species (25)	4 (16)
Escherichia coli (45)	4 (9)
Neisseria gonorrhoeae (41)	2 (5)
Streptococcus species, group B (24)	2 (8)

[a]A total of 7 failures occurred in 104 cases caused by single pathogens, and 15 failures occurred in 146 cases due to multiple pathogens. Therapeutic failure was defined as the failure of the patient's signs and symptoms to disappear or decrease during therapy.

24, and lung abscess in 12. Microorganisms isolated from patients with lower respiratory tract infections are listed in Table 7. Most frequently isolated microorganisms were *Streptococcus pneumoniae* (126 strains), *Hemophilus influenzae* (49 strains), and *Pseudomonas* species (46 strains). A total of 124 cases of respiratory infections due to *Strep. pneumoniae* responded to moxalactam therapy. The results with *Pseudomonas* species were significantly less favorable, with 16 of 46 patients failing to respond satisfactorily.

6. Skin and Skin Structure Infections

Therapy could be evaluated in 464 cases of skin and skin structure infections treated with moxalactam. Most of these were cellulitis (157 cases), subcutaneous abscesses (81 cases), and postoperative wound infections (83 cases). A total of 92% of these patients responded satisfactorily to moxalactam therapy and appropriate adjunctive surgical procedures designed to drain purulent material when necessary. As anticipated, virtually all of these infections were due to *Staphylococcus aureus*, streptococci, and *P. aeruginosa.*

Table 7 Bacteriological Response of Lower Respiratory Tract Infections Due to Various Organisms to Moxalactam Therapy

Organism (number isolated)	Number of bacteriological failures (%)[a]
Streptococcus pneumoniae (126)	2 (1.5)
Hemophilus influenzae (49)	3 (6)
Pseudomonas species (46)	16 (35)
Klebsiella species (22)	1 (5)
Serratia species (13)	4 (31)
Escherichia coli (13)	2 (15)
Staphylococcus aureus (13)	4 (31)

[a]Bacteriological failure was defined as the failure to eradicate the causative pathogen or reduce the number of colony-forming units to an insignificant value.

7. Bone and Joint Infections

Moxalactam was evaluated in the treatment of bone and joint infections in 122 patients. The clinical diagnosis was osteomyelitis in 92 patients, 82 of which responded satisfactorily to moxalactam therapy. There were 19 cases of infective arthritis treated. Of these, 16 responded favorably to antibiotic therapy. *Staphylococcus aureus* was the most frequently encountered pathogen (38 cases), of which 35 cases responded to moxalactam therapy. *Pseudomonas aeruginosa* was isolated in 24 cases, 17 of which responded to therapy. The remainder of cases was caused by gram-negative enteric bacilli.

8. Bacteremia and Endocarditis

Therapy could be evaluated in 232 episodes of bacteremia and 9 cases of bacterial endocarditis treated with moxalactam. Concomitant infections resulting in bacteremia were identifiable in 138 of these cases. Of these, 57 originated in the urinary tract, 31 in the lower respiratory tract, 23 from intra-abdominal sites, 22 from skin and skin structures, and 5 from bone and joint infections. A total of 227 patients responded satisfactorily to treatment with moxalactam. Gram-positive clinical pathogens isolated from multiple blood cultures in these patients are listed in Table 8. *Staphylococcus aureus, Strep. pneumoniae,* and other *Streptococcus* species were most frequently isolated. All patients with *Staph. aureus* bacteremia responded to moxalactam therapy.

Table 8 Bacteriological Response to Moxalactam Therapy for Gram-Positive and Gram-Negative Blood Culture Isolates from Patients with Bacteremia

Organism (number isolated)	Number of bacteriological failures[a]
Gram-positive bacteria	
Staphylococcus aureus (21)	0
Staphylococcus epidermidis (5)	1
Streptococcus species (13)	2
Streptococcus pneumoniae (18)	0
Peptococcus species (1)	0
Peptostreptococcus species (1)	0
Clostridium perfringens (1)	0
Gram-negative bacteria	
Escherichia coli (76)	1
Pseudomonas aeruginosa (25)	4
Serratia marcescens (21)	2
Klebsiella species (14)	0
Proteus species (10)	0
Enterobacter species (8)	1
Hemophilus influenzae (6)	0
Bacteroides fragilis (5)	0
Miscellaneous (17)	3

[a]Bacteriological failure was defined as failure to eradicate the causative pathogen.

Gram-negative bacteria causing bacteremia in moxalactam-treated patients are also listed in Table 8. *Escherichia coli, P. aeruginosa,* and *Serratia marcescens* were the most frequently isolated gram-negative pathogens. All but one *E. coli* strain were eradicated from the blood, as were 21 of 25 infections due to *P.aeruginosa.* Of 21 patients bacteremic with *S. marcescens*, 2 failed therapy. There were five bacteremias due to *B. fragilis,* all of which responded to therapy.

Moxalactam failed to eradicate bacteria from the blood of three patients with endocarditis. One was infected with a strain of *P. aeruginosa,* the second with a *Streptococcus* group H (minimal inhibitory concentration, 3.12 μg/ml), and the third with a strain of *Alcaligenes.*

9. Central Nervous System Infections

Moxalactam was used as a single agent in the treatment of 260 cases of gram-negative meningitis; 241 (93%) patients had a satisfactory response to antibiotic therapy. Patients ranged in age from neonates to the elderly. The largest single group of cases was due to *H. influenzae,* with 146 of 148 children responding to therapy. Of 105 patients treated for meningitis due to Enterobacteriaceae (*E. coli, Klebsiella pneumoniae, S. marcescens, Enterobacter* species, and *Citrobacter* species), 87% had a satisfactory response to therapy with moxalactam. Meningitis due to *P. aeruginosa* did not respond to moxalactam therapy. Three of four cases had an unsatisfactory outcome.

C. Adverse Reactions Associated with the Administration of Moxalactam

Clinical investigators were asked to assess adverse reactions occurring during these clinical evaluations. Events were classified as either (a) related to antimicrobial therapy, (b) unrelated to antimicrobial therapy, or (c) impossible to assess or of unknown relationship. Of the 3558 patients treated with moxalactam, 223 had adverse reactions considered to be related to antibiotic therapy. An additional 311 patients had reactions that were classified as of unknown relationship to therapy.

The most frequently reported adverse effects were hematopoietic and these occurred in 165 patients (4.6%). Eosinophilia was reported most frequently, followed by reversible leukopenia and thrombocytopenia. In this group of clinical cases hypoprothrombinemia was reported in 25 patients. Prothrombin determinations were not a routine part of the moxalactam safety battery. It is therefore impossible to adequately assess the frequency of hypoprothrombinemia in these studies. Five patients had a prolongation of bleeding time during moxalactam therapy. Clinical bleeding occurred in approximately 2.3% of clinical trial patients treated with this drug.

Drug-induced hypoprothrombinemia is reversed by administration of vitamin K. However, platelet dysfunction or immune-mediated thrombocytopenia are not reversible by vitamin K and constitute grounds for discontinuing moxalactam therapy. Hepatic and renal dysfunction and the use of other drugs that affect hemostasis may increase the risk of bleeding during moxalactam therapy.

After hematopoietic events, the next most frequently reported adverse effects were hypersensitivity reactions, which occurred in 104 patients. Local pain was observed in 102 patients and gastrointestinal adverse effects were encountered in 74. Diarrhea was the most frequently encountered gastrointestinal side effect with this drug. Sixty-four patients were noted to have some abnormality of renal function associated with drug therapy (however, only two were considered to be related to moxalactam therapy). Four patients experienced disulfuram-like reactions following the ingestion of alcohol and/or alcohol-containing medications during moxalactam therapy. *Clostridium difficile* and its toxin were demonstrated in one patient experiencing colitis while receiving moxalactam.

D. Cross-Allergenicity with Penicillins and Cephalosporins

Moxalactam was administered to 344 patients who had historical allergy to penicillin or cephalosporins. Of these patients, 4.1% experienced hypersensitivity reactions to moxalactam. These included nine incidences of skin rash, three of drug fever, one positive Coombs' test, and one case of anaphylaxis.

IV. PHARMACOKINETICS OF MOXALACTAM

Moxalactam is not absorbed orally and should be given parenterally. Pharmacokinetic studies of moxalactam have been done in healthy subjects and adult or pediatric patients after intramuscular injection and intravenous bolus or slow infusion. Concentrations of moxalactam in plasma, serum, urine, and other biological specimens have been determined by either microbiological assay (18) or high-performance liquid chromatography (HPLC) (19-23). No active metabolite has been detected by thin-layer chromatographic bioautography of plasma (24), urine (24), and feces (25) collected from healthy volunteers given moxalactam.

Plasma or serum concentrations are usually analyzed by the one-compartment open model with a first-order absorption process for an intramuscular injection, and by the two-compartment open model for an intravenous bolus or slow infusion (26).

A. Blood Concentration and Urinary Excretion

1. Healthy Volunteers

Intramuscular Injection. An intramuscular dose of moxalactam is rapidly absorbed (24,25). Mean peak concentrations in plasma or serum observed 0.5–1.0 hr (rarely 2 hr) after single intramuscular injections of 0.25, 0.5, and 1.0 g of moxalactam were 10–13.3 (24,25,27), 15–23.6 (24,25,28,29), and 27–61.4 μg/ml (25,30–35), respectively. Examples are shown in Figure 10 (24). Pharmacokinetic properties are summarized in Table 9. Average values of elimination half-life and urinary recovery after intramuscular injection of moxalactam were 2.3 hr and 71%, respectively.

Results from multiple injection studies (25,28) indicate that little or no accumulation is observed after intramuscular administration of 0.25, 0.5, and 1.0 g of moxalactam every 8 or 12 hr.

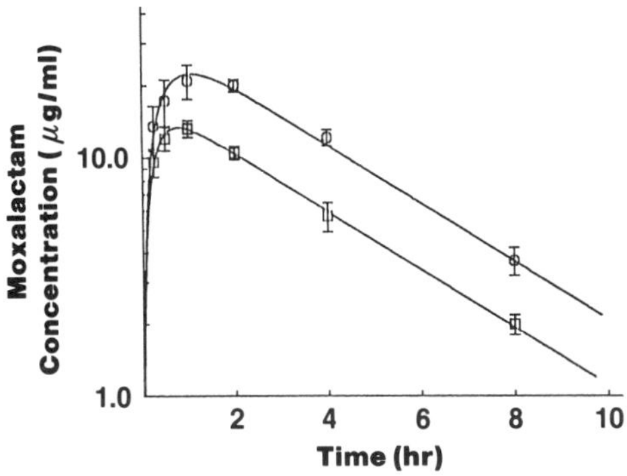

Figure 10 Plasma concentrations after intramuscular injections of 0.25 and 0.5 g of moxalactam in healthy volunteers (□, 0.25 g; ○, 0.5 g). Each plot represents a mean ± SD (n = 4).

Intravenous Bolus Injection. Mean concentrations in plasma or serum after intravenous bolus injections of 0.5, 1.0, and 2.0 g of moxalactam have been reported (24,30,33,36–45). Average values of plasma or serum half-life of the terminal phase and urinary recovery after intravenous bolus injections were 2.2 hr and 80%, respectively, as shown in Table 10.

Blood concentration and urinary excretion of moxalactam after intravenous administration with and without probenecid have been measured (37,38,43). These results indicate that there are little or no effects of probenecid on the blood concentration, elimination half-life, and urinary excretion. Based on these facts and its high urinary recovery, moxalactam appears to be eliminated primarily by kidney via glomerular filtration.

Results of multiple intravenous injections of 1.0 g of moxalactam every 12 hr show no accumulation in plasma concentration (24) (Fig. 11).

Intravenous Slow Infusion. Plasma or serum concentrations after 15-, 20-, and 4.0 g of moxalactam have been reported (24,25,29,31,32,34,35,46–50). Plasma concentrations during and after slow intravenous infusion over the same period are proportional to the dose (Fig. 12). Pharmacokinetic properties are summarized in Table 11.

Plasma concentrations after multiple 20-min intravenous infusions of 0.25, 0.5, 1.0, and 2.0 g every 8 hr for 28 doses and of 3.0 and 4.0 g every 8 hr for 7 doses indicated no accumulation (25).

Table 9 Pharmacokinetic Properties of Moxalactam After Intramuscular Injection in Healthy Volunteers

Dose (g)	Number of subjects	C_{max}[a] (μg/ml)	t_{max}[b] (hr)	$t_{1/2}$[c] (hr)	UR(t)[d] (%)	Reference
0.25	4	13.3	1	2.5	97.9 (24)[e]	7
	5	10	1	2.4	65 (24)	8
	3	11.4	0.5	1.8	49.2 (6)	10
0.5	4	21.0	1	2.8	97.1 (24)	7
	5	15-16[f]	1	2.3	59 (24)	8
	7	17.8	1.3	2.4	–	11
	5	23.6	1	–	86.8 (24)	12
1.0	5	27	2	2.1	55 (24)	8
	10	23.0	1.2	2.5	53 (24)	13
	6	49	0.5	2.3	76 (24)	14
	4	52.3	1.0	2.3	71 (24)	15
	8	38.6	0.7	1.9	78.6 (24)	16
	10	47.6	1.7	2.1	76.4 (24)	17
	3	61.4	0.5	1.9	68.8 (6)	18
Mean[g] ± SD				2.3 ± 0.3	71.2 ± 14.4	

[a]Maximum of mean concentration of moxalactam in plasma or serum.
[b]Time at which C_{max} occurred.
[c]Elimination half-life.
[d]Cumulative urinary recovery to time t.
[e]Time t is in hours.
[f]Read on the graph.
[g]Mean weighted by the number of subjects.

Protein Binding. Protein binding of moxalactam in plasma from healthy volunteers is 52-60% (50,51). The extent of plasma protein binding of R and S epimers is discussed later.

2. Patients with Renal Failure

Moxalactam is excreted mostly in the urine. Therefore elimination of this drug is delayed in patients with renal failure. The relationship between creatinine clearance and moxalactam elimination has been studied (38,50,52-64). The elimination half-life of moxalactam increases with decrease in creatinine clearance (Table 12) (52).

Table 10 Half-Life and Urinary Recovery of Moxalactam After Intravenous Bolus Injection in Healthy Volunteers

Dose (g)	Number of subjects	$t_{1/2}(\beta)^a$ (hr)	$UR(t)^b$ (%)	Reference
0.5	4	1.6	97.4 (24)[c]	7
	4	1.5[d]	79.8 (6)	19
	6	2.35	79 (24)	20
1.0	4	1.3	94.1 (24)	7
	11	3.47	76.0 (∞)[e]	13
	8	1.97	79.0 (24)	16
	6	2.25	71 (24)	20
	4	1.6	86.7 (8)	21
	4	1.7	77.4 (8)	21
	4	2.1[d]	80.1 (8)	22
	6	1.5	76.7 (8)	23
	3	1.7	55.2 (6)	24
	5	2.1[d]	90.5 (10)	25
	5	2.28	73.0 (24)	26
	6	2.85	87.5 (24)	27
2.0	6	2.42	73 (24)	20
Mean[f] ± SD		2.19 ± 0.6	80.0 ± 9.0	

[a]Elimination half-life at the terminal phase.
[b]Cumulative urinary recovery to time t.
[c]Time t is in hours.
[d]Calculated by the reviewers.
[e]Corrected to time infinity by the authors, based on the data to 12 hr.
[f]Mean weighted by the number of subjects.

The effect of hemodialysis on moxalactam elimination has been reported (38,51,54,56,60,61). An investigation of serum half-lives of moxalactam in renal insufficiency patients given doses both during and between hemodialysis treatment shows that there is a moderate removal of moxalactam by hemodialysis (Table 13) (50).

An investigation in uremic patients indicated that protein binding of moxalactam was 36 ± 6.4% (mean ± SD), which was less than in normal subjects (52 ± 7.8%) (50).

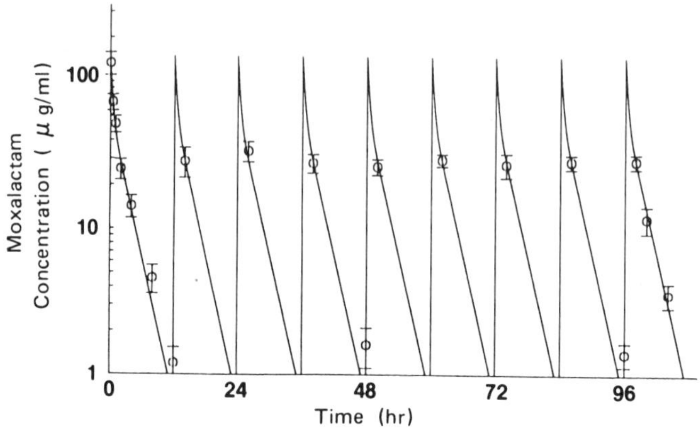

Figure 11 Plasma concentrations after multiple intravenous injections of 1.0 g of Moxalactam every 12 hr for 9 doses in healthy volunteers. The simulation curve was calculated using pharmacokinetic parameters obtained from the data of the first dose. Each plot represents a mean ± SD (n = 4).

3. Elderly Patients

Creatinine clearance in elderly patients, even if showing normal serum creatinine levels, is usually lower than in healthy young subjects. Therefore elimination of moxalactam excreted mainly by kidneys is slower in elderly subjects than in healthy young subjects. Wittmann and Schassan (65) reported that the mean elimination half-life in elderly patients showing normal serum creatinine

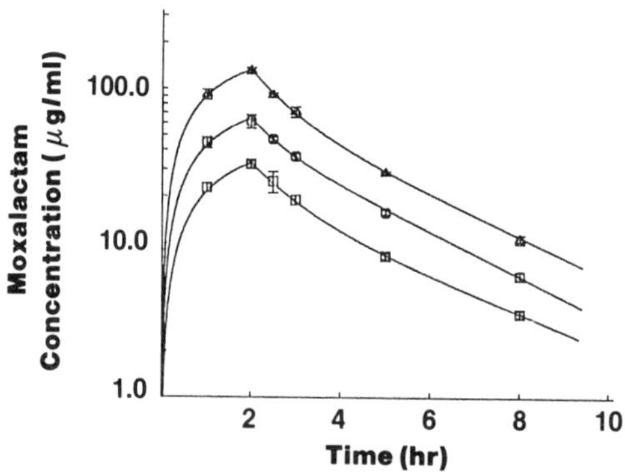

Figure 12 Plasma concentrations during and after 2-hr slow intravenous infusions of 0.5, 1.0, and 2.0 g of moxalactam in healthy volunteers (□, 0.5 g; ○, 1.0 g; △, 2.0 g). Each plot represents a mean ± SD (n = 4).

Table 11 Pharmacokinetic Properties of Moxalactam After Slow Intravenous Infusion in Healthy Volunteers

T[a] (hr)	Dose (g)	Number of subjects	C_T[b] (μg/ml)	$t_{1/2}(\beta)$[c] (hr)	UR(t)[d] (%)	Reference
1/4	2	10	244.8	2.2	80.3 (24)[e]	29
1/3	0.25	4	20	1.84	49 (24)	8
	0.5	4	28–30[f]	1.68	73 (24)	8
	1.0	4	70	1.98	92 (24)	8
	1.0	4	70.7	2.3	71 (24)	15
	2.0	4	120	2.01	80 (24)	8
	3.0	4	260–270[f]	1.61	74 (24)	8
	4.0	4	443	1.86	71 (24)	8
1/2	1.0	6	49	2.3	76 (12)	14
	1.0	10	68.5	1.94	76.4 (24)	17
	1.0	5	75–80[f]	2.1	69.3 (12)	33
	2.0	6	180–200[f]	2.51	70.5 (24)	12
	2.0	5	150–170[f]	2.3	60.2 (12)	33
1	1.0	4	85.0	2.2	96.5 (24)	7
	1.0	3	76.4	1.8	76.9 (7)	18
	1.0	6	72.0	2.23	80.4 (6)	30
	2.0	6	133.8	3.60	83.1 (6)	30
2	0.5	4	32.2	2.6	102.7 (24)	7
	1.0	4	61.4	2.1	100.8 (24)	7
	2.0	4	131.3	1.7	98.1 (24)	7
	Mean[g] ± SD			2.18 ± 0.44	78.5 ± 12.1	

[a]Infusion period.
[b]Plasma or serum concentration of moxalactam at the end of infusion.
[c]Elimination half-life at the terminal phase.
[d]Cumulative urinary recovery to time t.
[e]Time t is in hours.
[f]Read on the graph.
[g]Mean weighted by the number of subjects.

Table 12 Relationship Between Creatinine Clearance and Moxalactam Elimination Half-Life

C_{cr}[a] (ml/min per 1.73 m^2)	$t_{1/2}$[b] (hr)
>80	
110.2	2.0
95.0	2.0
89.3	2.9
82.2	2.2
80.8	2.4
40–80	
72.3	3.7
70.9	2.6
67.8	2.6
64.2	3.9
61.1	4.3
46.9	4.6
<40	
37.0	5.3
15.8	5.7

[a]Creatinine clearance.
[b]Moxalactam elimination half-life.

levels (3.1 hr; mean age, 71.5 years) was longer than in young volunteers (2.2 hr; mean age, 22.8 years). Similar results were reported by Shimada et al. (66).

4. Pediatric Patients

Many pharmacokinetic studies of moxalactam in pediatric patients have been published (67–84). Schaad et al. (67) found that mean elimination half-lives were 6.2 hr in neonates less than 1 week of age, 4.4 hr in those 1–4 weeks, and 1.6 hr in infants 1–24 months of age. Recently, similar results were reported by Motohiro et al. (68) (Fig. 13). Reed et al. (69) reported that in children 0.2–16 years old the mean elimination half-life of moxalactam (1.5 hr) was significantly shorter than in adults. Latif et al. (70) have shown that plasma concentration versus time curves after the first and subsequent 10-min intravenous infusions

Table 13 Effect of Hemodialysis on the Elimination Half-Life of Moxalactam in Renal Failure Patients

Hemodialysis	Dose (g)	Number of patients	$t_{1/2}$[a] (hr)
Off	0.5	5[b]	13.9
	1.0	5[c]	13.3
On	0.5	5[b]	4.4
	1.0	5[c]	5.7

[a]Half-life of the mean serum concentration of moxalactam in these patients.
[b]Same patients.
[c]Same patients.

of 25 mg/kg moxalactam every 8 hr in children 9 months to 1.4 years were virtually superimposable, indicating no change in the pharmacokinetics of this drug after repeated administration.

B. Distribution of Moxalactam

1. Concentration in Body Fluids and Tissues

Information about the concentration of a drug in body fluids and tissues where the drug action is expected is clinically more important than blood concentra-

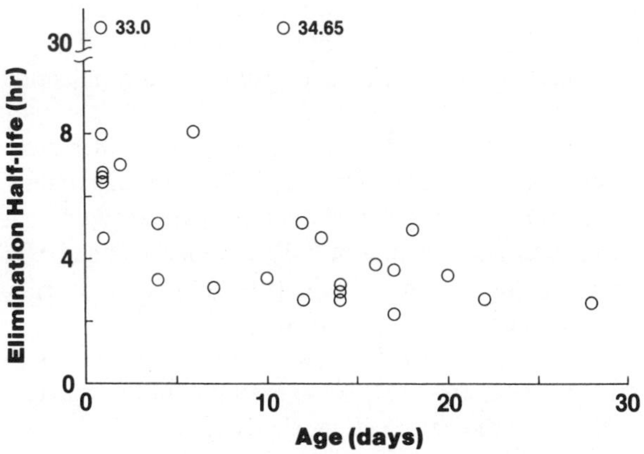

Figure 13 Elimination half-lives of moxalactam in neonates.

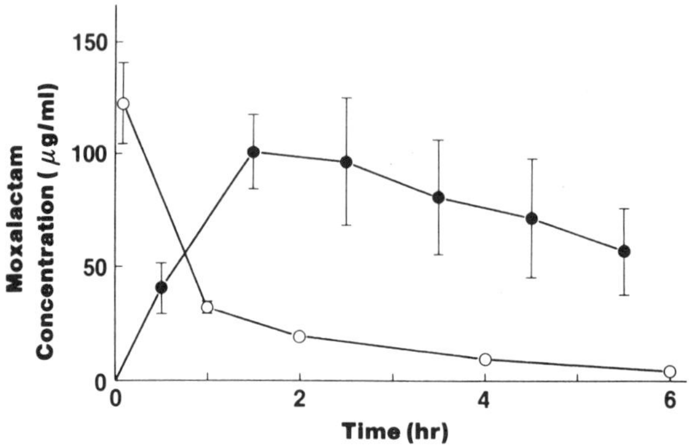

Figure 14 Serum and bile concentration in patients with biliary tract infections after intravenous injection of 1.0 g of moxalactam: ○, serum (n = 6); ●, bile (n = 9). Each plot represents a mean ± SE.

tion. Moxalactam concentrations in body fluids and tissues have been reported by many researchers (73,74,85-126).

Penetration of moxalactam into the cerebrospinal fluid has been investigated (73,74,85-91). Landesman et al. (85) reported that the peak cerebrospinal fluid levels of moxalactam in patients with meningitis who received 2.0 g of the drug intravenously ranged from 25 to 39 μg/ml. Kaplan et al. (86) observed that the mean cerebrospinal fluid concentration as a percentage of serum concentration for moxalactam in children with meningitis after three 50-mg/kg doses at 8-hr intervals was 18.5% (range, 2.0-61%).

Data on biliary excretion of moxalactam have been published (91-105). Tanimura et al. (98) reported the concentrations in the serum and bile of patients with biliary tract infections after intravenous bolus injections of 1.0 g moxalactam (Fig. 14). Biliary recovery of moxalactam within 6 hr after injection was 0.24-1.58%.

Moxalactam concentrations in peritoneal fluid after intravenous or intramuscular administration have been reported (92,100,106,107). The mean maximum concentration in fluid samples taken from peritoneal drains of patients was about 50 μg/ml 1-2 hr after intravenous injection of 2.0 g of moxalactam (107).

Peak levels of moxalactam in sputum reported by Matsumoto et al. were 1.84 and 2.11 μg/ml after intravenous injection of 1.0 g (108).

Concentrations of moxalactam in maternal serum, umbilical serum, and amniotic fluid have been investigated (22,109-117). Some examples of moxalactam level in these fluids are mentioned in the next section. Concentrations in mother's milk after intravenous administration of 1.0 g of moxalactam were 1 μg/ml or less (110,111,117).

With respect to aqueous humor, Axelrod and Kochman (118) reported that moxalactam concentrations were 0.92, 0.87, 1.98, 2.13, and 1.24 μg/ml 0.5, 1, 2, 4, and 6 hr, respectively, after 2.0-g intravenous dosages. Giamarellou et al. (91) obtained 2.4–3.25, 2.5–3.0, and 9.5–10.0 μg/ml 3.5, 4.5, and 5.0 hr, respectively, after a 2.0-g intravenous infusion over 30 min.

Kaplan et al. (119) reported moxalactam concentrations in joint fluid (9.1–19.8 and 2.1 μg/ml 5 and 7 hr after dose) and pleural fluid (11.4 μg/ml 0.75 hr after dose) for pediatric patients given 113–200 mg/kg daily in three or four divided doses (119).

Moxalactam levels in the uterus, oviduct, and ovary were 6.5-52.7, 5.1-39.0, and 12.2–24.3 μg/g, respectively, about 1 hr after intravenous injection of 1.0 g (109,120); 7.1-30.4, 12.3-29.9, and 16.5-31.8 μg/g, respectively, about 2.5 hr after intravenous administration of 2.0 g (111); and 5.1–17.2, 5.33–12.0, and 5.75–12.5 μg/g, respectively, about 50 min after intramuscular injection of 1.0 g (121).

Concentrations of moxalactam in retroperitoneal exudate ranged from 10.31 ± 3.58 (mean ± SD, n = 10) to 25.11 ± 4.79 μg/ml (n = 8) over 3 days when 1.0 g was injected intravenously every 6 hr (122).

Moxalactam concentrations in tonsil have been reported (123,124). The concentrations 1 hr after intravenous injection of 0.5 g were 5.8–6.4 μg/g (n = 4) (123).

Maximum levels in lung tissue (alveoli) observed directly after the end of a 1-hr intravenous infusion of 1.0 g of moxalactam were 34.5 ± 8.5 μg/g (mean ± SD; n = 3) (125). In appendix moxalactam concentrations in serum collected within 5 hr after intramuscular injection of 0.5 g were 1.55–5.34 μg/g in normal and slight catarrhal cases, 3.15–7.30 μg/g in moderate phlegmous cases, and 5.35–8.05 μg/g in serious gangrenous perforate cases (92). Moxalactam levels in normal intestinal tissue 1, 1.5, 2, and 2.5 hr after intravenous injection of 1.0 g were 14.8 ± 9.8 (mean ± SD, n = 4), 11.0 ± 2.9 (n = 5), 10.9 ± 5.0 (n = 4), and 10.5 ± 2.8 μg/g (n = 4), respectively (126).

The concentrations in rib bone marrow 0.5, 1, and 1.5 hr after the start of 1-hr intravenous infusion of 1.0 g of moxalactam were 3.4 ± 1.1 (mean ± SD, n = 3), 5.9 ± 2.5 (n = 9), and 4.8 ± 1.8 μg/g (n = 4), respectively (125).

These data indicate that moxalactam is widely distributed to various body fluids and tissues in humans.

2. Modified Compartment Analysis for Concentration in Body Fluids and Tissues

In some cases moxalactam concentrations in body fluids and tissues conform to modified compartment models (127–129). For example, the concentration versus time curves for maternal serum, umbilical serum, and amniotic fluid after intravenous injection of 2.0 g of moxalactam were calculated by such a model (129) and fit the observed values (Fig. 15).

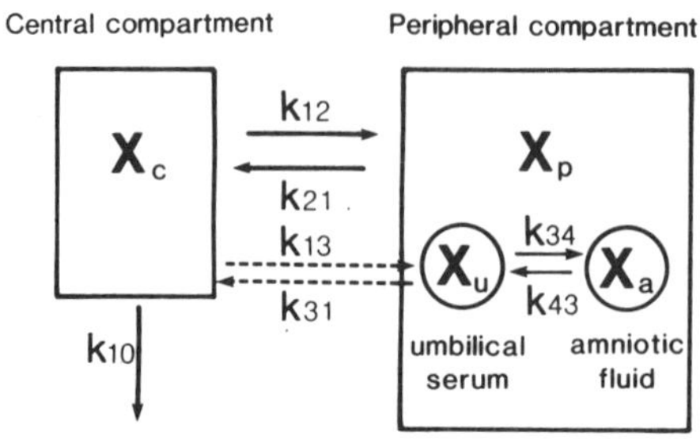

$$C_c = \frac{(k_{21}-\alpha)D_0}{(\beta-\alpha)V_c}e^{-\alpha t} + \frac{(k_{21}-\beta)D_0}{(\alpha-\beta)V_c}e^{-\beta t}$$

$$C_u = \frac{k_{13}(k_{21}-\alpha)(k_{43}-\alpha)D_0}{(\beta-\alpha)(\gamma-\alpha)(\delta-\alpha)V_u}e^{-\alpha t} + \frac{k_{13}(k_{21}-\beta)(k_{43}-\beta)D_0}{(\alpha-\beta)(\gamma-\beta)(\delta-\beta)V_u}e^{-\beta t} + \frac{k_{13}(k_{21}-\gamma)(k_{43}-\gamma)D_0}{(\alpha-\gamma)(\beta-\gamma)(\delta-\gamma)V_u}e^{-\gamma t} + \frac{k_{13}(k_{21}-\delta)(k_{43}-\delta)D_0}{(\alpha-\delta)(\beta-\delta)(\gamma-\delta)V_u}e^{-\delta t}$$

$$C_a = \frac{k_{13}k_{34}(k_{21}-\alpha)D_0}{(\beta-\alpha)(\gamma-\alpha)(\delta-\alpha)V_a}e^{-\alpha t} + \frac{k_{13}k_{34}(k_{21}-\beta)D_0}{(\alpha-\beta)(\gamma-\beta)(\delta-\beta)V_a}e^{-\beta t} + \frac{k_{13}k_{34}(k_{21}-\gamma)D_0}{(\alpha-\gamma)(\beta-\gamma)(\delta-\gamma)V_a}e^{-\gamma t} + \frac{k_{13}k_{34}(k_{21}-\delta)D_0}{(\alpha-\delta)(\beta-\delta)(\gamma-\delta)V_a}e^{-\delta t}$$

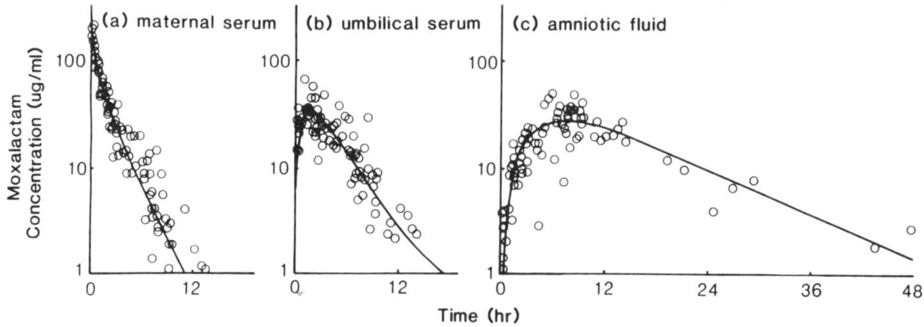

Figure 15 Moxalactam concentrations in maternal serum, umbilical serum, and amniotic fluid after intravenous injection of 2.0 g: (a) maternal serum, (b) Umbilical serum, and (c) amniotic fluid. The curves were calculated using Eqs. (1)–(3), where V_A was assumed to be 500 ml.

C. Pharmacokinetics of R and S Epimers of Moxalactam

Pharmacokinetic studies of R and S epimers of moxalactam have been reported (21,22,37,61,93,98,130-133). The concentrations of R and S epimers of moxalactam in body fluids and tissues were determined separately by high-performance liquid chromatography (19-23).

1. Healthy Volunteers

There is a significant difference in the plasma concentration versus time curves for R and S epimers (130). The ratio of R to S epimers was 0.84 in plasma 10 min after administration and it decreased to 0.5 at 5 hr (37). Renal clearances for the epimers were measured and found to be 61-67 and 41-48 ml/min per 1.48 m^2 for R and S, respectively. The fractions unbound to plasma protein were found to be 47 and 33% for R and S, respectively. The renal clearances of unbound R and S epimers calculated from these results were 130-147 and 124-146 ml/min per 1.48 m^2, respectively. There is no significant difference.

Table 14 Serum R/S Ratios After Intravenous Bolus Injection of 1.0 g of Moxalactam in Patients with Various Degrees of Creatinine Clearance

C_{cr}[a] (ml/min)	$t_{1/2}$[b] (hr)	R/S ratios after dosing 1 hr	2 hr	4 hr	6 hr
4	20	0.86	0.86	0.81	0.81
3	19.3	0.87	0.98	0.96	0.91
9	13.4	1.02	0.93	1.0	0.86
35	4.5	NT[c]	0.81	0.77	0.67
120	2.6	NT[c]	0.69	0.65	0.55

[a]Creatinine clearance.
[b]Moxalactam elimination half-life.
[c]Not tested.

These facts suggest that the difference in the pharmacokinetic behaviors of R and S epimers of moxalactam is mainly due to the difference in the plasma protein binding of these epimers.

2. Patients with Renal Failure

Wise et al. (131) reported serial R/S ratios of moxalactam in the serum of patients with various degrees of renal dysfunction. As shown in Table 14, equilibrium ratios of R/S in serum (0.82) was maintained in patients with more severe renal impairment, possibly because elimination in these patients was slower than conversion of the S to the R epimer.

3. Pediatric Patients

The difference of total clearance between the R and S epimers of moxalactam was observed also in 8- to 45-month-old children (132). The paired t-test showed that the total clearance of R epimer (mean, 69.59 ml/min per square meter) was significantly higher than that of S epimer (mean, 41.55 ml/min per square meter).

Mean values of the total clearance of R and S epimers of moxalactam after multiple doses in children (15-min intravenous infusions of 50 mg/kg every 8 hr for at least 3 days) were 124 and 85 ml/min per 1.73 m^2, respectively (133). These values were the same as those after the first dose (123 and 86 ml/min per 1.73 m^2 for R and S, respectively). It seems that multiple dosing does not change the pharmacokinetic behavior of R and S epimers.

4. Concentrations in Body Fluids and Tissues

Mean R/S ratios in umbilical cord serum and uterine tissue obtained 15-130 min after 20-min intravenous infusions of moxalactam (2 g) were 0.93 and 1.22, respectively (22). The high R/S ratio in the uterine tissue may indicate that the R epimer has a greater diffusibility to tissues, because of its lower protein binding in maternal blood serum.

V SUMMARY

In conclusion, moxalactam is a unique antibiotic, possessing an oxazine- rather than the naturally occurring thiazine-azetidinone ring system. Because of its different chemical constitution, synthesis of the substance is difficult, and development of new chemical methodologies was a necessary prerequisite for commercial production. Following parenteral administration, the substance is widely distributed, achieving therapeutically significant levels in many fluids and tissues, most notably in the cerebrospinal fluid. The clinical efficacy of moxalactam has been demonstrated by successful treatment of a variety of infections in each of the major organ systems. Incidence of side-effects during therapy with moxalactam is low, but serious hematopoietic effects have been observed in some patients.

REFERENCES

1. K. Murakami, M. Takasuka, K. Motokawa, and T. Yoshida. 1-Oxacephalosporins: Enhancement of β-lactam reactivity and antibacterial activity. *J. Med. Chem., 24*:88-93 (1981).
2. T. Yoshida. Structural requirements for antibacterial activity and β-lactamase stability of 7β-arylmalonylamino-7α-methoxy-1-oxacephems. *Philos. Trans. R. Soc. London, B289*:231-237 (1980).
3. N. Hashimoto, T. Tasaki, and H. Tanaka. Degradation and epimerization kinetics of moxalactam in aqueous solution. *J. Pharm. Sci., 73*:369 (1984).
4. M. Narisada and W. Nagata. Arylmalonamido-1-oxadethiacephalosporins. U.S. patent 4,323,567 (1982).
5. P. G. Sammes. *Topics in Antibiotic Chemistry,* Ellis Horwood, Chichester, West Sussex, 1980, pp. 61-79.
6. W. Nagata, M. Narisada, and T. Yoshida. Partial synthesis of nuclear analogs of cephalosporins, in *Chemistry and Biology of β-Lactam Antibiotics,* Vol. 2 (R. B. Morin and M. Gorman, eds.), Academic, New York, 1982, pp. 1-42.
7. H. Otsuka, W. Nagata, M. Yoshioka, M. Narisada, T. Yoshida, Y. Harada, and H. Yamada. Discovery and development of moxalactam (6059-S): The chemistry and biology of 1-oxacephems, in *Medicinal Research Reviews* (ed: G. de Stevens), Vol. 1, Wiley, New York, 1981, pp. 221-226.
8. W. Nagata. Synthetic aspects of 1-oxacephem antibiotics, in *IUPAC Current*

Trends in Organic Synthesis (H. Nozaki, ed.), Pergamon, Oxford, 1983, p. 83.

9. M. Narisada, H. Onoue, and W. Nagata. Synthetic studies on β-lactam antibiotics. Part 5. A synthesis of 7β-acylamino-3-methyl-1-oxadethia-3-cephem-4-carboxylic acids. *Heterocycles, 7*:839 (1977).
10. M. Narisada, T. Yoshida, H. Onoue, M. Ohtani, T. Okada, T. Tsuji, I. Kikkawa, N. Haga, H. Satoh, H. Itani, and W. Nagata. Synthetic studies on β-lactam antibiotics. Part 10. Synthesis of 7β-[2-carboxy-2-(4-hydroxyphenyl)acetamido]-7α-methoxy-3-[[(1-methyl-1H-tetrazol-5-yl)thio]-methyl]-1-oxa-1-dethia-3-cephem-4-carboxylic acid disodium salt (6059-S) and its related 1-oxacephems. *J. Med. Chem., 22*:757 (1979).
11. M. Yoshioka, I. Kikkawa, T. Tsuji, Y. Nishitani, S. Mori, K. Okada, M. Murakami, F. Matsubara, M. Yamaguchi, and W. Nagata. Synthetic studies on β-lactam antibiotics. Part 11. Completely stereocontrolled synthesis of 7α-unsubstituted 1-oxacephems from penicillins. *Tetrahedr. Lett.*, 4287 (1979).
12. S. Uyeo, I. Kikkawa, Y. Hamashima, H. Ona, Y. Nishitani, K. Okada, T. Kubota, K. Ishikura, Y. Ide, K. Nakano, and W. Nagata. Stereocontrolled synthesis of 7α-methoxy-1-oxacephems from 6-epipenicillin G. *J. Am. Chem. Soc., 101*:4403 (1979).
13. M. Yoshioka, T. Tsuji, S. Uyeo, S. Yamamoto, T. Aoki, Y. Nishitani, S. Mori, H. Satoh, Y. Hamada, H. Ishitobi, and W. Nagata. Stereocontrolled, straightforward synthesis of 3-substituted methyl 7α-methoxy-1-oxacephems. *Tetrahedr. Lett., 21*:351 (1980).
14. T. Tsuji, T. Kataoka, M. Yoshioka, Y. Sendo, Y. Nishitani, S. Hirai, T. Maeda, and W. Nagata. Synthetic studies on β-lactam antibiotics. VII. Mild removal of the benzyl ester protecting group with aluminum trichloride. *Tetrahedr. Lett.*, 2793 (1979).
15. H. Yanagisawa and A. Ando. Conversion of cephem-1-oxide into 1-oxadethiacepham. *Tetrahedr. Lett., 23*:3379 (1982).
16. S. Yamamoto, H. Itani, T. Tsuji, and W. Nagata. Oxidatively assisted hydrolysis of allylic iodides to rearrange allylic alcohols. A new example of [2,3] sigmatropic rearrangement. *J. Am. Chem. Soc., 105*:2908 (1983).
17. T. Aoki, T. Konoike, H. Itani, T. Tsuji, M. Yoshioka, and W. Nagata. New route to 3-(substituted) methyl 1-oxa- and (1-thia)cephems from 3-exomethylene intermediates via sulfenyl chloride adducts. *Tetrahedron, 39*: 2515 (1983).
18. Y. Kimura and T. Yoshida. Microbiological assay methods of 6059-S concentrations in body fluids. *Chemotherapy Tokyo Suppl., 7*:178 (1980).
19. R. Konaka, K. Kuruma, R. Nishimura, Y. Kimura, and T. Yoshida. High-performance liquid chromatographic analysis of a new β-lactam antibiotic, 6059-S (moxalactam). *J. Chromatogr., 225*:169 (1981).
20. W. F. Diven, B. D. Obermeyer, R. L. Wolen, V. L. Yu, J. Lyon, and J. Zuravleff. Measurement of serum and tissue concentration of moxalactam using high pressure liquid chromatography. *Ther. Drug Monitor, 3*:291 (1981).

21. J. A. Ziemniak, D. A. Chiarmonte, D. J. Miner, and J. J. Schentag. HPLC determination of D and L moxalactam in human serum and urine. *J. Pharm. Sci., 71*:399 (1982).
22. R. E. Bawdon, F. G. Cunningham, J. G. Quirk, and M. L. Roark. Maternal and fetal pharmacokinetics of moxalactam given intrapartum. *Am. J. Obstet. Gynecol., 144*:546 (1982).
23. D. J. Miner, D. L. Coleman, A. M. M. Shepherd, and T. C. Hardin. Determination of moxalactam in human body fluids by liquid chromatographic and microbiological methods. *Antimicrob. Agents Chemother., 20*:252 (1981).
24. H. Yamada, T. Yoshida, T. Oguma, Y. Kimura, Y. Tochino, J. Kurihara, K. Matsumoto, Y. Uzuka, H. Shishido, and T. Nagatake. Clinical pharmacology of 6059-S in healthy volunteers. *Chemotherapy Tokyo Suppl., 7*: 251 (1980).
25. K. S. Israel, H. R. Black, G. L. Brier, J. D. Wolny, and K. A. DeSante. Single- and multiple-dose pharmacokinetics of moxalactam in normal subjects. *Antimicrob. Agents Chemother., 22*:94 (1982).
26. M. Gibaldi and D. Perrier. *Pharmacokinetics,* Marcel Dekker, New York, 1975.
27. K. Suzuki, Y. Naide, T. Fujita, N. Okisio, H. Asano, and T. Yamagoe. Basic and clinical studies on the use of 6059-S against infections in the urological field. *Chemotherapy Tokyo Suppl., 7*:783 (1980).
28. A. M. M. Shepherd, T. C. Hardin, T. M. Ludden, and D. J. Miner. Pharmacokinetics of a new β-lactam antibiotic, moxalactam. *Clin. Pharmacol. Ther., 29*:283 (1981).
29. H. C. Standiford, G. L. Drusano, W. B. McNamee, B. Tatem, P. A. Ryan, and S. C. Schimpff. Comparative pharmacokinetics of moxalactam, cefoperazone, and cefotaxime in normal volunteers. *Rev. Infect. Dis. Suppl., 4*: S585 (1982).
30. W. M. Scheld, D. A. Spyker, G. R. Donowitz, W. K. Bolton, and M. A. Sande. Moxalactam and cefazolin: Comparative pharmacokinetics in normal subjects. *Antimicrob. Agents Chemother., 19*:613 (1981).
31. S. Srinivasan, K. P. Fu, and H. C. Neu. Pharmacokinetics of moxalactam and cefazolin compared in normal volunteers. *Antimicrob. Agents Chemother., 19*:302 (1981).
32. J. N. Parsons, J. M. Romano, and M. E. Levison. Pharmacology of a new 1-oxa-β-lactam (LY127935) in normal volunteers. *Antimicrob. Agents Chemother., 17*:226 (1980).
33. T. B. Tjandramaga, A. Van Hecken, A. Mullie, R. Verbesselt, P. J. De Schepper, and L. Verbist. Comparative pharmacokinetics of ceftazidime and moxalactam. *Antimicrob. Agents Chemother., 22*:237 (1982).
34. B. R. Meyers, S. Z. Hirschman, J. Giron, and E. S. Srulevitch. Pharmacokinetic studies of single and multiple doses of moxalactam (Moxam) in normal volunteers. *Clin. Trials J., 19*:63 (1982).
35. Y. Sawae, K. Okada, T. Yanase, T. Yokoi, K. Takemori, and H. Yokota. Laboratory and clinical studies on 6059-S. *Chemotherapy Tokyo Suppl., 7*: 530 (1980).

36. K. Hikosaka, M. Hazama, Y. Kuroda, S. Kamidono, and J. Ishigami. Fundamental and clinical studies on 6059-S in urological field. *Chemotherapy Tokyo Suppl.,* 7:808 (1980).
37. R. Lüthy, J. Blaser, A. Bonetti, H. Simmen, R. Wise, and W. Siegenthaler. Comparative multiple-dose pharmacokinetics of cefotaxime, moxalactam, and ceftazidime. *Rev. Infect. Dis. Suppl., 4*:S581 (1982).
38. Y. Ueda, J. Shimada, F. Matsumoto, A. Saito, M. Ohmori, K. Shiba, T. Yamaji, H. Ihara, T. Hojo, and T. Miyahara. Clinical studies on 6059-S, a new semisynthetic oxacephem for parenteral use. *Chemotherapy Tokyo Suppl.,* 7:370 (1980).
39. O. Kunii, K. Fukaya, S. Nakamura, T. Komatsu, and K. Iwata. Studies on 6059-S. *Chemotherapy Tokyo Suppl.,* 7:388 (1980).
40. K. Nakagawa, K. Watanabe, H. Hukui, Y. Kawaguchi, H. Nakazawa, N. Kihara, T. Suzuki, M. Koyama, Y. Hoshihara, and M. Yokozawa. Fundamental and clinical studies on 6059-S. *Chemotherapy Tokyo Suppl.,* 7:420 (1980).
41. I. Nakayama, Y. Akieda, K. Tajima, S. Iwai, H. Kawamura, H. Kawaguchi, D. Jinno, T. Sakabe, and S. Ishiyama. Studies on 6059-S, a new oxacephem antibiotic, in surgery – Antibacterial activity, pharmacokinetics, tissue distribution, metabolism and its clinical application. *Chemotherapy Tokyo Suppl.,* 7:606 (1980).
42. T. Tominaga, H. Kishi, T. Niijima, Y. Nishimura, S. Minowada, M. Asano, A. Miyashita, and O. Tukada. Laboratory and clinical evaluation of 6059-S in the field of urology. *Chemotherapy Tokyo Suppl.,* 7:717 (1980).
43. K. A. DeSante, K. S. Israel, G. L. Brier, J. D. Wolny, and B. L. Hatcher. Effect of probenecid on the pharmacokinetics of moxalactam. *Antimicrob. Agents Chemother., 21*:58 (1982).
44. R. Wise, S. Baker, and R. Livingston. Comparison of cefotaxime and moxalactam pharmacokinetics and tissue levels. *Antimicrob. Agents Chemother., 18*:369 (1980).
45. B. Kemmerich, H. Lode, G. Belmega, T. Jendroschek, K. Borner, and P. Koeppe. Comparative pharmacokinetics of cefoperazone, cefotaxime, and moxalactam. *Antimicrob. Agents Chemother., 23*:429 (1983).
46. H. Lode, V. Madey, G. Dzwillo, K. Borner, and P. Koeppe. Serum bactericidal activity and kinetics of azlocillin and moxalactam after single and combined administration. *J. Antimicrob. Chemother. Suppl. B, 11*:121 (1983).
47. A. Saito, Y. Kato, K. Ishikawa, H. Uemura, E. Odagaki, M. Shinohara, M. Tomizawa, I. Nakayama, Y. Kinoshita, and K. Sato. Studies on 6059-S. *Chemotherapy Tokyo Suppl., 7*:279 (1980).
48. K. Sakai, M. Fujimoto, T. Ueda, N. Kawabata, T. Sasaki, S. Maeda, A. Sawada, A. Masada, M. Kawashima, F. Kitano, and S. Doi. A clinical study on 6059-S in the field of surgery. *Chemotherapy Tokyo Suppl.,* 7:681 (1980).
49. R. E. Polk, B. J. Kline, and S. M. Markowitz. Cefazolin and moxalactam pharmacokinetics after simultaneous intravenous infusion. *Antimicrob. Agents Chemother., 20*:576 (1981).
50. L. R. Peterson, B. Bean, C. E. Fasching, W. P. Korchik, and D. N. Gerding. Pharmacokinetics, protein binding, and predicted extravascular distribution

of moxalactam in normal and renal failure subjects. *Antimicrob. Agents Chemother., 20*:378 (1981).

51. T. Yoshida, Y. Kimura, and Y. Tochino. Pharmacokinetics of 6059-S in experimental animals. *Chemotherapy Tokyo Suppl.,* 7:194 (1980).
52. P. Garzone, J. Lyon, V. L. Yu, J. Zuravleff, W. Diven, and W. Pasculle. Steady-state moxalactam kinetics: Comparisons with other cephalosporins. *Clin. Pharmacol. Ther., 30*:86 (1981).
53. E. Singlas, H. F. Boutron, H. Merdjan, J. F. Brocard, M. Pocheville, and D. Fries. Moxalactam kinetics during chronic ambulatory peritoneal dialysis. *Clin. Pharmacol. Ther., 34*:403 (1983).
54. S. Srinivasan and H. C. Neu. Pharmacokinetics of moxalactam in patients with renal failure and during hemodialysis. *Antimicrob. Agents Chemother., 20*:398 (1981).
55. M. Lam, C. V. Manion, and A. W. Czerwinski. Pharmacokinetics of moxalactam in patients with renal insufficiency. *Antimicrob. Agents Chemother., 19*:461 (1981).
56. G. R. Aronoff, R. S. Sloan, S. A. Mong, F. C. Luft, and S. A. Kleit. Moxalactam pharmacokinetics during hemodialysis. *Antimicrob. Agents Chemother., 19*:575 (1981).
57. W. K. Bolton, W. M. Scheld, D. A. Spyker, T. L. Overby, and M. A. Sande. Pharmacokinetics of moxalactam in subjects with various degrees of renal dysfunction. *Antimicrob. Agents Chemother., 18*:933 (1980).
58. A. Leroy, G. Humbert, and J. P. Fillastre. Pharmacokinetics of moxalactam in subjects with normal and impaired renal function. *Antimicrob. Agents Chemother., 19*:965 (1981).
59. G. R. Aronoff, R. S. Sloan, and F. C. Luft. Pharmacokinetics of moxalactam in patients with normal and impaired renal function. *J. Infect. Dis., 145*:365 (1982).
60. E. J. Jacobson, J. J. Zahrowski, and A. R. Nissenson. Moxalactam kinetics in hemodialysis. *Clin. Pharmacol. Ther., 30*:487 (1981).
61. N. Wright, P. J. Wills, and R. Wise. The pharmacokinetics of moxalactam in renal failure. *J. Antimicrob. Chemother., 8*:395 (1981).
62. R. Ukai, K. Hatachi, M. Fujii, H. Nihira, S. Matsuki, and M. Hirayama. Laboratory and clinical evaluations of 6059-S in the field of urology. *Chemotherapy Tokyo Suppl.,* 7:840 (1980).
63. N. Aoki, O. Sekine, Y. Usuda, Y. Yuasa, T. Shimizu, N. Wakabayashi, S. Hayashi, and K. Watanabe. Clinical studies on 6059-S. *Chemotherapy Tokyo Suppl.,* 7:361 (1980).
64. Y. Nishimoto, M. Yamakido, M. Kuwabara, and T. Watanabe. Clinical studies on 6059-S, with special reference to the treatment of respiratory infections. *Chemotherapy Tokyo Suppl.,* 7:523 (1980).
65. D. H. Wittmann and H.-H. Schassan. Distribution of moxalactam in serum, bone, tissue fluid, and peritoneal fluid. *Rev. Infect. Dis. Suppl., 4*:S610 (1982).
66. K. Shimada, T. Inamatsu, K. Urayama, and K. Adachi. Evaluation on 6059-S, its antimicrobial activity, pharmacokinetic and clinical response. *Chemotherapy Tokyo Suppl.,* 7:435 (1980).

67. U. B. Schaad, G. H. McCracken, Jr., N. Threlkeld, and M. L. Thomas. Clinical evaluation of a new broad-spectrum oxa-beta-lactam antibiotic, moxalactam, in neonates and infants. *J. Pediatr., 98*:129 (1981).
68. T. Motohiro, K. Tanaka, T. Koga, Y. Shimada, N. Tomita, Y. Sakata, T. Fujimoto, T. Nishiyama, K. Ishimoto, K. Tominaga, F. Yamashita, T. Tanaka, H. Watari, N. Takajō, H. Araki, Y. Odajima, S. Imai, K. Ichikawa, T. Yokoyama, O. Inoue, A. Kawakami, Y. Kimura, K. Nagayama, T. Yuasa, Y. Tanaka, S. Tsugawa, T. Hashimoto, H. Nakajima, S. Fukuda, S. Kinoshita, K. Yuge, E. Ootaki, T. Takemura, H. Nagano, J. Kameyama, H. Matsuo, M. Matsuyama, Y. Eto, Y. Koga, and M. Matsuyuki. Fundamental and clinical studies of latamoxef in the neonates and immature infants. *Jpn. J. Antibiot., 36*:2364 (1983).
69. M. D. Reed, J. S. Bertino, S. C. Aronoff, C. M. Myers, W. T. Speck, and J. L. Blumer. Pharmacokinetics of moxalactam in children. *Clin. Pharmacol. Ther., 31*:262 (1982).
70. R. Latif, M. C. Thirumoorthi, J. A. Buckley, D. M. Kobos, M. K. Aravind, R. E. Kauffman, and A. S. Dajani. Pharmacokinetic and clinical evaluation of moxalactam in infants and children. *Dev. Pharmacol. Ther., 3*:222 (1981).
71. G. H. McCracken, Jr., and U. B. Schaad. Pharmacokinetics of moxalactam in neonates and young infants. *Rev. Infect. Dis. Suppl., 4*:S595 (1982).
72. R. Fujii. Absorption, excretion, and clinical efficacy of moxalactam in pediatric patients. *Rev. Infect. Dis. Suppl., 4*:S656 (1982).
73. Y. Toyonaga, M. Sugita, Y. Kurosu, K. Kumagai, M. Hori, and T. Takahashi. Experimental and clinical studies on 6059-S. *Jpn. J. Antibiot., 34*:764 (1981).
74. Y. Toyonaga, Y. Kurosu, M. Sugita, M. Kitagawa, and M. Hori. Basic and clinical studies on use of latamoxef in neonates. *Jpn. J. Antibiot., 36*: 2322 (1983).
75. S. Nakazawa, H. Sato, K. Niino, Y. Hirama, A. Narita, S. Nakazawa, and H. Chikaoka. Fundamental and clinical studies in neonates and infants on latamoxef. *Jpn. J. Antibiot., 36*:2302 (1983).
76. N. Yamashita, K. Sunakawa, N. Hara, S. Nanri, Y. Morikawa, H. Akita, M. Hotta, M. Tojo, Y. Ichihashi, and M. Hirose. Basic and clinical examinations of 6059-S in pediatrics. *Jpn. J. Antibiot., 34*:576 (1981).
77. M. Varghese, A. J. Khan, G. Quaye, U. Patel, K. Kumar, and H. E. Evans. Clinical and pharmacokinetic evaluation of moxalactam in infants and children. *Chemotherapy Basel, 28*:417 (1982).
78. P. Bégué, C. Safran, J. Fleurette, Y. Brun, D. Floret, and P. Monnet. Le moxalactam en pédiatrie, expérience clinique et pharmacocinétique. A propos de trente-sept observations. *Sem. Hop. Paris, 59*:1972 (1983).
79. H. Keyserling, W. E. Feldman, S. Moffitt, N. Manning, and M. Hollins. Clinical and pharmacokinetic evaluation of parenteral moxalactam in infants and children. *Antimicrob. Agents Chemother., 21*:898 (1982).
80. M. Takimoto, T. Oka, H. Yoshioka, A. Tsuchida, N. Sanae, and S. Maruyama. Clinical and pharmacokinetic evaluation of latamoxef in newborn infants. *Jpn. J. Antibiot., 36*:2297 (1983).

81. M. Tojo, K. Sunakawa, S. Nanri, H. Akita, S. Iwata, Y. Iwasaki, T. Kanemitsu, Y. Satoh, T. Oikawa, M. Osano, Y. Ichihashi, K. Ishikawa, K. Shirane, M. Hirose, H. Tsuchiya, and Y. Taguchi. Basic and clinical examinations of latamoxef in neonates and immature infants. *Jpn. J. Antibiot., 36*:2312 (1983).
82. N. Iwai, A. Sasaki, Y. Taneda, F. Mizoguchi, H. Nakamura, N. Tauchi, M. Kawamura, and T. Ozaki. Study on the use of latamoxef in neonates. *Jpn. J. Antibiot., 36*:2336 (1983).
83. Y. Kobayashi, T. Haruta, S. Kuroki, and K. Okura. Evaluation of latamoxef in treatment of infections in newborns. *Jpn. J. Antibiot., 36*:2359 (1983).
84. T. Nishimura, K. Tabuki, and T. Takashima. Pharmacokinetic and clinical studies of latamoxef in neonates. *Jpn. J. Antibiot., 36*:2349 (1983).
85. S. H. Landesman, M. L. Corrado, C. C. Cherubin, M. Gombert, and D. Cleri. Diffusion of a new beta-lactam (LY127935) into cerebrospinal fluid. Implications for therapy of gram-negative bacillary meningitis. *Am. J. Med., 69*:92 (1980).
86. S. L. Kaplan, E. O. Mason, Jr., H. Garcia, S. J. Kvernland, E. M. Loiselle, D. C. Anderson, A. A. Mintz, and R. D. Feigin. Pharmacokinetics and cerebrospinal fluid penetration of moxalactam in children with bacterial meningitis. *J. Pediatr., 98*:152 (1981).
87. M. C. Thirumoorthi, J. A. Buckley, M. K. Aravind, R. E. Kauffman, and A. S. Dajani. Diffusion of moxalactam into the cerebrospinal fluid in children with bacterial meningitis. *J. Pediatr., 99*:975 (1981).
88. S. Nakazawa, H. Sato, K. Niino, S. Nakazawa, H. Suzuki, A. Iwasaki, H. Chikaoka, S. Oka, Y. Hirama, and A. Narita. Fundamental and clinical studies in pediatric field on 6059-S. *Jpn. J. Antibiot., 34*:562 (1981).
89. S. L. Kaplan, E. O. Mason, Jr., S. J. Kvernland, E. L. Calaway, and R. D. Feigin. Pharmacology and cerebrospinal fluid penetration of moxalactam in children and dosage recommendations. *Rev. Infect. Dis. Suppl., 4*:S597 (1982).
90. J. Modai, M. Wolff, J. Lebas, A. Meulemans, and C. Manuel. Moxalactam penetration into cerebrospinal fluid in patients with bacterial meningitis. *Antimicrob. Agents Chemother., 21*:551 (1982).
91. H. Giamarellou, J. Tsagarakis, and G. K. Daikos. Moxalactam in serious infections: Clinical, bacteriologic, and pharmacokinetic studies. *Rev. Infect. Dis. Suppl., 4*:S629 (1982).
92. T. Nakamura, I. Hashimoto, Y. Sawada, J. Mikami, E. Bekki, S. Hirasawa, H. Abe, H. Katoh, and S. Matsuda. Clinical pharmacokinetics of 6059-S in infected tissues following intramuscular administration. *Chemotherapy Tokyo Suppl., 7*:263 (1980).
93. W. Takahashi, S. Onochi, I. Uematsu, H. Kimura, Y. Takazawa, H. Ise, N. Suzuki, and T. Sato. Studies on biliary excretion and gallbladder tissue concentrations of 6059-S. *Chemotherapy Tokyo Suppl., 7*:274 (1980).
94. Y. Nonoshita, M. Yoshida, and M. Menjo. Concentration in serum, bile and gallbladder tissue, and clinical effect of 6059-S. *Chemotherapy Tokyo Suppl., 7*:627 (1980).

95. S. Katoh, T. Tanaka, M. Ishida, and N. Takenaka. Fundamental and clinical studies of 6059-S in surgical field. *Chemotherapy Tokyo Suppl., 7*: 636 (1980).
96. Y. Yamada and T. Saito. Laboratory and clinical study of 6059-S in surgery. *Chemotherapy Tokyo Suppl., 7*:640 (1980).
97. J. Yura, N. Shinagawa, M. Emina, T. Doi, S. Ishikawa, T. Hanai, K. Matsugaki, K. Shibata, and T. Ito. Fundamental and clinical studies of 6059-S in the surgical field. *Chemotherapy Tokyo Suppl., 7*:650 (1980).
98. H. Tanimura, T. Sekiya, K. Miki, Y. Hikasa, M. Okamoto, T. Yasutomi, H. Kawaguchi, H. Matsumoto, H. Ohtani, H. Miyake, H. Awane, K. Fukuchi, Y. Takahashi, Y. Nishijima, S. Kido, T. Nishikawa, K. Nishikawa, M. Kurahashi, K. Konishi, R. Fujita, Y. Ueyama, Y. Naito, F. Rai, and H. Hashino. Chemotherapy of biliary tract infection (X) with special reference on biliary excretion, tissue concentration in gallbladder and clinical effects in patients treated with 6059-S. *Chemotherapy Tokyo Suppl., 7*: 661 (1980).
99. K. Sakai, M. Fujimoto, T. Ueda, N. Kawabata, T. Sasaki, S. Maeda, A. Sawada, A. Masada, M. Kawashima, F. Kitano, and S. Doi. A clinical study on 6059-S in the field of surgery. *Chemotherapy Tokyo Suppl., 7*: 681 (1980).
100. T. Yokoyama, T. Ichikawa, N. Miyoshi, T. Hijikata, and T. Sueda. Fundamental and clinical studies on 6059-S in surgical field. *Chemotherapy Tokyo Suppl., 7*:694 (1980).
101. H. Shimura and Y. Yamamoto. Laboratory and clinical study of 6059-S in surgical field. *Chemotherapy Tokyo Suppl., 7*:699 (1980).
102. O. V. Martinez, J. U. Levi, A. Livingstone, T. I. Malinin, R. Zeppa, D. Hutson, and N. Einhorn. Biliary excretion of moxalactam. *Antimicrob. Agents Chemother., 20*:231 (1981).
103. J. Shimada and Y. Ueda. Moxalactam – Absorption, excretion, distribution, and metabolism. *Rev. Infect. Dis. Suppl., 4*:S569 (1982).
104. D. N. Gerding and L. R. Peterson. Comparative tissue and extravascular fluid concentrations of ceftizoxime. *J. Antimicrob. Chemother. Suppl. C, 10*:105 (1982).
105. J. Yura, S. Hayashi, N. Tsuruga, T. Hashimoto, Y. Murata, and Y. Kamiya. Fundamental and clinical studies of latamoxef in the pediatric surgery. *Jpn. J. Antibiot., 36*:2383 (1983).
106. Y. Yamada, Y. Hanatani, and K. Ishibiki. Basic and clinical studies on a new oxacephem antibiotic, 6059-S. *Chemotherapy Tokyo Suppl., 7*:621 (1980).
107. D. H. Wittman and H.-H. Schassan. Penetration of eight β-lactam antibiotics into the peritoneal fluid. *Arch. Surg., 118*:205 (1983).
108. K. Matsumoto, Y. Uzuka, T. Nagatake, H. Shishido, H. Suzuki, and K. Watanabe. Laboratory and clinical studies on 6059-S, a new oxacephem antibiotic. *Chemotherapy Tokyo Suppl., 7*:578 (1980).
109. N. Cho, K. Fukunaga, and K. Kunii. Fundamental and clinical studies on 6059-S in the field of obstetrics and gynecology. *Chemotherapy Tokyo Suppl., 7*:892 (1980).

110. Z. Takase, K. Inoue, H. Shirafuji, and M. Uchida. Clinical and laboratory studies on 6059-S in the field of obstetrics and gynecology. *Chemotherapy Tokyo Suppl., 7*:924 (1980).
111. R. Motomura, K. Nakanishi, C. Teramoto, Y. Ichinose, Y. Nishimura, and T. Yamabe. Basic and clinical studies on 6059-S in the field of obstetrics and gynecology. *Chemotherapy Tokyo Suppl., 7*:953 (1980).
112. M. Ishikawa, M. Sakuraba, and T. Shimizu. Clinical studies of latamoxef on perinatal infections. *Jpn. J. Antibiot., 36*:2391 (1983).
113. N. Cho, H. Suzuki, T. Akiyama, E. Kawamura, M. Togo, S. Nishimoto, T. Hidaka, K. Fukunaga, and K. Kunii. A study of clinical application of latamoxef in perinatal period. *Jpn. J. Antibiot., 36*:2395 (1983).
114. K. Ninomiya, Y. Hasegawa, T. Kanamoto, T. Yoshimoto, K. Hamaya, K. Niwa, and T. Nishio. Fundamental and clinical studies of latamoxef during periparturient period. *Jpn. J. Antibiot., 36*:2409 (1983).
115. T. Yamamoto, J. Yasuda, M. Kanao, and H. Okada. Fundamental and clinical studies on latamoxef in the perinatal period. *Jpn. J. Antibiot., 36*: 2423 (1983).
116. Z. Takase, Y. Komoto, M. Nakayama, T. Miyoshi, M. Hujiwara, M. Seto, and H. Shirafuji. Study on latamoxef in the perinatal period. *Jpn. J. Antibiot., 36*:2431 (1983).
117. M. Hayasaki, Y. Takada, H. Kondoh, K. Itoh, K. Noda, M. Iida, C. Chin, Y. Yamada, S. Ohsugi, R. Katoh, Y. Lin, Y. Baba, and K. Wakita. Pharmacokinetics and clinical studies on latamoxef in the perinatal period. *Jpn. J. Antibiot., 36*:2437 (1983).
118. J. L. Axelrod and R. S. Kochman. Moxalactam concentration in human aqueous humor after intravenous administration. *Arch. Ophthalmol., 100*:1334 (1982).
119. S. L. Kaplan, E. O. Mason, Jr., S. J. Kvernland, E. M. Loiselle, and R. D. Feigin. Moxalactam treatment of serious infections primarily due to *Haemophilus influenzae* type b in children. *Pediatrics, 71*:187 (1983).
120. H. Nakamura, S. Hayashi, K. Seki, T. Fukuda, S. Aoyama, and S. Kurasawa. Laboratory and clinical study of 6059-S, drug concentrations in uterus and adnexa tissues and clinical results. *Chemotherapy Tokyo Suppl., 7*:902 (1980).
121. K. Hirabayashi and E. Okada. Fundamental and clinical studies of 6059-S in the field of obstetrics and gynecology. *Chemotherapy Tokyo Suppl., 7*: 935 (1980).
122. E. Yamada, T. Hira, H. Haraguchi, and I. Mori. Fundamental and clinical studies on 6059-S in the gynecological field. *Chemotherapy Tokyo Suppl., 7*:966 (1980).
123. T. Iwasawa. Fundamental and clinical studies on 6059-S in the otorhinolaryngologic field. *Chemotherapy Tokyo Suppl., 7*:983 (1980).
124. J. Hondoh, S. Baba, K. Wada, T. Hatano, K. Murai, and Y. Suzuki. Laboratory and clinical studies on 6059-S in oto-rhino-laryngological field. *Chemotherapy Tokyo Suppl., 7*:996 (1980).
125. M. Imaizumi, J. Kimura, S. Akiyama, T. Uchida, I. Ichimura, K. Hirai, K.

Kawahara, and T. Kondo. Clinical studies on latamoxef of oxacephem antibiotics, especially concentration of latamoxef in lung tissues and prophylaxis of infections after thoracotomy. *Jpn. J. Antibiot., 36*:2081 (1983).

126. Y. Mori, T. Hirayama, and K. Kikuchi. Fundamental and clinical studies of latamoxef in intestinal surgery. *Jpn. J. Antibiot., 36*:2093 (1983).
127. T. Uoi, Y. Masubuchi, K. Hayashi, and Y. Inoue. A trial of pharmacokinetic analysis of tissue concentrations of drugs. *Jpn. J. Clin. Pharmacol. Ther., 14*:67 (1983).
128. D. A. Noe and K. M. Kumor. Drug kinetics in low-flux (small) anatomic compartments. *J. Pharm. Sci., 72*:718 (1983).
129. H. Okada, M. Kanao, T. Yamamoto, J. Yasuda, T. Oguma, and H. Yamada. Pharmacokinetic analysis of latamoxef in tissues. *Jpn. J. Clin. Pharmacol. Ther.*, (in press).
130. H. Yamada, T. Ichihashi, K. Hirano, and H. Kinoshita. Plasma protein binding and urinary excretion of R- and S-epimers of an arylmalonylamino 1-oxacephem I: In humans. *J. Pharm. Sci., 70*:112 (1981).
131. R. Wise, N. Wright, and P. J. Wills. Activity, stability, and pharmacology of the epimers of moxalactam. *Rev. Infect. Dis. Suppl., 4*:S564 (1982).
132. M. C. Nahata, D. E. Durrell, and W. J. Barson. Moxalactam epimer kinetics in children. *Clin. Pharmacol. Ther., 31*:528 (1982).
133. M. D. Reed, S. C. Aronoff, C. M. Myers, M. P. Husak, J. S. Bertino, Jr., and J. L. Blumer. Developmental pharmacokinetics of moxalactam. *Antimicrob. Agents Chemother., 24*:383 (1983).

13

Cefoxitin and Other Cephamycins

EDWARD O. STAPLEY
Merck Institute for Therapeutic Research, Rahway, New Jersey
EDWARD S. INAMINE and CHRISTOPHER M. MARTIN
Merck Sharp & Dohme Research Laboratories, Rahway, New Jersey and West Point, Pennsylvania

I. DISCOVERY AND DEVELOPMENT OF CEPHAMYCINS

A. Introduction

The discovery of the cephamycins represents the finding of a third valuable group of beta-lactam antibiotics differentiated from the first group, the penicillins, by the presence of an additional carbon in the bicyclic ring system as seen in the cephalosporins and differentiated from the cephalosporins by the presence of an α-methoxyl group in the 7-position as shown in Figure 1. The finding of various members of the cephamycin family was reported independently by Nagarajan et al. (1) and Stapley et al. (2) with Miller et al. (3). The first four compounds shown in Figure 1 were identified in these early reports. All of these natural products shared the α-aminoadipoyl moiety in the 7β-position. The differences, as shown in Figure 1, between the various natural cephamycins are found in the substitutions to the 3-position. These were the first cephem compounds discovered as products of actinomycetes. As such, they heralded the discovery of many new beta-lactam antibiotics, as recently reviewed by Cassidy (4), and it is now clear that the actinomycetes have the capacity to produce a very wide variety of beta-lactam antibiotics. Additional members of the naturally occurring cephamycins have been subsequently reported and are shown in Figure 1 (1,2,5–8).

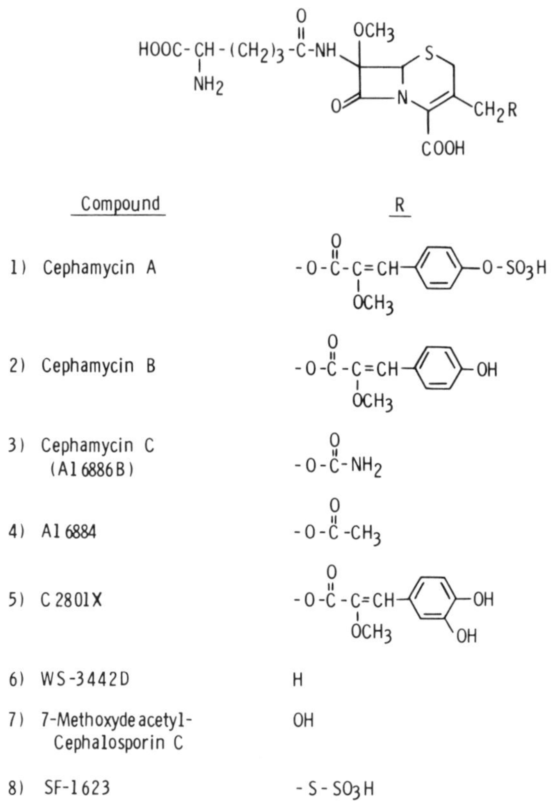

Figure 1 Cephamycins: natural actinomycete products.

B. Natural Cephamycin Products

1. In Vitro Studies

Data on the comparative characteristics of the natural cephamycin products are very limited. The most detailed studies available are on cephamycins A, B, and C. The characteristics of these substances will be discussed here as the basis for the development of cefoxitin and other semisynthetic cephamycin antibiotics. The antibacterial spectrum of cephamycins A, B, and C reported by Stapley et al. (2) is shown in Table 1 and a comparison of cephamycins A, B, and C-2801X reported by Fukase et al. (5) is shown in Table 2. The different substitutions at the 3-position change the antibacterial spectrum and potency of these materials considerably. Cephamycin A is a broad-spectrum antibiotic active on both gram-positive and gram-negative cultures, but of low potency and poor chemical sta-

Table 1 Antibacterial Spectrum of Cephamycins A, B, and C

Test organism	Inhibition zone with 7-mm paper disks (mm)		
	Cephamycin A, 5 mg/ml	Cephamycin B, 1 mg/ml	Cephamycin C, 0.166 mg/ml
Bacillus sp.	22	16	8
Staphylococcus aureus	26	18	0
Bacillus subtilis	33	25	13
Sarcina lutea	26	23	10
Streptococcus faecalis	0	0	0
Proteus vulgaris	29	21	22
Pseudomonas aeruginosa	0	0	0
Serratia marcescens	0	0	0
Alcaligenes faecalis	25	25	27
Bordetella bronchiseptica	21	7	24
Salmonella gallinarum	15	7	21
Vibrio percolans	36	24	30
Xanthomonas vesicatoria	15	0	19
Escherichia coli	15	0	20

Source: Ref. 2.

bility. Cephamycin B is also a relatively unstable and low-potency compound, with its best activity against gram-positive bacteria and only very limited activity against selected gram-negative organisms. Cephamycin C is much more potent and stable than either cephamycin A or B, but its antibacterial activity is almost completely limited to the gram-negative organisms. The only other comparative data available, shown in Table 2, confirm the importance of variations in structure, since C-2801X is much more potent and stable than either cephamycin A or B, although it differs only slightly in structure. The lesson from these early studies is clear; the characteristics, both chemical and microbiological, of cephamycins are very much dependent on the substitutions to the basic chemical structure.

2. In Vivo Studies

In vivo studies undertaken by Miller et al. (9) confirm the characteristics shown in vitro with regard to antimicrobial spectrum.

Table 2 Antibacterial Spectrum of Cephamycins A, B, and C-2801X

Test organism	Minimal inhibitory concentration (μg/ml) Cephamycin A	Cephamycin B	Cephamycin C-2801X
Staphylococcus aureus	50	50	50
Bacillus subtilis	25	25	12.5
Escherichia coli	⩾100	⩾100	25
Proteus vulgaris	6.25	50	12.5
Proteus mirabilis	6.25	50	3.13
Klebsiella pneumoniae	⩾100	25	6.25
Pseudomonas aeruginosa	⩾100	⩾100	⩾100
Salmonella enteritidis	⩾100	⩾100	6.25
Alcaligenes faecalis	50	25	12.5

Source: Ref. 5.

Cephamycin A was shown to be active in vivo in the protection of mice against both gram-positive and gram-negative infections, but was poorly absorbed orally and low in potency. Cephamycin B was even less potent than cephamycin A. All three cephamycins were found to be active in vivo in the protection of mice against various bacterial infections, without evidence for toxicity when given parenterally. Cephamycin C, although its in vivo activity was chiefly limited to protection against gram-negative infections in mice, was a stable potent agent with activity equal or superior to that of the cephalosporin cephalothin. Mice were found to tolerate up to 10 g/kg, indicating remarkably little toxicity for this antibiotic.

3. Beta-Lactamase Resistance

A very important characteristic of the cephamycins is their resistance to beta-lactamase degradation. Data shown in Table 3 were presented in the first reports on this family of compounds: Cephamycins A and C were completely resistant to various beta-lactamase enzymes capable of rapid and complete destruction of cephalosporin C. Subsequent studies by Daoust et al. (10), reported in Table 4, clearly show that all three cephamycins studied are orders of magnitude more resistant to the potent beta-lactamase from *Enterobacter cloacae* than cephalosporin C. These differences in susceptibility to beta-lactamase were suspected to be related to the presence of the 7α-methoxyl group, pointed out earlier as the salient difference between the cephamycins and the cephalosporins.

Table 3 Beta-Lactamase Resistance of Cephamycins A and C

Antibiotic substrate	*Alcaligenes faecalis*; washed cells inactivation (%)
Cephamycin A	0
Cephamycin C	0
Cephalosporin C	⩾99

Source: Ref. 2.

4. Chemical Modification

The characteristics observed in the cephamycins, as well as the history of modification of the cephalosporins, suggested that chemical modification of the naturally occurring cephamycins might lead to a very valuable antimicrobial agent. Cephamycin C was selected as the starting point because of its stability and high potency. The objective was to substitute new groups for the α-aminoadipic acid found in the 7β-position of the natural compound. This task proved to be much harder than anticipated because the chemistry which applied to analogous change in the cephalosporin series did not work in the presence of the 7α-methoxyl substitution. Preparation of new cephamycins required the development of new chemical procedures. Karady et al. (11) developed a method for exchange of the side-chain, and Cama et al. (12) developed a procedure for stereospecific introduction of the 7-methoxyl group to the cephem molecule. With this new chemistry, it became possible to prepare a wide variety of semisynthetic cephamycins.

Table 4 Degradation of Cephem Antibiotics by Beta-Lactamase from *Enterobacter cloacae* 18410/62

Substrate	$V_{max} \times 10^{-3}$ (μM/min per mg protein)	$K_m \times 10^{-2}$ (μM)
Cephamycin A	1.2	9.5
Cephamycin B	1.0	6.2
Cephamycin C	3.3	2.4
Cephalosporin C	200	14.3

Source: Ref. 10.

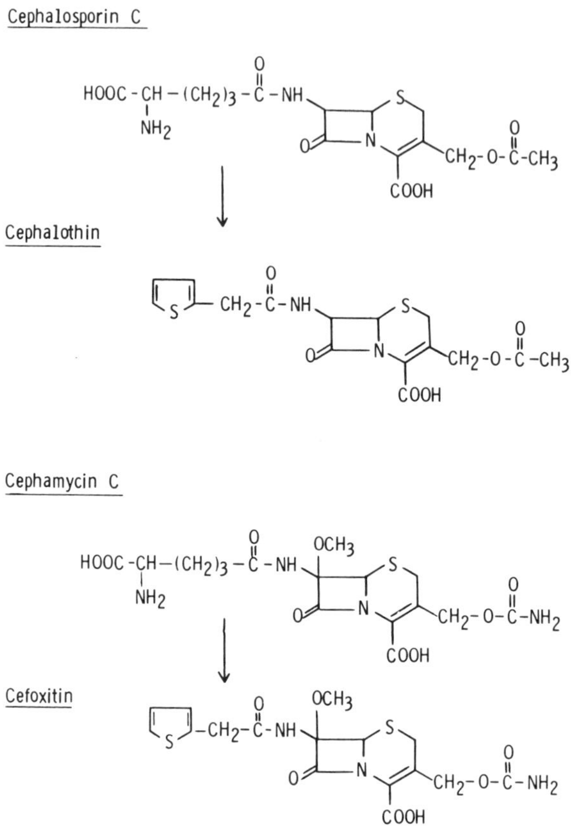

Figure 2 Comparison of natural and semisynthetic cephamycin and cephalosporin.

C. Cefoxitin: A Semisynthetic Product

Cefoxitin is prepared from cephamycin C in a manner analogous to the preparation of cephalothin from the natural product cephalosporin C as shown in Figure 2. The introduction of the 7β-thienyl group in place of the natural α-aminoadipic acid in cephamycin C results in the formation of cefoxitin. The new molecule differs from the analogous cephalosporin, cephalothin, by the presence of the 7α-methoxyl group and the 3-carbamoyl group in place of the 3-acetyl group found in cephalosporin C and the semisynthetic compound cephalothin. Thus cefoxitin and cephalothin differ from each other in exactly the same way as cephamycin C and cephalosporin C, from which they can be prepared.

Table 5 Effect of the Thienyl Group on Antimicrobial Activity

Test organism	Minimal inhibitory concentration (μg/ml)	
	Cephamycin C, 7β-adipoyl	Cefoxitin, 7β-thienyl
Staphylococcus aureus	>100	6.25
Streptococcus pneumoniae	>100	3.12
Escherichia coli	25	6.25
Klebsiella pneumoniae	12.5	3.12
Proteus mirabilis	3.12	6.25

Source: Ref. 13.

1. Effect of the Thienyl Group on Antimicrobial Activity

As discussed earlier, cephamycin C and cefoxitin differ in the substitution of the 7β-thienyl for the naturally occurring 7β-adipoyl group. The data in Table 5 (13) are representative of the difference in antimicrobial spectrum observed between these two compounds. Cefoxitin acquires potent antibiotic activity against gram-positive organisms such as *Staphylococcus aureus* and *Streptococcus pneumoniae* by virtue of the presence of the 7β-thienyl group. This change in spectrum is accompanied by retention, and even some enhancement, of the activity against gram-negative organisms. Thus the thienyl group confers broad-spectrum activity covering both gram-positive and gram-negative bacteria.

2. Effect of the Thienyl Group on Beta-Lactamase Sensitivity

Onishi et al. (14) studied the beta-lactamase sensitivity of cefoxitin compared to that of cephamycin C. Some data from these studies are reported in Table 6, where it may be seen that the thienyl group results in increasing the already impressive resistance of cephamycin C to beta-lactamase. Cefoxitin is about 175 times more resistant to the beta-lactamase, in this example, compared with cephamycin C.

3. Effect of the 7α-Methoxy Group on Beta-Lactamase Resistance

Comparison of cefoxitin to the analogous compound lacking the methoxyl group is reported in Table 7 (13). The compound cefoxitin is completely resis-

Table 6 Effect of the Thienyl Group on Beta-Lactamase Sensitivity

Antibiotic	$V_{max} \times 10^{-3}$ (μM/min per mg protein)	$K_m \times 10^{-2}$ (μM)
Cephamycin C, 7β-adipoyl	3.3	2.4
Cefoxitin, 7β-thienyl	0.019	0.6

Source: Ref. 14.

tant to two potent beta-lactamases under conditions where the analogous compound lacking the 7α-methoxyl group is completely destroyed. Thus it is clear that the 7α-methoxyl group is responsible for conferring beta-lactamase resistance on this family of compounds.

4. Effect of the 3-Carbamoyl Group

The 3-position of the cefoxitin molecule has a carbamoyl group as found in the natural product cephamycin C. The cephalosporin natural product has an acetoxy group in this position which is retained in the semisynthetic compound cephalothin (see Fig. 2). Comparison of cefoxitin with the analogous compound having the 3-acetoxy group is shown in the data of Table 8 (13). This change has very little effect on the in vitro activity of cefoxitin. Both compounds have comparable activity against *Staph. aureus* and *Morganella morganii*. However, although cefoxitin shows good activity in vivo by protecting mice against infections produced with these two pathogens, the 3-acetoxy analog has little in vivo potency. The carbamoyl group is resistant to the deacetylase enzymes found in vivo which remove the acetyl group from the 3-position of cefoxitin. In the case of the mouse this enzyme is very active and, in the example given here, results in the formation of a deacetylated compound which is not potent enough to protect the mice against these two infections. Similar metabolism is known to occur

Table 7 Effect of the 7α-Methoxy Group on Beta-Lactamase Resistance

Antibiotic	Inactivation (%) by beta-lactamase from	
	Enterobacter cloacae	*Escherichia coli*
Cefoxitin, 7α-OCH_3	0	0
Cefoxitin analog, 7α-H	>99	>99

Source: Ref. 13.

Table 8 Effect of the 3-Carbamoyl Group

Organism	Test	Cefoxitin, 3-carbamoyl	Analog, 3-acetoxy
Staphylococcus aureus	MIC[a] (μg/ml)	6.25	6.25
	ED_{50}[b] (mg/kg)	12.5	>100
Morganella morganii	MIC (μg/ml)	6.25	12.5
	ED_{50} (mg/kg)	7.55	>100

[a]Minimal inhibitory concentrations.
[b]Median effective dose.
Source: Ref. 13.

in humans, though to a much lesser extent than in the mouse, as discussed by Wick (15). Urinary recovery in various species is almost quantitative for cefoxitin, but much lower for the 3-acetoxy analog, which is degraded in vivo (13).

5. Structure Activity Summary for Cefoxitin

On the basis of the characteristics discussed and more extensive studies available in the literature (13), the structure-activity relationships for cefoxitin have been conclusively demonstrated. These are illustrated in Figure 3. The basic cephem structure becomes a true broad-spectrum antibiotic having activity of an equivalent nature in vitro and in vivo against gram-positive and gram-negative bacteria by substitution of the thienyl group for the α-aminoadipic group. The high beta-lactamase resistance is a result of the presence of the methoxyl group and the excellent metabolic stability is conferred by the presence of the carbamoyl

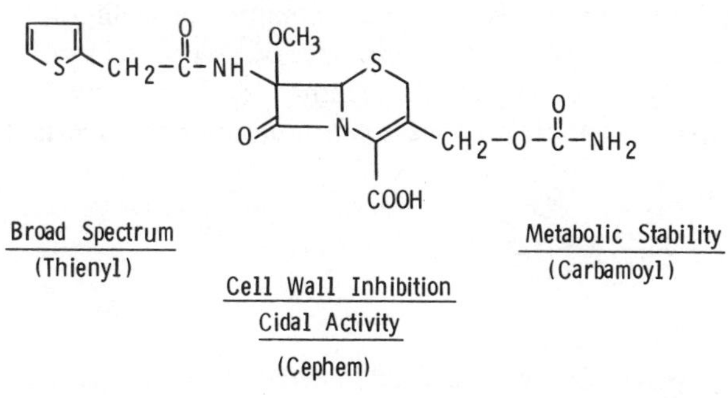

Figure 3 Structure-activity relationships for cefoxitin.

group. Cefoxitin is a cell wall-active antibiotic, as are the cephalosporin compounds, as shown from the studies of Onishi et al. (16). This activity must be attributed basically to the cephem nucleus found in both cephalosporin and cephamycin. It is interesting that the 7β-thienyl group not only conferred breadth of spectrum but also intensified the beta-lactamase resistance found in the natural cephamycins.

II. CEFOXITIN MODE OF ACTION

Both natural cephamycins, reported by Stapley et al. (2), and semisynthetic compounds, reported by Onishi et al. (16), are cell wall-active antibiotics that cause the formation of filaments and osmotically sensitive spheroplasts. A desirable result of this mode of action is a bactericidal effect which has been confirmed in many studies. Miller et al. (17) reported excellent correlation between in vitro susceptibility and in vivo efficacy in mouse protection studies for cefoxitin. One of the reasons for this good correlation is the bactericidal activity of cefoxitin as shown from the studies of Wallick and Hendlin (18) and Jones et al. (19). There is very little difference between the minimal inhibitory concentration (MIC) and minimal bactericidal concentration (MBC) for cefoxitin. Another reason for the excellent agreement between in vitro and in vivo data may well be the almost complete resistance to beta-lactamase exhibited by cefoxitin (14,20-22).

Since the initial studies on the penicillin-binding proteins of *E. coli* reported by Spratt (23,24), the characteristics associated with the penicillin-binding proteins have been well defined. Curtis et al. (25) found the binding of cefoxitin to be similar to that seen with another semisynthetic cephamycin, cefmetazole. The cephamycins are apparently strongly bound to penicillin-binding proteins 4 and 5/6, as well as 1A, 1B, and 3, which are clearly associated with bactericidal and lytic effects on the cell. Cephamycins appear not to be bound to penicillin-binding protein 2. Onishi et al. (16) demonstrated that cefoxitin was bound unusually tightly to the bacterial cell, which agrees with the work of Spratt (24), who reported that cefoxitin was essentially irreversibly bound to penicillin-binding proteins, especially 1 and 3. While the significance of observations on the penicillin-binding proteins is not completely established, the apparently irreversible binding of cefoxitin to these proteins is perceived to be an important characteristic.

III. MICROBIOLOGY OF CEFOXITIN

A. In Vitro Studies

The antimicrobial activity of cefoxitin was reported in detail by Wallick and Hendlin (18). They found it to be a broad-spectrum agent with activity against gram-positive aerobes, with the exception of *Enterococcus*, and gram-negative aerobes, with the exception of *Pseudomonas.* Data were developed by them to support the use of a 30-μg disk in the Kirby–Bauer sensitivity test (26), with susceptibility at 16 μg/ml or less chosen as the break point. Resistance was attributed to cultures showing an MIC of 32 μg/ml or more. They found cefoxitin to be more active than cephalothin against *Escherichia coli, Proteus mirabilis, Klebsiella,* indole-positive *Proteus,* and *Providencia.* There was even some activity against *Serratia,* an unusually resistant pathogen. In a study of clinical isolates selected because of their resistance to cephalothin, the authors found 66% of 174 of such cultures to be susceptible to cefoxitin.

Wallick and Hendlin (18) also showed that the gram-positive pathogens *Staph. aureus, Strep. pneumoniae,* and some other streptococci, excluding *Enterococcus* and methicillin-resistant *Staphylococcus,* were sensitive to cefoxitin.

The results of a survey of clinical isolates for susceptibility to cefoxitin and cephalothin conducted at several major hospitals were reported by Stapley et al. (27), as summarized in Table 9. The survey covered nearly 25,000 clinical isolates and showed a clear overall superiority for cefoxitin over cephalothin for the gram-negative aerobes and essentially equivalent activity against gram-positive aerobes. Neither cephem antibiotic showed very good activity against *Enterococcus* or *Pseudomonas.* Cefoxitin was clearly superior against gram-negative anaerobic organisms. The latter observation was expected based upon studies with anaerobes by Sutter and Finegold (28), Tally et al. (29), Ernst et al. (30), Darland and Birnbaum (22), and Olsson et al. (31) as summarized in Table 10. The important gram-negative anaerobic pathogen *Bacteroides fragilis* was found to be quite sensitive to cefoxitin in contrast to its resistance to cephalothin. Thus, of 531 clinical isolates of *B. fragilis,* 92% were found susceptible to cefoxitin and

Table 9 Survey of Clinical Isolates for Susceptibility to Cefoxitin and Cephalothin

		Percent susceptible to	
Cultures	Number	Cefoxitin	Cephalothin
Gram-positive anaerobes	4,948	95	98
Enterococcus	1,767	6	16
Gram-negative aerobes	16,004	81	63
Pseudomonas	1,469	4	1
Gram-negative anaerobes	362	76	19
	24,550	74	62

Source: Ref. 27.

Table 10 Summary of Five Studies of the Susceptibility of *Bacteroides fragilis* to Cefoxitin and Cephalothin

Number of clinical isolates	MIC ≤ 16 μg/ml	
	Cefoxitin	Cephalothin
531	92%	9%

Source: Data summarized from Refs. 22 and 28-31.

only 9% to cephalothin. *Bacteroides fragilis* has been reported by DelBene and Farrar (32), Anderson and Sykes (33), and Olsson et al. (34) to produce a beta-lactamase with characteristics typical of a cephalosporinase. Darland and Birnbaum (22) studied the importance of this enzyme to the resistance of *B. fragilis* to beta-lactam antibiotics. They found that at least two different types of enzymes may be produced by *B. fragilis.* Cefoxitin was resistant to both enzymes but acted as a competitive inhibitor. While there was no significant association between the presence of beta-lactamase activity by *B. fragilis* and susceptibility or resistance to cefoxitin, a significant correlation with the presence of beta-lactamase and resistance to cephalosporins such as cefamandole, cefazolin, and cephaloridine was observed. Beta-lactamase from *B. fragilis* degraded cephaloridine, cephalothin, cefazolin, cefamandole, and cefuroxime, but not cefoxitin. Thus the excellent resistance to beta-lactamase of cefoxitin is a very important factor in determining the susceptibility of pathogens. Cefoxitin is also active against other anaerobes, such as *Fusobacterium, Peptococcus, Peptostreptococcus, Veillonella,* and *Clostridium*, as shown by Tally et al. (29) and Sutter and Finegold (28).

The susceptibility of the *B. fragilis* group, based upon the resistance of cefoxitin and other cephamycins to *B. fragilis* beta-lactamase, is not absolute, as evidenced by the fact that Cuchural et al. (35) recently reported the isolation of a rare *B. fragilis* culture which could inactivate cefoxitin. Yotsuji et al. (36) purified a beta-lactamase from a clinical isolate of *B. fragilis* and found that it was capable of actively degrading cefoxitin and other cephamycin antibiotics.

B. In Vivo Studies

Evaluation of cefoxitin in experimental infections in laboratory animals was reported by Miller et al. (37). These studies confirmed the observations made in in vitro tests that the good gram-negative activity of cephamycin C was retained and intensified in cefoxitin while the lack of significant activity against gram-positive organisms observed with cephamycin C was overcome in cefoxitin. Indeed, cefoxitin appeared to have essentially the same level of activity in vitro and in vivo against both gram-positive and gram-negative pathogens. The exceptions to this sensitivity were the expected ones of *Pseudomonas* and *Enterococcus* and the methicillin-resistant *Staphylococcus.* Even such resistant pathogens as *Serratia* and *M. morganii* and some strains of *Ent. cloacae* could be protected against in mouse infection studies. Thus the favorable data observed for cefoxitin with regard to beta-lactamase resistance and extended spectrum of activity was confirmed in studies of protection of mice against experimental infections.

The importance of the high level of resistance of cefoxitin to beta-lactamase was also emphasized in a study by Miller et al. (17) which compared the relationship of in vitro activity to in vivo efficacy for experimental infections in mice. In vitro activity very accurately predicted in vivo efficacy with cefoxitin, but such was not the case with the cephalosporin cefamandole. Pathogens which produced beta-lactamase were less sensitive to cefamandole in vivo than would be predicted from the in vitro susceptibility testing.

IV. CEFOXITIN AND OTHER SEMISYNTHETIC CEPHAMYCINS

The discovery of the cephamycins and the subsequent development of the first semisynthetic product, cefoxitin, stimulated a considerable research effort in various organizations looking for other new variations on the cephamycin structure. From the large number of compounds that have been made and studied, seven substances have been reported as selected for superior characteristics (see Fig. 4). The first substance to be studied in detail and introduced into the market as a therapeutic for human infections was cefoxitin. This was followed by cefmetazole, developed in Japan. There are currently active evaluation studies in progress on cefotetan and cefbuperazone. Very little information has appeared about MT-141. Compounds SKF 73678 and SQ 14359 did receive preclinical evaluation and have been discussed in an earlier review (38) but apparently will not be developed as marketed products.

All of the cephamycins suggested as competitive or superior compared to cefoxitin share the same methyltetrazole substitution on the 3-carbon of the six-membered ring in contrast to the carbamoyl group of cefoxitin (Fig. 4). The differences between these various compounds are found in the changes in the 7β-side chain on the four-membered lactam ring. All of these semisynthetic cephamycins are broad-spectrum antibiotics with general characteristics similar to those of cefoxitin.

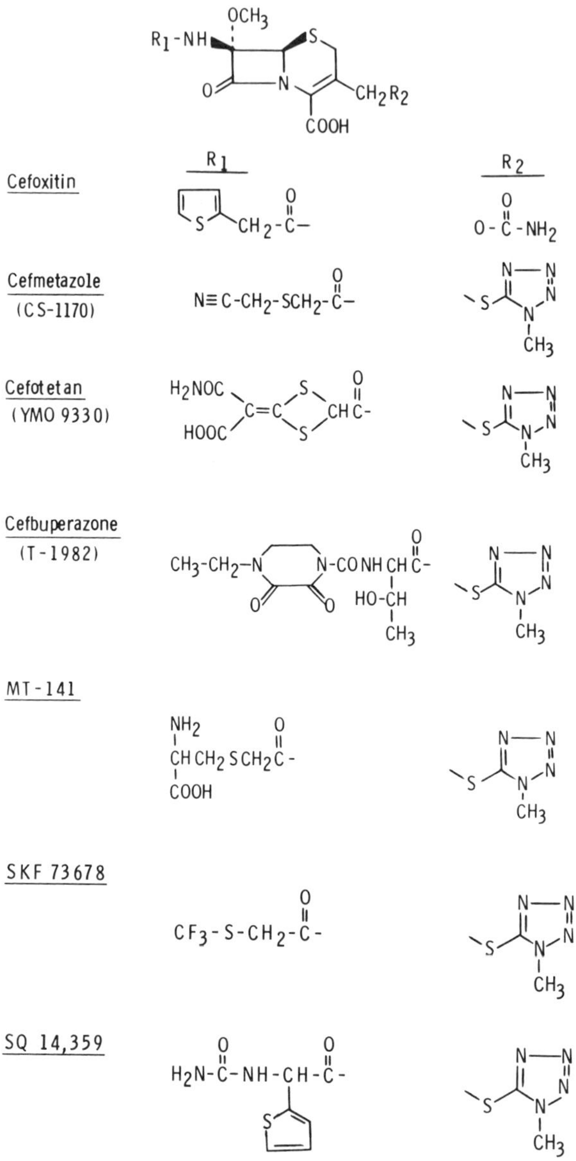

Figure 4 Cephamycins: semisynthetic products.

A. SKF 73678

The in vitro activities for SKF 73678 and cefmetazole are very similar to that of cefoxitin against selected test organisms, with in vitro activity two to four times greater than that of cefoxitin (39). The three cephamycins were considered almost equivalent, with a slight potency advantage for SKF 73678 and CS-1170 but a better pharmacokinetic profile, in mice, for cefoxitin. The MIC values for 213 clinical isolates comparing cefoxitin and SKF 73678 confirmed the spectrum comparison. The overall spectrum against the clinical isolates was very similar for cefoxitin and SKF 73678, with a higher in vitro potency, usually two- to four-fold for SKF 73678. In vivo data in the protection of mice against experimental infections were reported for this same comparison, with results roughly parallel to those observed in vitro. A susceptibility comparison from these studies of cefoxitin and SKF 73678 in vitro, is presented in Table 11. Surprisingly, these workers did not report anything about the activity of SKF 73678 versus anaerobes, one of the most important characteristic activities for the cephamycins.

Table 11 In Vitro Susceptibility Comparison for Cefoxitin and SKF 73678

Culture identity	Number of strains	Percent susceptible to 12.5 μg/ml or less	
		Cefoxitin	SKF 73678
Staphylococcus aureus	25	100	100
Escherichia coli	24	88	100
Enterobacter aerogenes	21	19	90
Enterobacter cloacae	21	10	67
Klebsiella pneumoniae	25	100	100
Proteus mirabilis	24	92	92
Proteus, indole positive	25	88	92
Serratia marcescens	25	56	56
Citrobacter spp.	10	80	90
Providencia spp.	9	89	89

Source: Data from Ref. 39.

B. SQ 14359

The general characteristics of SQ 14359 have been compared by Gadebusch et al. (40) with cefmetazole and cefoxitin. All three compounds were similar in potency against gram-positive organisms *Streptococcus pyogenes* and *Strep. pneumoniae* and the two gram-negative cultures *Neisseria gonorrhoeae* and *B. fragilis.* Cefmetazole and SQ 14359 were more potent than cefoxitin against *Staph. aureus, Klebsiella, Shigella, E. coli,* and *Salmonella.* In susceptibility determinations similar percentages of gram-positive and gram-negative pathogens fell within the susceptibility range of all three antibiotics for these organisms. The compound SQ 14359 was somewhat more potent against *Ent. cloacae, Citrobacter,* and *Serratia.* A comparison of the performance of SQ 14359, cefoxitin, and cefmetazole in experimental infections in mice confirms the similarity in their antimicrobial spectrum based upon in vivo efficacy (Table 12). In parallel with the general observations on in vitro potency, cefmetazole and SQ 14359 were somewhat more potent than cefoxitin. All three of these antibiotics were resistant to beta-lactamase and bactericidal, as would be expected. In experiments comparing the pharmacology of these agents in mice and rats, cefoxitin gave a somewhat higher serum concentration and a considerably higher urinary recovery. It may be inferred from these observations that both SQ 14359 and cefmetazole were excreted to a much greater extent than cefoxitin by the biliary route, since no metabolites of these two agents were reported. The signi-

Table 12 Efficacy of Cefoxitin, Cefmetazole, and SQ 14359 in Experimental Infections in Mice

Infection	ED_{50} (mg/kg)		
	Cefoxitin	Cefmetazole	SQ 14359
Staphylococcus aureus	20	9.8	6.9
Escherichia coli	4	2	2
Salmonella schottmuelleri	11	4	0.6
Klebsiella pneumoniae	6	2.6	1.7
Morganella morganii	25	13.4	55
Proteus rettgeri	78	111	55
Citrobacter freundii	186	80	89
Serratia marcescens	26	16	7.4
Enterobacter cloacae	193	182	76

Source: Data from Ref. 40.

ficance of these pharmacokinetic differences is important in evaluating animal protection experiments but may not be reflected in humans. In general, it appears that SQ 14359 is very similar in its biological characteristics to cefoxitin, with a somewhat higher in vitro potency which appears to carry over to animal protection experiments. As in the case of SKF 73678, in vitro differences in potency are not as obvious in in vivo experiments, which may well be the result of pharmacokinetic differences favoring cefoxitin in mice.

C. Cefmetazole

It has already been pointed out that cefmetazole is very similar to cefoxitin in its antibacterial spectrum but appears to be more potent in vitro by a factor of 2-4. The difference seen in in vivo experiments in animals is not as marked as that seen in in vitro tests (see Table 12). This pattern is attributed to differences in the pharmacokinetics between cefmetazole and cefoxitin which favor cefoxitin (41). One of the factors may be increased excretion of cefmetazole by the biliary route. In vitro data on cefmetazole are reported in Table 14 in comparison with cefoxitin and cefbuperazone. Tai et al. (42) confirmed the results of other workers to show that cefmetazole is generally more active than cefoxitin by a factor of about 2. The antibacterial spectrum is very nearly identical. Both cefoxitin and cefmetazole are broad-spectrum agents with almost complete resistance to beta-lactamase but lack effective activity against the gram-negative bacteria *Enterobacter* and *Pseudomonas* as well as the gram-positive pathogens *Enterococcus* and methicillin-resistant *Staphylococcus.* These comparisons in vitro have been confirmed by the work of Benlloch et al. (43), who found that cefmetazole was more active than cefoxitin in a study with 322 clinical isolates, with the important exception of *B. fragilis.* In the case of *B. fragilis* these workers found the potency advantage to be with cefoxitin.

D. Cefotetan

Some of the biological characteristics of this new substance were first reported by Saito et al. (44) in comparison with cefoxitin, cefmetazole, and cefazolin. Cefotetan (YM09330) was two to four times less active than cefoxitin against gram-positive bacteria but more potent than cefoxitin against gram-negative bacteria, except *Pseudomonas aeruginosa* and *Acinetobacter calcoaceticus,* which were not sensitive. Cefotetan had activity equivalent to cefoxitin against *Bacteroides* spp. Antibacterial spectrum data were reported in support of these observations except for the anaerobe cultures. From these data it appears that cefotetan has acquired somewhat increased gram-negative potency at the expense of activity against the gram-positive pathogens. As would be expected, cefotetan is a cell wall-active antibiotic binding to cell membrane proteins, including four novel binding proteins in a strain of *E. coli.* Cefotetan has a stronger

Table 13 In Vitro Activity of Consecutive Clinical Isolates to Cefoxitin and Cefotetan

Organism group	Number of isolates	Antibiotic	Cumulative percent susceptible at μg/ml						
			0.125 μg/ml	0.5 μg/ml	1 μg/ml	2 μg/ml	4 μg/ml	8 μg/ml	32 μg/ml
Enterobacteriaceae	7474	Cefoxitin	0	1	12	39	66	75	82
		Cefotetan	66	81	86	89	91	93	97
Other gram-negative bacilli	2040	Cefoxitin	0	1	1	2	3	4	7
		Cefotetan	2	3	3	4	5	7	14
Gram-positive cocci, except enterococci	1714	Cefoxitin	2	6	17	32	87	94	98
		Cefotetan	1	2	4	6	22	72	92
Enterococci	1032	Cefoxitin	0	0	0	1	2	2	5
		Cefotetan	0	0	0	0	1	1	2

Source: Data from Ref. 45.

lytic activity than cefoxitin, perhaps explaining the higher gram-negative potency of cefotetan. Ayers et al. (45) reported antibacterial spectrum data based on a survey of over 12,000 consecutive clinical isolates. The results of their studies comparing cefoxitin and cefotetan are summarized in Table 13. These data confirm the observations of Saito et al. (44) for the Enterobacteriaceae. Both agents are active, with a potency advantage for cefotetan. Neither antibiotic is very active against other gram-negative bacilli such as *Pseudomonas,* nor are they active against the enterococci. In the case of gram-negative cocci, except enterococci, the potency advantage lies with cefoxitin. The data indicated that cefotetan resembles the "third-generation" cephems versus gram-negative bacteria but is less active against the gram-positive pathogens. Bauernfeind (46) found similar results and reported cefotetan to be the least active of six cephem antibiotics tested against *Staphylococcus.* These observations have been repeated and confirmed by numerous workers. An additional important observation which has been repeatedly made is that cefotetan is less active than cefoxitin against *B. fragilis,* in contrast to the original report of Saito et al.

The general picture for antimicrobial activity for cefotetan compared with cefoxitin is that it is more active on Enterobacteriaceae and less active against gram-positive bacteria and *B. fragilis.* Reports to that effect have come from Chattopadhyay and Teli (47), Clarke and Zemcov (48), Grassi et al. (49), and Ruckdeschel (50). Owens and Finegold (51) found 98% of *B. fragilis* susceptible to cefoxitin at clinically achievable concentrations, compared to 53% for cefotetan. This difference may be attributable to the difference in stability to beta-lactamase produced by *B. fragilis,* since Moosdeen et al. (52) found cefoxitin to be more stable to *Bacteroides* beta-lactamase than cefotetan and also reported that cefoxitin was more active than cefotetan versus *B. fragilis* clinical isolates. These observations suggest that cefotetan may have achieved increased potency against gram-negative cultures at the expense of activity against both gram-positive pathogens and gram-negative anaerobes. The activity of cephamycins against *B. fragilis* is a salient characteristic important to their clinical utility.

E. Cefbuperazone

The antibacterial activity of cefbuperazone (T-1982) was reported in 1982 by Tai et al. (42). Representative data on the in vitro activity of cefbuperazone compared to that of cefmetazole and cefoxitin from the work of these investigators is presented in Table 14. Cefbuperazone has superior activity compared with the other two cephamycins against gram-negative bacteria, especially *Serratia marcescens, Enterobacter,* and *Citrobacter.* As in the case of cefotetan, cefbuperazone has achieved this improved gram-negative activity at the expense of a loss in potency against gram-positive organisms. This drop in gram-positive activity may be great enough so that cefbuperazone should be considered essentially a gram-negative-active antibiotic. It is interesting that it appears to have re-

Table 14 In Vitro Activity of Cefbuperazone Compared to That of Cefmetazole and Cefoxitin

Organism	Number of isolates	MIC$_{50}$ (μg/ml)		
		Cefbuperazone	Cefmetazole	Cefoxitin
Staphylococcus sp.	25	12.5	0.78	3.13
Escherichia coli	25	0.2	0.78	6.25
Klebsiella pneumonia	15	0.2	1.56	6.25
Proteus mirabilis	25	1.56	3.13	12.5
Proteus vulgaris	20	1.56	3.13	6.25
Proteus rettgeri	25	1.56	1.56	3.13
Morganella morganii	25	3.13	6.25	12.5
Serratia marcescens	20	6.25	100	100
Enterobacter sp.	14	0.39	⩾100	⩾100
Citrobacter freundii	20	6.25	50	⩾100
Hemophilus influenzae	25	1.56	3.13	6.25
Bacteroides fragilis	29	1.56	6.25	6.25

Source: Data from Ref. 42.

tained and perhaps even have superior activity against the gram-negative anaerobe *B. fragilis.* The other characteristics reported for cefbuperazone are those to be expected of a cephamycin. Little or no inoculum effect was observed, with results similar to those seen for cefoxitin and cefmetazole and much better than those observed with cefazolin and cefoperazone. In experiments on bactericidal activity, the MBC was approximately the same as the MIC, except versus *Staphylococcus* at a high inoculum level, where the results were equivalent to those observed with cefmetazole and cefoxitin. All three cephamycins were reported quite stable to a variety of beta-lactamase enzymes, both plasmid mediated and chromosomal. In a study of the protection of mice against experimental infections, the results were in good relation to the MIC values observed, and hence cefbuperazone was the least active of the three cephamycins versus *Staphylococcus* but the most active versus *E. coli, Klebsiella pneumoniae, Proteus vulgaris,* and *Ser. marcescens.* Overall, on the basis of this early report, cefbuperazone appears to be a superior cephamycin versus gram-negative bacteria, including anaerobes, but distinctly inferior versus gram-positive organisms such as *Staphylococcus.*

F. MT-141

The preparation of a new semisynthetic cephamycin, MT-141, from the natural product SF-1623 was reported by Iwamatsu et al. (53) in 1983. The data in this report have not been compared with those for established antibiotics in the cephamycin series, so there is no frame of reference for the evaluation of MT-141. The MIC values compared with those of the parent compound SF-1623 show that MT-141 has reasonably good activity against *Staph. aureus, E. coli, Prot. vulgaris,* and *Ser. marcescens.* Its in vivo activity is better than expected based upon the in vitro potency compared with other analogs studied. The significance of these observations and a true evaluation of MT-141 must await more extensive testing in comparison with established agents.

V. BIOSYNTHESIS OF THE CEPHAMYCINS

A. Introduction

Biosynthetic pathways of the cephamycins, cephalosporins, and penicillins have many reactions in common. Thus the pioneering studies on the latter two antibiotics have contributed significantly to the rapid progress seen with the cephamycins. The reader is referred to recent reviews for a comprehensive coverage of beta-lactam antibiotics in general (54,55).

B. Immediate Precursors of Cephamycin C

Incorporation studies with labeled substrates have established that L-α-aminoadipic acid, L-cysteine, and L-valine are precursors of the cephamycin molecule in *Nocardia* (formerly *Streptomyces*) *lactamdurans* (56) and in *Streptomyces clavuligerus* (57). The sites of incorporation of these amino acids are identical to that observed in the fungal synthesis of cephalosporin C. The methyl moiety of the 7α-methoxyl group is derived from the methyl of methionine (57). The oxygen attached to the C-3' methylene group and the oxygen in the 7α-methoxyl group are both derived from molecular oxygen (58). Carbamoyl phosphate serves as the precursor to the carbamoyl moiety attached to C-3' (59,60). Various cephamycins produced by other microorganisms differ from cephamycin C only with respect to the acyl group attached to C-3'.

In contrast to fungi, where L-α-aminoadipic acid is an obligate intermediate of lysine biosynthesis, the streptomycetes derive L-α-aminoadipic acid via the degradation of L-lysine (61). The enzyme, identified as L-lysine ε-aminotrans-

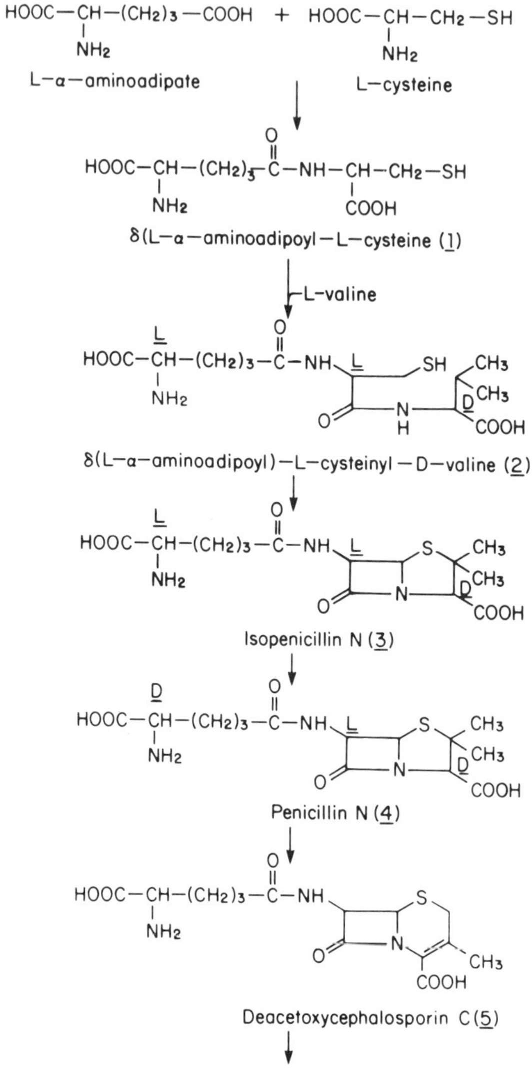

Figure 5 Scheme for the biosynthesis of the cephamycins.

ferase, converts L-lysine to L-1-piperideine-6-carboxylate (62). The subsequent oxidation to L-α-aminoadipic acid is catalyzed presumably by an NAD-linked enzyme. Studies with *N. lactamdurans* (63) suggest that cysteine for cephamycin C biosynthesis is preferentially derived from cystathionine via the trans-sulfuration pathway. The likely involvement of the pathway in antibiotic synthesis was

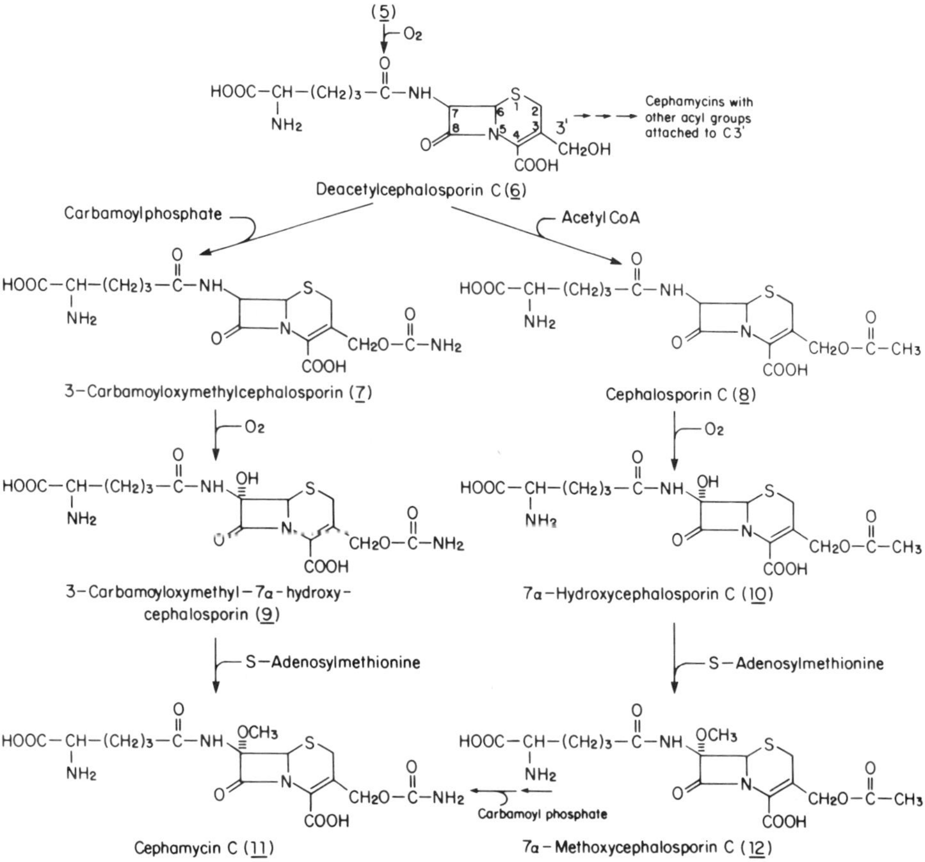

Figure 5 (continued).

indicated by the observation that propargylglycine, a potent mechanism-based inhibitor of the γ-lyase, is also a strong inhibitor of cephamycin C biosynthesis.

C. Sequence of Biosynthetic Reactions

The pathway of cephamycin C biosynthesis is outlined in Figure 5. Individual steps are discussed below.

1. δ-(L-α-Aminoadipoyl)-L-Cysteine, Compound 1

The dipeptide derived from the condensation of L-α-aminoadipate and L-cysteine has been found in the cells of the 7α-methoxycephalosporin producers *S. clavuligerus* and *Streptomyces lipmanii* (64). Synthesis of the dipeptide from the component amino acids by cell-free extracts of the cephalosporin C-producing fungus *Cephalosporium acremonium* was reported recently by Adlington et al. (65).

2. δ-(L-α-Aminoadipoyl)-L-Cysteinyl-D-Valine, Compound 2

The product derived from the condensation of δ-L-α-aminoadipoyl-L-cysteine and L-valine has been referred to as LLD-ACV and LLD-tripeptide. The compound has been detected in the mycelia of *S. clavuligerus* and *S. lipmanii* (64). It has also been found after incubation of *S. clavuligerus* washed cells with [1-^{14}C] valine (66).

3. Isopenicillin N, Compound 3

Conversion of the LLD-tripeptide to penicillin by a cell-free preparation of *S. clavuligerus* in about 10% yield was reported by Jensen et al. (67). The antibacterial spectrum of the reaction mixture indicated the production of both isopenicillin N and penicillin N. Cyclization of the tripeptide yields isopenicillin N while an epimerase (discussed elsewhere) converts isopenicillin N to penicillin N. Dithiothreitol and oxygen were absolutely required for the cylase activity while ascorbic acid and Fe^{2+} stimulated the reaction.

High-performance liquid chromatography has been employed to improve the quantification of the cyclization reaction (68). The disappearance of the LLD-tripeptide coincided with the appearance of isopenicillin N and penicillin N (antibiotics were not resolved). The conversion was 39.5% with a crude cell-free extract and 35.5% with an ammonium sulfate precipitate of the extract. Properties of the purified isopenicillin N synthetase from the cephalosporin C-producing fungus *C. acremonium* has been reported (69). The cyclization enzymes of the two organisms share similar properties with respect to dithiothreitol and cofactor requirements, pH, and temperature optima, and so on.

4. Penicillin N, Compound 4

The conversion of isopenicillin N to penicillin N involves the epimerization of the L-α-aminoadipoyl side chain to the D isomer. The epimerase activity in a cell-free extract of *S. clavuligerus* has been demonstrated with isopenicillin N as substrate (70). Penicillin N, the product, was bioassayed with *E. coli* Ess. The assay organism is about 30-fold more sensitive to penicillin N than to isopenicillin N. The streptomycete enzyme was found to be much more stable than the comparable epimerase enzyme of the fungus *C. acremonium.*

Partial purification and characterization of the *S. clavuligerus* epimerase have been reported by Jensen et al. (71). No cofactor requirements were demonstrated for the enzyme. However, although pyridoxal phosphate failed to stimulate activity, its presence during enzyme purification prevented the otherwise rapid and irreversible inactivation of the epimerase. The results imply that pyridoxal phosphate is tightly bound to the enzyme and that it is slowly lost during purification.

5. Deacetoxycephalosporin C, Compound 5

The conversion of penicillin N to deacetoxycephalosporin C has been demonstrated in cell-free extracts of *S. clavuligerus* (70). The requirements for 2-ketoglutarate, Fe^{2+}, and ascorbic acid indicate that the ring expansion enzyme is an intermolecular dioxygenase. Some enhancement of the activity was observed by the addition of Mg^{2+} while ATP was inhibitory. LLD-Tripeptide, isopenicillin N, and penicillin N were the only substrates that were transformed by the crude enzyme system. More recently Jensen et al. (72) have examined the ring expansion activity of a purified enzyme preparation from *S. clavuligerus* by high-performance liquid chromatography. Penicillin N was converted to deacetoxycephalosporin C in 85% yield after a 2-hr incubation. Purification of the comparable enzyme from the cephalosporin C-producing fungus *C. acremonium* was reported recently by Kupka et al. (73). The latter enzyme has a molecular weight of about 31,000 and its activity was inhibited by phosphate.

6. Deacetylcephalosporin C, Compound 6

Turner et al. (74) have demonstrated that cell-free extracts of *S. clavuligerus* oxidize the 3-methyl group of deacetoxycephalosporin C to a 3-hydroxymethyl group. The partially purified enzyme required ascorbate, dithiothreitol, Fe^{2+}, and 2-ketoglutarate for full activity. Its behavior is that expected of a 2-ketoglutarate-coupled intermolecular dioxygenase. The origin of the oxygen atom has been established by O'Sullivan et al. (58). Washed cells of *S. clavuligerus* incubated in the presence of $^{18}O_2$ showed that the oxygen linked to the exocyclic methylene at C-3' in cephamycin C is derived from molecular oxygen.

7. 3-O-Carbamoyloxymethylcephalosporin, Compound 7

Brewer et al. (60) have shown that cell-free extracts of *S. clavuligerus* transfer a carbamoyl group from carbamoyl phosphate to deacetylcephalosporin C to give 3-O-carbamoyloxymethylcephalosporin. The purified enzyme required ATP and a mixture of Mn^{2+} and Mg^{2+} for full activity. Phosphate stabilized the enzyme while pyrophosphate at 5 mM inhibited the reaction by 85%. High concentrations of ammonium sulfate and sodium chloride were found to inhibit the enzyme. The O-carbamoylphosphate transferase enzyme was found to accept an array of 7β-acylamino-3-hydroxymethylcephalosporins as substrate. An earlier study by Brewer et al. (59) with crude cell-free extracts of *S. clavuligerus* demonstrated the conversion of deacetyl-7α-methoxycephalosporin C and 7α-methoxycephalosporin C to cephamycin C in the presence of carbamoylphosphate. Brannon et al. (75) have reported that *S. clavuligerus* produces an extracellular esterase which hydrolyzes cephalosporin C to deacetylcephalosporin C. This result suggests that in the previous reaction 7α-methoxycephalosporin C was converted first to its deacetyl derivative, which then served as the substrate in the carbamoylation reaction.

8. 7α-Hydroxy-3-Carbamoyloxymethylcephalosporin, Compound 9; 7α-Hydroxycephalosporin C, Compound 10

To date only the conversion of cephalosporin C, compound 8, to 7α-hydroxycephalosporin C has been demonstrated. Hood et al. (76) isolated 7α-hydroxycephalosporin C after incubation of cephalosporin C with a cell-free extract of *S. clavuligerus.* O'Sullivan et al. (58) have shown that the oxygen in the 7α-methoxyl group of cephamycin C is derived from molecular oxygen.

9. 7α-Methoxycephalosporins, Compounds 11 and 12

Hood et al. (76) demonstrated that incubation of synthetic 7α-hydroxycephalosporin C with cell-free extracts of *S. clavuligerus* supplemented with S-adenosylmethionine gives rise to 7α-methoxycephalosporin C, compound 12. The latter compound is a normal metabolite of *S. lipmanii* (1). In other studies O'Sullivan and Abraham (66) demonstrated the ready conversion of 3-carbamoyloxymethylcephalosporin and cephalosporin C to cephamycin C, compound 11, and to 7α-methoxycephalosporin C, compound 12, respectively, by cell-free extracts of *S. clavuligerus.* Deacetylcephalosporin C was not a substrate, while deacetoxycephalosporin C, compound 5, was methoxylated only poorly. The crude enzyme preparation required 2-keto-glutarate, Fe^{2+}, ascorbic acid, and S-adenosylmethionine for full activity. The results of these studies strongly suggest that introduction of the methoxyl group via a hydroxylation-methylation sequence represents the final step in the biosynthesis of cephamycin C.

VI. REGULATION OF CEPHAMYCIN C BIOSYNTHESIS

A. Carbon Catabolite Regulation

Carbon regulation of cephamycin C production in *S. clavuligerus* has been reported by Aharonowitz and Demain (77). Preferred carbon sources supported good growth but decreased antibiotic production, while less readily metabolized carbon sources supported high specific production. It is not known whether the control mechanism involves inactivation, repression, or inhibition of the antibiotic–synthesizing machinery.

Recent studies by Braña et al. (78) with resting cells of *S. clavuligerus* indicate that the inhibitory effect of carbon sources is related to aeration. Glycerol at 1% strongly inhibited antibiotic production, but this effect was reversed by increased aeration. A similar release from carbon regulation was achieved at normal aeration conditions when cell density was decreased fivefold from normal.

Since several reactions in the pathway of cephem biosynthesis require molecular oxygen, the authors suggested that the observed effect may be due to competition for oxygen between product synthesis and respiration.

B. Nitrogen Metabolite Regulation

Ammonium salts as sole nitrogen source are reported to support growth but to strongly inhibit the production of cephamycin C by *S. clavuligerus* (79). When excess ammonium was added to growing cells, the repressive effect was dependent on the time of its addition. Severe inhibition was observed only when the addition was made during the growth phase, and later additions had essentially no effect. Lilley et al. (80) have reported that cephamycin C synthesis by *Streptomyces cattleya* is under nitrogen control. Optimum titers were obtained only under nitrogen-limited conditions.

Involvement of glutamine synthetase in ammonium regulation has been suggested by the results of Aharonowitz (81) with *S. clavuligerus*. A positive correlation was found between high specific productivity and high levels of glutamine synthetase. Cells grown in the presence of excess ammonium exhibited low titer and low glutamine synthetase activity. Additionally, extracellular serine protease levels were also found to be depressed. Ginther (82) has reported that production of cephamycin C and serine protease is coordinately regulated in *N. lactamdurans*. Strains that produced high levels of drug formed equally high levels of the protease.

C. Other Regulatory Processes

Regulation of lysine biosynthesis via the aspartate pathway in *S. clavuligerus* has been examined by Mendelovitz and Aharonowitz (83). Their results suggested that flow of carbon from aspartate to lysine is rate limiting in cephamycin C biosynthesis. Thus the addition of lysine, α-aminoadipate, or diaminopimelate to a fermentation stimulated antibiotic production by twofold.

These authors have isolated mutants resistant to the lysine analog S-(2-aminoethyl)-L-cysteine, whose aspartokinase was no longer sensitive to concerted feedback inhibition by threonine and lysine (84). Many of the mutants produced up to six-fold more antibiotic. Intracellular pools of free amino acids of these superior mutants showed considerable elevation of diaminopimelate, and the lysine level was also increased significantly. Accumulation of diaminopimelate implies that the decarboxylase is under regulation as suggested by Kirkpatrick et al. (85). An S-(2-aminoethyl)-L-cysteine-resistant mutant of *S. lipmanii* which produced 30% more 7α-methoxycephalosporin C than its parent has been reported by Godfrey (86).

Lysine ε-aminotransferase, the first enzyme involved in the transformation of lysine, is reported to be inhibited by α-aminoadipate, the end product of the reaction sequence (87).

D-Lysine is reported to greatly stimulate cephamycin C production by *N. lactamdurans* (88). The amino acid is not a precursor of the antibiotic and its regulatory role is not known.

VII. CEPHAMYCIN C FERMENTATION

Production of the antibiotic by fermentation of *S. clavuligerus* has been described by Nagarajan (89), and that of *N. lactamdurans* by Stapley et al. (2).

The seed medium for *N. lactamdurans* contained (in grams per liter) ardamine (10.0), dextrose (10.0), $MgSO_4 \cdot 7H_2O$ (0.05), and phosphate buffer (2.0 ml of a solution containing KH_2PO_4, 91.0 g, and Na_2HPO_4, 95.0 g, in a liter of water). The best production medium reported contained (in grams per liter) amber 300 yeast (10.0) and distiller's solubles (20.0). Inamine and Birnbaum (90) have described an improved production medium for this culture. It contained (in grams per liter) distiller's solubles (30.0), dried yeast (7.5), glycerol (12.5), dimethylformamide (10.0), glycine (0.5), L-phenylalanine (3.0), Mobil Par S defoamer (2.5), and DL-lysine (1.0).

VIII. ISOLATION OF CEPHAMYCIN C

Methods of cephamycin C isolation from fermentation broths have been described for *N. lactamdurans* (3), *S. clavuligerus* (89), and *Streptomyces jumonjinensis* (91). Miller et al. (3) employed the following sequence of steps with *N. lactamdurans*: (a) Filtered broth was passed through a column of Dowex 1 x 2 chloride cycle resin and the adsorbate eluted with 5% sodium chloride, (b) active fractions were pooled, adjusted to pH 2 with hydrochloric acid, charged onto a column of Dowex 50 x 2 hydrogen cycle resin, and the adsorbate eluted with 2% pyridine, (c) active fractions were pooled, neutralized with dilute NaOH, concentrated, chromatographed on Dowex 1 x 2 chloride cycle resin, and the activity eluted with pyridine hydrochloride buffer (0.1 M, pH 5.0), and (d) active fractions were pooled, adjusted to pH 8, concentrated to remove pyridine, and finally desalted on Bio-Gel P-2 to give the sodium salt of cephamycin C.

IX. CHEMICAL CONVERSION OF CEPHAMYCIN C TO CEFOXITIN

Semisynthetic cephalosporin C derivatives are prepared by first chemically removing the D-aminoadipoyl group of cephalosporin C to give 7-aminocephalosporanic acid. New cephalosporins are generated by derivatizing the latter compound with various acyl groups. Application of such chemistry to cephamycin C was prevented by the inherent instability of the 7-amino-7α-methoxycephalosporanic acid derivative. In order to circumvent this problem, a novel transacylation reaction sequence was developed for the synthesis of cefoxitin and other derivatives of cephamycin C (11,92). Cefoxitin is the generic name assigned to 7α-methoxy-7-[2-(2-thienyl)acetamido]-3-carbamoyloxymethyl-3-cephem-4-carboxylate.

The N-trichloroethoxycarbonyl derivative of cephamycin C was prepared followed by esterification with diphenyldiazomethane to give the N-trichloroethoxycarbonyl dibenzyl ester of the antibiotic. Treatment of the latter compound with thienylacetyl chloride and N-trimethylsilyltrifluoroacetamide gave the N-diacylated imide. On treatment of the imide with Zn in 90% acetic acid, the aminoadipoyl group was preferentially removed by transacylation. Cefoxitin free acid was then produced by deesterification of N-thienylacetylcephamycin C benzhydryl ester by treatment with trifluoroacetic acid and anisole.

X. PHARMACOLOGY

Preliminary information regarding the pharmacology of cefoxitin in laboratory animals was reported by Miller et al. (37). Their studies showed that the serum concentrations and the urinary recovery in mice after a 24-mg/kg subcutaneous dose of cefoxitin were two- to three-fold higher than for cephalothin. Tissue concentrations in mice tended to parallel the serum levels, so that the observed concentrations with cefoxitin were from 2- to 10-fold higher than those seen with cephalothin. Differences in the concentrations of the two drugs were attributed to the difference in the metabolic stabilities of these two antibiotics. As described earlier, cefoxitin undergoes very little metabolism to the descarbamoyl form, whereas appreciable amounts of cephalothin are metabolized in the mouse to the much less active desacetyl cephalothin. These investigators also showed that administration of probenecid resulted in higher and more prolonged serum concentrations of cefoxitin. Since probenecid is known to block the tubular excretion of beta-lactam antibiotics, these observations lead to the conclusion that cefoxitin is excreted by both tubular secretion and glomerular filtration. The significance of these observations for therapeutic applications was demonstrated in the treatment of experimental infections in mice. The ED_{50} values for infected mice treated with cefoxitin plus probenecid were one-half or less than those treated with the antibiotic alone. Studies on the oral administration of cefoxitin in laboratory animals, reported by Schrogie et al. (93), indicated that very little absorption took place in rats, mice, and monkeys. No serum concentrations could be detected in animals treated in this fashion and only 2–10% of the dose could be recovered in urine. These results are similar to the data which had been reported earlier for the natural cephamycins A and C by Miller et al. (9). Consequently, all studies in human subjects have involved the parenteral application of the drug.

Table 15 Mean Serum Concentrations of Cefoxitin or Cephalothin After a 3-min, 1-g Intravenous Infusion, with or Without Prior Probenecid Treatment[a]

Time after administration (min)	Serum concentration (μg/ml)			
	Cefoxitin	Cefoxitin + probenecid	Cephalothin[b]	Cephalothin + probenecid
5	124.77	115.33	101.80	103.05
10	62.82	89.23	58.30	75.92
20	38.66	68.91	24.57	56.60
40	19.16	52.73	11.28	39.43
60	12.09	40.39	5.89	26.08
90	7.23	33.04	3.11	14.75
120	4.21	25.83	1.50	9.51
180	<1.83	17.18	<1.0	5.56
240	<1.0	9.64	<1.0	2.32
360	<1.0	3.38	<1.0	<1.0

[a]Mean dose = 14.6 mg/kg cefoxitin or 14.7 mg/kg cephalothin, with or without 1 g of probenecid intravenously.
[b]Cephalothin-like activity is the sum of cephalothin plus desacetylcephalothin, which has about one-fourth the potency of cephalothin versus the assay organism.
Source: Data from Ref. 94.

Goodwin et al. (94) reported on the pharmacology of intravenous cefoxitin compared to cephalothin in humans. Their observations are in agreement with those reported for laboratory animal experiments. As shown in Table 15, cefoxitin gives somewhat higher and more prolonged blood levels than cephalothin and both drugs show increased and prolonged serum concentrations when administered following a dose of probenecid. The half-life ($T_{1/2}$) of cefoxitin was increased from 41 min with the drug alone to 83 min when probenecid was administered. Cephalothin had a half-life of 31 min, which increased to 59 min with probenecid. These studies suggest that cefoxitin is excreted by both tubular secretion and glomerular filtration.

Cefoxitin can be administered be either the intravenous or the intramuscular route. Some typical data from three different dosage regimens are shown in Table 16 from the studies of Brumfitt et al. (95). These results show that high serum levels are obtained by either intramuscular or intravenous dosage and that the half-life of the antibiotic is essentially the same by either route. Urinary re-

Table 16 Pharmacokinetic Observations for Three Dosage Regimens with Cefoxitin or Cephalothin

	Cefoxitin			Cephalothin		
Dosage (g)	Serum levels, mean peak (μg/ml)	T½ (hr)	Urinary recovery (%)	Serum levels, mean peak (μg/ml)	T½ (hr)	Urinary recovery (%)
0.5, i.m.	10.9	46	87.1	6.3	27	47.9
1.0, i.m.	22.5	45	90.1	20.8	28	55.5
2.0, i.v.	222.6	47	99.0	161.4	32	54.3

Source: Data from Ref. 95.

Table 17 Pharmacokinetics of Cefoxitin Related to Renal Function After a 30-min, 30-mg/kg Intravenous Infusion

Creatinine clearance (ml/min)	Serum concentration (μg/ml)	Serum $T_{1/2}$ (hr)	K_e[a] (hr^{-1})	V_{ad}[b] (liter)	Cefoxitin clearance (ml/min)	Urinary recovery of cefoxitin (%)		
						12 hr	24 hr	48 hr
Normal	125	0.78	0.894	7.70	329	86		
30–80	168	1.15	0.604	8.34	109	82	84	
10–30	151	6.31	0.110	12.26	19.8		55	60
10	158	13.18	0.053	11.33	6.2		27	36
Hemodialysis	189	21.56	0.032	12.58	–			

Source: Data from Ref. 132.
[a]Elimination constant rate per hour.
[b]Apparent volume of distribution of central compartment.

covery of cefoxitin is excellent, while that of cephalothin is much lower, a difference which can be attributed to metabolism to the desacetyl form (96-98). These pharmacokinetic observations have been confirmed and extended by several groups (99-102).

The pharmacology of cefoxitin has been reviewed by Schrogie et al. (103). Various reports have indicated serum binding in the range of 65-75% for cefoxitin. Less than 2% of cefoxitin is metabolized to the inactive descarbamoyl form, with recovery of 95% or more of the administered dose in urine after either intramuscular or intravenous administration. High concentrations of cefoxitin have been shown after recommended doses in virtually all body fluids studied (104-115), abnormal and/or infected body fluids (116-121), and tissues (122-129). The notable exception is the cerebrospinal fluid. Although regimens in the range of 2 g intravenously every 6 hr produce cerebrospinal levels of cefoxitin active against many strains of bacterial pathogens, these levels are probably inadequate to eradicate a substantial number of meningeal pathogens (130,131).

Administration of cefoxitin by intramuscular injection has been reported to be painful. The use of lidocaine with intramuscular injections prevents the pain on injection without any significant effect on the serum concentrations or excretion of the antibiotic (99).

Serum half-lives have been observed to increase rapidly with decrease in renal function (132-135). Fillastre et al. (132) studied the relationship of cefoxitin pharmacokinetics to renal function as shown in Table 17. Cefoxitin recoveries are still high, although necessarily prolonged, even with reduced renal function. The normal serum half-life was observed to increase from 0.78 to 21.6 hr with severe renal impairment (134,135).

Although the disposition of cefoxitin in pregnant women (136-138), patients with ascites (139), children (140), and premature and newborn babies (141) differs from that in normal, nonpregnant adults, the pharmacokinetics is similar.

Several investigators have concluded that the pharmacokinetics of cefoxitin fits a two-compartment open model as described by Schrogie et al. (103). Less than 1% of the cefoxitin dose is excreted into bile.

Cefoxitin is rarely dialyzed, as shown in studies with patients undergoing peritoneal dialysis (142,143) and hemodialysis (144).

Careful serial measures of glomerular filtration rate, renal enzymuria, and other parameters of renal function by Trollfors et al. (145) and Ormrod and Miller (146) failed to produce evidence that cefoxitin has nephrotoxic properties in recommended doses.

The concurrent presence of substantial concentrations of cefoxitin falsely elevates serum and urine levels of creatinine, as measured by the Jaffé reaction (147-149).

In summary, cefoxitin is well absorbed and distributed after either intramuscular or intravenous administration. It is rapidly excreted, with high tissue and urine concentrations and almost complete urinary recovery of the unaltered drug. Repeated administration does not result in drug accumulation.

XI. CLINICAL EXPERIENCE

A. Introduction

The results of in vitro studies, the resistance of cefoxitin to bacterial beta-lactamases, and the results of chemotherapeutic studies in a wide variety of experimental animal models of infection all suggest that cefoxitin would be clinically useful (150). The most valuable property of cefoxitin is the ability to both prevent and treat mixed aerobic-anaerobic infections (151-157). Cefoxitin has also been suggested for initial therapy of presumed bacterial infections of community origin, pending the results of culture and susceptibility studies (151).

B. Surgical Infections

The usefulness of cefoxitin in surgical infections (particularly intra-abdominal infections) was projected from the extensive studies of Bartlett et al. using the rat model for mixed aerobic-anaerobic infections (158). In this model of peritonitis, septicemia, and intra-abdominal abscesses, cefoxitin was as effective as any combination of antibiotics used in the model. Therefore it was anticipated that cefoxitin would find great utility as a single agent in infections involving multiple organisms—whether these were all aerobic, all anaerobic, or mixed aerobes and anaerobes.

The properties of cefoxitin responsible for its activity against anaerobes—particularly *B. fragilis*—have been reviewed by Tally (159).

Early clinical evidence of the effectiveness of cefoxitin in the management of surgical infections, including peritonitis and intra-abdominal abscess, was provided by several investigators (160-165). Their favorable observations have since been widely confirmed and extended (166-175).

C. Obstetric and Gynecological Infections

Since the flora of the female genital tract is complex and consists of both facultative as well as obligate anaerobes, combined therapy to cover a multiplicity of organisms has been used in the treatment of infections at this site. In both comparative and noncomparative studies, cefoxitin alone was used in the treatment of various infections such as endomyometritis, pelvic abscess, and pelvic inflammatory disease. Sweet et al. (176) treated 42 patients with acute salpingitis, endoparametritis, pelvic cellulitis, or pelvic abscess with cefoxitin in a dose of 3-6 g/day for a period of 5-10 days. Even though drainage is ordinarily required for the treatment of pelvic abscesses, three of seven patients with pelvic abscesses responded without drainage. The overall favorable clinical response to cefoxitin alone was 88%. Gonzalez-Enders et al. (177) reported a clinical cure rate of 100% in 70 cases of postpartum endometritis treated with cefoxitin and eradication of 95% of the strains of bacteria isolated. In 27 women with soft tissue pelvic infections treated with intravenous cefoxitin, White et al. (178) reported the clinical response was excellent, with a rate of 93%. Their favorable observations have been extensively confirmed and extended (167,179–185).

D. Skin and Skin Structure Infections

When skin and soft tissue infections are deep or in patients with poor vascular supply (such as in diabetes mellitus), they may be very difficult to treat. Fierer et al. (186) found that more than half of these infections in patients with diabetes were due to mixed aerobes and anaerobes and that *B. fragilis* was the most frequently isolated anaerobe. These authors were able to substitute cefoxitin for a combination of chloramphenicol or clindamycin plus an aminoglycoside; it was their impression that the clinical response was such that some extremities were salvaged owing to the rapid and relatively complete healing. Similarly, Perkins (187) combined the use of cefoxitin with incision and drainage in the treatment of soft tissue infections in patients with vascular compromise and noted a favorable response without resorting to amputation. McCloskey, in a treatment series of 35 patients with skin and soft tissue infections, noted a failure rate of only 3% (188).

Subsequent reports have confirmed these findings and identified new areas for successful application of cefoxitin therapy (171,189–192).

E. Urinary Tract Infections

In contrast to cephalothin, cefoxitin is excreted essentially unchanged into the urine; 70–95% of the administered dose is recovered unchanged in 24 hr. Neu (193) reviewed the clinical experience with cefoxitin in the treatment of urinary tract infections and noted a rate of favorable response of 94%; the most frequently recovered organisms were *E. coli* and other common members of the Enterobacteriaceae. Cox (194), in a study of infections in both complicated and uncomplicated urinary tract disease, found an overall cure rate of 87%; this included patients with indole-positive *Proteus* strains, which are always resistant to the first-generation cephalosporins. In general, the eradication rate for cephalosporin-resistant organisms treated with cefoxitin has been as good as that for cephalosporin-susceptible organisms. This ability to treat infections caused by cephalosporin-resistant organisms appears to be related to the extraordinary resistance of cefoxitin to beta-lactamases. In contrast to most of the first- and second-generation cephalosporins, cefoxitin has been shown to be active against many strains of *Ser. marcescens* (195), an important cause of urinary tract infections acquired in hospitals.

More recent reports (196-199) indicate the continuing efficacy of cefoxitin, without emergence of resistant bacterial strains.

F. Respiratory Tract Infections

Although active against most common lower respiratory tract pathogens, cefoxitin has proven particularly valuable in the management of infections characterized by mixed aerobic-anaerobic flora, such as aspiration pneumonia (200,201), and by polymicrobial sputum flora (202,203).

G. Bone and Joint Infections

In their clinical evaluation of cefoxitin on an orthopedic service, Schurman and Dillingham (204) treated 40 patients for moderate to severe infections. Of these, 15 had either osteomyelitis or joint infections, and most of these were caused by *Staph. aureus.* The cure rate was 80%. Similarly, Liu and Hinthorn (205) treated eight patients with osteomyelitis from 14 to 28 days. The dosage used was 4-12 g/day and a favorable clinical and bacteriological response occurred in all eight patients.

H. Septicemia and Endocarditis

Septicemia, that is, a positive blood culture in a patient with clinical sepsis, carries a high fatality rate. It is frequently treated with several antibiotics, particularly if the etiology at the time of patient admission is unknown. Pazin et al. (206) reviewed the clinical experience of 135 patients treated with cefoxitin for septicemia or bacteremia. The most commonly isolated organism was *E. coli*; the favorable outcome in that group of patients was 96%, while the overall rate of favorable outcome for all organisms was 83%.

Webb et al. (207) reported their experience with the use of cefoxitin in seven patients who had bacterial endocarditis. Five of these were caused by *Staph. aureus,* one by *Staphylococcus epidermidis,* and one by a beta-hemolytic *Streptococcus.* Blood cultures turned negative in less than 3 days; one patient had to be switched to alternate therapy after 10 days because of an adverse reaction. In none of the patients was there a recurrence after therapy was completed.

More recent reports (208,209) confirmed the earlier findings.

I. Infections in Immunosuppressed Patients

Partly because of its reliably bactericidal nature, cefoxitin may be used in the treatment of infections in immunosuppressed patients, particularly patients with cancer (210-215).

J. Gonorrhea

Extensive experience with the use of cefoxitin in the treatment of patients with uncomplicated gonorrhea caused by penicillin-susceptible or penicillin-resistant gonococci (216,217) demonstrated that the drug was highly efficacious in effecting clinical cure with eradication of the organisms. Because penicillin is still active against most strains of the gonococcus, cefoxitin should be used for cases in which resistance to penicillin and/or spectinomycin is suspected or shown to be present.

The steady spread of penicillin-resistant gonococci bearing plasmid-mediated beta-lactamase production capability has widened the use of cefoxitin for this indication and confirmed its usefulness (218,219).

K. Pediatric Infections

Increased recognition of the frequency of polymicrobial and mixed aerobic-anaerobic infections in children has led to wider use of cefoxitin in infants and children (220-224). Second-generation cephalosporins are also effective against *H. influenzae,* a common pathogen in pediatric patients.

L. Cefoxitin in Surgical Prophylaxis

For the same reasons that underlie the use of cefoxitin in the therapy of surgical infections (see above), the antibiotic has found wide use as a surgical prophylactic, significantly reducing the frequency of postoperative infection when utilized perioperatively for brief periods in operations classified as contaminated or potentially contaminated.

The preventative use of antibiotics in surgery has been controversial; more recently such use of antibiotics has gained a great deal of attention. Mickal et al. (225) reported in 1980 that cefoxitin was highly effective in reducing the infectious morbidity in patients undergoing vaginal hysterectomy when the drug was given perioperatively and for a short time postoperatively. Similarly, Larson et al. (226) demonstrated that cefoxitin was effective in reducing maternal infectious morbidity in women undergoing cesarean section, with the drug being given after the cord clamping and for not more than 24 hr. Additional studies have demonstrated the efficacy of cefoxitin in the prevention of wound infections in gastrointestinal surgery (227) and of site-related infections in surgery involving orthopedic prostheses (228).

Recent reviews of this topic discuss the role of cefoxitin (229-231).

Multiple studies confirm the earlier observations of the effectiveness of prophylactic cefoxitin in gastrointestinal surgery (232-242), vaginal hysterectomy (243-246), abdominal hysterectomy (247-249), cesarean section (250-254), transurethral prostatectomy (255,256), and orthopedic prosthetic surgery (257, 258).

M. Tolerance

Comparative studies of intravenous cefoxitin and cephalothin revealed that both were tolerated equally well; intolerance which did occur was almost always injection-site related and, interestingly, significantly related to the presence of a plastic indwelling catheter rather than to one of the drugs per se. The incidence of intolerance was extremely low in patients whose drugs were administered by small-gauge steel needles and changed every 24 hr or so. Thus the tolerance of this new cephamycin is comparable to that of the first-generation cephalosporins. When given intramuscularly, cefoxitin appears to be about as painful as the other cephalosporins (except cephaloridine, which is a zwitterion) and this pain is readily alleviated with the use of 0.5 or 1.0% lidocaine as a diluent (259).

N. Safety

Cefoxitin exhibits the same high degree of safety enjoyed by the penicillins and cephalosporins.

In their review of the experience with 1749 patients who received cefoxitin, Norrby et al. (260) noted that the most common reaction was the development of a rash. This occurred in 2.2% of the patients. Other reactions which occurred in those patients and which cefoxitin shares with other beta-lactam antibiotics include thrombophlebitis, diarrhea, and pruritus. Some patients receiving beta-lactams such as cefoxitin develop transient elevations of liver enzymes such as SGOT and SGPT, and a wide variety of hematological reactions have been described, some of which may be drug related. These include transient leukopenia and neutropenia. False-positive Coombs' tests have occurred and one case of hemolytic anemia was attributed to the drug.

Elevations of blood urea nitrogen and/or serum creatinine have occurred in patients treated with cefoxitin, but, as is the case for other beta-lactam antibiotics, these reactions occur in a setting in which the etiology of such changes is difficult to assess. In 153 patients treated concomitantly with gentamicin and cefoxitin, drug-related elevations of creatinine or blood urea nitrogen were not observed.

Approximately 3% of the 1749 patients treated with cefoxitin developed a clinically apparent superinfection (260). The organisms recovered most frequently from these patients were *Pseudomonas* species and *Enterobacter* species. The frequency of these superinfections parallels that reported in other studies (261).

XII. CONCLUSIONS

Cefoxitin is a semisynthetic cephamycin which, by virtue of an OCH_3 group in the 7α-position, exhibits almost absolute resistance to destruction by beta-lactamases, whether derived from gram-positive bacteria such as *Staph. aureus* or gram-negative organisms and whether aerobic such as *E. coli* or obligatory anaerobic such as *B. fragilis.* The pharmacokinetics, including tissue penetration, serum half-life, and urinary excretion, is similar to that of the first- and second-generation cephalosporins. The major pathogenic organisms routinely resistant to cefoxitin are *Ps. aeruginosa,* some *Enterobacter* species, and group D streptococci such as *Enterococcus.*

In clinical trials cefoxitin was shown to be comparable in efficacy to cephalothin against relatively uncomplicated infections. Situations in which cefoxitin may be superior to cephalosporins include the mixed infections commonly found in gynecological patients, intra-abdominal infections due to mixed organisms, and a broad variety of other kinds of infections in which one might expect to find multiple organisms including both aerobic and anaerobic isolates. On occasion, in appropriate patients cefoxitin may be substituted for combinations of antibiotics such as clindamycin and gentamicin, or penicillin and streptomycin, and so on. It should be recognized that although cefoxitin is one of the most active beta-lactams against anaerobic organisms (especially *B. fragilis*), drugs of other types (e.g., clindamycin, chloramphenicol, and metronidazole) are generally considered more reliable, although they may also be more toxic. The role of cefoxitin as a preoperative adjunct to surgery in the prevention of infections has been defined in gynecology, obstetrics, gastrointestinal surgery, urological surgery, and orthopedics, but it requires further study before widespread use in other fields.

REFERENCES

1. R. Nagarajan, L. D. Boeck, M. Gorman, R. L. Hamill, C. E. Higgins, M. M. Hoehn, W. M. Stark, and J. G. Whitney. β-Lactam Antibiotics from *Streptomyces. J. Am. Chem. Soc., 93*:2308–2310 (1971).
2. E. O. Stapley, M. Jackson, S. Hernandez, S. B. Zimmerman, S. A. Currie, S. Mochales, J. M. Mata, H. B. Woodruff, and D. Hendlin. Cephamycins, a new family of β-lactam antibiotics. I. Production by actinomycetes, including *Streptomyces lactamdurans* sp. *Antimicrob. Agents Chemother., 2*:122–131 (1972).
3. T. W. Miller, R. T. Goegelman, R. G. Weston, I. Putter, and F. J. Wolf. Cephamycins, a new family of β-lactam antibiotics. II. Isolation and chemical characterization. *Antimicrob. Agents Chemother., 2*:132–135 (1972).
4. P. J. Cassidy. Novel naturally occurring β-lactam antibiotics – A review. *Dev. Ind. Microbiol., 22*:181–209 (1981).

5. H. Fukase, T. Hasegawa, K. Hatano, H. Iwasaki, and M. Yoneda. C-2801X, a new cephamycin-type antibiotic. II. Isolation and characterization. *J. Antibiot., 29*:113–120 (1976).
6. Meiji Seika Kaisha, Ltd. U.S. patent 3,974,035. August 10 (1976).
7. Fujisawa Pharmaceutical Co., Ltd. British patent 1,425,081. February 18 (1976).
8. S. Inouye, M. Kojima, T. Shomura, K. Iwamotsu, T. Niwa, Y. Kondo, T. Niida, Y. Ogawa, and K. Kusama. Discovery, isolation and structure of novel cephamycins of *Streptomyces chartreusis. J. Antibiot., 36*:115–124 (1983).
9. A. K. Miller, E. Celozzi, Y. Kong, B. A. Pelak, H. Kropp, E. O. Stapley, and D. Hendlin. Cephamycins, a new family of β-lactam antibiotics. IV. *In vivo* studies. *Antimicrob. Agents Chemother., 2*:287–290 (1972).
10. D. R. Daoust, H. R. Onishi, H. Wallick, D. Hendlin, and E. O. Stapley. Cephamycins, a new family of β-lactam antibiotics: Antibacterial activity and resistance to β-lactamase degradation. *Antimicrob. Agents Chemother., 3*: 254–261 (1973).
11. S. Karady, S. H. Pines, L. M. Weinstock, F. E. Roberts, G. S. Brenner, A. M. Hoinowski, T. Y. Cheng, and M. Sletzinger. Semisynthetic cephalosporins via a novel acyl exchange reaction. *J. Am. Chem. Soc., 94*:1410–1411 (1972).
12. L. D. Cama, W. J. Leanza, T. R. Beattie, and B. G. Christensen. Substituted penicillin and cephalosporin derivatives. I. Stereospecific introduction of the C-6 (7) methoxyl group. *J. Am. Chem. Soc., 94*:1408–1410 (1972).
13. E. O. Stapley, D. R. Daoust, D. Hendlin, A. K. Miller, S. B. Zimmerman, J. Birnbaum, L. D. Cama, and B. G. Christensen. Cefoxitin: Mechanism of activity against cephalosporin-resistant bacteria. *Microb. Drug Resis., 2*:405–417 (1979).
14. H. R. Onishi, D. R. Daoust, S. B. Zimmerman, D. Hendlin, and E. O. Stapley. Cefoxitin, a semi-synthetic cephamycin antibiotic. Resistance to β-lactamase inactivation. *Antimicrob. Agents Chemother., 5*:38–48 (1974).
15. W. E. Wick. *In vitro* and *in vivo* laboratory comparison of cephalothin and desacetylcephalothin. *Antimicrob. Agents Chemother.,* 870–875 (1965).
16. H. R. Onishi, S. B. Zimmerman, and E. O. Stapley. Observations on the mode of action of cefoxitin. *Ann. N.Y. Acad. Sci., 235*:406–425 (1974).
17. A. K. Miller, E. Celozzi, B. A. Pelak, J. Birnbaum, and E. O. Stapley. Correlation of *in vitro* susceptibility with *in vivo* efficacy in mice for cefoxitin in comparison with cephalosporins. *J. Antimicrob. Chemother., 5*:569–579 (1979).
18. H. Wallick and D. Hendlin. Cefoxitin, a semi-synthetic cephamycin antibiotic: Susceptibility studies. *Antimicrob. Agents Chemother., 5*:25–32 (1974).
19. R. N. Jones, C. Thornsberry, A. L. Barry, P. C. Fuchs, T. L. Gavan, and E. H. Gerlach. BL-S786, a new parenteral cephalosporin. II. *In vitro* antimicrobial activity in comparison with six related cephalosporins. *J. Antibiot., 30*:583–592 (1977).
20. W. E. Farrar, Jr., and P. K. Gramling. Antistaphylococcal activity and β-lactamase resistance of newer cephalosporins. *J. Infect. Dis., 133*:691–695 (1976).

21. I. W. Fong, E. R. Engelking, and W. M. M. Kirby. Relative inactivation by *Staphylococcus aureus* of eight cephalosporin antibiotics. *Antimicrob. Agents Chemother., 9*:939–944 (1976).
22. G. Darland and J. Birnbaum. Cefoxitin resistance to beta-lactamase a major factor for susceptibility of *Bacteroides fragilis* to the antibiotic. *Antimicrob. Agents Chemother., 11*:725–734 (1977).
23. B. G. Spratt. Distinct penicillin binding proteins involved in the division, elongation and shape of *Escherichia coli* K12. *Proc. Nat. Acad. Sci. U.S.A., 92*:2999–3003 (1975).
24. B. G. Spratt. Properties of the penicillin-binding protein of *Escherichia coli* K12. *Eur. J. Biochem., 72*:341–352 (1977).
25. N. A. C. Curtis, G. W. Ross, and M. G. Boulton. Effect of 7α-methoxy substitution of cephalosporins upon their affinity for the penicillin-binding proteins of *E. coli* K12. Comparison with antibacterial activity and inhibition of membrane bound model transpeptidase activity. *J. Antimicrob. Chemother., 5*:391–398 (1979).
26. A. W. Bauer, W. M. M. Kirby, J. C. Sherris, and M. Turck. Antibiotic susceptibility testing by a standardized single disc method. *Am. J. Clin. Pathol., 45*:493–496 (1966).
27. E. O. Stapley, J. Birnbaum, A. K. Miller, H. Wallick, D. Hendlin, and H. B. Woodruff. Cefoxitin and cephamycins: Microbiological studies. *Rev. Infect. Dis., 1*:73–87 (1979).
28. V. L. Sutter and S. M. Finegold. Susceptibility of anaerobic bacteria to 23 antimicrobial agents. *Antimicrob. Agents Chemother., 10*:736–752 (1976).
29. F. P. Tally, N. V. Jacobus, J. G. Bartlett, and S. L. Gorbach. Susceptibility of anaerobes to cefoxitin and other cephalosporins. *Antimicrob. Agents Chemother., 7*:128–132 (1975).
30. E. C. Ernst, S. Berger, M. Barza, N. V. Jacobus, and F. P. Tally. Activity of cefamandole and other cephalosporins against aerobic and anaerobic bacteria. *Antimicrob. Agents Chemother., 9*:852–855 (1976).
31. B. Olsson, K. Dornbusch, and C. F. Nord. Susceptibility to beta-lactam antibiotics and production of β-lactamases in *Bacteroides fragilis. Med. Microbiol. Immunol., 163*:183–194 (1977).
32. V. E. DelBene and W. E. Farrar. Cephalosporinase activity in *Bacteroides fragilis. Antimicrob. Agents Chemother., 3*:369–372 (1973).
33. J. D. Anderson and R. B. Sykes. Characterization of a β-lactamase obtained from a strain of *Bacteroides fragilis* resistant to β-lactam antibiotics. *J. Med. Microbiol., 6*:201–206 (1973).
34. B. Olsson, C. E. Nord, and T. Wadstrom. Formation of beta-lactamase in *Bacteroides fragilis*: Cell-bound and extracellular activity. *Antimicrob. Agents Chemother., 9*:727–735 (1976).
35. G. J. Cuchural, Jr., F. P. Tally, N. V. Jacobus, P. K. Marsh, and J. W. Mayhew. Cefoxitin inactivation by *Bacteroides fragilis. Antimicrob. Agents Chemother., 24*:936–940 (1983).
36. A. Yotsuji, S. Minami, M. Inoue, and S. Mitsuhashi. Properties of novel β-lactamase produced by *Bacteroides fragilis. Antimicrob. Agents Chemother., 24*:925–929 (1983).

37. A. K. Miller, E. Celozzi, Y. Kong, B. A. Pelak, D. Hendlin, and E. O. Stapley. Cefoxitin, a semi-synthetic cephamycin antibiotic: *In vivo* evaluation. *Antimicrob. Agents Chemother.*, *5*:33–37 (1974).
38. E. O. Stapley and J. Birnbaum. Chemistry and microbiological properties of the cephamycins, in *β-Lactam Antibiotics* (M. Salton and G. D. Shockman, eds.), Academic, New York, 1981, pp. 327–351.
39. J. V. Uri, P. Actor, J. R. Guarini, L. Phillips, D. Pitkin, R. M. Demarinis, and J. A. Weisbach. Biological and chemotherapeutic studies on three semisynthetic cephamycins. *J. Antibiot.*, *31*:82–91 (1978).
40. H. H. Gadebusch, R. Schwind, P. Lukassow, R. Whitney, and R. J. McRipley. Cephamycin derivatives: Comparison of the *in vitro* and *in vivo* antibacterial activities of SQ14,359, CS-1170 and cefoxitin. *J. Antibiot.*, *31*: 1046–1058 (1978).
41. I. Nakayama, H. Iwamoto, S. Iwai, H. Mizuoshi, and S. Ishiyama. Comparative study of CS1170 and cefoxitin: Absorption, distribution, and metabolism. *Curr. Chemother.*, *2*:851–852 (1978).
42. M. Tai, Y. Fukuoka, A. Yotsuji, K. Kumano, M. Takahata, H. Mikami, T. Yasuda, I. Saikawa, and S. Mitsuhashi. *In vitro* and *in vivo* antibacterial activity of T-1982, a new semisynthetic cephamycin antibiotic. *Antimicrob. Agents Chemother.*, *22*:728–734 (1982).
43. M. Benlloch, A. Torres, and F. Soriano. Cefmetazole (CS1170): A new cephamycin with activity against gram-negative bacilli and staphylococci. *J. Antimicrob. Chemother.*, *10*:347–350 (1982).
44. T. Saito, M. Toda, M. Inoue, M. Saito, K. Suzaki, K. Yano, T. Isono, and S. Mitsuhashi. YM09330, a new broad-spectrum semisynthetic cephamycin antibiotic, antibacterial activities and some biochemical approaches, in *Antibiotic Resistance, Transposition and Other Mechanisms* (S. Mitsuhashi, J. Roswal, and V. Kremery, eds.), Springer-Verlag, Berlin, 1980, pp. 223–227.
45. L. W. Ayers, R. N. Jones, A. L. Barry, C. Thornsberry, P. C. Fuchs, T. L. Gavan, E. H. Gerlach, and H. M. Sommers. Cefotetan, a new cephamycin: Comparison of *in vitro* antimicrobial activity with other cephems, betalactamase stability, and preliminary recommendations for disk diffusion testing. *Antimicrob. Agents Chemother.*, *22*:859–877 (1982).
46. A. Bauernfeind. Cefotetan: Profile of *in vitro* activity. *J. Antimicrob. Chemother. Suppl. A*, *11*:19–29 (1983).
47. B. Chattopadhyay and J. C. Teli. Comparison of *in vitro* activity of cefotetan (ICI 156834), a new cephamycin derivative, with that of cefoxitin. *J. Antimicrob. Chemother.*, *10*:151–154 (1982).
48. A. M. Clarke and S. J. V. Zemcov. Antibacterial activity of the cephamycin cefotetan: An *in vitro* comparison with other β-lactam antibiotics. *J. Antimicrob. Chemother. Suppl. A*, *11*:67–72 (1983).
49. G. G. Grassi, R. A. Alesina, A. Ferrara, and V. Peona. *In vitro* antibacterial activity of cefotetan. *J. Antimicrob. Chemother. Suppl. A*, *11*:45–58 (1983).
50. G. Ruckdeschel. Activity *in vitro* of cefotetan against non-sporing anaerobes: A comparative study. *J. Antimicrob. Chemother. Suppl. A*, *11*:117–124 (1983).

51. W. E. Owens and S. M. Finegold. Comparative *in vitro* susceptibilities of anaerobic bacteria to cefmenoxime, cefotetan and N-formidoyl thienamycin. *Antimicrob. Agents Chemother., 23*:626–629 (1983).
52. F. Moosdeen, J. Maskell, J. Philpott-Howard, and J. D. Williams. Cefotetan activity against gram-negative aerobes and anaerobes. *J. Antimicrob. Chemother. Suppl. A, 11*:59–65 (1983).
53. K. Iwamatsu, S. Inouye, T. Tsuruoka, K. Mizutami, S. Omoto, H. Ogino, K. Miyauchi, T. Watanabe, and T. Nida. Synthesis and biological activity of 7β-(2-amino-2-carboxy)-ethylthioacetamido-7α-methoxycephalosporin derivatives. *J. Antibiot., 36*:229–241 (1983).
54. A. L. Demain. Biosynthesis of β-lactam antibiotics, in *Antibiotics Containing the β-Lactam Structure,* Vol. 1 (A. L. Demain and N. A. Solomon, eds.), Springer-Verlag, New York, 1983, pp. 189–228.
55. S. W. Queener and N. Neuss. The biosynthesis of β-lactam antibiotics, in *Chemistry and Biology of β-Lactam Antibiotics,* Vol. 3 (R. B. Morin and M. Gorman, eds.), Academic, New York, 1982, pp. 1–81.
56. E. Inamine and J. Birnbaum. Cephamycin C biosynthesis: Isotope incorporation studies, in *Abstracts of the Annual Meeting of the American Society for Microbiology,* American Society for Microbiology, Washington, D.C., 1972, p. 12.
57. J. G. Whitney, D. R. Brannon, J. A. Mabe, and K. J. Wicker. Incorporation of labeled precursors into A16886B, a novel β-lactam antibiotic produced by *Streptomyces clavuligerus. Antimicrob. Agents Chemother., 1*:247–251 (1972).
58. J. O'Sullivan, R. T. Aplin, C. M. Stevens, and E. P. Abraham. Biosynthesis of a 7α-methoxycephalosporin. Incorporation of molecular oxygen. *Biochem. J., 179*:47–52 (1979).
59. S. J. Brewer, T. T. Boyle, and M. K. Turner. The carbamoylation of the 3-hydroxymethyl group of 7α-methoxy-7β-(5-D-aminoadipamido)-3-hydroxymethylceph-3-em-4-carboxylic acid (desacetyl-7α-methoxycephalosporin C) by homogenates of *Streptomyces clavuligerus. Biochem. Soc. Trans., 5*:1024–1026 (1977).
60. S. J. Brewer, P. M. Taylor, and M. K. Turner. An adenosine triphosphate-dependent carbamoylphosphate-3-hydroxymethylcepham-O-carbamoyltransferase from *Streptomyces clavuligerus. Biochem. J., 185*:555–564 (1980).
61. J. R. Kirkpatrick, J. L. Doolin, and O. W. Godfrey. The role of lysine in antibiotic biosynthesis in *Streptomyces lipmanii,* in *Abstracts of the Annual Meeting of the American Society for Microbiology,* American Society for Microbiology, Washington, D.C., 1973, p. 13.
62. B. A. Kern, D. Hendlin, and E. Inamine. L-lysine ε-aminotransferase involved in cephamycin C synthesis in *Streptomyces lactamdurans. Antimicrob. Agents Chemother., 17*:679–685 (1980).
63. B. A. Kern and E. Inamine. Cystathionine γ-lyase activity in the cephamycin C producer *Streptomyces lactamdurans. J. Antibiot., 34*:583–589 (1981).
64. E. P. Abraham. β-Lactam antibiotics and related substances. *Jpn. J. Antibiot., 30*:S1–S26 (1977).

65. R. M. Adlington, J. E. Baldwin, M. Lopez-Nieto, A. A. Murphy, and N. Patel. A study of the biosynthesis of the tripeptide δ-(L-α-aminoadipyl)-L-cysteinyl-D-valine in a β-lactam-negative mutant of *Cephalosporium acremonium. Biochem. J., 213*:573–576 (1983).
66. J. O'Sullivan and E. P. Abraham. The conversion of cephalosporins to 7α-methoxycephalosporins by cell-free extracts of *Streptomyces clavuligerus. Biochem. J., 186*:613–616 (1980).
67. S. E. Jensen, D. W. S. Westlake, and S. Wolfe. Cyclization of δ-(L-α-amino-adipyl)-L-cysteinyl-D-valine to penicillins by cell-free extracts of *Streptomyces clavuligerus. J. Antibiot., 35*:483–490 (1982).
68. S. W. Jensen, D. W. S. Westlake, and S. Wolfe. High performance liquid chromatographic assay of cyclization activity in cell-free systems from *Streptomyces clavuligerus. J. Antibiot., 35*:1026–1032 (1982).
69. J. Kupka, Y.-Q. Shen, S. Wolfe, and A. L. Demain. Studies on the ring-cyclization and ring-expansion enzymes of β-lactam biosynthesis in *Cephalosporium acremonium. Can. J. Microbiol., 29*:488–496 (1983).
70. S. E. Jensen, D. W. S. Westlake, R. J. Bowers, and S. Wolfe. Cephalosporin formation by cell-free extracts from *Streptomyces clavuligerus. J. Antibiot., 35*:1351–1359 (1982).
71. S. E. Jensen, D. W. S. Westlake, and S. Wolfe. Partial purification and characterization of isopenicillin N epimerase activity from *Streptomyces clavuligerus. Can. J. Microbiol., 29*:1526–1531 (1983).
72. S. E. Jensen, D. W. S. Westlake, and S. Wolfe. Analysis of penicillin N ring expansion activity from *Streptomyces clavuligerus* by ion-pair high-pressure liquid chromatography. *Antimicrob. Agents Chemother., 24*:307–312 (1983).
73. J. Kupka, Y.-Q. Shen, S. Wolfe, and A. L. Demain. Partial purification and properties of the α-ketoglutarate-linked ring-expansion enzyme of β-lactam biosynthesis of *Cephalosporium acremonium. FEMS Microbiol. Lett., 16*: 1–6 (1983).
74. M. K. Turner, J. E. Farthing, and S. J. Brewer. The oxygenation of [3-methyl-^{3}H] desacetylcephalosporin C by 2-oxoglutarate-linked dioxygenases from *Acremonium chrysogenum* and *Streptomyces clavuligerus. Biochem. J., 173*:839–850 (1978).
75. D. R. Brannon, D. S. Fukuda, J. A. Mabe, F. M. Huber, and J. G. Whitney. Detection of a cephalosporin C acetyl esterase in the carbamate cephalosporin antibiotic-producing culture, *Streptomyces clavuligerus. Antimicrob. Agents Chemother., 1*:237–241 (1972).
76. J. D. Hood, A. Elson, M. L. Gilpin, and A. G. Brown. Identification of 7α-hydroxycephalosporin C as an intermediate in the methoxylation of cephalosporin C by a cell-free extract of *Streptomyces clavuligerus. J. Chem. Soc. Chem. Commun.*, 1187–1188 (1983).
77. Y. Aharonowitz and A. L. Demain. Carbon catabolite regulation of cephalosporin production in *Streptomyces clavuligerus. Antimicrob. Agents Chemother., 14*:159–164 (1978).

78. A. F. Braña, W.-S. Hu, and A. L. Demain. Involvement of aeration in carbon source regulation of cephem antibiotic biosynthesis in *Streptomyces clavuligerus. Biotechnol. Lett., 5*:791–794 (1983).
79. Y. Aharonowitz and A. L. Demain. Nitrogen nutrition and regulation of cephalosporin production in *Streptomyces clavuligerus. Can. J. Microbiol., 25*:61-67 (1979).
80. G. Lilley, A. E. Clarke, and G. C. Lawrence. Control of the production of cephamycin C and thienamycin by *Streptomyces cattleya* NRRL 8057. *J. Chem. Technol. Biotechnol., 31*:127–134 (1981).
81. Y. Aharonowitz. Regulatory interrelationships of nitrogen metabolism and cephalosporin biosynthesis, in *Genetics of Industrial Microorganisms* (O. K. Sebek and A. I. Laskin, eds.), American Society for Microbiology, Washington, D.C., 1979, p. 210.
82. C. L. Ginther. Sporulation and the production of serine protease and cephamycin C by *Streptomyces lactamdurans. Antimicrob. Agents Chemother., 15*:522–526 (1979).
83. S. Mendelovitz and Y. Aharonowitz. Regulation of cephamycin C synthesis, aspartokinase, dihydrodipicolinic acid synthetase and homoserine dehydrogenase by aspartic acid family amino acids in *Streptomyces clavuligerus. Antimicrob. Agents Chemother., 21*:74–84 (1982).
84. S. Mendelovitz and Y. Aharonowitz. β-Lactam antibiotic production by *Streptomyces clavuligerus* mutants impaired in regulation of aspartokinase. *J. Gen. Microbiol., 129*:2063–2069 (1983).
85. J. R. Kirkpatrick, L. E. Doolin, and O. W. Godfrey. Lysine biosynthesis in *Streptomyces lipmanii*: Implication in antibiotic biosynthesis. *Antimicrob. Agents Chemother., 4*:542–550 (1973).
86. O. W. Godfrey. Isolation of regulatory mutants of the aspartic and pyruvic acid families and their effect on antibiotic production in *Streptomyces lipmanii. Antimicrob. Agents Chemother., 4*:73–79 (1973).
87. E. Inamine, B. A. Kern, and D. Hendlin. Paper presented at the Annual Meeting of the American Society for Microbiology, Miami, Florida, May 11–16, 1980.
88. E. Inamine and J. Birnbaum. Process of making cephamycin C by fermentation. U.S. patent 3,886,044 (1975).
89. R. Nagarajan. β-lactam antibiotic from *Streptomyces,* in *Cephalosporin and Penicillins, Chemistry and Biology* (E. H. Flynn, ed.), Academic, New York, 1972, pp. 637–661.
90. E. Inamine and J. Birnbaum. Fermentation of cephamycin C. U.S. patent 3,977,942 (1976).
91. M. Arai, Y. Itoh, M. Nakahara, H. Kayamori, and S. Sugaware. Process for the production of antibiotic substance cephemimycin. U.S. patent 3,865,693 (1975).
92. L. M. Weinstock, S. Karady, F. E. Roberts, A. M. Hoinowski, G. S. Brenner, T. B. K. Lee, W. C. Lumma, and M. Sletzinger. The chemistry of cephalosporins. IV. Acylation of amides in the presence of neutral acid scavengers. *Tetrahedr. Lett., 46*:3979–3982 (1975).

93. J. J. Schrogie, J. D. Rogers, K. C. Yeh, R. D. Davies, G. I. Holmes, H. Skeggs, and C. M. Martin. Pharmacokinetics and comparative pharmacology of cefoxitin and cephalosporins. *Rev. Infect. Dis., 1*:90–97 (1979).
94. C. S. Goodwin, E. B. Raftery, A. D. Goldberg, H. Skeggs, A. E. Till, and C. M. Martin. Effects of rate of infusion and probenecid on serum levels, renal excretion, and tolerance of intravenous doses of cefoxitin in humans: Comparison with cephalothin. *Antimicrob. Agents Chemother., 6*:338–346 (1974).
95. W. Brumfitt, J. Kosmidis, J. M. T. Hamilton-Miller, and J. N. Gilchrist. Cefoxitin and cephalothin: Antimicrobial activity, human pharmacokinetics, and toxicology. *Antimicrob. Agents Chemother., 6*:290–299 (1974).
96. R. P. Buhs, T. E. Maxim, N. Allen, T. A. Jacob, and F. J. Wolf. Analysis of cefoxitin, cephalothin and their deacylated metabolites in human urine by high-performance liquid chromatography. *J. Chromatogr., 99*:609–618 (1974).
97. W. M. M. Kirby, J. B. de Maine, and W. S. Serrill. Pharmacokinetics of the cephalosporins in healthy volunteers and uremic patients. *Postgrad. Med. J. Suppl., 47*:41–46 (1971).
98. P. F. Sonneville, R. R. Kartodirdjo, H. Skeggs, A. E. Till, and C. M. Martin. Comparative clinical pharmacology of intravenous cefoxitin and cephalothin. *Eur. J. Clin. Pharmacol., 9*:397–403 (1976).
99. P. F. Sonneville, K. S. Albert, H. Skeggs, H. Gentner, K. C. Kwan, and C. M. Martin. Effect of lidocaine on the absorption, disposition and tolerance of intramuscularly administered cefoxitin. *Eur. J. Clin. Pharmacol., 12*:273–279 (1977).
100. D. S. Reeves, A. J. Bint, H. A. Holt, and P. J. Stocks. Cefoxitin sodium: A clinical and pharmacological study. *J. Antimicrob. Chemother. Suppl. B, 4*:155–160 (1978).
101. R. Wise, B. Cadge, A. P. Gillett, and A. Bhamjee. The pharmacology of cefoxitin and the comparison of two human tissue models. *J. Infect. Suppl., 1*:49–56 (1979).
102. D. S. Reeves, D. W. Bullock, M. J. Bywater, H. A. Holt, L. O. White, and D. P. Thornhill. The effect of probenecid on the pharmacokinetics and distribution of cefoxitin in healthy volunteers. *Br. J. Clin. Pharmacol., 11*:353–359 (1981).
103. J. J. Schrogie, J. D. Rogers, K. C. Yeh, R. O. Davies, G. I. Holmes, H. Skeggs, and C. M. Martin. Pharmacokinetics and comparative pharmacology of cefoxitin and cephalosporins. *Rev. Infect. Dis., 1*:90–97 (1979).
104. J. J. Axelrod and R. S. Kochman. Cefoxitin levels in human aqueous humor. *Am. J. Ophthalmol., 90*:388–393 (1980).
105. A. P. Gillett and R. Wise. Penetration of four cephalosporins into tissue fluid in man. *Lancet, 1*:962–964 (1978).
106. J. F. Hansbrough and J. E. Clark. Concentrations of cefoxitin in gallbladder bile of cholecystectomy patients. *Antimicrob. Agents Chemother., 22*:709–710 (1982).

107. T. Ishii, T. Yokoyama, D. Kishi, M. Takeda, F. Furumoto, and T. Ichikawa. Laboratory and clinical evaluation of cefoxitin in surgical field. *Chemotherapy Tokyo Suppl., 1*:442–446 (1978).
108. M. N. Logan, R. Wise, and R. P. Grimley. Biliary levels of cefoxitin. *J. Antimicrob. Chemother., 5*:620–621 (1979).
109. S. Matsuda, M. Tanno, T. Kashiwakura, and H. Furuya. Laboratory and clinical studies on cefoxitin in the field of obstetrics and gynecology. *Chemotherapy Tokyo Suppl., 1*:462–467 (1978).
110. C. Nankun, K. Uehara, S. Sugizaki, F. Seo, J. Miyagami, H. Saito, and T. Nakayama. Clinical studies of cefoxitin in the field of obstetrics and gynecology. *Chemotherapy Tokyo Suppl., 1*:469–475 (1978).
111. G. H. Santo. Passage of cefoxitin into breast milk. *Eur. J. Clin. Study Treat. Infect. Suppl., 1*:90–91 (1979).
112. K. Seiga and M. Minagawa. Study on cefoxitin. *Chemotherapy Tokyo Suppl., 1*:494–495 (1978).
113. Z. Takase, H. Shirafuji, and M. Uchida. Clinical and laboratory studies on cefoxitin in the field of obstetrics and gynecology. *Chemotherapy Tokyo Suppl., 1*:502–505 (1978).
114. R. Wise, I. A. Donovan, N. S. Ambrose, and J. E. Allcock. Penetration of cefoxitin into peritoneal fluid, in *Current Chemotherapy and Immunotherapy,* (P. Periti and G. G. Grassi, eds.), American Society for Microbiology, Washington, D.C., 1982, pp. 380–381.
115. D. H. Wittman and H. Schassan. Penetration of eight β-lactam antibiotics into the peritoneal fluid: A pharmacokinetic investigation. *Arch. Surg., 118*:205–213 (1983).
116. E. Bergogne-Berezin, J. Pierre, G. Berthelot, J. Kafe, and C. Morel. Pharmacokinetics of cephalosporins in human bronchial secretions. *Drugs Exp. Clin. Res., 5*:159–165 (1979).
117. J. Bourreille, G. LeBihan, B. Beau, A. Leroy, and G. Humbert. Penetration of cefoxitin into ascitic fluid, in *Current Chemotherapy and Infectious Disease,* American Society for Microbiology, Washington, D.C., 1980, pp. 645–647.
118. R. Fujino, H. Yamamoto, and F. Nakayama. Laboratory and clinical study on cefoxitin in surgical field. *Chemotherapy Tokyo Suppl., 1*:447–452 (1978).
119. A. M. Geddes, L. P. Schnurr, A. P. Ball, D. McGhie, G. R. Brookes, R. Wise, and J. Andrews. Cefoxitin: A hospital study. *Br. Med. J., 1*:1126–1128 (1977).
120. H. Tanimura, M. Takenaka, K. Maruyama, S. Mukaihara, M. Setoyama, T. Kamata, M. Nagase, and Y. Hikasa. Chemotherapy of biliary infections (Report III): Biliary excretion and tissue concentration in the gallbladder in patients treated with cefoxitin. *Chemotherapy Tokyo Suppl., 1*:413–428 (1978).
121. T. Ueda, K. Morimoto, S. Hirao, M. Fujimoto, K. Sakai, and Y. Shiraha. A clinical trial of cefoxitin in the field of surgery. *Chemotherapy Tokyo Suppl., 1*:429–435 (1978).

122. F. Daschner, E. Petersen, H. Langmaack, and T. Trennhauser. Antibiotic prophylaxis in gynecology: Cefoxitin concentrations in serum, myometrium, endometrium and salpinges. *Infection, 10*:341–342 (1984).
123. K. Hirabayashi and E. Okada. Laboratory and clinical studies on cefoxitin in the field of obstetrics and gynecology. *Jpn. J. Antibiot., 31*:315-324 (1978).
124. D. Hutch, G. Richards, R. A. Brown, and D. S. Mulder. Bioactive antibiotic levels in the human aorta. *Surgery, 92*:1068–1071 (1982).
125. C. H. Nightingale, N. Olson, and R. Quintiliani. Penetration of cefoxitin into the right atrial appendage and pericardial fluid of patients undergoing open-heart operations. *Curr. Ther. Res., 29*:444–451 (1981).
126. E. J. Perea, M. C. Garcia-Iglesias, J. Ayarra, and J. Loscertales. Comparative concentrations of cefoxitin in human lungs and sera. *Antimicrob. Agents Chemother., 23*:323–324 (1983).
127. R. Plaue, O. Muller, V. Jenne, K. Fabricius, and R. O. Bethke. Investigation of the rate of diffusion of cefoxitin in various human tissues. *Med. Klin., 74*:481–487 (1979).
128. K. Saito, K. Michi, and K. Hashimoto. Concentration of cefoxitin in oral tissues and serum, in *Current Chemotherapy and Immunotherapy*, (P. Periti and G. G. Grassi, eds.), American Society for Microbiology, Washington, D.C., 1982, pp. 382–383.
129. J. T. Summersgill, L. G. Schupp, and M. J. Raff. Comparative penetration of metronidazole, clindamycin, cloramphenicol, cefoxitin, ticarcillin, and moxalactam into bone. *Antimicrob. Agents Chemother., 21*:601-603 (1982).
130. C. Liu, D. R. Hinthorn, G. R. Hodges, J. L. Harms, G. Couchonnal, and D. I. Dworzack. Penetration of cefoxitin into human cerebrospinal fluid: Comparison with cefamandole, ampicillin, and penicillin. *Rev. Infect. Dis., 1*:127–131 (1979).
131. P. A. Galvao, A. V. Lonar, W. Francisco, C. V. F. D. Godoy, and R. Norrby. Cefoxitin penetration to cerebrospinal fluid in patients with purulent meningitis, in *Current Chemotherapy and Infectious Disease*, (J. D. Helson and C. Grassi, eds.), American Society for Microbiology, Washington, D.C., 1980, pp. 632–634.
132. J. P. Fillastre, A. Leroy, M. Godin, G. Oksenhendler, and G. Humbert. Pharmacokinetics of cefoxitin sodium in normal subjects and in uraemic patients. *J. Antimicrob. Chemother. Suppl. B, 4*:79–83 (1978).
133. M. J. Garcia, A. Dominguez-Fil, J. M. Taberno, and J. A. Sanchez Tomera. Pharmacokinetics of cefoxitin in patients with normal or impaired renal function. *Eur. J. Clin. Pharmacol., 16*:119–124 (1979).
134. G. Humbert, J. P. Fillastre, A. Leroy, M. Godin, and C. van Winzum. Pharmacokinetics of cefoxitin in normal subjects and in patients with renal insufficiency. *Rev. Infect. Dis., 1*:118–125 (1979).
135. P. Wilson, T. Leung, and J. D. Williams. Antibacterial activity, pharmacokinetics and efficacy of cefoxitin in patients with abdominal sepsis and other infections. *J. Antimicrob. Chemother. Suppl. B, 4*:127–141 (1978).
136. J. F. Flaherty, G. W. Boswell, C. A. Winkel, and J. P. Elliot. Pharmacokinetics of cefoxitin in patients at term gestation: Lavage versus intra-

venous administration. *Am. J. Obstet. Gynecol., 146*:760–766 (1983).
137. M. Dubois, D. Delapierre, J. Demonty, R. Lambotte, and A. Dresse. Transplacental and mammary transfer of cefoxitin. Paper presented at the 11th International Congress of Chemotherapy and 19th Interscience Conference on Antimicrobial Agents and Chemotherapy, Boston, Mass., October 1–5, 1979, Abstract 118.
138. H. Giamarellou, J. Gazis, A. A. Petrikkos, D. Araventinos, and G. K. Daikos. A study of cefoxitin, moxalactam, and ceftazidime kinetics in pregnancy. *Am. J. Obstet. Gynecol., 147*:914–919 (1983).
139. M. J. Garcia, A. Dominguez-Gil, F. D. Perez, F. P. Rodriguez, and F. D. Moronta. Disposition of cefoxitin in patients with ascites. *Eur. J. Clin. Pharmacol., 20*:371–374 (1981).
140. R. Olegard, U. Jodal, J.-E. Brorson, J. Johnsson, P. Lincoln, J. Bjure, and R. Norrby. Pharmacokinetics of cefoxitin in children, in *Current Chemotherapy and Infectious Disease,* (J. D. Nelson and C. Grassi, eds.), American Society for Microbiology, Washington, D.C., 1980, pp. 1152–1154.
141. R. Roos, H. M. von Hattingberg, B. H. Belohradsky, and W. Marget. Pharmacokinetics of cefoxitin in premature and newborn babies: A method for measuring cefoxitin serum levels in combination therapy with penicillin G and amikacin, in *Current Chemotherapy and Infectious Disease,* (J. D. Nelson and C. Grassi, eds.), American Society for Microbiology, Washington, D.C., 1980, pp. 1159–1161.
142. P. H. Vlasses, H. D'Silva, M. L. Rocci, Jr., J. R. Koplin, J. A. Bland, and E. G. Siciliano. Disposition of intravenous and intraperitoneal cefoxitin during chronic intermittent peritoneal dialysis. *Clin. Pharmacol. Ther., 31*:277–278 (1982).
143. W. L. Greaves, J. H. Kreeft, R. I. Ogilvie, and G. K. Richards. Cefoxitin disposition during peritoneal dialysis. *Antimicrob. Agents Chemother., 19*:253–255 (1981).
144. M. J. Garcia, A. Dominguez-Gil, J. M. Taberno, and R. A. Bondia. Pharmacokinetics of cefoxitin in patients undergoing hemodialysis. *Int. J. Clin. Pharmacol. Biopharm., 17*:366–370 (1979).
145. B. Trollfors, S. Norrby, and K. Kristianson. Effects on renal function of treatment with cefoxitin alone or in combination with furosemide, in *Current Chemotherapy,* (W. Siegenthaler and R. Lüthy, eds.), American Society for Microbiology, Washington, D.C., 1978, pp. 760–762.
146. D. J. Ormrod and T. E. Miller. Evaluation of cefoxitin nephrotoxicity in experimentally induced renal failure. *Antimicrob. Agents Chemother., 19*:18–21 (1981).
147. R. R. Swain and S. L. Briggs. Positive interference with the Jaffé reaction by cephalosporin antibiotics. *Clin. Chem., 23*:1340–1342 (1977).
148. A. J. Saah, T. R. Koch, and G. L. Drusano. Cefoxitin falsely elevates creatinine levels. *J. Am. Med. Assoc., 247*:205–206 (1982).
149. D. R. P. Guay, R. C. Meatherall, and P. A. Macaulay. Interference of selected second- and third-generation cephalosporins with creatinine determination. *Am. J. Hosp. Pharm., 40*:435–438 (1983).

150. C. M. Martin, K. R. Brown, R. Norrby, and C. van Winzum. Cefoxitin, a new cephamycin antibiotic: Observations in 1,749 patients. Proceedings of the I Mediterranean Congress of Chemotherapy, Madrid, Spain, 1978.
151. R. V. McCloskey and R. C. Goren. Current status of therapy with cefoxitin. *Clin. Ther., 3*:66–79 (1980).
152. H. C. Neu. Clinical use of cephalosporins. *Lancet, 2*:252–255 (1982).
153. R. L. Sweet. Treatment of mixed aerobic–anaerobic infections of the female genital tract. *J. Antimicrob. Chemother. Suppl. D, 8*:105–114 (1981).
154. G. D. Brooks and S. L. Barriere. Clinical use of the new beta-lactam antimicrobial drugs: Practical considerations for physicians, microbiology laboratories, pharmacists, and formulary committees. *Ann. Intern. Med., 98*:530–535 (1983).
155. P. Garzone, J. Lyon, and V. L. Ye. Third-generation and investigational cephalosporins: I. Structure–activity relationships and pharmacokinetic review. *Drugs Intell. Clin. Pharm., 17*:507–515 (1983).
156. R. W. Bradsher and R. S. Abernathy. Parenteral cephalosporin antibiotics in clinical practice. *J. Ark. Med. Soc., 79*:130–135 (1982).
157. J. L. LeFrock, R. F. Shell, B. B. Carr, S. F. Kowalsky, and J. R. Tillotson. Cefoxitin therapy in aerobic, anaerobic, and mixed aerobic–anaerobic infections. *Drug Intell. Clin. Pharm., 16*:306–312 (1982).
158. J. G. Bartlett, T. J. Louie, S. L. Gorbach, D. L. Kasper, and A. B. Onderdonk. Comparative efficacy of three cephalosporins and cefoxitin in experimental intra-abdominal sepsis, in *Current Chemotherapy,* (W. Siegenthaler and R. Lüthy, eds.), American Society for Microbiology, Washington, D.C., 1978, pp. 298–299.
159. F. P. Tally. Antimicrobial activity against an important anaerobic bacterium: *Bacteroides fragilis. Curr. Ther. Res. Clin. Exp., 33*:1–7 (1983).
160. D. F. Busch, P. N. R. Heseltine, R. D. Meyer, V. L. Sutter, and S. M. Finegold. Cefoxitin sodium therapy of anaerobic infections. *J. Antimicrob. Chemother. Suppl. B, 4*:197–202 (1978).
161. S. R. Nair and C. E. Cherubin. Use of cefoxitin sodium in difficult-to-treat infections. *J. Antimicrob. Chemother. Suppl. B, 4*:167–178 (1978).
162. V. Speranza and G. Mennini. Clinical experience with cefoxitin sodium in abdominal surgery. *J. Antimicrob. Chemother. Suppl. B, 4*:143–149 (1978).
163. A. M. Geddes and R. M. L. Wilcox. Cefoxitin in abdominal sepsis. *J. Antimicrob. Chemother. Suppl. B, 4*:151–153 (1978).
164. L. Laplante, E. Bastien, Y. Giroux, and R. Girard. Intravenous treatment of systemic infections in 20 patients with cefoxitin sodium. *J. Antimicrob. Chemother. Suppl. B, 4*:219–222 (1978).
165. W. Schumer, R. L. Nichols, and A. Acharya. Use of cefoxitin sodium in moderate to severe surgical infections. *J. Antimicrob. Chemother. Suppl. B, 4*:231–233 (1978).
166. S. L. Gorbach and K. McGowan. Comparative clinical trials in treatment of intra-abdominal sepsis. *J. Antimicrob. Chemother. Suppl. D, 8*:95–104 (1981).

167. H. Vellend, M. G. Bergeron, G. Krip, and A. R. Ronald. Clinical evaluation of cefoxitin in the treatment of intra-abdominal and pelvic infections: A multi-centre study in Canada. *Curr. Ther. Res. Clin. Exp., 33*:528–538 (1983).
168. F. Mingolla and F. Feliciotti. Experience with cefoxitin in the intensive care department of surgery. *Chir. Ital., 34*:404–416 (1982).
169. T. Hirayama, K. Kikuchi, and K. Chiba. Clinical evaluation of cefoxitin in the treatment of infections in surgery. *Jpn. J. Antibiot., 33*:716–719 (1980).
170. H. Majkova, P. Havranek, and O. Prazan. Experience with the treatment of peritonitis of appendical origin with mefoxin. *Rozhl. Chir., 59*:474–477 (1980).
171. N. Asano. Experience in the use of cefoxitin in surgery. *Yakuri to Chiryo, 8*:3781–3784 (1980).
172. J. Shibata, M. Kodama, K. Yamakishi, F. Tsunoda, K. Naito, K. Hori, H. Kurioka, and I. Hashimoto. Clinical evaluation of cefoxitin in gastrointestinal surgery. *Kiso to Rinsho, 14*:2572–2578 (1980).
173. K. Shiramatsu, K. Sasaki, Y. Maruyama, K. Uchizawa, K. Hirata, and H. Hayasaka. The use of cefoxitin in abdominal surgery. *Jpn. J. Antibiot., 33*:1268–1273 (1980).
174. E. Bucci, F. Di Lauro, and R. Martina. Evaluation of cefoxitin sodium in oral surgery. *Arch. Stomatol., 22*:41–54 (1981).
175. G. Belcaro, R. Cotellese, A. D'Aulerio, A. Dell'Osa, G. Tenaglia, F. Radocchia, A. De Capite, N. Caizzi, and M. Santarelli. Treatment and prophylaxis of surgical infections. *Chir. Patol. Sper., 29*:151–157 (1982).
176. R. L. Sweet, K. W. Handley, J. Mills, and M. Robbie. Experience with intravenous cefoxitin sodium in obstetrics and gynecology. *J. Antimicrob. Chemother. Suppl. B, 4*:249–253 (1978).
177. R. Gonzalez-Enders, A. Yi, J. Calderon, and J. Trelles. Treatment of postpartum endometritis with cefoxitin, in *Current Chemotherapy,* (W. Siegenthaler and R. Lüthy, eds.), American Society for Microbiology, Washington, D.C., 1978, pp. 768–770.
178. J. S. White, C. Gee, and W. Ledger. The use of intravenous cefoxitin sodium in patients with obstetric/gynecologic infections. *J. Antimicrob. Chemother. Suppl. B, 4*:239–240 (1978).
179. R. L. Sweet. Mixed aerobic–anaerobic pelvic infection, in *Proceedings of a Symposium on Prophylaxis and Treatment of Pelvic Infections, Tokyo, Japan, October 29, 1979,* (K. Mashimo and W. J. Ledger, eds.), Biomedical Information, New York, 1981, pp. 129–141.
180. S. Matsuda. Clinical efficacy of cefoxitin against intrapelvic infections, in *Proceedings of a Symposium on Prophylaxis and Treatment of Pelvic Infections, Tokyo, Japan, October 29, 1979,* (K. Mashimo and W. J. Ledger, eds.), Biomedical Information, New York, 1981, pp. 99–118.
181. R. Gonzelez-Enders. Treatment of septic abortion with cefoxitin, in *Proceedings of a Symposium on Prophylaxis and Treatment of Pelvic Infections, Tokyo, Japan, October 29, 1979,* (K. Mashimo and W. J. Ledger, eds.), Biomedical Information, New York, 1981, pp. 119–128.

182. M. J. Gribble and A. W. Chow. Gynecologic infections: A management approach. *Drug Ther., 11*:67–76 (1981).
183. N. Cho, H. Araki, H. Saito, Y. Sanai, S. Oishi, K. Komatsuzaki, K. Takasaki, and I. Matsumura. Clinical evaluation of cefoxitin in treatment of infections in obstetric and gynecologic field. *Jpn. J. Antibiot., 35*:884–891 (1982).
184. K. Hagiwara and K. Ueno. Cefoxitin in treatment of obstetric and gynecologic infections caused by anaerobes and mixed aerobes and anaerobes. *Chemotherapy Tokyo, 30*:514–531 (1982).
185. P. Duff, J. F. Keiser, and S. L. Strong. A comparative study of two antibiotic regimens for the treatment of operative site infections. *Am. J. Obstet. Gynecol., 142*:996–1003 (1982).
186. J. Fierer, D. Daniel, and C. Davis. The fetid foot: Lower extremity infections in patients with diabetes mellitus. *Rev. Infect. Dis., 1*:210–217 (1979).
187. R. L. Perkins. Surgical considerations in skin and soft tissue infections and osteomyelitis treated with cefoxitin sodium. *J. Antimicrob. Chemother. Suppl. B, 4*:183–187 (1978).
188. R. V. McCloskey. Cefoxitin sodium treatment of anaerobic and polymicrobial aerobic infections. *J. Antimicrob. Chemother. Suppl. B, 4*:223–225 (1978).
189. H. Thadepalli, D. Webb, I. Roy, and V. Bach. Evaluation of cefoxitin sodium therapy in anaerobic infections. *J. Antimicrob. Chemother. Suppl. B, 4*:203–208 (1978).
190. T. A. Narsete, G. E. Omer, and M. S. Moneim. Hand infections from human saliva. *Orthop. Rev., 12*:81–85 (1983).
191. J. L. LeFrock, A. Molavi, K. Rolston, B. Smith, R. Schell, P. Chandrasekar, and B. Carr. *In vitro* and *in vivo* comparisons of mezlocillin and cefoxitin. *J. Antimicrob. Chemother. Suppl. C, 11*:83–90 (1983).
192. J. LeFrock, F. Blais, R. F. Schell, B. B. Carr, R. L. Jacobs, C. R. Wirth, S. F. Kowalsky, and J. R. Tillotson. Cefoxitin in the treatment of diabetic patients with lower extremity infections. *Infect. Surg., 1*:361–374 (1983).
193. H. C. Neu. Cefoxitin: An overview of clinical studies in the United States. *Rev. Infect. Dis., 1*:233–239 (1979).
194. C. Cox. Intravenous cefoxitin sodium in the treatment of urinary tract infections. *J. Antimicrob. Chemother. Suppl. B, 4*:193 (1978).
195. J. C. Tsang, G. A. Sansing, and M. A. Miller. Relation of β-lactamase activity to antimicrobial susceptibility in *Serratia marcescens*. *Antimicrob. Agents Chemother., 8*:277–281 (1975).
196. T. Asahi, M. Hirano, N. Irie, T. Kohama, Y. Ohbashi, M. Mizuno, T. Akaki, Y. Ozaki, and H. Ohmori. Clinical results of cefoxitin therapy in complicated urinary tract infections. *Shinyaku to Rinsho, 30*:827–830 (1981).
197. C. E. Cox, S. J. Childs, W. G. Wells, S. Mirelmant, and W. C. Lesky. Preliminary report on a comparative trial of cefotetan and cefoxitin in the treatment of urinary tract infections. *J. Antimicrob. Chemother. Suppl. A, 11*:227–232 (1983).

198. K. Naber. Urinary-tract infections: Side effects of chemotherapy. *Med. Monatsschr. Pharm., 6*:108–116 (1983).
199. J. Y. Gillenwater. Use of beta-lactam antibiotics in urinary tract infections. *J. Urol., 129*:457–460 (1983).
200. R. V. McCloskey. Antibiotic treatment of aspiration pneumonia: Results with cefoxitin sodium. *Curr. Ther. Res. Clin. Exp., 33*:740–744 (1983).
201. I. Brook. Anaerobic bacteria in pediatric respiratory infection: Progress in diagnosis and treatment. *South. Med. J., 74*:719–726 (1981).
202. Y. Hiraga, M. Abe, K. Kikuchi, and M. Nakahashi. Study of cefoxitin in chronic respiratory tract infections not responding to other antibiotics. *Jpn. J. Antibiot., 33*:1111–1124 (1980).
203. S. Yaguchi, M. Ogi, K. Yamahina, T. Kobayashi, Y. Takuchi, H. Kagaya, T. Matsushima, and K. Kitahama. Clinical evaluation of cefoxitin in intractable bronchopulmonary infections. *Jpn. J. Antibiot., 33*:1259–1267 (1980).
204. D. J. Schurman and M. Dillingham. A clinical evaluation of cefoxitin sodium in extensive trials. *J. Antimicrob. Chemother. Suppl. B, 4*:227–229 (1978).
205. C. Liu and D. R. Hinthorn. Osteomyelitis treated with cefoxitin sodium. *J. Antimicrob. Chemother. Suppl. B, 4*:235–237 (1978).
206. G. J. Pazin, S. N. Schwartz, M. Ho, J. A. Lyon, and A. W. Pasculle. Treatment of septicemic patients with cefoxitin: Pharmacokinetics in renal insufficiency. *Rev. Infect. Dis., 1*:189–194 (1979).
207. D. Webb, H. Thadepalli, V. Bach, and I. Roy. Clinical and experimental evaluation of cefoxitin therapy. *Chemotherapy, 25*:233–242 (1979).
208. R. Gleckman and A. Esposito. Gram-negative bacteremic shock: Pathophysiology, clinical features, and treatment. *South. Med. J., 74*:335–341 (1981).
209. D. Webb and H. Thadepalli. Evaluation of cefoxitin, cefazolin and cephradine in comparison with methicillin in the treatment of bacterial endocarditis. *Curr. Ther. Res. Clin. Exp., 34*:311–318 (1983).
210. H. Yamaguchi and M. Ichimaru. Treatment of bacterial infections during acute leukemia. *Jpn. J. Antibiot., 33*:1215–1222 (1980).
211. R. Giura, C. Epifani, and L. Boncinelli. Cefoxitin in the treatment of infections in patients with neoplastic and other serious diseases. *Drugs Exp. Clin. Res., 7*:435–437 (1981).
212. D. Tanphaichitra. Cefoxitin sodium in immunocompromised patients. *Clin. Res., 29*:679A (1981).
213. H. Lagast and J. Klastersky. Anaerobic infections in cancer patients—A retrospective analysis of clindamycin, tinidazole, doxycycline, cefoxitin and lamoxactam. *Infection, 10*:144–148 (1982).
214. S. Dreizen, K. B. McCredie, M. J. Kresting, and G. P. Bodey. Oral infections associated with chemotherapy in adults with acute leukemia. *Postgrad. Med., 71*:133–146 (1982).
215. O. Quesada, A. E. Brown, and D. Armstrong. Efficacy and safety of cefoxitin in combination with gentamicin and carbenicillin as empiric therapy

of febrile, neutropenic pediatric patients with cancer. *Clin. Res., 31*:373A (1983).

216. S. W. Berg, M. E. Kilpatrick, W. O. Harrison, and J. A. McCutchan. Cefoxitin as a single-dose treatment for urethritis caused by penicillinase-producing *Neisseria gonorrhoeae. N. Engl. J. Med., 301*:509–511 (1979).
217. M. S. Siegel, S. E. Thompson, P. L. Perrine, S. T. Brown, G. Reynolds, and C. Thornsberry. Treatment of uncomplicated gonococcal urethritis with cefoxtin: Comparison with penicillin. *Rev. Infect. Dis., 1*:183-187 (1979).
218. Y. M. Felman. Penicillinase-producing *Neisseria gonorrhoeae* in New York City: Recommendations for treatment and control. *N.Y. State J. Med., 82*:1559–1561 (1982).
219. Editorial. Penicillinase-producing gonococci: Further complications. *Lancet, 2*:912–913 (1982).
220. E. J. Perez-Stable. Urethritis in men. *West. J. Med., 138*:426–429 (1983).
221. T. Okazaki, K. Mitsui, and I. Suzuno. Bacteriological and clinical evaluation of a single 2-g administration of cefoxitin on male gonococcal urethritis (especially on β-lactamase-producing gonococci). *Chemotherapy Tokyo, 31*:717–722 (1983).
222. J. A. Jacobsen, J. J. Santos, and W. M. Palmer. Clinical and bacteriological evaluation of cefoxitin therapy in children. *Antimicrob. Agents Chemother., 16*:183–185 (1979).
223. H. E. Gnehm, R. A. Seger, and C. M. Boyle. The efficacy and tolerance of cefoxitin in the treatment of pediatric infections. *Curr. Med. Res. Opin., 8*:44–50 (1982).
224. K. H. Rhodes and C. M. Johnson. Antibiotic therapy for severe infections in infants and children. *Mayo Clin. Proc., 58*:158–164 (1983).
225. A. Mickal, D. Curole, and C. Lewis. Cefoxitin sodium: Double-blind vaginal hysterectomy prophylaxis in premenopausal patients. *Obstet. Gynecol., 56*:222–225 (1980).
226. P. Larson, K. E. Nelson, M. Ismail, and P. J. Geiseler. Double-blind study of cefoxitin prophylaxis of post-cesarean section infection, in *Current Chemotherapy and Infectious Disease,* (J. D. Nelson and C. Grassi, eds.), American Society for Microbiology, Washington, D.C., 1980, pp. 1212–1214.
227. C. E. J. Hoffman, P. J. McDonald, and J. McK. Watts. Use of preoperative cefoxitin to prevent infection after colonic and rectal surgery. *Ann. Surg., 193*:353–356 (1981).
228. D. J. Schurman, D. Burton, K. Moser, and G. Kajiyama. Efficacy and pharmacology of perioperative cefoxitin in the prevention of infections complicating total joint replacement. Paper presented at the 11th International Congress of Chemotherapy, Boston, Mass., October 1–5, 1979, Abstract 342.
229. Anonymous. Antimicrobial prophylaxis for surgery. *Med. Lett. Drugs Ther., 23*:77–80 (1981).
230. J. T. DiPiro, K. E. Record, K. S. Schanzenbach, and B. A. Bivins. Antimicrobial prophylaxis in surgery: Part 1. *Am. J. Hosp. Pharm., 38*:320–334 (1981).

231. B. J. Guglielmo, D. C. Hohn, P. J. Koo, T. K. Hunt, R. L. Sweet, and J. E. Conte, Jr. Antibiotic prophylaxis in surgical procedures: A critical analysis of the literature. *Arch. Surg., 118*:943–955 (1983).
232. R. J. Utley, R. Scott, and W. A. A. G. Macbeth. Double-blind prospective trial using prophylactic cefoxitin preoperatively in the prevention of wound infections complicating abdominal surgery. *N.Z. Med. J., 90*:517 (1979).
233. C. J. L. Strachan. Biliary microflora, postsurgical infection and antibiotic prophylaxis, in *Proceedings of the Symposium on Antibiotic Prophylaxis in Surgery: Current Concepts. XXII Meeting of the International College of Surgeons, Mexico City, July 1980,* (H. C. Neu and A. Percival, eds.), Merck Sharp & Dohme, Rahway, N.J., 1981, pp. 12–19.
234. T. C. Fabian, E. C. Mangiante, and S. J. Boldreghini. Prophylactic antibiotics in patients undergoing elective colorectal surgery or operation for acute bowel obstruction: A double-blind comparative study between cefonicid and cefoxitin. Paper presented at the 22nd Interscience Conference on Antimicrobial Agents and Chemotherapy, Miami Beach, Fla., October 4–6, 1982, Abstract 761.
235. G. Panichi, A. Pantosti, G. Giunchi, F. Tonelli, P. O'Amicis, G. Fegiz, P. Gianfrilli Mastrantonio, I. Luzzi, and M. E. Grandolfi. Cephalothin, cefoxitin, or metronidazole in elective colonic surgery? A single-blind randomized trial. *Dis. Colon Rectum, 25*:783–786 (1982).
236. A. Liegeois, M. A. Brieu, M. C. Gervais, and J. Loygue. Prevention of infectious complications in digestive tract surgery by preoperative cefoxitin: A milti-center study of 582 patients. *Ann. Chir., 36*:545–553 (1982).
237. D. G. Maki and D. R. Aughey. Comparative study of cefazolin, cefoxitin and ceftizoxime for surgical prophylaxis in colo-rectal surgery. *J. Antimicrob. Chemother. Suppl. C, 10*:281–287 (1982).
238. G. F. Coppa, K. Eng, T. H. Gouge, J. H. C. Ranson, and S. A. Localio. Parenteral and oral antibiotics in elective colon and rectal surgery. *Am. J. Surg., 145*:62–65 (1983).
239. R. E. Winslow, R. E. Dean, and J. W. Harley. Acute nonperforating appendicitis: Efficacy of brief antibiotic prophylaxis. *Arch. Surg., 118*:651–655 (1983).
240. L. Kager, A. S. Malmborg, and C. E. Nord. Impact of short-term as compared with long-term prophylaxis with cefoxitin on the colonic microflora in patients undergoing colorectal surgery. *Drugs Exp. Clin. Res., 9*:387–392 (1983).
241. R. J. Baker, A. P. Robin, and K. W. Anderson. Perioperative piperacillin and cefoxitin prophylaxis in elective abdominal operations. Paper presented at the Proceedings of the 13th International Congress of Chemotherapy, Vienna, Austria, August 28 to September 2, 1983.
242. S. E. Wilson, R. A. Williams, and S. A. Finegold. A comparative study of piperacillin and cefoxitin for perioperative prophylaxis in biliary and upper gastrointestinal surgery. Paper presented at the Proceedings of the 13th International Congress of Chemotherapy, Vienna, Austria, August 28 to September 2, 1983.

243. D. L. Hemsell, F. G. Cunningham, S. Kappus, and B. Nobles. Cefoxitin for prophylaxis in premenopausal women undergoing vaginal hysterectomy. *Obstet. Gynecol., 56*:629–634 (1980).
244. J. Pretorius. Cefoxitin prophylaxis in vaginal hysterectomy, in *Proceedings of a Symposium on Prophylaxis and Treatment of Pelvic Infections, Tokyo, Japan, October 29, 1979,* (K. Mashimo and A. Percival, eds.), Biomedical Information, New York, 1981, pp. 29–37.
245. G. K. M. Harding, C. K. Yuen, and B. Lank. Cefoxitin sodium for prophylaxis in premenopausal women undergoing vaginal hysterectomy: Results of a placebo-controlled randomized double-blind study, in *Proceedings of a Symposium on Prophylaxis and Treatment of Pelvic Infections, Tokyo, Japan, October 29, 1979,* (K. Mashimo and A. Percival, eds.), Biomedical Information, New York, 1981, pp. 39–51.
246. O. Hayakawa, T. Kusangi, T. Noda, H. Ito, and R. Etoh. Clinical effect of cefoxitin in treating and preventing gynecological postoperative infections. *Kiso to Rinsho, 15*:287–290 (1981).
247. J. P. Schepers and F. W. H. M. Merkus. Cefoxitin sodium: Double-blind, placebo-controlled, prophylactic study in premenopausal patients undergoing abdominal hysterectomy. *Clin. Pharmacol. Ther., 29*:281 (1981).
248. D. L. Hemsell and F. G. Cunningham. Prophylactic use of antibiotics in abdominal hysterectomy, in *Proceedings of the Symposium on Antibiotic Prophylaxis in Surgery: Current Concepts. XXII Meeting of the International College of Surgeons, Mexico City, July 1980,* (H. C. Neu and A. Percival, eds.), Merck Sharp & Dohme, Rahway, N.J., 1981, pp. 110–117.
249. D. L. Hemsell, E. R. Johnson, R. E. Bawdon, P. G. Hemsell, M. L. Heard, and B. J. Nobles. Cefoperazone and cefoxitin prophylaxis for abdominal hysterectomy. *Obstet. Gynecol., 63*:467–472 (1984).
250. E. Siciliano, M. Aziz, K. Brown, and F. Ricci. Multiclinic, double-blind trial of cefoxitin in the prevention of infectious morbidity of cesarean sections. Paper presented at the World Conference on Clinical Pharmacology and Therapeutics, London, England, August 3–9, 1980, Abstract 0672.
251. W. P. Dillon, M. S. Seigel, A. S. Lele, and J. A. O'Leary. Evaluation of cefoxitin prophylaxis for cesarean section. *Int. J. Gynaecol. Obstet., 19*: 133–139 (1982).
252. H. G. Stiver, K. R. Forward, R. A. Livingstone, P. Fugere, M. Lemay, G. Verschelden, J. D. W. Hunter, G. D. Carson, P. Beresford, and D. L. Tyrrell. Multicenter comparison of cefoxitin versus cefazolin for prevention of infectious morbidity after nonelective cesarean section. *Am. J. Obstet. Gynecol., 145*:158–163 (1983).
253. P. A. Hawrylyshyn, P. Bernstein, and F. R. Papsin. Short-term antibiotic prophylaxis in high-risk patients following cesarean section. *Am. J. Obstet. Gynecol.,* 285–289 (1983).
254. R. Young, L. Platt, and W. Ledger. Prophylactic cefoxitin in cesarean section. *Surg. Gynecol. Obstet., 157*:11–14 (1983).
255. P. O. Madsen, N. Frimodt-Moller, O. S. Nielsen, and S. Maigaard. Prophylaxis of infection in transurethral prostatectomy: A double-blind study

with cefoxitin versus placebo, in *Current Chemotherapy and Infectious Disease,* (J. D. Nelson and C. Grassi, eds.), American Society for Microbiology, Washington, D.C., 1980, pp. 1209–1210.

256. R. R. Landes. Perioperative antibiotic prophylaxis in urologic surgery: A double-blind controlled trial using transurethral prostatectomy as a model, in *Proceedings of the Symposium on Antibiotic Prophylaxis in Surgery: Current Concepts. XXII Meeting of the International College of Surgeons, Mexico City, July 1980,* (H. C. Neu and A. Percival, eds.), Merck Sharp & Dohme, Rahway, N.J., 1981, pp. 91–99.
257. M. B. Rosenfeld, J. Campos, K. R. Ratzan, and I. Uredo. Chemoprophylaxis with cefoxitin and cephalothin in orthopedic surgery: A comparison. *Antimicrob. Agents Chemother., 19*:826–830 (1981).
258. D. J. Schurman, D. S. Burton, and G. Kajiyama. Cefoxitin antibiotic concentration in bone and synovial fluid. *Clin. Orthop. Related Res., 168*:64–68 (1982).
259. C. van Winzum. Clinical safety and tolerance of cefoxitin sodium: An overview. *J. Antimicrob. Chemother. Suppl. B, 4*:91–104 (1978).
260. R. Norrby, C. M. Martin, C. van Winzum, and K. R. Brown. The toxicity of cefoxitin in man. *J. Infect. Suppl., 1*:57–65 (1979).
261. E. Appelbaum and W. A. Leff. Occurrence of superinfections during antibiotic therapy. *J. Am. Med. Assoc., 138*:119 (1948).

PART 4

NEW TYPES OF BETA-LACTAM ANTIBIOTICS

14

Imipenem - Cilastatin

HELMUT KROPP, FREDERICK M. KAHAN,
JAMES S. MacDONALD, and JEROME BIRNBAUM
Merck Sharp & Dohme Research Laboratories, Rahway, New Jersey, and West Point, Pennsylvania

I. INTRODUCTION

This review highlights the in vitro and in vivo activity, pharmacokinetics, and metabolism of two new drugs to be administered in a 1:1 ratio as an injectable antimicrobial. One of the components, imipenem, is the N-formimidoyl derivative of thienamycin and the first of this new class of beta-lactam antibiotics to be used clinically. Imipenem has an unusually broad antibacterial spectrum, including pathogens resistant to most other antimicrobial agents. The companion drug, cilastatin sodium, is a specific inhibitor of a renal dipeptidase, designated dehydropeptidase-I (DHP-I), an enzyme responsible for the metabolism of imipenem and which is present in all mammalian species, including humans. The extensive metabolism of imipenem observed in the kidney results in low urinary recovery of intact antibiotic. Cilastatin is devoid of antimicrobial activity and does not interfere with the antibacterial activity of imipenem; however, when cilastatin or other inhibitors of DHP-I are coadministered with imipenem, the level of intact antibiotic recovered in the urine is greatly increased. In addition, cilastatin eliminates the nephrotoxic potential of imipenem by preventing tubular necrosis induced by high dose rates of antibiotic in the rabbit and the rhesus monkey.

The exceptional antibacterial properties of imipenem coupled with improved urinary tract bioavailability and safety provided by cilastatin have made this combination a clinically useful antibiotic preparation for treatment of serious infections (1).

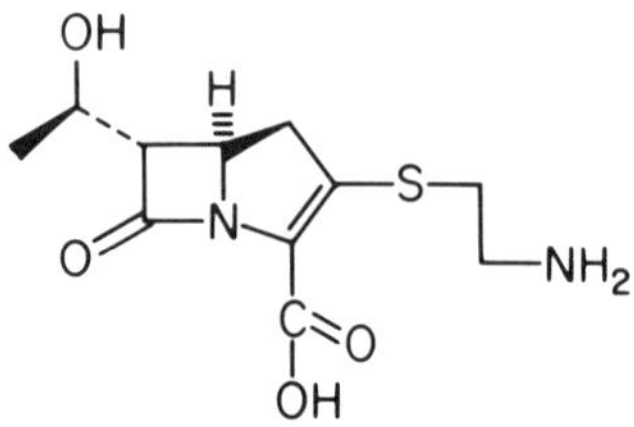

Figure 1 Thienamycin.

II. MICROBIOLOGY

A. Background of Thienamycin Leading to Imipenem

Thienamycin was discovered as a member of a complex of beta-lactam antibiotics produced in fermentation broths by the soil actinomycete, *Streptomyces cattlyea,* itself a hitherto undescribed species (2). Thienamycin is structurally dissimilar (Fig. 1) (3) from all other natural and synthetic beta-lactam antibiotics in the following respects: The five-membered, fused ring lacks sulfur and, unlike the five-membered penicillins, has an enamine system typical of the six-

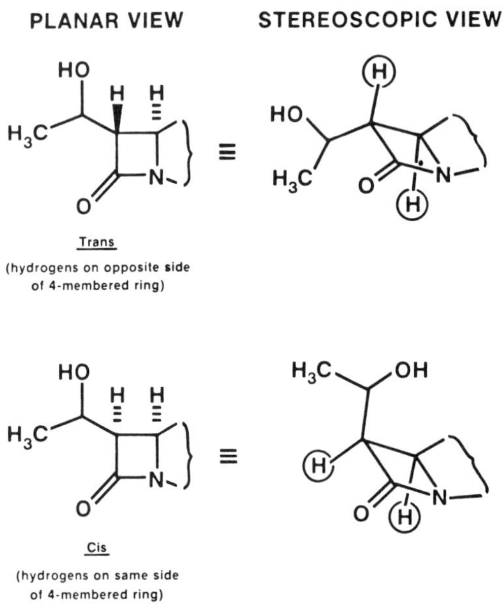

Figure 2

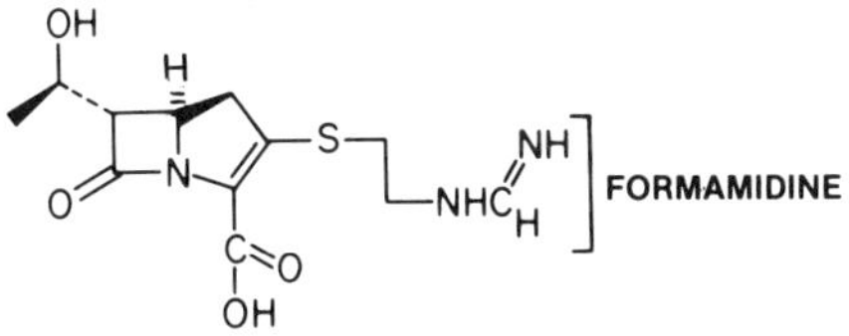

Figure 3 Imipenem (N-formimidoyl thienamycin, MK0787).

membered cephalosporins (it is from the exocyclic S-substituent at C-3 that thienamycin derives its name); the 6-position is directly alkylated by the side chain, in contrast to the acylamino group present at that position in all penicillins and cephalosporins; the configuration of the C-6 side chain is trans with respect to the five-membered ring, where in all other beta-lactam antibiotics the relative configuration is cis (Fig. 2).

Thienamycin resembles the classic beta-lactam antibiotics in its mode of action, being a specific inhibitor of bacterial peptidoglycan "cell wall" biosynthesis. At inhibitory concentrations, it induces the formation of bacterial spheroplasts, whose subsequent lysis accounts for the bactericidal nature of thienamycin action. Biochemical studies indicate thienamycin acts at a late stage of cell wall synthesis, probably by inactivating one or more of the transpeptidases that have been implicated in the mode of action of penicillins (Chapter 2, this volume; 4).

As described below, thienamycin and its derivative, imipenem (IPM) (Fig. 3), have a remarkably comprehensive spectrum of activity that includes important species inherently resistant to most beta-lactam antibiotics, such as *Pseudomonas aeruginosa,* the gram-negative anaerobes, and enterococci (5,6). Furthermore, the antibiotic potency is virtually unaffected by the presence of beta-lactamases directed against one or more of the penicillins and cephalosporins. The high order of potency exhibited in vitro by thienamycin and imipenem is accompanied by an equally high in vivo activity when evaluated parenterally by standard protective efficacy tests in experimentally infected mice (5).

Practical use of thienamycin was limited by inactivation of the antibiotic in solutions at concentrations greater than 3.0 mg/ml (2). Of the many derivatives and analogs synthesized, N-formimidoyl thienamycin proved to have overcome this problem (7) while retaining – and, indeed, improving upon – the desirable antimicrobial properties of the parent antibiotic (5).

Imipenem is a crystalline monohydrate of N-formimidoyl thienamycin and has a solubility of about 11.0 mg/ml in water at room temperature. The solubility limit decreases even further the ability of imipenem to undergo concentration-dependent self-inactivation.

Table 1 Comparison of the Antibacterial Activity of Imipenem to That of Other Antibiotics[a]

Strain (10^5 CFU[b])	MIC (μg/ml)[c]					
	IPM	THM	CFX	CEF	CAB	GEN
Staphylococcus aureus 2985	0.01	0.02	3.2	0.2	0.63	0.32
Staphylococcus aureus 210	0.02	0.04	3.2	0.4	1.3	0.32
Staphylococcus aureus 2874	0.02	0.04	3.2	0.2	1.3	0.16
Staphylococcus aureus 2314	0.04	0.04	6.3	0.8	20.0	0.63
Staphylococcus aureus 2867	0.02	0.04	6.3	0.8	20.0	0.63
Staphylococcus aureus 4428[d]	20.0	40.0	>100	>100	80.0	5.0
Enterococcus 2864	0.63	1.3	>100	25.0	40.0	10.0
Enterococcus 2862	1.3	2.5	>100	25.0	40.0	>20
Enterococcus 2863	40.0	40.0	>100	>100	>80	20.0
Escherichia coli 2482	0.32	0.63	6.3	12.5	5.0	0.32
Escherichia coli 2884	0.08	0.16	6.3	6.3	5.0	1.3
Escherichia coli 2964	0.32	0.32	6.3	100	>80	>20
Escherichia coli 2891	0.16	0.16	50.0	>100	40.0	2.5
Escherichia coli 2895	0.32	0.63	25.0	>100	>80	1.3
Shigella spp. 2880	0.16	0.32	3.2	6.3	5.0	1.3
Salmonella typhimurium 826	0.32	0.32	3.2	6.3	20.0	2.5
Enterobacter cloacae 2647[e]	0.16	0.32	12.5	12.5	20.0	1.3
Enterobacter cloacae 2646	0.63	0.63	>100	>100	>80.0	1.3

Enterobacter cloacae 2828	1.3	2.5	>100	>100	20.0	0.63
Enterobacter spp. 2903	0.63	1.3	>100	>100	5.0	1.3
Enterobacter spp. 2902	1.3	2.5	>100	>100	20.0	1.3
Enterobacter aerogenes 2906	2.5	5.0	>100	>100	5.0	1.3
Klebsiella pneumoniae 2921	0.63	0.63	6.3	12.5	>80	1.3
Klebsiella pneumoniae 2922	0.63	0.63	6.3	100	>80	>20
Klebsiella spp. 2888	0.63	1.3	>100	>100	10.0	1.3
Klebsiella spp. 2890	1.3	1.3	>100	>100	10.0	1.3
Klebsiella spp. 2889	2.5	5.0	>100	>100	10.0	1.3
Serratia spp. 2840	0.63	2.5	25.0	>100	10.0	2.5
Serratia spp. 2855	0.63	2.5	12.5	>100	>80	1.3
Proteus mirabilis 3125	5.0	10.0	3.2	6.3	1.3	5.0
Proteus mirabilis 2831	2.5	5.0	25.0	50.0	2.5	10.0
Proteus mirabilis 2830	5.0	10.0	6.3	>100	>80	2.5
Proteus morganii 2833	5.0	5.0	12.5	>100	>80	2.5
Proteus morganii 2834	2.5	10.0	12.5	>100	1.3	0.32
Providencia spp. 2851	1.3	2.5	1.6	>100	1.3	0.63

[a]Agar dilution study.
[b]CFU, colony-forming unit.
[c]Antibiotic abbreviations: IPM, imipenem, formerly N-formimidoyl thienamycin; THM, thienamycin; CFX, cefoxitin; CEF, cephalothin; CAB, carbenicillin; GEN, gentamicin.
[d]Methicillin resistant.
[e]Beta-lactamase-negative mutant (HSC 18410/M62) derived from parent strain 2646 (HSC 18410/62).
Source: Ref. 5.

Table 2 Susceptibility of *Pseudomonas* Isolates to Imipenem and Other Antibiotics[a]

P. aeruginosa strain number (10^5 CFU)	MIC (μg/ml)[b]							
	IPM	THM	CAB	GEN	AMK	MOX	CTX	PIP
40	1.6	3.1	50	50	6.3	12.5	12.5	3.1
2824	0.63	0.63	80	2.5				
2835	2.5	5	80	5.0				
3350[c]	10	20	>80	>20				
3286	2.5	10	80	5.0	6.3	50	25	6.3
3287[d]	2.5	10	>80	5.0				
3288[e]	20	40	80	5.0				
4293	6.3	25	100	12.5	25	25	25	6.3
4294	12.5	50	100	25	50	25	25	6.3

[a]Agar dilution study.
[b]Antibiotic abbreviations: IPM, imipenem, formerly N-formimidoyl thienamycin; THM, thienamycin; CAB, carbenicillin; GEN, gentamicin; AMK, amikacin; PIP, piperacillin; MOX, moxalactam; CTX, cefotaxime.
[c]Strain 3350 bears plasmid-mediated carbenicillin and gentamicin resistance.
[d]Laboratory isolate from strain 3286 showing spontaneous resistance to carbenicillin.
[e]Laboratory isolate from strain 3286 showing spontaneous resistance to thienamycin.
Source: Ref. 5.

B. Antibacterial Spectrum and Potency of Imipenem

Early during the microbiological evaluation of imipenem, this derivative was noted to retain the desirable broad-spectrum antibacterial properties of the parent antibiotic thienamycin (5). Against some important pathogens such as *P. aeruginosa,* the activity actually improved. Against aerobic organisms, comparative in vitro studies of imipenem, thienamycin, and several reference antibiotics clearly demonstrated the superior antibacterial spectra and potencies of the thienamycin antibiotics (Tables 1 and 2). The activity exceeds that of other beta-lactam antibiotics against both gram-positive species, including enterococci, and gram-negative species, such as *Pseudomonas.* This activity was also retained against isolates exhibiting beta-lactamase-mediated resistance to one or more penicillins and cephalosporins. The minimal inhibitory concentration (MIC) values of imipenem against such isolates were close to the inhibitory levels found for strains susceptible to beta-lactam antibiotics from the same species. Cross-resistance between imipenem and carbenicillin for *P. aeruginosa* isolates has not been observed, nor was carbenicillin resistance found for a thienamycin-

Table 3 Susceptibility of Gram-Negative Aerobes to Imipenem[a]

Pathogen	Number of isolates	MIC_{50} (μg/ml)	MIC_{90} (μg/ml)
Escherichia coli	1122	0.14	0.26
Enterobacter spp.	1276	0.34	1.30
Klebsiella spp.	952	0.18	0.41
Serratia spp.	805	0.76	1.93
Proteus spp. (indole +ve and -ve)	1655	1.3	2.90
Pseudomonas aeruginosa	2278	1.57	3.54
Carbenicillin resistant	142	1.70	3.70
Aminocyclitol resistant	317	2.10	3.80
Acinetobacter spp.	436	0.22	0.47
Alcaligenes spp.	86	0.97	2.0
Brucella melitensis	98	1.0	2.0
Eikenella corrodens	56	0.15	0.22
Hemophilus influenzae	302	0.95	1.82
Moraxella spp.	37	0.08	0.37
Neisseria gonorrhoeae	387	0.10	0.30
Neisseria meningitidis	266	0.05	0.11
Shigella spp.	33	0.17	0.27
Yersinia enterocolitica	234	0.23	0.44
Citrobacter spp.	370	0.30	0.62

[a]Values presented are the geometric means of broth or agar dilution susceptibility distributions measured at inoculum densities of about 10^5 CFU. Results are a composite prepared from the references cited in the text.
Source: Ref. 9.

resistant variant of *P. aeruginosa* (Table 2). During the same evaluation, a methicillin-resistant *Staphylococcus* isolate (#4428) was found to be the single exception to this general absence of cross-resistance. The mechanism of methicillin resistance is known to be unrelated to beta-lactamase activity (see Ref. 8 and Chap. 3).

A large number of independent studies of imipenem have been performed by both university and hospital microbiological laboratories around the world. This evaluation has generated a large number of publications (9) that describe

Table 4 Susceptibility of Gram-Positive Aerobes to Imipenem[a]

Pathogen	Number of isolates	MIC_{50} (μg/ml)	MIC_{90} (μg/ml)
Staphylococcus aureus	1290	≤0.07	≤0.13
Penicillin resistant	110	0.06	0.08
Methicillin resistant	161	0.72	4.70
Staphylococcus epidermidis	509	0.09	1.33
Streptococcus spp. (groups A, B, C, and G)	1293	≤0.03	≤0.05
Streptococcus faecalis	795	0.93	1.58
Listeria monocytogenes	36	0.08	0.11
Nocardia asteroides	45	1.15	2.66

[a]Values presented are the geometric means of broth or agar dilution susceptibility distributions measured at inoculum densities of about 10^5 CFU. Results are a composite prepared from the references cited in the text.
Source: Ref. 9.

the antibacterial properties of imipenem and confirm the initial finding of the Merck Laboratories. Summaries of the composite susceptibility surveys show that the comprehensive scope of activity is matched by no other antibiotic, including the extended-spectrum beta-lactams (Tables 3 and 4). The data include all bacterial species found susceptible to imipenem based on the susceptibility criteria of ≤8.0 μg/ml. By this criterion, three species would be considered resistant: *Pseudomonas maltophilia* (the only species that is uniformly resistant to imipenem), *Pseudomonas cepacia,* and *Streptococcus faecium.*

An additional distinctive feature of imipenem and one which is unequaled by the newer extended-spectrum beta-lactams is its good activity against all isolates of gram-positive cocci (Table 4). Against these organisms, the activity of imipenem approaches the potency displayed by the penicillins against susceptible isolates, an activity uncompromised by bacterial lactamases present in penicillin-resistant staphylococci. On occasion, a given gram-negative species is found more sensitive to a comparative antibiotic in vitro; however, the overall potency of imipenem against the total spectrum is unequaled. A survey of reported in vitro comparative susceptibility studies (5-27) demonstrates the overall superior activity of imipenem when compared to that of other beta-lactam agents and aminoglycoside antibiotics (Table 5).

In general, the activity of beta-lactam antibiotics against group D streptococci is minimal and in most instances completely absent. Though the mean

Table 5 Comparative In Vitro Activities of Imipenem and Beta-Lactam and Aminoglycoside Antibiotics[a]

Organism	Antibiotic	Number of isolates	Geometric mean MIC	
			MIC_{50} (μg/ml)	MIC_{90} (μg/ml)
Gram-positive organisms				
Staphylococcus aureus	Imipenem	379	≤0.04	≤0.06
	Cefotaxime	150	2.1	3.7
	Cefoxitin	35	3.3	8.8
	Cephalothin	199	0.34	0.7
	Ceftazidime	37	19.2	>30.0
	Moxalactam	160	9.2	>12.5
	Piperacillin	160	5.8	30.2
	Tobramycin	69	0.12	0.5
Staphylococcus epidermidis	Imipenem	163	≤0.06	0.44
	Cephalothin	105	≤0.16	1.2
	Ceftazidime	12	8.0	32.0
	Moxalactam	40	16.6	>45.0
	Penicillin G	117	0.69	5.8
	Tobramycin	18	0.25	>32.0
Streptococcus spp. (groups A, B, C, G, and H)	Imipenem	265	≤0.02	≤0.04
	Cephalothin	136	≤0.16	≤0.03
	Moxalactam	215	2.6	4.9
	Oxacillin	32	0.13	0.21
	Penicillin G	170	≤0.02	≤0.05
	Piperacillin	95	≤0.06	≤0.2
	Tobramycin	95	>32.0	>32.0
Streptococcus group D (enterococci)	Imipenem	307	1.17	2.1
	Ampicillin	94	1.15	1.4
	Carbenicillin	29	50.0	50.0
	Cefoperazone	126	>34.0	>50.0
	Piperacillin	110	5.4	20.5
	Ticarcillin	29	100.0	200.0
	Tobramycin	26	>32.0	>32.0
	Vancomycin	29	1.0	2.0

Table 5 (continued)

Organism	Antibiotic	Number of isolates	Geometric mean MIC	
			MIC_{50} (μg/ml)	MIC_{90} (μg/ml)
Gram-negative organisms				
Escherichia coli	Imipenem	446	≤0.16	0.35
	Cefoperazone	80	0.13	1.5
	Cefotaxime	160	≤0.05	0.10
	Cefoxitin	97	3.5	6.4
	Ceftazidime	60	0.12	0.5
	Moxalactam	243	0.10	0.21
	Piperacillin	206	1.82	>45.0
	Amikacin	88	2.4	8.0
Enterobacter spp.	Imipenem	518	0.36	1.04
	Cefotaxime	371	0.09	0.61
	Cefoxitin	281	>12.0	>124.0
	Ceftazidime	34	0.5	16.0
	Moxalactam	313	0.13	0.76
	Carbenicillin	106	5.7	47.0
	Piperacillin	171	2.3	15.1
	Ticarcillin	134	>5.3	>87.0
	Amikacin	51	2.0	4.0
	Tobramycin	27	0.5	0.73
Klebsiella spp.	Imipenem	315	≤0.17	0.47
	Cefotaxime	139	≤0.02	≤0.09
	Cefoxitin	48	2.7	4.8
	Ceftazidime	57	0.25	1.0
	Moxalactam	141	0.10	0.30
	Carbenicillin	96	>631.0	>631.0
	Piperacillin	174	6.3	>22.0
	Amikacin	48	1.3	4.6

Table 5 (continued)

Organism	Antibiotic	Number of isolates	Geometric mean MIC: MIC_{50} (μg/ml)	Geometric mean MIC: MIC_{90} (μg/ml)
Serratia spp.	Imipenem	214	0.68	1.3
	Cefotaxime	102	0.26	2.0
	Cefoxitin	47	20.0	>55.0
	Ceftazidime	30	0.25	0.25
	Moxalactam	77	0.76	2.1
	Carbenicillin	70	22.0	>578.0
	Gentamicin	47	4.2	51.0
Proteus mirabilis	Imipenem	210	1.4	3.0
	Cefoperazone	74	0.61	2.0
	Cefotaxime	146	0.02	0.03
	Cefoxitin	26	4.6	8.0
	Ceftazidime	60	0.06	0.06
	Moxalactam	101	≤0.12	0.16
	Carbenicillin	33	0.78	0.78
	Piperacillin	101	≤0.41	≤1.33
	Ticarcillin	121	0.68	>14.0
	Tobramycin	38	0.86	3.0
Proteus spp. indole (+)	Imipenem	386	1.8	3.3
	Cefoperazone	82	1.5	6.5
	Cefotaxime	318	≤0.04	0.4
	Cefoxitin	215	4.3	>15.0
	Ceftazidime	60	0.12	0.21
	Moxalactam	265	0.11	0.20
	Piperacillin	95	0.77	6.0
	Ticarcillin	110	>4.5	>48.0
	Amikacin	38	2.3	5.8

Table 5 (continued)

Organism	Antibiotic	Number of isolates	Geometric mean MIC: MIC_{50} (μg/ml)	MIC_{90} (μg/ml)
Pseudomonas aeruginosa	Imipenem	590	1.5	4.9
	Cefoperazone	254	3.9	22.4
	Cefotaxime	372	12.2	>43.4
	Ceftazidime	59	2.0	4.0
	Ceftizoxime	100	64.0	>64.0
	Moxalactam	389	13.0	>42.4
	Carbenicillin	198	75.0	563.0
	Piperacillin	230	5.2	19.6
	Gentamicin	237	2.3	>11.0
	Tobramycin	138	1.4	10.2

[a]Results are a composite prepared from the references cited in the text.

MIC of imipenem against the major portion of such clinical isolates was found to be low (MIC_{90} ∼2.0 μg/ml), the minimal bactericidal concentrations (MBC) were found to be several-fold higher for a significant number of the isolates examined (28,29). This observation is not unexpected, since incomplete killing of enterococci by cell-wall-active agents may indicate an inherent ability by this organism to resist these agents. Despite the fact that some strains of *Streptococcus faecalis* are tolerant to imipenem, the potential of this new antibiotic to be used as a single agent and in combination with other antibiotics in the treatment of certain enterococcal infections appears quite promising.

No discrepancies in inhibitory endpoints have been encountered between agar dilution and broth dilution (microtiter) susceptibility testing methods (5). Comparative studies were conducted while measuring the effect of inoculum on imipenem endpoints of clinical isolates of *P. aeruginosa* (Table 6) and the bacteriostatic and bactericidal activities of imipenem against a representative group of gram-positive and gram-negative species (Table 7). The clinical *Pseudomonas* isolates, half of which were considered resistant to carbenicillin, were uniformly susceptible to imipenem at both inoculum levels. The generally small inoculum effect on imipenem activity observed with most gram-negative enteric strains is considered an added advantage in comparison to other agents. Imipenem, as ex-

Table 6 Effect of Inoculum Levels on the Susceptibility of 13 Clinical *P. aeruginosa* Isolates to Imipenem and Seven Reference Antibiotics[a]

	MIC					
	10^5 CFU inoculum			10^7 CFU inoculum		
Compound	Range	MIC_{50} (μg/ml)	MIC_{90} (μg/ml)	Range	MIC_{50} (μg/ml)	MIC_{90} (μg/ml)
Imipenem	0.8–12.5	3.1	6.3	3.1–12.5	6.3	12.5
Thienamycin	1.6–50	6.3	25	3.1–50	12.5	25
Moxalactam	12.5–>50	25	50	50–>50	>50	>50
Cefotaxime	12.5–>100	25	100	50–>100	>100	>100
Carbenicillin	50–>400	100	400	100–>400	200	>400
Piperacillin	3.1–>100	6.3	25	25–>100	100	>100
Gentamicin	1.6–>50	6.3	50	6.3–>50	6.3	>50
Amikacin	1.6–50	6.3	25	6.3–50	12.5	50

[a]Agar dilution study.
Source: Ref. 5.

pected for a cell wall antibiotic, was shown to be bactericidal, with MBC values equal to or only two- to fourfold higher than the MIC values against several genera of organisms. Other investigators have reported similar results, with only a minor fraction of their bacterial isolates displaying MBC values exceeding the MIC for imipenem (22,30).

The antibacterial properties of imipenem shown for anaerobic bacteria are similar to those observed for the aerobic species. The activity against *Bacteroides fragilis* in particular (Table 8) is unmatched by any other beta-lactam antibiotic and equals and in some instances exceeds the activity of metronidazole, clindamycin, and chloramphenicol (5,14,16,23,24,31,34,35). The anaerobe activity of imipenem covers essentially all species, including *Clostridium difficile* (Table 9), as well as bacteroides and clostridia isolates found resistant to clindamycin and cefoxitin (13,18). Based on a significant collection of in vitro data, imipenem clearly emerges as a most promising new beta-lactam antibiotic for the treatment of bacterial infections involving anaerobes as well as those involving a mixed flora of aerobes and anaerobes.

Indifference of imipenem to beta-lactamase activity was observed during the initial in vitro evaluation of this new antibiotic (5). Subsequent studies by numerous investigators (13,30,32,33) have established the stability of imipenem to

Table 7 Comparative Bacteriostatic and Bactericidal Activities of Imipenem at Increasing Inoculum Levels[a]

Organism	Inoculum (CFU)	Imipenem MIC (μg/ml)	Imipenem MBC (μg/ml)	Cephalothin MIC (μg/ml)	Cephalothin MBC (μg/ml)
Staphylococcus aureus 2985	10^3	0.012	0.012	0.4	0.4
	10^5	0.012	0.025	0.4	0.4
	10^7	0.025	0.025	0.4	0.4
Escherichia coli 2891	10^3	0.1	0.2	>200	
	10^5	0.2	0.4		
	10^7	0.8	6.3		
Enterobacter cloacae 2646	10^3	0.4	0.4	>200	
	10^5	0.4	0.8		
	10^7	6.3	12.5		
Klebsiella pneumoniae 2888	10^3	0.8	0.8	>200	
	10^5	0.8	0.8		
	10^7	3.1	6.3		
Proteus morganii 2833	10^3	0.8	0.8	>200	
	10^5	1.6	3.1		
	10^7	6.3	6.3		
Serratia marcescens 3548	10^3	0.4	0.4	>200	
	10^5	1.6	1.6		
	10^7	1.6	>50		
Pseudomonas aeruginosa 40	10^3	0.8	0.8	>200	
	10^5	0.8	0.8		
	10^7	3.1	6.3		
Pseudomonas aeruginosa 3286	10^3	1.6	1.6	>200	
	10^5	3.1	3.1		
	10^7	12.5	12.5		

[a]The MIC and MBC values were determined using the broth dilution (MH) microtiter technique.
Source: Ref. 5.

Carbenicillin		Cefotaxime		Moxalactam	
MIC (μg/ml)	MBC (μg/ml)	MIC (μg/ml)	MBC (μg/ml)	MIC (μg/ml)	MBC (μg/ml)
0.8	0.8	0.8	0.8	6.3	6.3
0.8	1.6	1.6	1.6	6.3	12.5
0.8	1.6	1.6	1.6	6.3	12.5
25	25	1.6	1.6	0.4	0.8
50	50	3.1	6.3	0.8	1.6
50	>200	12.5	50	12.5	100
200	200	50	50	3.1	3.1
200	200	>100		12.5	50
>200				50	50
6.3	6.3	0.2	0.2	0.1	0.2
100	200	25	25	1.6	25
>200		>100		25	50
>200		0.025	0.025	0.2	0.2
		3.1	3.1	0.2	0.4
		25	25	12.5	12.5
>200		0.4	0.4	0.8	0.8
		0.8	3.1	1.6	1.6
		25	>100	25	>100
25	50	6.3	6.3	6.3	6.3
50	50	12.5	50	12.5	12.5
100	200	50	>100	50	>100
50	50	6.3	12.5	12.5	12.5
100	100	12.5	50	25	25
200	>200	>100		>100	

Table 8 Comparative Susceptibility Studies on *B. fragilis* Strains to Imipenem and Reference Antibiotics[a]

Antibiotic	Number of isolates	Geometric mean MIC: MIC_{50} (μg/ml)	Geometric mean MIC: MIC_{90} (μg/ml)
Imipenem	345	0.15	0.4
Cefotaxime	47	4.8	≤25.0
Cefoxitin	203	9.3	20.2
Moxalactam	180	0.6	4.8
Chloramphenicol	100	4.0	8.0
Clindamycin	156	≤0.47	1.6
Metronidazole	56	0.5	1.0

[a]Results are a composite prepared from the references cited in the text.

hydrolysis by all common beta-lactamases and most unusual, rare beta-lactamases (see Chap. 3). As a result, the full antibacterial activity of imipenem is retained against strains carrying beta-lactamase resistance to one or more penicillins and cephalosporins (33,36–38). Beta-lactamase resistance is not the only factor which determines the lack of cross-resistance of imipenem with other beta-lactam antibiotics. Imipenem activity is also impressive against the majority of multiply-resistant gram-negative and gram-positive strains, including strains with acquired resistance to carbenicillin, the newer ureidopenicillins, and aminoglycoside antibiotics (13,17,21,24,38–43). Of particular interest is the uniform response of imipenem against isolates of *P. aeruginosa* exhibiting increased carbenicillin resistance unrelated to the production of carbenicillinase (44). Imipenem differs significantly from the newer extended-spectrum cephalosporins by maintaining full sensitivity to carbenicillin-resistant isolates, while cefotaxime, moxalactam, cefoperazone, cefsulodin, ceftriaxone, and ceftazidime show a correlated increase in resistance to these isolates. Changes in cell permeability and/or affinity for target proteins are proposed as the possible basis for this carbenicillin and cephalosporin resistance.

The mode of action of imipenem has been studied in several bacteria (reviewed in Ref. 9). Imipenem interferes with murein synthesis and crosslinking by interacting with numerous sites in the cell responsible for these functions, accounting in part for its exceptional potency. Dramatic morphological and surface disruptions of the cell are observed. These cellular aberations are brought about by preferential action of imipenem on the penicillin-binding protein PBP-

Table 9 Susceptibility of Anaerobes to Imipenem[a]

Pathogen	Number of isolates	MIC_{50} (μg/ml)	MIC_{90} (μg/ml)
Gram-negative organisms			
Bacteroides fragilis	907	≤0.08	≤0.33
Fusobacterium spp.	57	0.03	0.50
Viellonella spp.	23	0.05	0.25
Campylobacter fetus	92	0.07	0.07
Gram-positive organisms			
Clostridium perfringens	31	0.06	0.54
Clostridium difficile	80	4.06	6.05
Clostridium spp.	133	0.09	0.28
Eubacterium spp.	6	0.06	2.0
Peptococcus spp.	55	0.03	0.07
Peptostreptococcus spp.	32	0.01	0.05

[a]Values presented are the geometric means of broth or agar dilution susceptibility distributions measured at inoculum densities of about 10^5 CFU. Results are a composite prepared from the references cited in the text.
Source: Ref. 9.

2, thereby preventing filament formation and leading to cell death and lysis. Excellent cell penetration coupled with the high affinity for a multitude of penicillin-binding proteins and potent inhibition of cell wall crosslinking enzymes accounts for the superior antibacterial activity of imipenem.

As indicated earlier, although a large portion of methicillin-resistant *Staphylococcus aureus* (MRSA) strains are sensitive to imipenem (Table 4), these isolates show a wide distribution of sensitivities, with major differences in MIC values observed among the published studies (12,45–47). Additional laboratory studies and clinical experience will decide the utility of imipenem against MRSA strains. In contrast, coagulase-negative staphylococci are generally very sensitive to imipenem (MIC, <0.1 μg/ml). Though high MIC values have been occasionally reported for *Staphylococcus epidermidis* (48), the majority of isolates that were examined have been found to be susceptible (10,20,24,30). Less prevalent and generally antibiotic-resistant species such as *Acinetobacter* and *Nocardia asteroides* have been reported to be sensitive to imipenem (49–61). An alphabetical listing of the full spectrum of bacterial species found susceptible to imipenem is presented in Table 10. The data are compiled from reports of 16,000 isolates

Table 10 Alphabetical Listing of Bacterial Susceptibility to Imipenem

Bacterial strain	Gram (+/-)	N	Geometric mean MIC MIC_{50} (μg/ml)	MIC_{90} (μg/ml)
Achromobacter Vd-1, Vd-2		10	2.0	2.0
Achromobacter xylosoxidans		7	2.0	4.0
Actinomyces odontolyticus		5	0.06	0.13
Acinetobacter calcoaceticus (includes subspecies *anitratus, lwoffii, haemolyticus, alcaligenes*)	–	436	≤0.22	0.47
Aeromonas hydrophilia	–	5	0.05	0.10
Alcaligenes spp. (incl. *faecalis*)	–	86	≤0.97	2.04
Bacteroides spp. (incl. *fragilis, disiens, distasonis, melanin, melaninogenicus, oralis, ruminocola brevis, thetaiotaomicron, vulgatus, ovatus, uniformis*)	–	997	≤0.08	<0.33
Bordetella bronchiseptica		5	0.5	4.0
Bordetella bronchicanis	–	13	4.0	4.0
Brucella melitensis	–	98	1.0	2.0
Campylobacter (incl. *fetus, jejuni, intestinalis*)	–	92	≤0.07	≤0.07
Citrobacter/Salmonella (incl. *C. freundii, diversus, Arizona hinshawii*)	–	370	≤0.30	≤0.62
Clostridia spp. (incl. *septicum, difficile, perfringens, bifermentans, botulinum*)	+	292	≤0.31	≤1.14
Escherichia coli	–	1122	≤0.14	≤0.26
Eikenella corrodens	–	56	0.15	0.22

Table 10 (continued)

Bacterial strain	Gram (+/-)	N	Geometric mean MIC: MIC_{50} (μg/ml)	MIC_{90} (μg/ml)
Enterobacter spp. (incl. *cloacae, aerogenes, agglomerans*)	–	1276	0.34	1.30
Erysipelothrix rhusiopathiae	+	2	≤0.02	≤0.02
Eubacterium sp.	+	6	≤0.06	2.0
Flavobacterium spp. (incl. IIb)	–	59	5.04	28.0
Fusobacterium sp.	–	57	0.03	0.50
Gardnerella vaginalis	–	25	–	0.50
Hemophilus influenzae	–	302	0.95	1.82
Hafnia spp. (incl. *alvei*)	–	14	≤0.28	≤0.46
Klebsiella spp. (incl. *pneumoniae, oxytoca*)	–	952	≤0.18	≤0.41
Listeria monocytogenes	+	36	≤0.08	≤0.11
Moraxella spp. (incl. *osloensis*)	–	37	≤0.08	0.37
Mycobacterium avium intracellulare	–	22		0.48
Mycobacterium fortuitum	+	12	3.12	12.50*
Neisseria gonorrhoeae	–	387	≤0.10	≤0.30
Neisseria meningitidis	–	266	0.05	0.11
Nocardia spp. (incl. *asteroides*)	+	83	≤0.91	2.00
Pasteurella multocida	–	10	0.50	1.00
Peptococcus/Peptostreptococcus (incl. *Peptococcus asaccharolyticus, magnus*)	+	87	≤0.02	≤0.06
Plesiomonas shigelloides	–	15	≤0.13	0.25
Propionibacterium acnes	+	26	0.01	0.02

Table 10 (continued)

			Geometric mean MIC	
Bacterial strain	Gram (+/-)	N	MIC_{50} (μg/ml)	MIC_{90} (μg/ml)
Proteus/Providencia spp. (incl. *Proteus vulgaris, mirabilis, morganii, rettgeri* and *Prov. stuartii*)	–	1655	1.30	2.90
Pseudomonas spp. (incl. *aeruginosa, acidovorans, putrefaciens, stutzeri, fluorescens*)	–	2278	1.57	3.54
Pseudomonas cepacia		40	4.5	>50.0
Rhodococcus spp.	–	11	≤0.39	≤0.39
Staphylococcus aureus	+	1290	≤0.07	≤0.13
Staphylococcus epidermidis	+	509	≤0.09	≤1.33
Serratia spp. (incl. *marcescens*)	–	806	≤0.76	1.93
Shigella spp.	–	33	0.17	0.27
Streptococcus spp. (incl. groups A, B, C, G, and H)	+	1293	≤0.03	≤0.05
Streptococcus faecalis (group D)	+	795	0.93	1.58
Streptococcus viridans	+	51	≤0.06	≤0.11
Veillonella spp. (incl. *parvula*)	–	23	0.05	0.25
Yersinia spp. (incl. *enterocolitica, pseudotuberculosis*)	–	234	≤0.23	0.44

*MIC_{70}

cited in the literature and is presented to serve as a convenient reference chart for the overall activity of imipenem.

Successful treatment of certain bacteria, including *P. aeruginosa* and tolerant gram-positive cocci such as *Strep. faecalis,* have in some instances required the use of beta-lactam antibiotics in combination with aminoglycosides. Synergistic combinations of imipenem and aminoglycosides have been reported in susceptibility surveys of gram-positive and gram-negative bacterial species, including multiple-resistant *P. aeruginosa* (30,63,64,66–68), *Strep. faecalis* (28,62,65,69), *Listeria monocytogenes* (65), and *Serratia* spp. (64,67). The degree of synergy not only varies with the aminoglycoside used in combination with imipenem but also is dependent on the relative sensitivity of a given isolate to imipenem alone, a phenomenon more frequently observed with *P. aeruginosa* strains. In general, a lack of synergism against such organisms was in most instances attributable to the efficiency of killing by imipenem as a single agent. Many investigators also commented on the significant increase in magnitude and rate of killing when imipenem was combined with an aminoglycoside. Rapid bactericidal action was observed by a combination of imipenem and tobramycin against several strains of *P. aeruginosa* and *Staph. aureus* isolated from patients with endocarditis (66). A high degree of synergistic interaction was reported on combinations of imipenem with amikacin and gentamicin against isolates of *Strep. faecalis* (65) and *N. asteroides* (59); antagonistic interactions were observed only rarely in the majority of the published studies.

Though full synergy (defined as a fourfold or greater reduction in the MIC values of both antibiotics) is in general not readily predictable in all cases with combinations of imipenem and aminoglycosides, more rapid bactericidal effects almost invariably result from the combination. A demonstration of this beneficial effect of synergy in animal models will be discussed below.

C. Protective Efficacy of Imipenem Against Experimental Infections

Evidence for protective efficacy in vivo was first established in the mouse septicemia model (5) when imipenem was evaluated against comparative antibiotics in gram-positive and gram-negative experimental infections. The same advantage in spectrum and potency over established therapeutics observed earlier in vitro was also demonstrated in vivo. The in vivo activity was explored further in a variety of additional studies employing experimental animal models that were designed to predict the effectiveness of imipenem in the clinic.

Many investigators have reported on the outstanding bactericidal effectiveness of imipenem in animals. Imipenem was found highly effective in peritonitis and intra-abdominal sepsis against mixed aerobe and anaerobe infections in the rat (71,72). In this model the activity of imipenem was greater than that of comparative antibiotics, such as cefoxitin and a combination of gentamicin plus clindamycin. Effective therapy was also demonstrated against *P. aeruginosa* in a guinea pig pneumonia model (70) and bacteremia in neutropenic rats (73). The activity was further enhanced when imipenem was combined with amikacin, resulting in a 95% survival rate of neutropenic rats, and suggests a promising therapeutic potential of imipenem in immunocompromised patients. In a model of acute pyelonephritis the antibacterial efficacy of imipenem surpassed the comparison agent cefotaxime against both *Escherichia coli* and *P. aeruginosa* infections (74). Imipenem was also found to be strikingly efficacious in the treatment of *Staph. aureus* pyelonephritis in the rat, regardless of the methicillin sensitivity of the infecting organism (75). Several investigators have reported on the ability of imipenem to penetrate into the cerebrospinal fluid (CSF) of animals with normal as well as inflamed meninges (76,78–80). Though antibiotic levels in the CSF of uninfected animals were expectedly low ($\leq$1% = CSF to plasma ratio), comparison of areas under the curves showed good penetration ranging from 10 to 31%. Striking reductions in bacterial counts resulting in most cases in sterile CSF were observed in rabbits with inflamed meninges induced by *E. coli* (78), *Hemophilus influenzae* (80), and *Streptococcus pneumoniae* (79) infections. Imipenem was found to be more effective than penicillin G against group B *Streptococcus* bacteremia and meningitis in an infant rat model (76). The investigator reported greater bactericidal activity in both blood and CSF and enhanced clearance of bacteria from these sites leading to more rapid sterilization of the blood. The potential of imipenem in the treatment of bacterial endocarditis was evaluated in rat and rabbit models. Against strains of *Staph. aureus* isolated from endocarditis patients, imipenem was significantly more potent and more rapid in its bactericidal action when compared with nafcillin in a rabbit model (81). Other investigators measured the effectiveness of imipenem as a single agent in the treatment of enterococcal endocarditis using an isolate of *Strep. faecalis* expressing tolerance to this antibiotic (MIC, 1.56; MBC, >128 μg/ml). In this rabbit model, designed to simulate streptococcal prosthetic valve infections in humans, the activity of imipenem was equal to that of penicillin G but not as bactericidal as a combination of penicillin G plus gentamicin (29), which was in agreement with the in vitro results. The combination of imipenem plus gentamicin (or amikacin), which was synergistic and bactericidal against *Strep. faecalis* isolates in several in vitro studies (28,65,69), was not tested for comparison in this rabbit model. Equivalent activity to a combination of cloxacillin and gentamicin was, however, demonstrated against *Staph. aureus* endocarditis in the rat, following a 5-day treatment. Antibiotic serum levels comparable to those achieved in humans after an intravenous injection of a 750-mg dose of imipenem were obtained (77).

For the convenience of the reader, a summary (Table 11) has been prepared to briefly list the observations and results achieved with the infection models described.

Judging from its impressive performance in these infectious disease models, often showing better activity than comparison agents with established records of clinical efficacy, it is anticipated that imipenem will play a major role in the treatment and control of difficult clinical infections.

Table 11 Efficacy of Imipenem Against Experimental Infections

Animal species	Infection model	Results and observations	Reference
Mouse	Septicemia	Outstanding efficacy of IPM versus gram-positive and gram-negative pathogens; often up to 10 times more effective than reference antibiotics	5
Guinea pig	*P. aeruginosa* pneumonia	IPM highly effective in preventing mortality and clearing organism from the lung; equal to tobramycin and superior to ticarcillin	70
Rat	Peritonitis induced by injection of human fecal suspensions	IPM was more effective than cefoxitin or gentamicin plus clindamycin	71
Rat	Intra-abdominal infection simulating intra-abdominal sepsis in patients	Cefoxitin and IPM only antibiotics to give cures as single agents; IPM more potent than cefoxitin	72
Rat	*P. aeruginosa* bacteremia in neutropenic rats	IPM superior to amikacin; IPM with amikacin gave 95% cures	73
Rat	*E. coli* and *P. aeruginosa* pyelonephritis	IPM demonstrated antibacterial effects superior to cefotaxime	74
Rat	Methicillin-sensitive and methicillin-resistant staphylococcal pyelonephritis	IPM very efficacious, regardless of methicillin sensitivity	75
Infant rat	Group B *Streptococcus* bacteremia and meningitis	IPM more effective than penicillin G; greater bactericidal activity in blood and CSF and more rapid bacterial clearing from these sites, as well as quick sterilization of the blood	76

Table 11 (continued)

Animal species	Infection model	Results and observations	Reference
Rat	*Staph. aureus* endocarditis	IPM found equivalent in activity to combination of cloxacillin and gentamicin following 5-day treatment	77
Rabbit	*E. coli* meningitis	IPM penetrated CSF to 31% of plasma peak; large killing effect of infecting organism in CSF observed	78
Rabbit	*Strep. pneumoniae* meningitis	IPM penetrated CSF to 10% of plasma peak	79
Rabbit	*H. influenzae* meningitis	IPM penetration into CSF ranged from 18 to 23% of plasma peak	80
Rabbit	Enterococcus endocarditis	IPM equal to penicillin G in efficacy; however, not as effective as penicillin G plus gentamicin	29
Rabbit	*Staph. aureus* endocarditis	IPM more rapidly bactericidal than nafcillin	81

III. BIOCHEMICAL, METABOLIC, AND PHARMACOLOGICAL STUDIES

A. Location of Thienamycin Metabolism in the Kidney

Thienamycin, imipenem, and related carbapenem antibiotics are subject to extensive and species-variable metabolism, evident from the generally low urinary recovery of antibiotic in animals and humans (Table 12). Disposition studies in the mouse and dog showed that incomplete recovery is also not attributable to a significant biliary clearance pathway, an observation later confirmed in humans (84a). Measures of the systemic bioavailability of imipenem and thienamycin, for example half-life and area under the curve (AUC), compare favorably in the species listed in Table 12 with those of nonmetabolized antibiotics and to those that undergo only minor metabolism. However, renal clearance rates of imipenem were found to be unusually low; for example, the renal clearance in the dog is 0.49 ml/min per kilogram, which is far below the glomerular filtration rate for this animal. An analogous low rate of renal

Table 12 Disposition of Imipenem and Related Antibiotics in Laboratory Species and Humans

Species	Antibiotic[a]	$T_{1/2}$ (min)	Urinary recovery (%)	Clearance rates: Plasma (ml/min per kg)	Clearance rates: Renal (ml/min per kg)	Glomerular filtration rate[b] (ml/min per kg)
Rabbit	IPM[c]	16.0	44.0	33.0	14.0	(2.7)
anephric[d]	IPM	86.0	—	1.4	—	—
Dog	IPM	31.0	8.0	5.2	0.5	4.9
	THM	17.0	5.0	3.6	0.4	—
Chimpanzee	IPM	45.0	14.0	4.4	0.6	2.0
	THM	36.0	12.3	3.4	1.0	—
Man	IPM[e]					
	High metabolism	55.0	14.0	2.8	0.39	(1.8)
	Low metabolism	—	30.0	3.2	0.96	—

[a]Abbreviations: IPM, imipenem (MK0787); THM, thienamycin.
[b]Inulin clearance rates; values in parentheses from handbook references to that species; values for the dog determined as creatinine clearance.
[c]Kropp et al., (82). Dose rates were 5.0 mg/kg and administered as an intravenous bolus.
[d]Rabbit was rendered anephric by bilateral ligation of renal arteries.
[e]Data from Norrby et al. (90) for two panels of eight subjects each, grouped according to urinary recovery of imipenem. Individuals with high metabolism showed a range of recoveries of 7–17%. Individuals with low metabolism had urinary recoveries of 20–37%. Imipenem was administered intravenously at a dose of 500 or 1000 mg.
Source: Ref. 9.

clearance of imipenem was observed in the chimpanzee, a species having an excretion pattern similar to that of humans.

This inconsistency between persistent antibiotic levels in the circulation and low renal clearance rates suggested that metabolism of the antibiotic occurs primarily in the kidney. Biochemical studies subsequently confirmed that the major metabolic inactivation of imipenem and other carbapenem and penem antibiotics results from the hydrolysis of the beta-lactam ring by a renal dipeptidase, dehydropeptidase-I (DHP-I) (82).

B. Role of a Specific Renal Dipeptidase, Dehydropeptidase-I, in Thienamycin Metabolism

Low renal clearance rates suggested that the antibiotic is destroyed during the process of excretion. In the rat, where urinary recovery of thienamycin is 20%, plasma clearance rates are reduced from 11.7 ml/min per kilogram in a sham-operated control to 6.1 ml/min per kilogram in the animal with ligated renal arteries. In rabbits, which exhibit urinary recoveries from 40 to 50%, plasma clearance is reduced by more than 95% following bilateral ligation. Importantly, the major role of the kidney in metabolism was confirmed by the finding of prolonged plasma levels of antibiotic following bilateral ligation of the renal arteries in the rat and the rabbit (82).

These experiments pointed directly to the kidney as the major site of metabolism and prompted the examination of inactivation of thienamycin by tissue homogenates of kidney and other organs from several species, including humans (82). Significant hydrolysis of thienamycin was detected only in kidney extracts, an observation consistent with the results obtained from the disposition studies. Loss of antibiotic activity was matched by an equivalent decline in the specific absorbance of thienamycin measurable at 297 nm. Heat inactivation of tissue homogenates or treatment with EDTA eliminated the activity, while the degradative activity of kidney homogenates was retained following extensive dialysis and was independent of oxygen. These results suggested a hydrolytic reaction. Involvement of a specific membrane-bound Zn-metallopeptidase appeared likely, since the activity of preparations inhibited by EDTA was restored only by the addition of Zn^{2+} (Mg^{2+} and Co^{2+} had no effect) and since other (soluble) Zn-metalloenzymes (e.g., carboxypeptidase-A, carboxypeptidase-B, leucine-aminopeptidase and acylase-I) had no effect on the antibiotic (82).

A review of the known renal metallopeptidases, matched with the properties observed with homogenates, suggested that the responsible enzyme was the renal dipeptidase, dehydropeptidase-I (EC 3.4.13.11), so named by its original discoverer Greenstein (83) based on a broad and general specificity for substrates, including unnatural LD and L-dehydro dipeptides. The structural similarity of the susceptible bond in thienamycin and dehydropeptides [e.g., glycyldehydro-

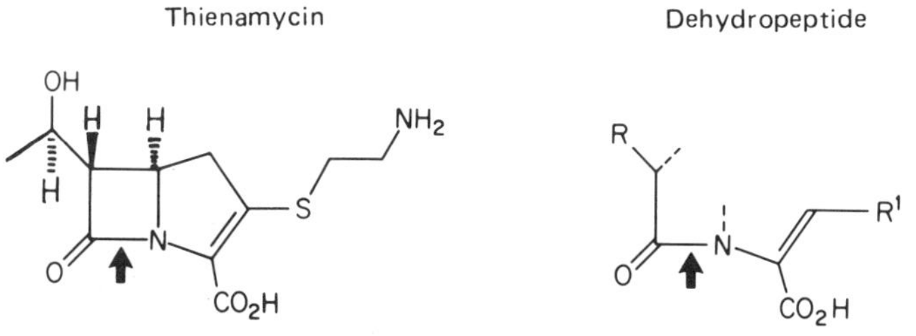

Figure 4 Structural homology postulated between THM and dehydropeptide substrates of DHP-I. The site of hydrolysis is indicated by an arrow. For Gly-dh-Phe, R = NH_2, R^1 = Phenyl. (Source, Ref. 82.)

phenylalanine (Gly-dh-Phe) Fig. 4] reinforced the attempts to isolate and purify this enzyme from pig kidney according to published procedures (84).

C. In Vitro and In Vivo Studies Confirming Imipenem Inactivation by Dehydropeptidase-I

Proof of the identity of the thienamycin-degrading enzyme with DHP-I was provided by the parallel increase in specific activity for Gly-dh-Phe (a suitable substrate for DHP-I) and thienamycin during solubilization and a 162-fold purification of the enzyme from porcine kidney. The 10-fold reduction in the catalytic rate with thienamycin and imipenem compared with the dipeptide substrate Gly-dh-Phe may be due to the 10-fold lower affinity of thienamycin (K_m = 5.7 mM versus 0.6 mM for Gly-dh-Phe) for this enzyme. Tested at equivalent concentrations, the relative rates of hydrolysis by DHP-I were found to be 100-fold lower for the thienamycin antibiotics (Fig. 5) than for the dipeptide substrate. The products formed by enzyme catalysis or controlled acid hydrolysis are identical (82). This finding revealed that DHP-I acts as a mammalian beta-lactamase on this new class of antibiotics, a unique and surprising feature, considering its proven resistance to hydrolysis by the standard bacterial beta-lactamases (30,32). Studies determining the metabolic disposition of radiolabeled imipenem conducted in the rat and the rabbit (82) and in humans as shown by Norrby et al. (84a) show that more than 90% of radioactivity is recovered in the urine, present in part as the unchanged parent antibiotic together with a major fraction of a metabolite found to be equivalent to the product formed by DHP-I hydrolysis in vitro. Importantly, the metabolite has no antibacterial activity of its own. Excretion via the bile appears to play no significant role in the metabolic disposition of imipenem, since less than 1% of the labeled imipenem dose was detected in the feces. Finally, loss of active antibiotic from the urine measured under controlled pH and temperature conditions

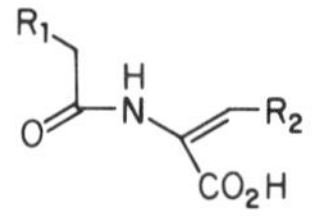

dehydropeptide

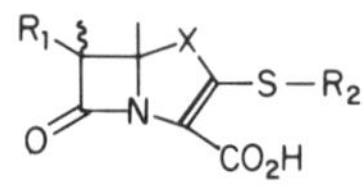

antibiotic

Substrates	R_1	X	R_2	Relative rate of hydrolysis by DHP	
Gly-dehydro-Phe	$CHNH_2$	–	C_6H_5	100	
thienamycin	*(8R, 6S)* CH_3CHOH	C	$(CH_2)_2NH_2$	1.0	
imipenem	*(8R,6S)* CH_3CHOH	C	$(CH_2)_2NHCH=NH$	0.85	
MM 13902	*(8S,6R)* CH_3CHOSO_3H	C	$CH=CH\text{-}NHAc$	30.	
SCH 29482	*(8R,6S)* CH_3CHOH	S	CH_2CH_3	0.6	
Inhibitors				I_{50} vs DHP, μM porcine	human
benzoyl-NH_2-acrylate	C_6H_5	–	CH_3	30	45
hexenoate	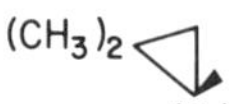 *(S)*	–	CH_2CH_3	0.11	—
MK0789	"	–	$(CH_2)_4CH_3$	0.08	0.08
MK0791 (cilastatin)	"		$(CH_2)_4SCH_2CH(NH_2)COOH$ *(L)*	0.11	0.13

Figure 5 Kinetic parameters for substrates and inhibitors of renal dehydropeptidase-I: Relative rates of hydrolysis (Gly-dehydro-Phe = 100) were determined at 0.1 mM of the indicated substrates employing dehydropeptidase-I purified 5100-fold from hog kidney using, as the final step, absorption to and elution from a sepharose column bearing immobilized MK0791 (Kropp et al., 1982). Inhibitory constants (I_{50}) are the concentrations of the indicated inhibitors which reduced by 50% the rate of hydrolysis of 0.05 mM Gly-dehydro-Phe. Human dehydropeptidase was solubilized and purified 162-fold from extracts of surplus donor kidneys from transplant centers. (Source, Ref. 9.)

accounts for less than 5% degradation and no evidence for enzymic inactivation of imipenem in the urine per se was detected (84b).

Urinary recoveries in mice of related carbapenems were reduced even further than thienamycin as a consequence of their acylated amino-alkylthio side chain (82). This finding underscores the efficiency with which the enzyme acts against these antibiotics, an in vivo response consistent with the increased in vitro susceptibility of these antibiotics to dehydropeptidase-I (Fig. 5). Exploratory pharmacokinetic and metabolic disposition studies of imipenem in the chimpanzee helped to further understand the phenomenon of "postexcretory metabolism." Awareness of the subcellular location of DHP-I in the brush border of the proximal renal tubule (85) led to the conclusion that the enzyme must have access not only to the glomerular ultrafiltrate but also to the secreted fraction as the antibiotic enters the tubular epithelium from the systemic circulation. A secretory pathway for imipenem, initially masked by postexcretory metabolism, does exist, as will be shown below in discussing dehydropeptidase inhibitors. Successful inhibition of DHP-I and the restoration of high and prolonged urinary concentrations were a desirable goal and, once attained by the development of cilastatin, provided convincing proof of the central role of the renal dipeptidase in the metabolism of carbapenem antibiotics.

IV. DEVELOPMENT OF CILASTATIN FOR COADMINISTRATION WITH IMIPENEM

A. Development of DHP-I Inhibitors: The Selection of Cilastatin

The extensive renal metabolism of imipenem resulting in low levels of intact antibiotic in the urine generated a concern that insufficient levels of antibiotic would compromise adequate treatment of severe infections of the urinary tract. Since the kidney is so often the primary site of infection in septicemia, it was considered possible that effective therapy of systemic infections with imipenem might be unreliable when the kidney is also involved. To overcome this potential deficiency, an inhibitor of DHP-I suitable for use in humans was developed for coadministration with imipenem. Based on reported observations (86) regarding the location and exterior orientation of DHP-I in the brush-border surface of proximal tubules, a minor salvaging role of dipeptide amino acids has been proposed for the function of this enzyme in normal metabolism. Therefore it was anticipated that the transient inhibition of DHP-I activity during the generally short period of antibiotic therapy would not result in any adverse effects. This presumption was later supported by the exceptionally good safety profile of DHP-I inhibitors established during animal toxicological studies and more recently confirmed in humans, specifically with cilastatin (87,88).

The search for specific and reversible inhibitors of DHP-I started with in vitro screens of compounds containing the dehydropeptide bond as a prominent feature. This screen uncovered the benzoyl-2-amino crotonate (Fig. 5) and led to the preparation of a series of selective inhibitors of the Z-2-acylaminopropenoate class (89). Inhibitory activity increased in parallel against both the porcine renal DHP-I and a solubilized DHP-I preparation from human kidney (Fig. 5). All the inhibitors share the S(+)-dimethylcyclopropyl carboxamido group, which confers maximum potency based on in vitro inhibitory activity. The propenoate substituents were varied from alkyl acids and diacids to polar,

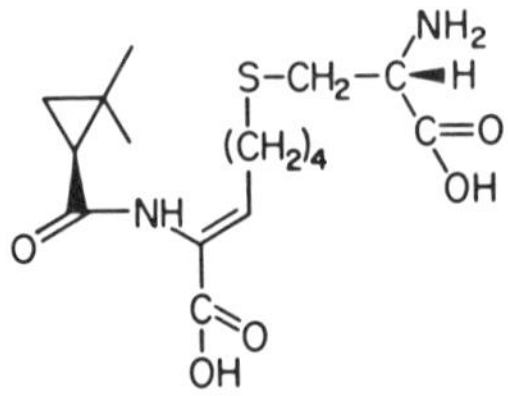

Figure 6 Cilastatin (MK0791).

zwitterionic groups, a modification that resulted in a reduction of in vitro potency. The loss of potency was well compensated by the gain in extended half-lives in vivo required to complement the pharmacokinetics of imipenem. Evidence of the efficacy of these inhibitors from studies performed in the chimpanzee suggested that coadministration of an appropriate inhibitor of DHP-I with imipenem would block renal metabolism of imipenem and thereby increase the concentration and persistence of the antibiotic in human urine.

B. Efficacy and Disposition of Cilastatin

Cilastatin sodium (the L-cysteinylthiohexenoate, MK0791; see Fig. 6) was chosen for development based on its good in vitro potency against both porcine and human DHP-I (K_I = 0.11 and 0.13 μM, respectively) and its excellent tolerance in animals following appropriate toxicological evaluations. For the selection of inhibitors with optimal properties, use was made of the chimpanzee, since the size (50-70 kg body weight) and excretion pattern of this species are very similar to those of humans. Coadministration of cilastatin with imipenem increased overall urinary recoveries of the antibiotic six- to eight-fold (Table 13). In the most favorable cases urinary recovery of active antibiotic approached a maximum of 75%, which is consistent with the observed ratio of incremental renal to plasma clearance rates. Quantitative measurements of imipenem administered intravenously, alone or in combination with cilastatin, are presented in Figure 7. Also compared is the performance of a suspension of imipenem administered by the intramuscular route.

The importance of continuously elevated incremental renal clearance rates obtained when cilastatin is combined with the antibiotic indicates effective inhibition of the imipenem metabolism, an effect achieved over the entire test period. Furthermore, it revealed the existence of a secretory pathway for imipenem previously masked during uncontrolled metabolism. Increasing the duration of inhibition of renal metabolism by DHP-I inhibitors has also been termed "effect time," as a measure of their effectiveness. Effect time represents the period during which renal clearance rates exceed the glomerular filtration rate

Table 13 Pharmacokinetic Parameters for Imipenem and Cilastatin Administered Separately or in Combination to a Chimpanzee

Component and route	Dose (mg/kg)		Plasma				Urinary recovery (%)		Clearance rates (ml/min per kg)	
					AUC (mg/liter x hr)					
	Imipenem	Cilastatin	C_{max} (mg/liter)	$T_{½}$ (hr)	0–4.5	0–∞	0–4.5	0–∞	CL_p	Cl_r
Imipenem										
Intravenous	5	0	20.0	0.70	18.5	19.0	12.2	13.0	4.75	0.6
Intravenous	5	4	30.0	0.73	21.4	22.0	75.8	77.8	3.8	2.9
Intramuscular	13	13	6.0	2.3	20.6	36.3	4.6	8.1	–	–
Intramuscular	13	13	9.0	2.4	28.6	44.8	42.5	63.3	–	–
Cilastatin[a]										
Intravenous	5	4	21.0	0.95	13.27	14.26	117.0	126.0	4.67	5.5
Intramuscular	13	13	12.6	1.2	25.9	26.0	97.4	⩾98.0	–	–

[a]Cilastatin levels were determined by measurement of inhibitory titer against porcine renal dehydropeptidase-I. This assay responds to both parent cilastatin and its N-acetyl metabolite. The latter has twice the inhibitory activity of cilastatin.

Source: Ref. 9.

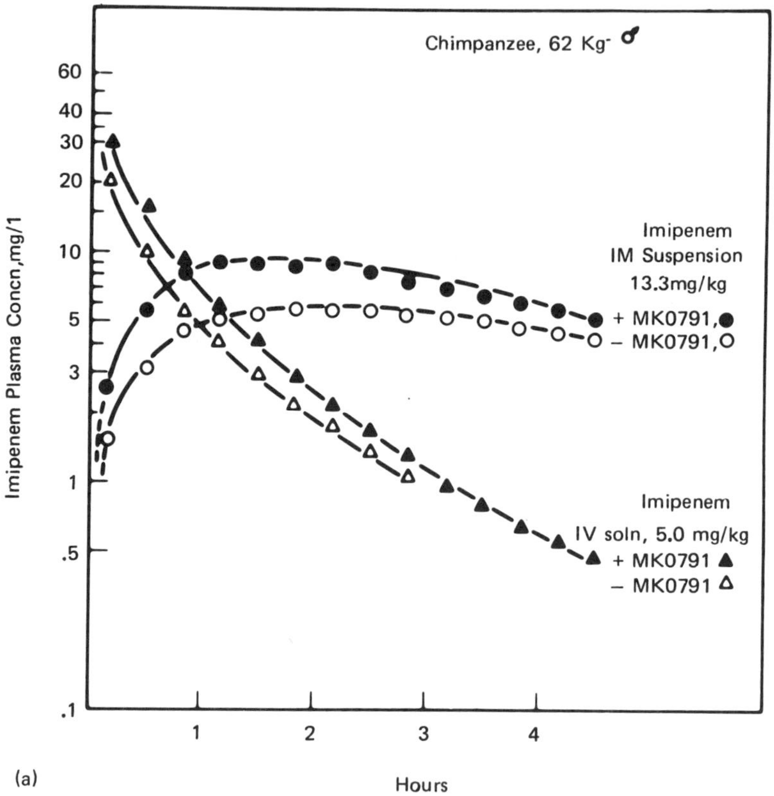

(a)

Figure 7 (a) Single-subject comparison of disposition in an anesthetized chimpanzee of imipenem (MK0787) injected as an intramuscular suspension or an intravenous bolus in each case with or without an equal weight of the renal dehydropeptidase inhibitor, cilastatin (MK0791). Intramuscular injections were 3.3 to 3.5 ml of a 250-mg/ml suspension of MK0787 in water or MK0791 solution. Intravenous injections were 15.5 ml of 20 mg/ml supersaturated solutions injected over 1–2 min. The chimpanzee received, 2 hr before drug administration, a loading dose of inulin (50 mg/kg) and a constant intravenous infusion of 5% mannitol in 0.45% saline supplemented with 22 mg inulin/ml and maintained at 3.0 ml min^{-1} from -1.5 to 4.7 hr. Each subject was catheterized for urine recovery at successive 20-min intervals. (Source, Ref. 9.) (b) Incremental clearance rates measured in successive 20-min urine collections for the single-subject comparison of the effect of cilastatin on the disposition of an intravenous or intramuscular dose of imipenem. Indicated to scale are the mean plasma clearance rates for imipenem determined from the intravenous study of imipenem plus cilastatin and the mean value for glomerular filtration rate determined in four chimpanzees utilizing continuously infused inulin (see Fig. 8). (Source, Ref. 9.)

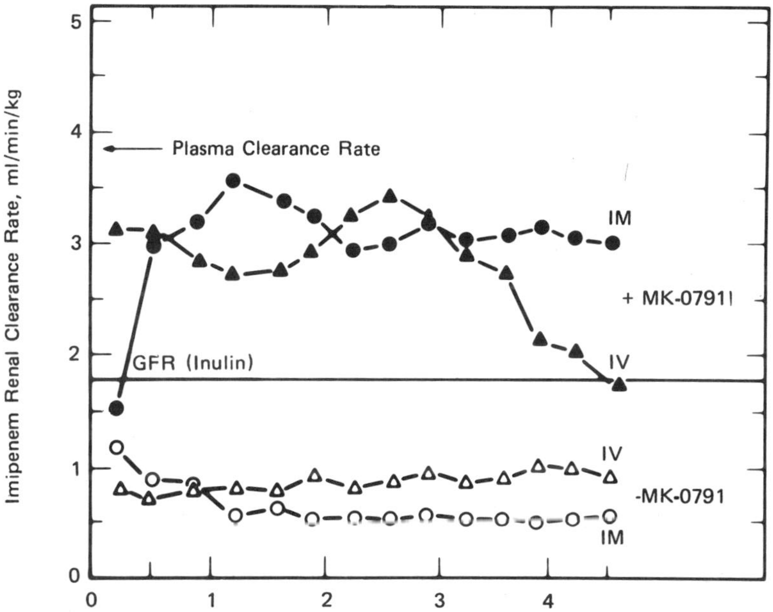

(b)

(GFR). It represents an index of both intrinsic potency and the persistence of inhibitor in the circulation. Inhibitors with effect times greater or equal to 3 hr achieve and maintain plasma concentrations from 3 to 5 μM (∿1.0–1.8 μg/ml) over that interval. For cilastatin this concentration is equivalent to 16-fold the K_I for DHP-I and provides a reflection of the intensity of tubular metabolism. This value suggests that the enzyme must be present in amounts 20-fold greater than necessary to degrade that fraction of imipenem that enters the renal tubule. The effect of cilastatin on the metabolic disposition of imipenem coadministered by the intravenous route was quite striking (Table 13). Not only did renal clearance rates of imipenem increase from a baseline of 13 to 80% of the plasma clearance rates but, most importantly, these rates were maintained at effective levels for the duration of the 4.5-hr test period (Fig. 7b). Studies in normal volunteers (90) confirmed these results previously observed in chimpanzees. Urinary recoveries were elevated consistently to 70% and, as observed in the chimpanzee, the coadministration of variable concentrations (250–1000 mg) of cilastatin with a fixed amount of imipenem caused a dose response elevation of plasma levels and plasma AUC (∿20% peak). These effects were more prevalent

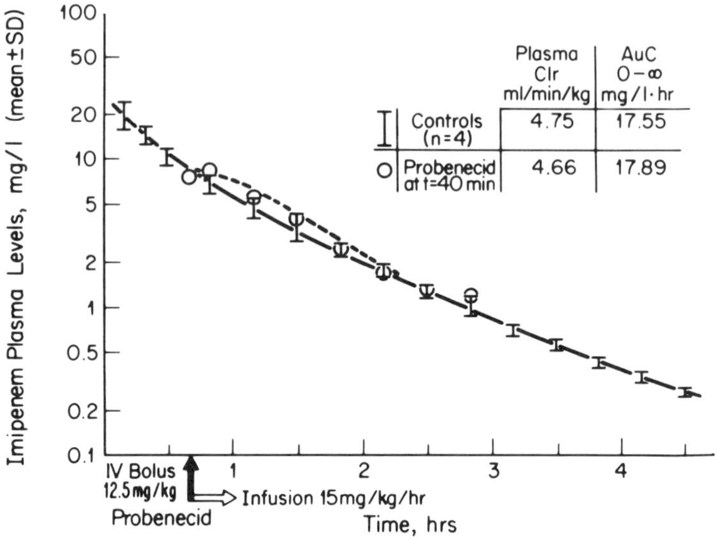

Figure 8 (a) Effect of an intercurrent probenecid administration on the plasma profile (a) and incremental renal clearance rate (b) of imipenem in the chimpanzee. Imipenem (5 mg/kg) was injected as an intravenous bolus followed at 40 min by probenecid. The latter was given as an intravenous bolus loading dose (12.5 mg/kg) and a maintenance infusion (15 mg/kg per hr). The average disposition of imipenem in four subjects (males, 60 ± 4 kg) is shown for comparison. (Source, Ref. 9.)

in the chimpanzee following intramuscular injection at a dosage three times higher than that administered intravenously (Fig. 7b). The resulting decline in plasma clearance of imipenem was, however, not constant over the entire test period, as the lack of increase in plasma half-lives during the beta-elimination phase indicates. In this regard the intramuscular route of administration of imipenem, which requires the injection of small-volume suspensions owing to the limited solubility of the antibiotic, may provide some additional advantages (Fig. 7a). The apparent half-life of imipenem administered intramuscularly increased to 2.5 hr, resulting in a substantial prolongation of blood levels in the therapeutic range of 3–8 μg/ml, sustained by a slow release of the antibiotic from the site of injection. A twice-daily regimen by the intramuscular route might thus match for most infections the effectiveness of imipenem administered three or four times daily by the intravenous route.

Initial studies on the disposition of cilastatin sodium conducted in primates indicated that the introduction of a zwitterionic substituent, L-cysteine, in cilastatin improved the systemic persistence of this inhibitor. This desirable function

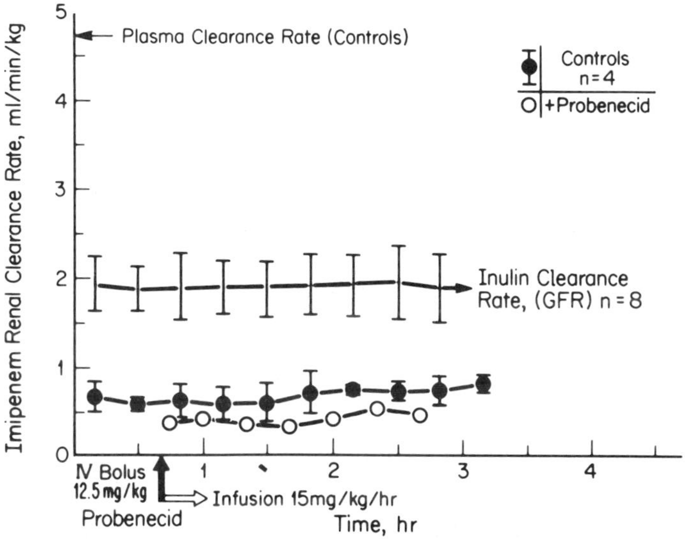

Figure 8 (b).

in turn extends the period of protection afforded by the inhibitor on imipenem during the passage of the antibiotic through the kidney. During pharmacokinetic studies of cilastatin in the chimpanzee it was observed that excess inhibitor activity (117–120%) was recovered in the urine not only of the chimpanzee but also during prior rhesus monkey studies (Kropp, unpublished). Speculation that cilastatin might undergo partial transformation in vivo to a more active metabolite was confirmed when an acidic compound with DHP-I inhibitory activity was isolated from urine. This inhibitor was identified as the N-acetyl derivative of cilastatin and its structure verified by comparison with a chemically synthesized sample. The N-acetyl derivative was shown to be approximately two times more potent against DHP-I (I_{50} = 0.06 μgM), when compared to the in vitro potency of cilastatin. Based on these differences in activity versus DHP-I and the amounts of metabolite extracted from urine specimens, it was possible to assign to each component its contribution to the overall inhibitor activity detected in the urine. Cilastatin made up 70% of the inhibitor dose recovered in the urine of chimpanzees, with the N-acetyl cilastatin metabolite contributing the remainder. A comparable degree of metabolism resulting in the formation of the same metabolite was found in man (R. Norrby, personal communication). The N-acetyl cilastatin was evaluated in the chimpanzee and found equally active in restoring overall urinary recovery of imipenem. Considerations to substitute cilastatin with the N-acetyl derivative of slightly higher in vitro potency were considered

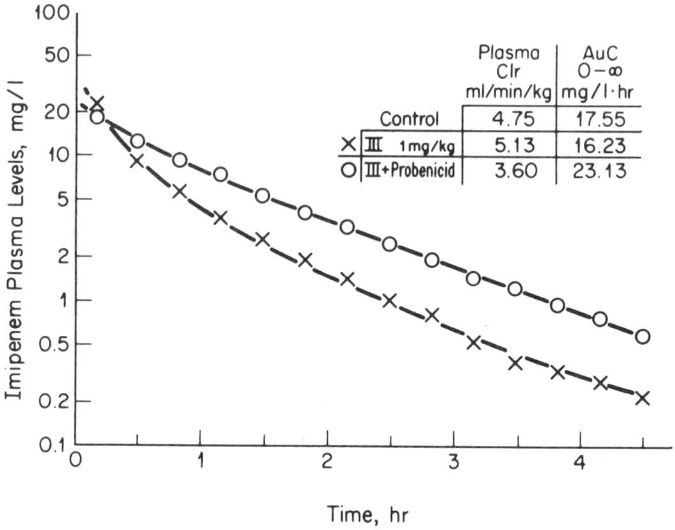

Figure 9 (a) Effect of probenecid infusion on the plasma profile (a) and incremental renal clearance rate (b) of imipenem coadministered with a renal dehydropeptidase inhibitor in a male chimpanzee. In both studies, imipenem (5 mg/kg) was coadministered as an intravenous bolus with 1 mg/kg of the hexenoate homologue (structure in Fig. 5) indicated as 'III' in these figures. Probenecid was administered starting with a loading dose of 12.5 mg/kg 10 min prior to the imipenem/inhibitor injection and was maintained by infusion at 15 mg/kg throughout the study. Control values for imipenem administered alone and for glomerular filtration rate were determined on four male chimpanzees. (Source, Ref. 9.)

only briefly, since it was shown that the persistence of this acyl derivative in the systemic circulation was decreased by more than 2.5 hr, a considerable reduction in the inhibitory effect time when compared with cilastatin administered at an equivalent dose. These pharmacokinetic studies in the chimpanzee also produced evidence that cilastatin is subject to tubular secretion. Based on the renal clearance rate of this inhibitor in the chimpanzee, which significantly exceeds the glomerular filtration rate, it was concluded that cilastatin is actively secreted. This observation is of considerable importance in interpreting the mechanism of protection provided by cilastatin against the nephrotoxic effect of high levels of imipenem observed in laboratory animals, a subject addressed later. Though the mechanism for transforming cilastatin in vivo to the acetylated metabolite has not yet been identified, evidence from studies in the rhesus monkey and chimpanzee (9) point once again to the kidney as the responsible

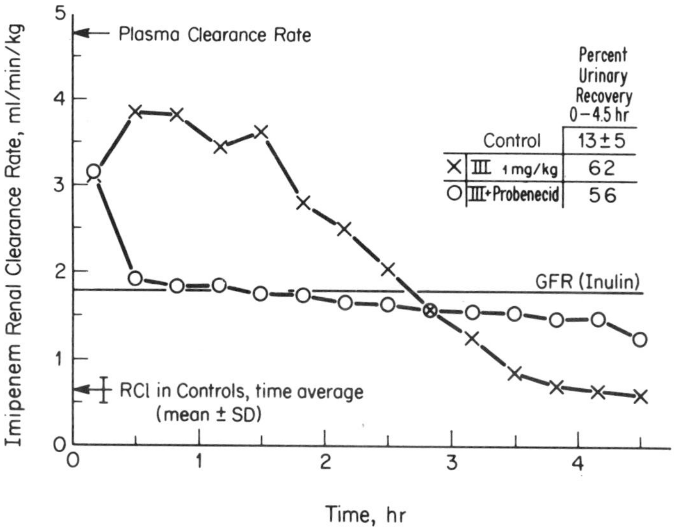

Figure 9 (b).

organ, a conclusion supported by the prolongation of cilastatin half-life in subjects with minimal renal function (91).

C. Renal Clearance Pathways of Imipenem Affected by Cilastatin

The extensive renal metabolism of imipenem observed during disposition studies in the chimpanzee with renal clearance rates well below the GFR seemed to rule out the involvement of a tubular secretory pathway in the overall excretion pattern of the antibiotic. When probenecid, an agent known to block tubular secretion, was added to imipenem, only minimal changes in the pharmacokinetic parameters were observed (Fig. 8), a finding later confirmed in humans (87). Not until inhibitors of renal metabolism were coadministered with the antibiotic was it possible to observe the presence of a proficient secretory pathway for imipenem. The hexenoate homolog (an inhibitor of DHP-I with a short half-life) was used in this study, resulting in the dramatic elevation of the renal clearance rate of imipenem (Fig. 9). This rate exceeded by twofold the GFR and continued to increase to peak at 75% of the plasma clearance rate before rapidly declining to baseline values by the fourth hour. The decline of imipenem to its (low) baseline renal clearance rate during the time course of the experiment signals the return of DHP-I activity and directly illustrates the reversible nature of the enzyme inhibitors in vivo. Further evidence for tubular secretion was pro-

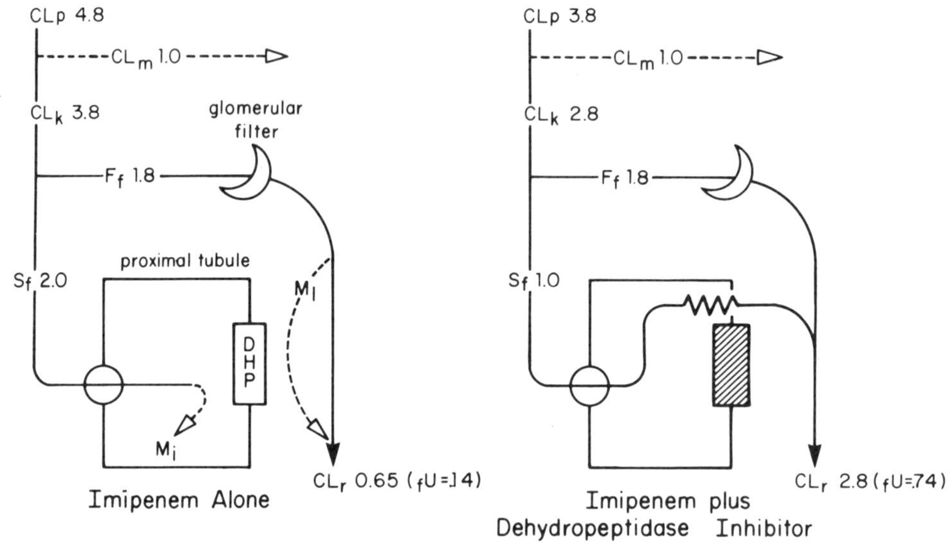

Figure 10 Model of renal clearance pathways accounting for the disposition of imipenem in the absence and presence of inhibitors of renal dehydropeptidase-I: The proximal tubule is shown with dehydropeptidase-I imbedded on the lumenal surface to the right. Designated clearance rates (ml/min per kg) were determined in the chimpanzee and apply, in the case of coadministered dehydropeptidase-I inhibitors, to the period of maximal inhibition. Metabolic pathways are indicated by open arrows. Symbols used are: Cl_p, plasma clearance rate; Cl_m, non-renal metabolism; Cl_k, input renal clearance; F_f, filtered fraction; S_f, secreted fraction; M_l, lumenal metabolism; M_i, intratubular metabolism; Cl_r, urinary clearance of intact antibiotic; fU, fraction of the dose recovered in urine. Entry of both imipenem and dehydropeptidase inhibitors is mediated by a probenecid sensitive anionic transport site shown at the contraluminal surface. The reduced secreted fraction resulting from inhibition of dehydropeptidase-I is suggested to result from impedance to net transtubular levels when imipenem accumulates to intratubular levels exceeding those in the circulation. (Source, Ref. 9.)

vided by the addition of probenecid to an imipenem–DHP-I inhibitor combination. In this study probenecid suppressed the renal clearance rate of imipenem to a level equivalent to the GFR for inulin in the chimpanzee (Fig. 9b). The expected effect of probenecid infusion, which resulted in the elevation of imipenem plasma levels and AUC values, as well as the observed increase in plasma half-life, provided direct evidence that, when protected from enzyme attack in the kidney, the antibiotic exits via both glomerular filtration and tubular secretion.

An attempt has been made to trace the pathways and metabolic encounters of imipenem as it is transported through the kidney in the absence or presence of cilastatin (Fig. 10). Pharmacokinetic studies in the chimpanzee (Table 13) and in human volunteers (90) have shown that urinary recovery of imipenem reaches a maximal level of 75%, regardless of the coadministered dose of the dehydropeptidase inhibitor (90). Similarly, the maximal renal clearance rate (Cl_r) of imipenem reaches only 75% of the plasma clearance rate (Cl_p); the 25% deficit is attributable to the extrarenal, cilastatin-insensitive, metabolic hydrolysis of imipenem. Support for the existence of an extrarenal metabolic pathway is evident from studies in volunteers with different degrees of preexisting renal insufficiency (91). In these studies an increase in plasma half-life associated with decreased renal function was limited to approximately 3 hr. Of the antibiotic undergoing renal clearance, approximately two-thirds exit by glomerular filtration and the remaining portion is cleared by tubular secretion. Imipenem concentrations in the absence of inhibitor must be lower at the tubular level than in the circulation, causing a passive flow of the antibiotic toward the site of metabolism, leading to continued degradation of imipenem mediated by dehydropeptidase-I. The lack of active transport is evident from the minimal effect of probenecid on the pharmacokinetics of imipenem when the antibiotic is administered alone. Active transport is, however, required in the presence of DHP-I inhibitors in order to promote the net secretion of imipenem, a precondition that allows expression of the classic probenecid effect. When cilastatin is coadministered, a twofold reduction in the secreted fraction of imipenem occurs as a result of the elimination of dehydropeptidase-mediated degradation of the antibiotic entering the tubule. This effect can account for the diminished plasma clearance rates and elevated plasma levels observed early. During inhibition of DHP-I by cilastatin, the imipenem concentration increases in the tubule owing to its slower egress from this site, rising to levels that exceed those of the circulation and thereby causing the minor elevations observed in plasma. However, as the plasma level of the inhibitor declines, the dehydropeptidase activity is restored and the enzyme acts on intratubular levels of imipenem, leading to the elimination of net secretion. Thus the plasma clearance rate returns to its higher baseline value observed when imipenem is administered alone. Based on this interpretation of the metabolic events, it is clear that coadministration of cilastatin can elevate plasma AUC of imipenem without affecting its plasma half-life. The data also indicate that the intense intratubular activity of DHP-I has the ability to fully degrade the antibiotic within the cell in the absence of inhibitor and thereby establish a passive flow for additional imipenem to enter the cell. However, a portion of imipenem cleared via filtration is not metabolized, even in the absence of inhibitor, because DHP-I activity on the filtered fraction is limited. This readily explains why the lower levels of cilastatin present later effectively protect the filtered fraction of the antibiotic from enzyme attack. Application of the pharma-

Table 14 Comparative Nephrotoxicity of Imipenem in the Rabbit

Dosage level[a] (mg/kg)	Route	Serum biochemistry[b] Urea nitrogen (mg/100 ml)	Serum biochemistry[b] Creatinine (mg/100 ml)	Tubular necrosis[c] (mean grade)
150	Intravenous	48.7 ± 8.7	3.9 ± 0.9	3.5 ± 0.6
150	Intramuscular[d]	15.9 ± 6.5	1.5 ± 0.7	1.0 ± 0.8
140	Subcutaneous	68.0 ± 22.0	3.3 ± 0.9	3.25 ± 0.5
Cephaloridine (120)	Intravenous	76.6 ± 11.3	3.9 ± 1.3	4.0
Control (0.9% saline)	Intravenous	17.5 ± 1.2	1.4 ± 0.1	0

[a]A rapid high-temperature dissolution procedure is required for the preparation of high-dose injection solutions of imipenem. The antibiotic is quickly dissolved at 70–75°C in saline or with appropriate solutions of cilastatin, followed by quick cooling to 37°C for prompt injection by the selected routes.
[b]Values shown, including (±) standard deviations, represents 48-hr postdose measurements just prior to termination of the study. All animals were subjected to necropsy and microscopic examination of kidney tissue.
[c]The degree of renal tubular necrosis was rated on a scale (grades 1–5) of increasing severity. The results represent the mean (grade) value for animals within each group (n = 2–6), made up of male and female New Zealand white rabbits weighing ≥3.0 kg.
[d]The intramuscular injection consisted of a suspension of imipenem at a stock concentration of 250 mg/ml.

cokinetic parameters for imipenem obtained in chimpanzees (Table 13) to the proposed model of renal clearance pathways (Fig. 10) therefore establishes a basis for appropriate interpretation of similar results observed in humans (90).

D. Prevention of Imipenem-Induced Nephrotoxicity by Cilastatin

Studies performed in rabbits revealed that imipenem administered parenterally at high dosage levels (>100 mg/kg) induces acute necrosis of proximal tubular epithelial cells (Table 14). Experimentation was undertaken to explain the nephrotoxic effect of imipenem and the possible prevention by dehydropeptidase-I inhibitors. It was assumed from the outset that imipenem per se could not be the toxic agent based on its short survival time in the kideny, as a consequence of its extensive metabolism by DHP-I.

Single-dose studies in rabbits of cilastatin coadministered with imipenem showed a dose-related reduction in the severity of renal damage (Table 15). Complete protection against renal damage was obtained when the dose of cila-

Table 15 Prevention of Imipenem Nephrotoxicity by Coadministration of Cilastatin in the Rabbit[a]

Dosage level (mg/kg)	Serum biochemistry: Urea nitrogen (mg/100 ml)	Serum biochemistry: Creatinine (mg/100 ml)	Tubular necrosis (mean grade)
Control (saline, 0.9%)	21.5 ± 3.2	1.8 ± 0.2	0
IPM, 140 alone	75.0 ± 9.1	4.8 ± 0.5	4.00 ± 0
Plus cilastatin			
10	78.3 ± 22.4	4.7 ± 1.5	3.75 ± 0.43
30	37.3 ± 4.2	2.7 ± 0.4	3.00 ± 0
60	29.2 ± 6.3	1.7 ± 0.3	1.75 ± 0.83
90	35.4 ± 11.4	2.1 ± 0.7	2.00 ± 1.41
140	22.5 ± 4.1	2.4 ± 0.4	0
IPM, 360 alone	61.0 ± 10.5	8.0 ± 1.2	5.00 ± 0
Plus cilastatin			
90	48.6 ± 4.6	3.3 ± 0.6	3.25 ± 0.43
180	35.0 ± 8.8	2.6 ± 0.6	2.25 ± 0.43
360	21.8 ± 3.8	1.5 ± 0.2	0
720	22.5 ± 4.8	1.7 ± 0.2	0

[a]See Table 14 for drug preparation and test procedures. Drugs were administered via single bolus intravenous injection.

statin and imipenem was administered at a weight ratio of 1:1. At the highest dose rate tested, that is, 360 mg/kg of imipenem plus 360 mg/kg of cilastatin, no functional or morphological evidence of renal damage was observed. Importantly, the protective effect of cilastatin is observed regardless of changes in dosing intervals, as seen in a rabbit experiment following a three times daily (50 mg/kg) split-dose schedule (Table 16). An initial approach to understanding the protective effect of cilastatin was to determine whether an inhibitor of DHP-I had similar effects on cephaloridine-induced nephrotoxicity in the rabbit. MK0789 (structure shown in Fig. 5) dramatically reduced cephaloridine-induced toxicity at a ratio of 2:1 (180 mg/kg of cephaloridine plus 90 mg/kg of MK0789). Probenecid, which has been shown to be an effective inhibitor of cephaloridine nephrotoxicity in rabbits (92,93) also prevented the nephrotoxicity of imipenem as well as that of cephaloridine (MacDonald, unpublished). These

Table 16 Effect of Coadministration of Cilastatin and Imipenem Following a Split-Dosage Regimen[a]

Dosage group	Serum biochemistry: Urea nitrogen (mg/100 ml)	Serum biochemistry: Creatinine (mg/100 ml)	Tubular necrosis (mean grade)
Control (0.9% saline)	15.5 ± 2.7	1.4 ± 0.2	0
Imipenem, 50 mg/kg three times daily	29.0 ± 10.5	2.1 ± 0.8	2 ± 0.8
Imipenem + cilastatin 50/50 mg/kg three times daily	17.2 ± 2.8	1.5 ± 0.2	0

[a]See Table 14 for drug preparation and test procedures. Drugs were administered every 6 hr three times daily by the intravenous route.

results suggested that the mechanism of prevention of imipenem-induced nephrotoxicity may not involve the inhibition of dehydropeptidase-I. Two additional observations further support this conclusion: For one, it has been shown that cephaloridine is not metabolized by DHP-I; secondly, the (-) enantiomer of MK0789, which lacks activity against dehydropeptidase-I, was as effective in preventing the nephrotoxicity induced by imipenem as was the (+) enantiomer of MK0789, a very potent inhibitor of DHP-I (Kropp and MacDonald, unpublished). This observation is consistent with the data gathered from additional studies in the rabbit where it was shown that cilastatin effectively reduces by approximately sixfold the cortical uptake of cephaloridine (Table 17). The values for cortical levels of cephaloridine presented here are quite similar to those obtained after coadministration of probenecid (92,93).

It has been proposed that cephaloridine nephrotoxicity is related to the attainment of high concentrations of the drug in proximal tubular epithelial cells (92). Although it has been shown that cephaloridine is actively transported into the tubular cells by the anionic transport system (94), it is said that the cationic charge may retard the exit from the cell, which leads to accumulation of the antibiotic (95). Accumulation of drug in the tubular cells is not, however, a necessary precondition for nephrotoxicity. Significant reduction in severity of renal damage from cephalosporin antibiotics can be achieved without sustained inhibition of cortical accumulation of drug (96).

At present, the mechanism of renal tubular cell injury by cephaloridine and other nephrotoxic beta-lactams is not firmly established; however, it is clear that exclusion of antibiotic from the renal tubular cells prevents damage (92,97).

Table 17 Effect of Cilastatin on Plasma and Renal Cortical Concentrations of Cephaloridine

Drug and dosage[a] administered	Time after drug administration (hr)	N	Mean concentration of cephaloridine[b] Plasma (μg/ml)	Kidney cortex (μg/g wet tissue weight)
Cephaloridine (150 mg/kg, I.V.)	0.5	3	344.8 ± 151.0	3078 ± 906
	3.0	4	29.7 ± 9.4	1340 ± 317
Cephaloridine (150 mg/kg, I.V.) + cilastatin (150 mg/kg, I.V.)	0.5	4	387.2 ± 57.0	584 ± 75
	3.0	4	21.6 ± 7.9	229 ± 80

[a]Drug was administered as a single dose by the intravenous route to New Zealand white rabbits weighing ≥ 3.0 kg.
[b]Plasma and cortical tissue concentrations of cephaloridine were determined by bioassay with use of a *Bacillus subtilis* MB32 tester strain.
N = Number of animals.

Data obtained thus far support the hypothesis that the prevention of imipenem-induced nephrotoxicity by cilastatin is a result of nonspecific competitive inhibition of transport of imipenem into the tubular epithelium.

Additional pharmacokinetic studies conducted in the chimpanzee indicate that cilastatin has the ability to suppress the tubular secretion of the antibiotic, even at use levels, when coadministered with imipenem, as observed after intramuscular administration (see Fig. 7). In the presence of cilastatin the incremental renal clearance rates of imipenem during the first 30-min period were held at the GFR, whereas during this same interval the plasma levels of imipenem noticably increased. This observation suggests a temporary blockade of imipenem's secretory pathway by cilastatin, which was extended further to more than 4 hr when probenecid was also added for coadministration (see Fig. 9b).

E. Accumulation of Imipenem-Related Metabolites in the Rabbit Kidney

The preceding sections have established that in the absence of an inhibitor of DHP-I, imipenem is substantially metabolized in the kidney. Furthermore, the data indicate that the antibiotic has a competent pathway to exit from the tubule and therefore, unlike cephaloridine, and surviving portion of imipenem would have little chance for intratubular accumulation. However, the accumulation of imipenem metabolites in the renal cortex, accounting for 8% of the ad-

Table 18 Effect of Coadministered Dehydropeptidase Inhibitor (MK0789) on Distribution and Clearance of [^{14}C]Imipenem[a] and Imipenem Metabolites in the Rabbit[b]

	Imipenem (142.0 mg/kg) + MK0789 (0.0 mg/kg)	Imipenem (128.0 mg/kg) + MK0789 (90.0 mg/kg)
Imipenem in plasma		
Concentration (mg/liter)		
30 min	140.0	230.0
60 min	10.0	20.0
AUC, 0–120 (mg/liter hr)	201.0	342.0
Cl_p (ml/min per kg)	11.8	6.3
Kidney cortex at 120 min (μg/g)		
Imipenem	60.0	8.0
Imipenem-OH[c]	1200.0	160.0
Imipenem-Cys[d]	1060.0	570.0
Urinary recovery (0–120 min)		
Imipenem, percent of dose	29.0	58.0
Imipenem-OH	58.0	17.0

[a]Labeled in formate carbon of formimidoyl side chain.
[b]Indicated dose rates of [^{14}C]imipenem were administered in supersaturated solution, 100 mg/ml, with or without MK0789 (structure shown in Fig. 5). Rabbits were male with body weights of 2.5 kg. Urine was collected by catheterization. At 120 min kidney was removed, cortex excised on ice and homogenized in 1 vol of 0.1 M MK0789, pH 7.0, to prevent further degradation by DHP-I. Metabolites in cortex homogenate and urine were separated by high-performance liquid chromatography using methods described for imipenem-OH (82). Imipenem-Cys was in two peaks, with retention times immediately preceding and coinciding with that of imipenem. The levels of imipenem were determined by $A_{310\ nm}$ during high-performance liquid chromatography and confirmed by bioassay in collected fractions.
[c]Hydrolyzed imipenem.
[d]7-Cysteinyl conjugate of imipenem.
Source: Ref. 9.

ministered dose, was detected in rabbits that had received nephrotoxic doses of [^{14}C]imipenem (Table 18). A major portion of the total radioactivity recovered was attributable to the primary metabolite (imipenem-OH) generated by the hydrolytic action of DHP-I on imipenem. A second metabolite, the cysteinyl conjugate of imipenem, found only in the kidney, was shown to be chromatographically identical with the initial and spontaneously rearranged products formed when imipenem reacts with cysteine. It is presumed that the lactam carbonyl reacts with cysteine to form the thiol ester, which subsequently forms the peptide.* As expected, only low levels of intact imipenem were detectable in the renal cortex homogenates.

Coadministration of the DHP-I inhibitor MK0789 with imipenem at a level which prevents nephrotoxicity, resulted in a sevenfold reduction of cortical levels of both the imipenem-OH (major metabolite) and the already low levels of imipenem. Interestingly, the cysteine adduct of imipenem was reduced only 1.7-fold, which suggests that neither this metabolite nor changes in intracellular levels of glutathione as a result of the formation of the cysteine adduct are responsible for the nephrotoxic effect.

Though the identity of the nephrotoxic agent is not yet defined and is the subject for further experimentation, the pharmacokinetic data in the rabbit (Table 18) show a definite secretory blockade of imipenem imposed by MK0789 and it is responsible for the prevention of nephrotoxicity. The observed threefold reduction in the plasma clearance rate of imipenem at nephrotoxic levels in the absence of MK0789 already indicates that tubular transport was partially saturated. Approximately 4 ml/min per kilogram was attributable to the sum of filtration and the extrarenal metabolism. The further reduction of 70% in the plasma clearance rate of imipenem by the coadministration of MK0789 thus indicates the effective blockade of the secreted fraction and supports the conclusion for the prevention of nephrotoxicity.

F. Rationale for the Imipenem-Cilastatin Combination

The definition of an antimicrobial combination generally infers the proper matching of two components, both with antibacterial activity, which is hopefully boosted by mutual potentiation; appropriate examples would be the fixed-ratio combination antimicrobials trimethoprim-sulfamethoxazole and amoxicillin-clavulanate. The customary benefits sought from these combinations are directed to broaden the spectrum of activity against a group of organisms either insensitive to both components or exhibiting preexistent resistance to one component only. The rationale for combining cilastatin with imipenem was not proposed in order to enhance the antibacterial activity of imipenem, since the sole antibacterial component of this new combination, imipenem, has outstanding breadth of spectrum, potency, and lack of cross-resistance with other agents.

---

*The reaction of imipenem with a beta-aminothiol such as cysteine is known to be rapid, yet a much slower response is observed with glutathione (2). The possibility exists that free cysteine or an N-terminal cysteine intermediate, such as cysteine-glycine formed in the glutathione cycle (98), plays a role in the formation of imipenem-cysteine.

The need for an antibacterial partner is therefore not necessary except in special clinical situations. The specific role of cilastatin in this combination is to control antibiotic inactivation encountered as a result of enzyme (DHP-I) action. In fact, the function of cilastatin closely resembles the role of carbidopa in the well-established carbidopa-levodopa combination. In both cases coadministration of an inhibitor prevents the undesirable metabolism of the active component, thereby requiring a lower dose that provides the obvious economic and safety benefits.

The prevention of metabolism by cilastatin provides effective antibiotic levels to combat bacterial persistence not only in the urinary tract but, more importantly, also at the site where bacteremia often originates, that is, in the kidney. Finally, cilastatin provides an additional margin of safety when coadministered with imipenem. The absence of renal damage in the rabbit receiving very high doses of imipenem in a 1:1 weight ratio with cilastatin attests to the safety benefit of this combination.

V. PRELIMINARY CLINICAL EXPERIENCE

Initial studies in normal volunteers explored the pharmacokinetics of imipenem administered as a single agent and combined with probenecid (87). Antibiotic plasma concentrations were found to be dose related and only slightly elevated by the addition of probenecid, which had no effect on the 1-hr plasma half-life of imipenem. Confirming previous observations in several animal species, the urinary recovery of intact imipenem varied substantially between subjects (6–38%), whereas the within-subject variation was minimal. The urinary recovery was further reduced upon coadministration of probenecid, resulting in a decrease of renal clearance rates of the antibiotic. The observation of a small increase in antibiotic plasma concentrations and a minimal effect on plasma half-life suggested that a modest secretory pathway for imipenem exists in humans.

Subsequent studies in volunteers confirmed that urinary concentrations and persistence of imipenem could be dramatically increased when inhibitors of dehydropeptidase-I, such as MK0789 or cilastatin, were coadministered with the antibiotic (90). The largest effect of the inhibitors was observed in individuals showing the highest degree of metabolizing activity. Urinary recovery increased to approximately 70% of the intact imipenem dose, with a maximum duration of inhibitory activity reached at a 1:1 dose ratio of cilastatin and imipenem. Similar results were obtained in a comparable study (99) where the effects of cilastatin on the pharmacokinetics of imipenem were explored. Here the coadministration of the inhibitor raised the urinary recovery from a baseline of 12% in the group of high metabolizers to 67% without significantly affecting the plasma AUC or half-life of imipenem. Thus studies with normal volunteers confirm the preclinical results on the effectiveness of cilastatin to prevent imipenem metabolism.

In patients with impaired renal function the elimination constant for imipenem decreased in proportion to the degree of renal insufficiency (91). The excretion of cilastatin was similarly decreased in these subjects, however, to a somewhat greater extent than it was for imipenem. Impairment of renal function resulted in prolongation of plasma half-life for both imipenem and cilastatin, with the inhibitor more affected than imipenem. For individuals with a GFR declining below 30 ml/min, residual clearance of the antibiotic results from the cilastatin-insensitive extrarenal metabolism of imipenem mentioned earlier. Thus, as with subjects of normal renal function, cilastatin does not significantly affect the kinetics of imipenem in the plasma of patients with renal failure.

The general safety and tolerability of imipenem-cilastatin was recently reviewed (88). In general, this new agent was as well tolerated as other beta-lactam agents, with a minimal number of clinical side effects.

Efficacy trials are ongoing and the results reported at formal scientific meetings are starting to appear in the literature (100–110). The uniformly favorable response to imipenem-cilastatin reported from these early studies indicate that this new antibiotic will be useful for the treatment of numerous severe infections. Based on its broad spectrum and safety, imipenem may be considered as a first-line antibiotic in the hospital setting. As clinical experience develops, the overall general utility of this new and promising agent will become apparent.

ACKNOWLEDGMENTS

The authors thank Jon G. Sundelof, Joann Huber, Richard Hajdu, and Dennis Bohn for their excellent technical assistance, and June Cieslarczyk for the preparation of this manuscript.

REFERENCES

1. G. B. Calandra, M. Hesney, V. I. Ahonkhai, and C. Grad. A multiclinic randomized study of the comparative efficacy, safety and tolerance of Primaxin and moxalactam. *Eur. J. Clin. Microbiol. 3*:478–487 (1984).
2. J. S. Kahan, F. M. Kahan, R. Goegelman, S. A. Currie, M. Jackson, E. O. Stapley, T. W. Miller, A. K. Miller, D. Hendlin, S. Mochales, S. Hernandez, H. B. Woodruff, and J. Birnbaum. Thienamycin, a new beta-lactam antibiotic: I. Discovery, taxonomy, isolation and physical properties. *J. Antibiot., 32*:1–12 (1979).
3. G. Albers-Schonberg, B. H. Arison, O. D. Hensens, J. Hirshfield, K. Hoogsteen, E. A. Kaczka, R. E. Rhodes, J. S. Kahan, F. M. Kahan, R. W. Ratcliffe, E. Walton, L. J. Ruswinkle, R. B. Morin, and B. G. Christensen. Structure

and absolute configuration of thienamycin. *J. Am. Chem. Soc., 100*:6491–6499 (1978).

4. J. S. Kahan, F. M. Kahan, R. Goegelman, S. A. Currie, M. Jackson, E. O. Stapley, T. W. Miller, A. K. Miller, D. Hendlin, S. Mochales, S. Hernandez, and H. B. Woodruff. Thienamycin. A new beta-lactam antibiotic. I. Discovery and isolation. Paper presented at the 16th Interscience Conference on Antimicrobial Agents and Chemotherapy, Chicago, Illinois, 1976, Abstract 227.
5. H. Kropp, J. G. Sundelof, J. S. Kahan, F. M. Kahan, and J. Birnbaum. MK0787 (N-formimidoyl thienamycin): Evaluation of *in vitro* and *in vivo* activities. *Antimicrob. Agents Chemother., 17*:993–1000 (1980).
6. T. Kesado, T. Hashizume, and Y. Asahi. Antibacterial activities of a new stabilized theinamycin, N-formimidoyl thienamycin in comparison with other antibiotics. *Antimicrob. Agents Chemother., 17*:912–917 (1980).
7. W. J. Leanza, K. J. Wildonger, T. W. Miller, and B. G. Christensen. N-Acetimidoyl- and N-formimidoyl thienamycin derivatives: Antipseudomonal beta-lactam antibiotics. *J. Med. Chem., 22*:1435–1436 (1979).
8. R. Sutherland and G. N. Rolinson. Characteristics of methicillin-resistant staphylococci. *J. Bacteriol., 87*:887 (1964).
9. F. M. Kahan, H. Kropp, J. G. Sundelof, and J. Birnbaum. Thienamycin: Development of imipenem–cilastatin. *J. Antimicrob. Chemother. Suppl. D, 12*:1–35 (1983).
10. V. W. Horadam, J. D. Smilack, C. L. Montgomery, and J. Werringloer. *In vitro* activity of N-formimidoyl thienamycin (MK0787), a crystalline derivative of thienamycin. *Antimicrob. Agents Chemother., 18*:557–561 (1980).
11. M. L. Corrado, S. H. Landesman, and C. E. Cherubin. Influence of inoculum size on activity of cefoperazone, cefotaxime, moxalactam, piperacillin and N-formimidoyl thienamycin (MK0787) against *Pseudomonas aeruginosa. Antimicrob. Agents Chemother., 18*:893–896 (1980).
12. C. E. Cherubin, M. L. Corrado, M. F. Sierra, M. E. Gombert, and M. Shulman. Susceptibility of gram-positive cocci to various antibiotics, including cefotaxime, moxalactam and N-formimidoyl thienamycin. *Antimicrob. Agents Chemother., 20*:553–555 (1981).
13. A. K. Hanslo, K. Shannon, C. Warren, and I. Phillips. N-Formimidoyl thienamycin (MK0787): *In vitro* antibacterial activity and susceptibility to beta-lactamases compared with that of cefotaxime, moxalactam and other beta-lactam antibiotics. *J. Antimicrob. Chemother.,7*:607–617 (1981).
14. F. P. Tally, N. V. Jacobus, and S. L. Gorbach. *In vitro* activity of N-formimidoyl thienamycin (MK0787). *Antimicrob. Agents Chemother., 18*:642–644 (1980).
15. W. K. Livingston, A. M. Elliott, and C. G. Cobbs. *In vitro* activity of N-formimidoyl thienamycin (MK0787) against resistant strains of *Pseudomonas aeruginosa, Staphylococcus epidermidis, Serratia marcescens* and *Enterococcus* spp. *Antimicrob. Agents Chemother., 19*:114–116 (1981).

16. M. Nasu, J. P. Maskell, R. J. Williams, and J. D. Williams. *In vitro* activity of MK0787 (N-formimidoyl thienamycin) and other beta-lactam compounds against *Bacteroides* spp. *Antimicrob. Agents Chemother., 20*:433–436 (1981).
17. A. S. Prince and H. C. Neu. Activities of new beta-lactam antibiotics against isolates of *Pseudomonas aeruginosa* from patients with cystic fibrosis. *Antimicrob. Agents Chemother., 20*:545–546 (1981).
18. R. D. Rolfe and S. M. Finegold. Comparative *in vitro* activity of new beta-lactam antibiotics against anaerobic bacteria. *Antimicrob. Agents Chemother., 20*:600–609 (1981).
19. S. Shadomy and R. S. May. N-Formimidoyl thienamycin (MK0787): *In vitro* study. *Antimicrob. Agents Chemother., 19*:201–204 (1981).
20. V. A. Tutlane, R. V. McCloskey, and J. A. Treat. *In vitro* comparison of N-formimidoyl thienamycin, piperacillin, cefotaxime and cefoperazone. *Antimicrob. Agents Chemother., 20*:140–143 (1981).
21. L. Verbist and J. Verhaegen. *In vitro* activity of N-formimidoyl thienamycin in comparison with cefotaxime, moxalactam and cefetazidime. *Antimicrob. Agents Chemother., 19*:402–406 (1981).
22. R. Wise, J. M. Andrews, and N. Patel. N-Formimidoyl thienamycin, a novel beta-lactam: An *in vitro* comparison with other beta-lactam antibiotics. *J. Antimicrob. Chemother., 7*:521–529 (1981).
23. T. Kesado, K. Watanabe, Y. Ashai, M. Isono, and K. Ueno. Susceptibilities of anaerobic bacteria to N-formimidoyl thienamycin (MK0787) and to other antibiotics. *Antimicrob. Agents Chemother., 21*:1016–1022 (1982).
24. H. L. Muytjens and J. Van Der Ros-Van De Repe. Comparative activities of 13 beta-lactam antibiotics. *Antimicrob. Agents Chemother., 21*:925–934 (1982).
25. D. L. Cohn, L. G. Reimer, and L. B. Reller. Comparative *in vitro* activity of MK0787 (N-formimidoyl thienamycin) against 540 blood culture isolates. *J. Antimicrob. Chemother., 9*:183–194 (1982).
26. M. R. Jacobs, F. Kelly, and W. T. Speck. Susceptibility of group B streptococci to 16 beta-lactam antibiotics, including new penicillin and cephalosporin derivatives. *Antimicrob. Agents Chemother., 22*:897–900 (1982).
27. J. E. Brown, V. E. Del Bene, and C. D. Collins. *In vitro* activity of N-formimidoyl thienamycin, moxalactam and other new beta-lactam agents against *Bacteroides fragilis*: Contribution of beta-lactamase to resistance. *Antimicrob. Agents Chemother., 19*:248–252 (1981).
28. G. M. Eliopoulos and R. C. Moellering, Jr. Susceptibility of *Enterococcus* and *Listeria monocytogenes* to N-formimidoyl thienamycin alone and in combination with an aminoglycoside. *Antimicrob. Agents Chemother., 19*:789–793 (1981).
29. R. Auckenthaler, W. R. Wilson, A. J. Wright, J. A. Washington II, D. T. Durack, and J. E. Geraci. Lack of *in vivo* and *in vitro* bactericidal activity of N-formimidoyl thienamycin against enterococci. *Antimicrob. Agents Chemother., 22*:448–452 (1982).

30. H. C. Neu and P. Labthavikul. Comparative *in vitro* activity of N-formimidoyl thienamycin against gram-positive and gram-negative aerobic and anaerobic species and its beta-lactamase stability. *Antimicrob. Agents Chemother., 21*:180–187 (1982).
31. J. Linares, J. L. Pérez, and R. Martin. Correspondance: Susceptibility studies in the *Bacteroides fragilis* group resistant to clindamycin. *J. Antimicrob. Chemother., 12*:293 (1983).
32. M. H. Richmond. The semi-synthetic thienamycin derivative MK0787 and its properties with respect to a range of beta-lactamases from clinically relevant bacterial species. *J. Antimicrob. Chemother., 7*:279–285 (1981).
33. A. Vuye. *In vitro* activity and beta-lactamase stability of N-formimidoyl thienamycin compared to that of second and third generation cephalosporins. *Chemotherapy, 28*:267–275 (1982).
34. R. W. Ryan, I. Kwasnik, and R. C. Tilton. The activity of five cephalosporins against *Bacteroides fragilis. Ann. Clin. Lab Sci., 12*:32–34 (1982).
35. C. C. Sanders, D. A. Martin, and R. L. Marier. N-Formimidoyl thienamycin (MK0787): *In vitro* activity against anaerobic bacteria. *Antimicrob. Agents Chemother., 21*:168–169 (1982).
36. S. B. Calderwood, A. Gardella, A. M. Philippon, G. A. Jacoby, and R. C. Moellering, Jr. Effects of azlocillin in combination with clavulanic acid, sulbactam and N-formimidoyl thienamycin against beta-lactamase-producing carbenicillin-resistant *Pseudomonas aerúginosa. Antimicrob. Agents Chemother., 22*:266–271 (1982).
37. A. Jaffe, Y. A. Chabbert, and E. Derlot. Selection and characterization of beta-lactam-resistant *Escherichia coli* K-12 mutants. *Antimicrob. Agents Chemother., 23*:622–625 (1982).
38. W. Cullmann and W. Dick. Investigations on beta-lactamase stability of recently developed beta-lactam compounds: Study of enzyme kinetics. *Zentralbl. Bakteriol. Mikrobiol. Hyg. Abt. Orig. A, 254*:413–422 (1983).
39. C. C. Sanders and W. E. Sanders, Jr. Sch 29482: Comparative activity against enterobacteriaceae multiply-resistant to beta-lactam antibiotics and mycobacteria. *J. Antimicrob. Chemother. Suppl. C, 9*:59–69 (1982).
40. R. H. Alford. Comparison of ceftazidime and N-formimidoyl thienamycin against gentamicin-susceptible and resistant *Pseudomonas aeruginosa. J. Antimicrob. Chemother., 11*:599–601 (1983).
41. S. D. R. Lang and D. T. Durack. *In vitro* efficacy of cefoperazone compared with cefotaxime, LY127935, and thienamycin. *Clin. Ther., 3*:112–116 (1980).
42. A. J. Matzkowitz, A. L. Baltch, R. P. Smith, N. T. Sutphen, M. C. Hammer, and J. V. Conroy. *In vitro* comparison of N-formimidoyl thienamycin (MK0787) and azlocillin with three aminoglycosides and ticarcillin against *Pseudomonas aeruginosa. Antimicrob. Agents Chemother., 21*:685–687 (1982).
43. P. R. Michael, R. H. Alford, and Z. A. McGee. Superior activity of N-formimidoyl thienamycin against gentamicin-resistant *Pseudomonas aeruginosa. Antimicrob. Agents Chemother., 20*:702–704 (1981).

44. D. M. Livermore, R. J. Williams, and J. D. Williams. *In vitro* activity of MK0787 (N-formimidoyl thienamycin) against *Pseudomonas aeruginosa* and other gram-negative organisms and its stability to their beta-lactamases. *J. Antimicrob. Chemother., 8*:355–362 (1981).
45. R. L. Thompson, K. A. Fisher, and R. P. Wenzel. *In vitro* activity of N-formimidoyl thienamycin and other beta-lactam antibiotics against methicillin-resistant *Staphylococcus aureus. Antimicrob. Agents Chemother., 21*:341–343 (1982).
46. J. L. Witte, F. L. Sapico, and H. N. Canawati. *In vitro* susceptibility of methicillin-resistant and methicillin-susceptible *Staphylococcus aureus* strains to N-formimidoyl thienamycin. *Antimicrob. Agents Chemother., 22*:906–908 (1982).
47. N. Markowitz, D. J. Pohlod, L. D. Saravolatz, and E. L. Quinn. *In vitro* susceptibility patterns of methicillin-resistant and -susceptible *Staphylococcus aureus* strains in a population of parenteral drug abusers from 1972 to 1981. *Antimicrob. Agents Chemother., 23*:450–457 (1983).
48. R. M. Blumentahl, R. Raeder, C. D. Takemoto, and E. H. Freimer. Occurrence and expression of imipemide (N-formimidoyl thienamycin) resistance in clinical isolates of coagulase-negative *Staphylococci. Antimicrob. Agents Chemother., 24*:61–69 (1983).
49. W. L. Dibb, V. A. Kjellevold, and A. Digranes. *Pseudomonas aeruginosa* and *Acinetobacter calcoaceticus*: *In vitro* susceptibility of 150 clinical isolates to five beta-lactam antibiotics and tobramycin. *Chemotherapy, 29*:332–336 (1983).
50. C. J. Fernandes, D. A. Stevens, S. I. Murray, and V. P. Ackerman. An evaluation of recently developed antibiotics. *J. Antimicrob. Chemother., 12*: 577–585 (1983).
51. I. Garcia, V. Fainstein, B. LeBlanc, and G. P. Bodey. *In vitro* activities of new beta-lactam antibiotics against *Acinetobacter* spp. antibiotics. *Antimicrob. Agents Chemother., 24*:297–299 (1983).
52. D. A. Strandberg, J. H. Jorgensen, and D. J. Drutz. Activities of aztreonam and new cephalosporins against infrequently isolated gram-negative bacilli. *Antimicrob. Agents Chemother., 24*:282–286 (1983).
53. G. Tischhauser and F. H. Kayser. The *in vitro* activity of N-formimidoyl thienamycin compared with other broad-spectrum cephalosporins and with clindamycin and metronidazole. *Infection, 11*:219–226 (1983).
54. E. Bergogne-Berezin, M. Joly-Guillou, F. Megraud, and C. Verin. *In vitro* activity of N-formimidoyl thienamycin compared with beta-lactamase-stable compounds against clinical strains of *Acinetobacter calcoaceticus. Curr. Chemother. Immunother., 1*:721–723 (1982).
55. M. H. Cynamon and G. S. Palmer. *In vitro* susceptibility of *Nocardia asteroides* to N-formimidoyl thienamycin and several cephalosporins. *Antimicrob. Agents Chemother., 20*:841–842 (1981).
56. D. H. Dewsnup and D. N. Wright. *In vitro* susceptibility of *Nocardia asteroides* to 25 antimicrobial agents. *Antimicrob. Agents Chemother., 25*: 165–167 (1984).

57. J. A. Garcia-Rodriguez, A. C. Gomez-Garcia, J. Aguero, and J. E. Garcia-Sanchez. *In vitro* susceptibility of *Nocardia* and *Rhodococcus* to fourteen beta-lactam antibiotics. *J. Antimicrob. Chemother., 10*:564–565 (1982).
58. M. E. Gombert. Susceptibility of *Nocardia asteroides* to various antibiotics, including newer beta-lactams, trimethoprim–sulfamethoxazole, amikacin and N-formimidoyl thienamycin. *Antimicrob. Agents Chemother., 21*: 1011–1012 (1982).
59. M. E. Gombert and T. M. Aulicino. Synergism of imipenem and amikacin in combination with other antibiotics against *Nocardia asteroides. Antimicrob. Agents Chemother., 24*:810–811 (1983).
60. L. Gutmann, F. W. Goldstein, M. D. Kitzis, B. Hautefort, C. Darmon, and J. F. Acar. Susceptibility of *Nocardia asteroides* to 46 antibiotics, including 22 beta-lactams. *Antimicrob. Agents Chemother., 23*:248–251 (1983).
61. L. Gutmann. *In vitro* susceptibility of 12 strains of *Norcardia asteroides* to 11 beta-lactam antibiotics alone or in combination with clavulanic acid and relationship to their beta-lactamase activity. *Fortschr. Med. Mikrobiol., 1*: 151–159 (1983).
62. J. Aznar, M. C. Garcia Iglesias, and E. J. Perea. Comparative activity of imipenem (N-formimidoyl thienamycin) on enterococci and its interactions with aminoglycosides. *J. Antimicrob. Chemother., 13*:129–132 (1984).
63. T. M. Hooton, A. D. Blair, M. Turck, and G. W. Counts. Synergism at clinically attainable concentrations of aminoglycoside and beta-lactam antibiotics. *Antimicrob. Agents Chemother., 26*:535–538 (1984).
64. M. Diez Enciso, M. L. Mateos Lindemann, and A. Gutierrez Altes. *In vitro* evaluation of N-formimidoyl thienamycin (MK0787) combined with amikacin against gram-negative bacilli and *Staphylococcus aureus. Antimicrob. Agents Chemother., 22*:1064–1066 (1982).
65. M. E. Gombert, L. B. Berkowitz, and M. C. Cummings. Synergistic effect of N-formimidoyl thienamycin with gentamicin and amikacin against *Streptococcus faecalis. Antimicrob. Agents Chemother., 23*:245–247 (1983).
66. C. Kallick, T. Rice, J. Norsen, K. Rajashekaraiah, D. Marsh, D. McCulley, and K. Thadhani. *In vitro* activity of N-formimidoyl thienamycin against *Pseudomonas* and staphylococci associated with endocarditis. *Curr. Chemother. Immunother., 1*:725–726 (1982).
67. R. D. Meyer and K. Pasiecznik. *In vitro* activity of newer beta-lactam agents in combination with amikacin against *Pseudomonas aeruginosa, Klebsiella pneumoniae* and *Serratia marcescens. Diagn. Microbiol. Infect. Dis., 1*:287–293 (1983).
68. G. Schroeter and A. Schrettenbrunner. Antibacterial activity of combinations of N-formimidoyl thienamycin with amikacin, cefoxitin or fosfomycin against *Klebsiella pneumoniae* and *Pseudomonas aeruginosa. Zentralbl. Bakteriol. Mikrobiol. Hyg. I Abt. Orig. A, 253*:355–357 (1982).
69. C. Watanakunakorn and J. C. Tisone. Synergism between N-formimidoyl thienamycin and gentamicin or tobramycin against enterococci. *Antimicrob. Agents Chemother., 22*:1082–1083 (1982).

70. J. E. Pennington and C. E. Johnson. Comparative activities of N-formimidoyl thienamycin, ticarcillin and tobramycin against experimental *Pseudomonas aeruginosa* pneumonia. *Antimicrob. Agents Chemother., 22*:406–408 (1982).
71. T. Hau, A. Phuangsab, and R. A. Nishikawa. MK0787 in the treatment of intraperitoneal polymicrobial infections. Paper presented at the Annual Meeting of the American Society of Microbiology, Dallas, Texas, 1982, Abstract A61.
72. G. Lahnborg, K. G. Hedstrom, and C. E. Nord. Efficacy of different antibiotics in the treatment of experimentally induced intra-abdominal sepsis. *J. Antimicrob. Chemother., 10*:497–504 (1982).
73. D. E. Johnson, F. M. Calia, M. J. Snyder, J. W. Warren, and S. C. Schimpff. Imipenem therapy of *Pseudomonas aeruginosa* bacteraemia in neutropenic rats. *J. Antimicrob. Chemother. Suppl. D, 12*:89–96 (1983).
74. V. W. Ritzerfeld. N-Formimidoyl thienamycin in animal studies. *Arzneim. Forsch., 33*:470–472 (1983).
75. P. A. Guze, G. M. Kalmanson, K. Ishida, L. R. Freedman, and L. B. Guze. Treatment of staphylococcal pyelonephritis in rats with N-formimidoyl thienamycin. *Chemotherapia, 3*:53–56 (1984).
76. S. K. Kim. Efficacy of imipenem in experimental group B streptococcal bacteremia and meningitis. *Chemotherapy 31*:304–309 (1985).
77. J. D. Baumgartner and M. P. Glauser. Comparative treatment of *Staphylococcus aureus* endocarditis in the rat. *J. Antimicrob. Chemother. Suppl. D, 12*:79–87 (1983).
78. P. Patamasucon and G. H. McCracken. Pharmacokinetics and bacteriological efficacy of N-formimidoyl thienamycin in experimental *Escherichia coli* meningitis. *Antimicrob. Agents Chemother., 21*:390–392 (1982).
79. E. A. Funk, P. R. Laun, and L. J. Strausbaugh. Penetration of N-formimidoyl thienamycin (NFT) into cerebrospinal fluid (CSF) in rabbits. Paper presented at the 22nd Interscience Conference on Antimicrobial Agents and Chemotherapy, Miami Beach, Florida, 1982, Abstract 233.
80. D. E. Washburn, J. R. Perfect, and D. T. Durack. Pharmacokinetics of N-formimidoyl thienamycin and influence of a renal dipeptidase inhibitor in experimental meningitis. *J. Antimicrob. Chemother., 12*:39–45 (1983).
81. W. M. Scheld and J. M. Keeley. Imipenem therapy of experimental *Staphylococcus aureus* and *Streptococcus faecalis* endocarditis. *J. Antimicrob. Chemother. Suppl. D, 12*:65–78 (1983).
82. H. Kropp, J. G. Sundelof, R. Hajdu, and F. M. Kahan. Metabolism of thienamycin and related carbapenem antibiotics by the renal dipeptidase: Dehydropeptidase-I. *Antimicrob. Agents Chemother., 22*:62–70 (1982).
83. J. P. Greenstein. Dehydropeptidases. In *Advances in Enzymology and Related Subjects of Biochemistry* (F. F. Nord, ed.), Interscience, New York, 1948, pp. 117–169.
84. B. J. Campbell. Renal dipeptidase, in *Methods in Enzymology,* Vol. 19 (S. P. Colowick and N. O. Kaplan, eds.), Academic, New York, 1970, pp. 722–729.

84a. S. R. Norrby, J. D. Rogers, F. Ferber, K. H. Jones, A. G. Zacchel, L. L. Weidner, J. L. Demetriades, D. A. Gravallese and J. Y.-K. Hsieh. Disposition of radio labeled imipenem and cilastatin in normal human volunteers. *Antimicrob. Agents Chemother., 26*:707-714 (1984).
84b. S. R. Norrby, B. Björnegard, F. Ferber, and K. H. Jones. Pharmacokinetics of imipenem in healthy volunteers. *J. Antimicrob. Chemother. Suppl. D, 12*:109–124 (1983).
85. H. S. P. Kim. Cellular orientation of renal dipeptidase in the microvilli and its catalytic activity on a novel beta-lactam antibiotic, N-formimidoyl thienamycin. Ph.D. dissertation, University of Missouri, Columbia (1982).
86. C. L. Welch and B. J. Campbell. Uptake of tritiated glycine from L-alanyl glycine into renal brush-border vesicles. *J. Membrane Biol., 54*:39 (1980).
87. S. R. Norrby, K. Alestig, F. Ferber, J. L. Huber, K. H. Jones, F. M. Kahan, M. A. P. Meisinger, and J. D. Rogers. Pharmacokinetics and tolerance of N-formimidoyl thienamycin (MK0787) in humans. *Antimicrob. Agents Chemother., 23*:293–299 (1983).
88. G. B. Calandra, F. M. Ricci, C. Wang, and K. R. Brown. Safety and tolerance comparison of imipenem–cilastatin to cephalothin and cefazolin. *J. Antimicrob. Chemother. Suppl. D, 12*:125–131 (1983).
89. W. T. Ashton, L. Barash, J. E. Brown, R. D. Brown, L. F. Canning, A. Chen, D. W. Graham, F. M. Kahan, H. Kropp, J. G. Sundelof, and E. F. Rogers. Z-2-Acylamino-3-substituted propenoates, inhibitors of the renal dipeptidase (dehydropeptidase-I) responsible for thienamycin metabolism. Paper presented at the 20th Interscience Conference on Antimicrobial Agents and Chemotherapy, New Orleans, Louisiana, 1980. Abstract 271.
90. S. R. Norrby, K. Alestig, B. Bjornegard, L. A. Burman, F. Ferber, J. L. Huber, K. H. Jones, F. M. Kahan, J. S. Kahan, H. Kropp, M. A. P. Meisinger, and J. G. Sundelof. Urinary recovery of N-formimidoyl thienamycin (MK0787) as affected by coadministration of N-formimidoyl thienamycin dehydropeptidase inhibitors. *Antimicrob. Agents Chemother., 23*:300–307 (1983).
91. G. A. Verpooten, L. Verbist, and M. E. DeBroe. The pharmacokinetics of MK0787 and a renal dehydropeptidase inhibitor (D.P.I.) in normal volunteers and in patients with differing degrees of renal failure, in *Proceedings of the 13th International Congress of Chemotherapy*, (K. H. Spitzy and K. Karrer, eds.), Egerman Druckerie, Vienna, 1983, pp. 38–45.
92. B. M. Tune. Relationship between the transport and toxicity of cephalosporins in the kidney. *J. Infect. Dis., 132*:189–194 (1975).
93. B. M. Tune, K. Y. Wu, and R. L. Kempson. Inhibition of transport and prevention of toxicity of cephaloridine in the kidney. Dose-responsiveness of the rabbit and the guinea pig to probenecid. *J. Pharmacol. Exp. Ther., 202*:466–471 (1977).
94. B. M. Tune, M. Finegold, and A. Schwartz. Mechanism of cephaloridine transport in the kidney. *J. Pharmacol. Exp. Ther., 191*:311–317 (1974).
95. J. S. Wold, S. A. Turnipseed, and B. L. Miller. The effect of renal cation transport inhibition on cephaloridine nephrotoxicity. *Toxicol. Appl. Pharmacol., 47*:115–122 (1979).

96. B. M. Tune, M. C. Browning, C. H. Hsu, and D. Fravert. Prevention of cephalosporin nephrotoxicity by other cephalosporins and by penicillins without significant inhibition of renal cortical uptake. *J. Infect. Dis., 145*: 174–180 (1982).
97. K. J. Child and M. G. Dodds. Mechanism of urinary excretion of cephaloridine and its effects on renal function in animals. *Br. J. Pharmacol. Chemother., 26*:108–119 (1966).
98. A. Meister. Selective modification of glutathione metabolism. *Science, 220*:472–477 (1983).
99. D. S. Reeves, S. T. Chapman, A. J. Davies, F. Ferber, and J. D. Rogers. Human pharmacokinetics of N-formimidoyl thienamycin alone and in combination with a dehydropeptidase inhibitor (MK0791) and probenecid in *Proceedings of the 13th International Congress of Chemotherapy,* (K. H. Spitzy and K. Karrer, eds.), Egerman Druckerie, Vienna, 1983, pp. 30–33.
100. L. J. Eron, D. L. Hixon, C. H. Park, R. I. Goldenberg, and D. M. Poretz. Imipenem versus moxalactam in the treatment of serious infections. *Antimicrob. Agents Chemother., 24*:841–846 (1983).
101. B. S. Ribner, R. Raeder, M. Hollstein, and E. H. Freimer. A randomized study comparing clinical efficacy and safety of thienamycin formamidine (MK0787)/renal dipeptidase inhibitor (MK0791) and cefazolin. *J. Antimicrob. Chemother., 12*:387–391 (1983).
102. F. Crokaert, J. P. Thys, Y. Glupczynski, C. Potuliege, E. Schoutens-Serruys, and E. Yourassowsky. A comparative evaluation of thienamycin (TH) and cefotaxime (CTx) in severe infections, in *Proceedings of the 13th International Congress of Chemotherapy,* (K. H. Spitzy and K. Karrer, eds.), Egerman Druckerie, Vienna, 1983, pp. 63–67.
103. G. K. Daikos, H. Giamarellou, and D. Voutsinas. Imipemide: A new approach in the treatment of multiresistant and serious infections, in *Proceedings of the 13th International Congress of Chemotherapy,* (K. H. Spitzy and K. Karrer, eds.), Egerman Druckerie, Vienna, 1983, pp. 19–22.
104. R. L. Marier, R. V. McCloskey, G. Dickinson, C. V. Sanders, T. Hoffman, D. Gutterman, and K. E. Aldridge. Comparative clinical trial of N-formimidoyl thienamycin – Dehydropeptide inhibitor (MK0787/MK0791) and cefazolin, in *Proceedings of the 13th International Congress of Chemotherapy,* (K. H. Spitzy and K. Karrer, eds.), Egerman Druckerie, Vienna, 1983, pp. 23–29.
105. F. P. Tally, J. L. Ho, and S. L. Gorbach. Thienamycin in the treatment of mixed infections; in *Proceedings of the 13th International Congress of Chemotherapy,* (K. H. Spitzy and K. Karrer, eds.), Egerman Druckerie, Vienna, 1983, pp. 30–33.
106. R. Jacobs, B. Marmer, A. Brown, G. Kearns, R. Kluza, J. Trang, F. Underwood, R. Steele, and T. Yamauchi. Thienamycin pharmacokinetics in children. Paper presented at the 23rd Interscience Conference on Antimicrobial Agents and Chemotherapy, Las Vegas, Nevada, 1983, Abstract 203.
107. M. S. Topiel, F. P. Paleologo, N. H. Goldstein, M. Vannes, C. June, J. Rosenstock, W. W. Karney, and G. L. Simon. A comparative evaluation

of MK0787/MK0791 and moxalactam in the treatment of serious bacterial infections. Paper presented at the 23rd Interscience Conference on Antimicrobial Agents and Chemotherapy, Las Vegas, Nevada, 1983, Abstract 206.

108. A. S. Berkeley, L. J. Strausbaugh, A. W. Cohen, K. S. Freedman, and W. J. Ledger. Randomized comparative trial of thienamycin formamidine/potentiator (MK0787/MK0791) and moxalactam in the treatment of serious obstetric and gynecologic infections. Paper presented at the 23rd Interscience Conference on Antimicrobial Agents and Chemotherapy, Las Vegas, Nevada, 1983, Abstract 207.

109. R. R. MacGregor, M. A. Fisher, B. A. Zajac, and G. Gibson. Efficacy and safety of high-dose treatment with MK0787/MK0791 (thienamycin). Paper presented at the 23rd Interscience Conference on Antimicrobial Agents and Chemotherapy, Las Vegas, Nevada, 1983, Abstract 208.

110. R. Norrby. Imipenem/cilastatin versus gentamicin/clindamycin for treatment of serious bacterial infections. *Lancet, 1*:868–871 (1984).

15

Augmentin: Clavulanate-Potentiated Amoxicillin

CHRISTOPHER READING and BRIAN SLOCOMBE
Beecham Pharmaceuticals Research Division, Chemotherapeutic Research Centre, Betchworth, Surrey, England

I. INTRODUCTION

A. Beta-Lactamase and Resistance

The development of new beta-lactam antibiotics over the last 20 years or so has been directed by two main considerations. First, there was a need to extend the spectrum of activity of the naturally occurring penicillins and cephalosporins and, second, a solution to the emergence of beta-lactamase-mediated resistance to these early beta-lactams was required. The discovery of the penicillin nucleus, 6α-aminopenicillanic acid (6-APA) was a major advance and led to the introduction of semisynthetic penicillins such as ampicillin and carbenicillin, penicillins with an extended spectrum of activity, including gram-negative bacteria and, in the case of carbenicillin, stability to some clinically important beta-lactamases. The discovery of methicillin and cloxacillin provided early success in the search for beta-lactams inherently stable to staphylococcal beta-lactamases, in this instance reducing the problem of penicillin-resistant staphylococci in the clinic.

In the case of broad-spectrum penicillins, their overall usefulness has slowly declined over the years as the incidence of beta-lactamase-producing gram-negative bacteria has increased, even in general practice. This has probably arisen through the selective pressures applied to the bacterial population by antibiotic usage over this period. The existence of plasmid-encoded beta-lactamases has greatly facilitated the rapid spread of antibiotic resistance. The reasons for this became even clearer with the discovery of transposons, which permit the rapid dissemination of genetic determinants between plasmids.

In the cephalosporin series the problem of beta-lactamase has become even greater than with the penicillins, in that virtually all gram-negative bacilli pro-

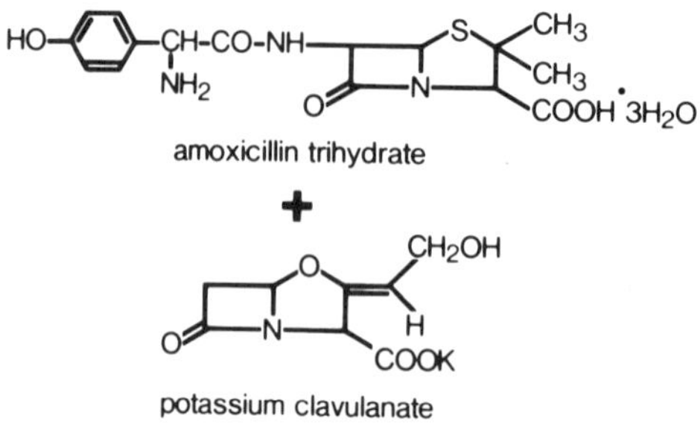

Figure 1 Components of Augmentin.

duce a chromosomally mediated cephalosporinase. The introduction of the α-methoxyimino- and 7-α-methoxy-substituted cephalosporin derivatives have represented further major successes in the search for beta-lactamase-stable beta-lactam antibiotics with an extended spectrum of antibacterial activity. The cephamycins (7-α-methoxycephalosporins) in fact illustrate how natural products can continue to provide useful leads in the beta-lactam field, and thienamycin and the monobactams are further notable examples. The rational synthetic approach has produced the oxacephem latamoxef; this, and the other recent developments mentioned above, are discussed in detail elsewhere in this volume.

This chapter deals with an alternative and highly successful approach to beta-lactamase-mediated resistance in that it reviews the properties of Augmentin,* a formulation of the α-aminopenicillin amoxicillin and the beta-lactamase inhibitor potassium clavulanate (Fig. 1). The concept of protecting a penicillin from degradation by beta-lactamase by combining it with an inhibitor of this enzyme provides an alternative strategy as well as some considerable advantages. The broad-spectrum penicillin amoxicillin is one of the most widely used beta-lactam antibiotics and, along with its earlier analog ampicillin, is the drug of choice for a wide range of clinical situations. As mentioned previously, the efficacy of these α-aminopenicillins has slowly declined in the face of an ever-increasing number of beta-lactamase-producing organisms. As a solution to this problem, what better than to retain all the well-documented intrinsic advantages of amoxicillin and yet extend its activity to cover beta-lactamase-producing organisms? This was made possible with the discovery of the beta-lactamase inhibitor clavulanic acid (1) which can protect amoxicillin from inactivation by bacterial beta-lactamases.

---

*Augmentin is a registered trademark of the Beecham Group plc.

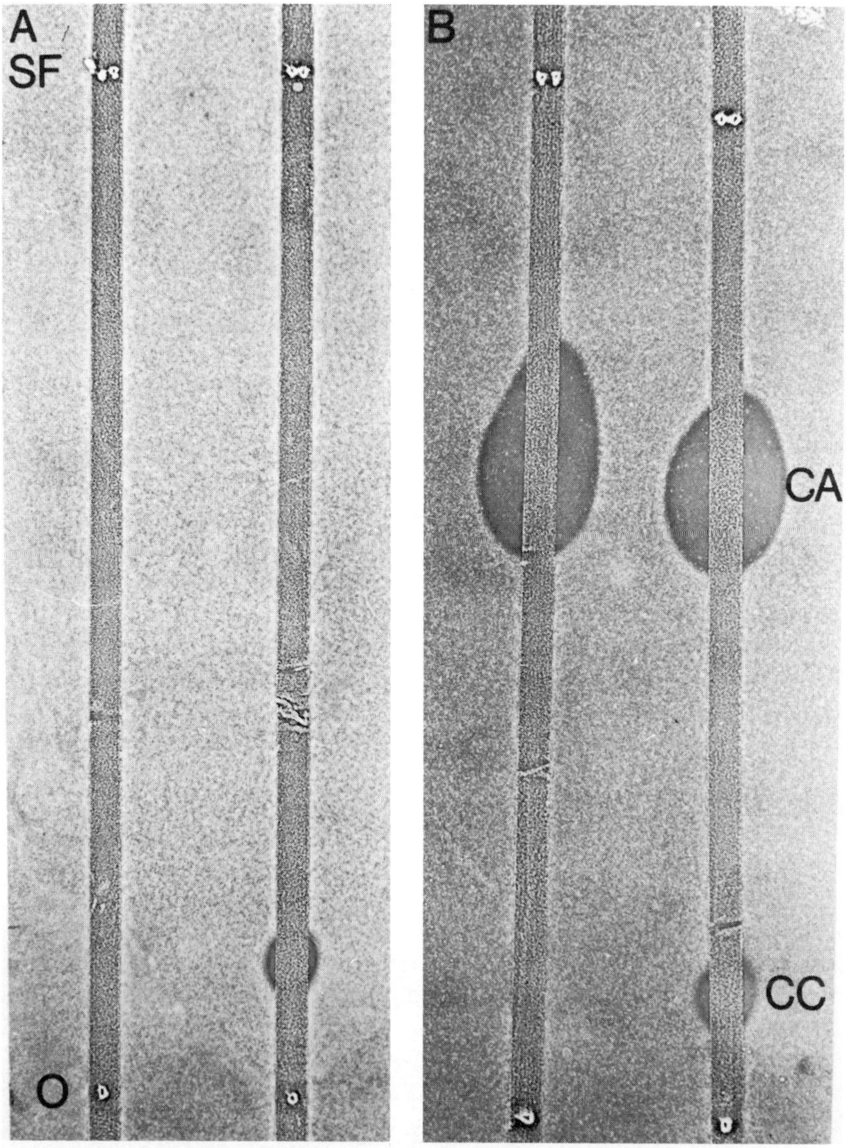

Figure 2 Paper-chromatographic detection of clavulanic acid in a 4-day fermentation sample of *Streptomyces clavuligerus.* The chromatograms were contacted with agar seeded with beta-lactamase-producing strains of *Klebsiella aerogenes* (A) without of (B) with the addition of a subinhibitory concentration of benzylpenicillin (6 μg/ml) to the agar. The second chromatogram of each pair was a fermentation sample supplemented with cephamycin C (10 μl of 1 mg/ml). The solvent system was n-butanol–acetic acid–water (12:3:5, vol./vol./vol.), the paper was Whatman grade 1, and the loading was 12 μl of sample. (SF, Solvent front; O, origin; CA, clavulanic acid; CC, cephamycin C). (Data from Ref. 1.)

B. Discovery of Clavulanic Acid

Many of the early semisynthetic penicillins, apart from having antibacterial activity, had also been shown to inhibit beta-lactamase; for instance, cloxacillin is a very potent inhibitor of class I cephalosporinases. This activity, however, did not extrapolate to in vitro antibacterial tests with any great success, mainly because these more hydrophobic penicillins fail to penetrate the outer membrane of gram-negative cells, as will be discussed later in more detail. These early results encouraged the start, some 16 years ago, of a systematic screening program in our laboratories to detect beta-lactamase inhibitors as natural products in the fermentation broths of microorganisms. The screen devised by Brown et al. (2) employed a simple plate test in which nutrient agar containing benzylpenicillin was seeded with *Klebsiella aerogenes,* which produced beta-lactamase. On incubation the penicillin in the agar is hydrolyzed by the bacterial beta-lactamase and the *Klebsiella* multiply to produce a confluent lawn of growth. If, however, a beta-lactamase inhibitor is applied to the agar before incubation, the penicillin is protected and produces a zone of inhibition of bacterial growth. After the screening of over 1000 isolates of actinomycetes, marked beta-lactamase inhibitory activity was detected in the culture filtrate of a strain of *Streptomyces olivaceus* (2). This was later found to be due to the presence of a family of beta-lactam compounds that have been called the olivanic acids (3). These are carbapenems related to thienamycin and have broad-spectrum antibacterial activity and are potent inhibitors of beta-lactamase as well.

Examination of further cultures led to the detection of activity in the culture filtrates of *Streptomyces clavuligerus.* Paper chromatography followed by bioautography on plates of nutrient agar containing benzylpenicillin seeded with *Klebsiella* (Fig. 2) showed the presence of a zone where $R_f = 0.63$ which was not present when identical chromatograms were plated on agar seeded with *Klebsiella* alone. This activity was distinct from cephamycin C, also produced by the culture and from the olivanic acids, which had lower R_f values in this particular chromatographic system. The compound responsible for this marked beta-lactamase inhibitory effect was isolated (1) and named clavulanic acid. Structure elucidation (4) revealed that the compound was a beta-lactam (Fig. 1) containing an oxazolidine ring, no 6-acylamino side chain as in the penicillins, and the penicillin gem-dimethyl being replaced by a 2-hydroxyethylidine side chain providing a novel beta-lactam with new and interesting properties.

II. BETA-LACTAMASE INHIBITORY ACTIVITY OF CLAVULANIC ACID

A. Spectrum of Clavulanic Acid

Clavulanic acid has been termed a progressive inhibitor in that the degree of inhibition increases with time. This is evident when the concentration required to in-

Table 1 Beta-Lactamase Inhibitory Activity of Clavulanic Acid

Type of beta-lactamase[a]	Example	I_{50} (μg/ml)[b] With preincubation, inhibitor added 5 min before substrate	I_{50} (μg/ml)[b] Without preincubation, inhibitor with substrate
Class I chromosomal cephalosporinase	Ia *Enterobacter cloacae* P99	110.0	>4000.0
	Ib *Escherichia coli* JT410	250.0	>400
	Id *Pseudomonas aeruginosa* A	>400	>400
	Ic *Proteus vulgaris* W091	0.001	0.3
	I *Escherichia coli* JD41	0.4	3.1
Class II penicillinase	*Proteus mirabilis* C889	0.015	10.0
Class IV broad-spectrum chromosomal	*Klebsiella pneumoniae* E70	0.007	0.63
	Klebsiella 1082E (K1)	0.025	3.0
	Branhamella catarrhalis (Ravasio)	0.04	–
Plasmid mediated	TEM-1	0.03	0.72
	TEM-2	0.01	0.5
	SHV-1	0.01	1.6
	OXA-1	0.6	>50
	OXA-2	0.15	>50
	OXA-3	0.37	>50
	PSE-1	0.004	2.0
	PSE-2	0.06	27.0
	PSE-4	0.007	2.5
Gram-positive penicillinase	*Staphylococcus aureus* (Russell)	0.03	75

[a]Data from Ref. 6.
[b]The I_{50} values were determined using an automated assay with nitrocefin as the substrate (5).
Source: Data from Ref. 5 and C. Reading (unpublished results).

hibit enzyme activity by 50% (I_{50} value) is determined with and without a preincubation stage. The results in Table 1 were obtained using an automated inhibition assay (5) where I_{50} values were determined using nitrocefin as the substrate. Enzyme and inhibitor were preincubated for 5 min at 37°C and then residual enzyme activity measured by adding the substrate and measuring hydrolysis after a further 5-min reaction period in comparison to an uninhibited control. The I_{50} values without the preincubation stage were obtained by adding enzyme to premixed substrate and inhibitor and measuring the extent of nitrocefin hydrolysis after a 5-min reaction period in comparison to an uninhibited control reaction. The results illustrate the time-dependent nature of the inhibition where I_{50} values with preincubation are significantly better than those obtained without the extra contact time. A simple competitive inhibitor would give identical I_{50} values both with and without preincubation.

Clavulanic acid inhibits a far wider range of beta-lactamase types than earlier penicillin and cephalosporin inhibitors. Chromasomally mediated enzymes such as the Richmond-Sykes (6) class II beta-lactamases (e.g., *Proteus mirabilis*) and broad-spectrum beta-lactamases of class IV (e.g., *Klebsiella* and *Branhamella* enzymes) are readily inhibited, as shown in Table 1.

Most importantly, the activity of clavulanic acid covers the plasmid-mediated enzymes, which are largely responsible for the spread of beta-lactamase-mediated resistance in the gram-negative bacteria. The widespread TEM beta-lactamases are inhibited by low concentrations of clavulanic acid, as is SHV-1, which is common in *Klebsiella.* The oxacillin-hydrolyzing enzymes OXA-1, OXA-2, and OXA-3 are also inhibited on incubation with clavulanic acid. In the presence of substrate (no preincubation) the I_{50} values are less favorable than those obtained with TEM beta-lactamase. This is an expression of the lower affinity of the inhibitor for the OXA-type beta-lactamases. Labia et al. (7) have shown the K_i values for clavulanic acid with these enzymes to range from 10 to 30 μM, while that for TEM-1 was 0.7 μM. The PSE group of beta-lactamases is also readily inhibited by clavulanic acid, as shown in Table 1. These enzymes, however, are mainly found in *Pseudomonas* and hence have little relevance to Augmentin.

The only beta-lactamase from a gram-positive bacterium which has major clinical significance is that produced by staphylococci. This beta-lactamase is also readily inhibited on preincubation with low concentrations of clavulanic acid, although the I_{50} values are less favorable without preincubation. As with the OXA type discussed above, this reflects the lower affinity of the inhibitor for this enzyme in comparison to some other beta-lactamase types. Although improvements in the affinity of clavulanic acid for certain enzymes would provide even more efficient protection of a beta-lactam antibiotic, the antibacterial activity of Augmentin is readily demonstrable with beta-lactamase-producing staphylococci and with *Escherichia coli* producing OXA-type enzymes. Clearly the affinity of the inhibitor, even with these enzymes, is sufficient to provide adequate protection of amoxicillin in both the in vitro and in vivo situations.

Clavulanic acid has a closer resemblance to the structure of the penicillin nucleus than to that of cephalosporins. It is perhaps not surprising, therefore, that the inhibitor has high activity against penicillinases while low concentrations have little inhibitory effect against most cephalosporinases (Table 1). High concentrations of clavulanic acid do, however, progressively inactivate cephalosporinases, as has been illustrated for *Enterobacter cloacae* P99 beta-lactamase (8). High concentrations of clavulanate can occur in urine following the administration of Augmentin. Under these circumstances it is possible to envisage protection of amoxicillin from even cephalosporinase-producing bacteria causing urinary tract infections. One group of enzymes, the Ic cephalosporinases, is in fact highly sensitive to inhibition by clavulanic acid. Because, unlike most cephalosporinases, these enzymes hydrolyze cefuroxime, Mitsuhashi and Inoue (9) have called them "cefuroximases." These enzymes are also unusual in that they hydrolyze amoxicillin at rates similar to that obtained with benzylpenicillin. Enzymes of this type are produced by the clinically important anaerobe *Bacteroides fragilis*, by *Proteus vulgaris*, and by *Pseudomonas cepacia.* The I_{50} values for the beta-lactamase of *Prot. vulgaris* are given in Table 1. *Pseudomonas cepacia* beta-lactamase is also sensitive, having a K_i value of 1.72 μM (10), while strains of *Bacteroides* produced enzymes with K_i values of 0.1-0.2 μM (11). Other species of *Bacteroides* produce beta-lactamases also readily inhibited by clavulanic acid (12-14). Another unusual cephalosporinase is produced by *E. coli* JD-41; this inducible beta-lactamase, like the Ic types, is also inhibited by clavulanate (Table 1).

Beta-lactamases which can hydrolyze carbapenems like thienamycin are relatively uncommon. *Bacillus cereus* II enzyme, a zinc-containing protein, is one example; the L-1 enzyme from *Pseudomonas maltophilia* (15), also a metalloprotein, is another. These types of beta-lactamase are not readily inhibited by clavulanic acid.

Legionella pneumophila is one of the few bacteria against which clavulanic acid has reasonable antibacterial activity in vitro. In tests (16) on nine strains, the minimum inhibitory concentration (MIC) values for clavulanic acid ranged from 0.2 to 0.4 μg/ml. Studies by Fu and Neu (17) on a further strain of *Legionella* showed that the organism produced a beta-lactamase which could hydrolyze cefamandole. Cell-free preparations of this enzyme were inhibited by clavulanate. Despite the production of beta-lactamase, *Legionella* remains highly sensitive to penicillin in vitro, which makes it difficult to explain the lack of clinical efficacy of penicillins in the treatment of these infections. Poor penetration into human cells is the likely reason.

The actinomycetes also produce beta-lactamase, and studies of clincial isolates of *Nocardia asteroides* (C. Reading, unpublished results) have shown that the beta-lactamases produced are highly sensitive to inhibition by clavulanic acid. The susceptibility of penicillin-resistant isolates of *Nocardia* to Augmentin (18) confirms the biochemical data. The inhibition of beta-lactamases from *Streptomyces* and *Actinomadura* has also been reported (19,20) but has little relevance to the clinical application of Augmentin.

B. Mode of Action of Clavulanic Acid

A system for the classification of beta-lactamases was first introduced by Richmond and Sykes (6), and this has proved most useful to those working with this large and diverse group of bacterial enzymes. In this system the beta-lactamases are categorized mainly on the basis of their ability to hydrolyze various beta-lactam antibiotics and their genetic location being either chromosomally or plasmid encoded. These two criteria of course have direct relevance to the clinical importance of beta-lactamase.

Studies on the structure (21,22) and active site (23-27) of beta-lactamases have recently shown that many of these enzymes are serine peptidases and hence bear similarities to some common proteolytic enzymes where the mechanism of action involves the formation of an acyl intermediate with a specific serine residue. These more recent data have allowed some beta-lactamases to be categorized on the basis of their structure and mechanism of action into classes A, B, and C (21,22). Class A beta-lactamases such as TEM and *B. cereus* I are serine enzymes. Class C beta-lactamases are structurally different from class A ones but also employ an acyl enzyme mechanism involving serine. Examples of class C are the chromosomal beta-lactamases of *E. coli* and *Pseudomonas* (27), which are normally described as "cephalosporinases," because under V_{max} conditions they hydrolyze some cephalosporins more readily than benzylpenicillin. Class B enzymes are metalloproteins and are uncommon; *B. cereus* II was the only example until the recent description (15) of the L-1 enzyme from *Ps. maltophila*, which is also a Zn-containing protein. Clavulanic acid readily inhibits class A beta-lactamases but, as we have seen earlier, has little activity at low concentrations against class C cephalosporinases. Class B beta-lactamases are also relatively insensitive to inhibition by clavulanic acid.

Clavulanic acid has high affinity for the active site of a large number of beta-lactamases and K_i values as low as 0.1 μM have been reported. Clavulanic acid can therefore compete efficiently with the substrate for the active site of the enzyme, but this competitive inhibition is only the first stage in its interaction. This is why assessment of enzyme inactivators such as clavulanic acid based solely on K_i values understates the inhibitory activity of the compound. Clavulanic acid is in fact accepted by the enzyme as a substrate and the peptide bond of the beta-lactam ring is cleaved with the formation of an acyl intermediate. Unlike normal substrates, further spontaneous reactions occur and the oxazoli-

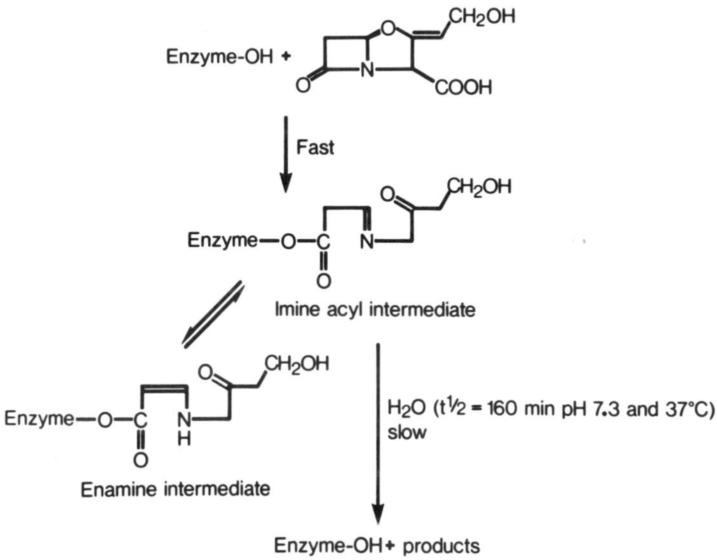

Figure 3 Possible scheme of interaction of staphylococcal beta-lactamase with clavulanic acid.

dine ring also opens, as illustrated in Figure 3. Whereas a normal substrate enzyme acyl intermediate rapidly breaks down to release a hydrolysis product, the straight-chain acyl intermediate formed in the clavulanate reaction either is relatively stable in its own right or achieves stability by further interaction with the enzyme. Such interactions are possible because the hydrolysis of the beta-lactam ring of clavulanic acid and subsequent oxazolidine ring opening unmasks reactive groups that can form stable covalent bonds at the active site. Compounds that produce this type of inhibition have been termed suicide inactivators (28) or, perhaps more scientifically, mechanism-based inactivators (29). These interactions are time dependent and hence the inhibitor can also be termed progressive.

The inhibitory mechanism of clavulanic acid therefore relies on adequate affinity for the active site and hydrolysis of its beta-lactam ring to produce a stable acyl intermediate. In some cases, however, the normal pathway of substrate hydrolysis and product release occurs at the same time as the formation of the stable enzyme-inhibitor complex. Because some inhibitor is lost by this route as hydrolysis product before the enzyme is inactivated, the stoichiometry of this reaction can be greater than unity. With TEM-2 beta-lactamase, for instance, 115 molecules of clavulanate are required in order to inactivate irreversibly 1 molecule of enzyme. The turnover number for some inactivators can be quite high, sulbactam, for instance, has a value of about 7000 with TEM-2 (30) and a significant loss of inhibitor occurs.

The interaction of clavulanic acid with various beta-lactamases has been studied in some detail. In the case of staphylococcal beta-lactamase (31,32) the pathway is linear (Fig. 3) and there is no detectable turnover, one molecule of inhibitor reacting with and inhibiting one molecule of enzyme. Because clavulanic acid has only moderate affinity for the staphylococcal enzyme, the rate of inactivation is concentration dependent over the concentration range that would be present under physiological conditions. The initial acyl intermediate after cleavage of the oxazolidine ring is the imine as illustrated in Figure 3. It has been suggested, however, that the imine would be in equilibrium with the enamine and that the enamine acyl intermediate would be sufficiently stable to account for the inactivation of the enzyme (31). Other interactions, however, are also possible (32) and could also account for the stability of the enzyme–clavulanate complex. The intermediate in the staphylococcal interaction is not completely stable and slowly decays ($t_{½}$ = 160 min at 37°C, pH 7.3) to release free enzyme and a product. The rate of reactivation increases at acid pH. The cephalosporinase produced by *Ent. cloacae* P99 reacts with clavulanic acid in a similar fashion, but far higher concentrations are required to achieve reasonable rates of inactivation. The moderately stable complex formed in this reaction has a half-life of 180 min at pH 7.3 and 37°C, which is also shortened at lower pH values.

The second type of mechanism involves a divergent pathway in which a number of different interactions between enzyme and inhibitor occur simultaneously. Studies with the plasmid-mediated TEM-2 beta-lactamase first revealed the existence of this type of complex interaction (33-35). Clavulanic acid has high affinity for TEM-2 (K_i = 0.7 μM), and this means that the initial interaction between enzyme and inhibitor proceeds at maximum velocity at concentrations likely to be present under physiological conditions. When the time course for inhibition of TEM-2 was followed at different molar ratios of inhibitor to enzyme (c/e), the results in Figure 4 were obtained. This and other experiments revealed that in order to obtain and maintain complete loss of activity, 115 molecules of clavulanic acid were required for every 1 molecule of beta-lactamase. At c/e ratios less than this, incomplete inhibition was obtained and, furthermore, there was a quite rapid return of activity ($t_{½}$ = 4 min). Not all the enzyme activity returned, and it appeared that some of the enzyme had been inhibited irreversibly, the extent of this inactivation being dependent on the c/e ratio. Further investigation led to a greater understanding of these events and allowed the interaction sequence in Figure 5 to be constructed.

It is proposed that the initial product of the interaction is the ring-opened acyl intermediate already described for the staphylococcal reaction. With TEM-2, however, three further and simultaneous reactions occur at this stage. The acyl enzyme intermediate breaks down to release free enzyme and products

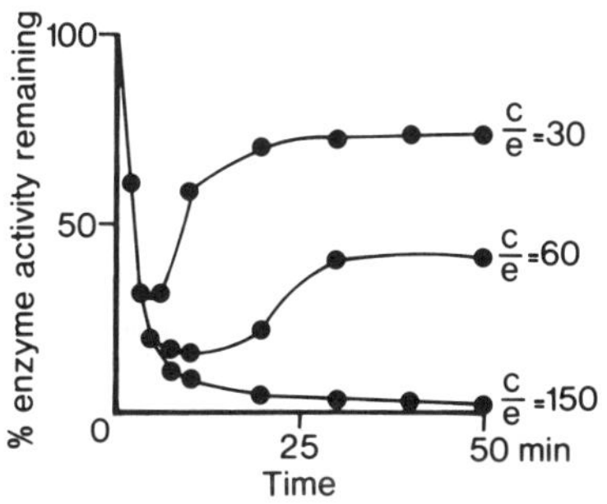

Figure 4 Time course of the inhibition of TEM-2 beta-lactamase by clavulanic acid. Clavulanate (c) and enzyme (e) were reacted at various ratios (c/e) and the enzyme activity followed with time; c = 2.0 mM and e varied between 13 and 66 μM. (Data from Ref. 33.)

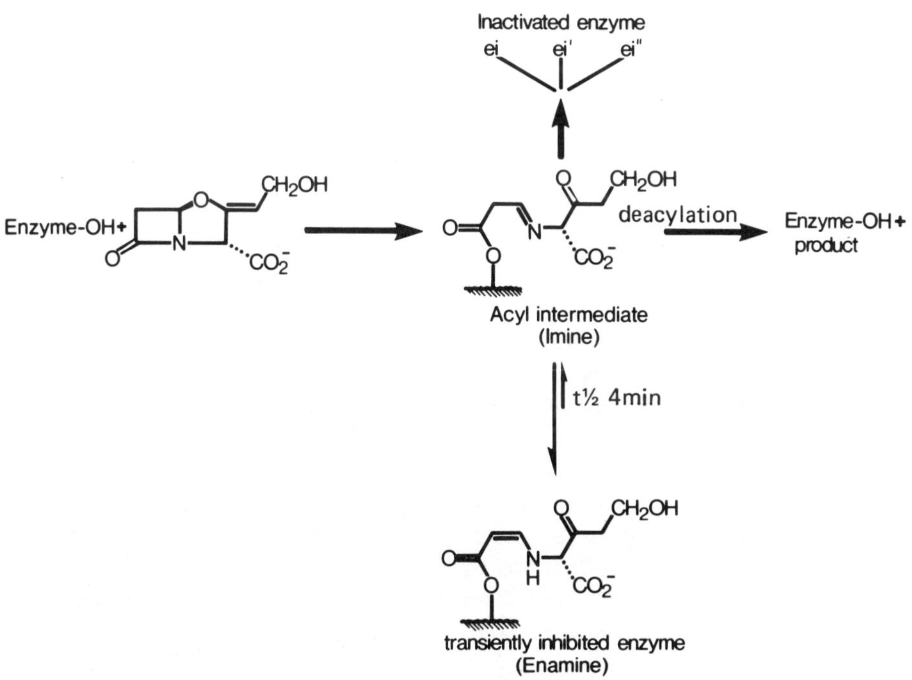

Figure 5 Possible scheme of interaction of TEM-2 beta-lactamase with clavulanic acid.

as would occur with a normal substrate, and this loss accounts for the majority of the excess clavulanate required to obtain complete inactivation. At the same time the acyl intermediate is converted into two other complexes. It has been suggested (30) that one of these, the transiently stable complex, arises by tautomerization of the initial imine structure to the more stable enamine as shown in Figure 5. The second type of complex results from further covalent interaction between the ring-opened clavulanate molecule and the enzyme to form irreversibly inactivated enzyme. This process is even more complex in that at least three types of irreversibly inactivated enzyme species have been detected (34). It has been suggested (30) that at least one of these irreversible species may result from fragmentation of the inhibitor and transimination involving the original beta-lactam nitrogen and an enzymic grouping. These initial events occur rapidly and the enzyme is soon captured as either the transient complex or the irreversible type complex in the proportions of 3:1, respectively. The transiently stable enamine slowly releases free enzyme and product by virtue of its being in equilibrium with the initial imine intermediate, which in turn feeds the product release pathway. The enzyme released by this route reacts with fresh clavulanic acid and the whole cycle is then repeated. With each cycle, more of the enzyme is irreversibly inactivated until all the enzyme activity has been permanently removed. Apart from the initial rapid partitioning between transient and irreversible complexes, the rate of inactivation is limited by the rate of tautomerization of the enamine to imine and subsequent release of free enzyme ($t_{1/2}$ = 4 min). This is why the time course for inactivation (as opposed to inhibition) is biphasic as illustrated in Figure 6 and why the second phase of inactivation is relatively slow. The complex mechanism of interaction with enzymes such as TEM can be confusing when considering the overall ability of clavulanic acid to protect a beta-lactam antibiotic such as amoxicillin from destruction. In this context it is worth remembering that as long as the enzyme is interacting with the inhibitor, in whatever way, it is unable to react with substrate. The high affinity of clavulanic acid for TEM beta-lactamase relative to that of amoxicillin ensures that beta-lactamase inhibition can occur even in the presence of amoxicillin. The degree of protection of amoxicillin depends, of course, on the relative concentrations of substrate and inhibitor and on the enzyme concentration.

The irreversible inactivation of beta-lactamase by clavulanic acid is not limited to the TEM-type enzymes (8). In Figure 6 the inactivation of a chromosomally mediated beta-lactamase from *Klebsiella aerogenes* (*pneumoniae*) is also illustrated. In this case the inactivation is more rapid than that obtained with TEM-2 beta-lactamase and is mainly due to the fact that the proportions of irreversible complex and transiently stable complex are equal, whereas with TEM-2 beta-lactamase the proportions were 3:1 in favor of the transient complex. With the penicillinase from *Prot. mirabilis* C889, the rate of irreversible inactivation is relatively slow. The inhibition of this enzyme by clavulanic acid depends mainly

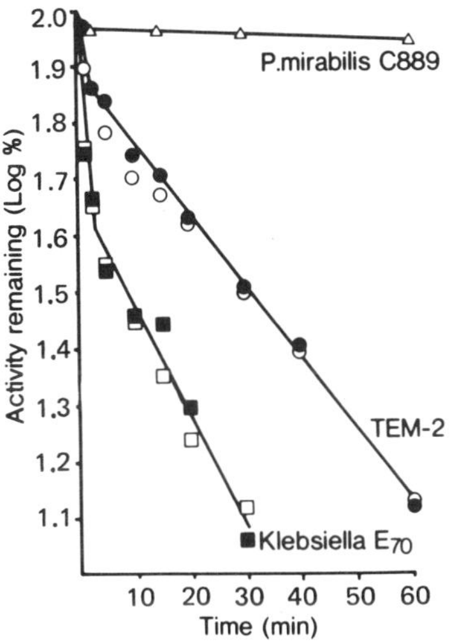

Figure 6 Time course for the irreversible inactivation of some beta-lactamases from gram-negative bacteria. The amount of irreversible inhibition was measured relative to an uninhibited enzyme control as the proportion of enzyme activity which did not return after any unstable complexes were allowed to decay. All reactions of enzyme and clavulanate were carried out at 37°C and pH 7.3. ●, 40 μM of clavulanic acid; ○, 100 μM of clavulanic acid; □, 3 μM of clavulanic acid; ■, 6 μM of clavulanic acid; △, 21 μM of clavulanic acid. (Data from Ref. 8.)

on the formation of a moderately stable complex of a type already seen in the reaction with staphylococcal beta-lactamase. Studies by Frère et al. (19) have also shown a complex interaction of clavulanate with *Streptomyces albus* and *Actinomadura* R39 beta-lactamases. *Streptomyces albus* produced significant turnover of the inhibitor before inactivation was complete (turnover number 21,600) while the R39 enzyme had a value of 200. The K_i values were also unimpressive, 29 and 97 μM, respectively, and a transiently stable complex was detected in the interaction with the R39 beta-lactamase.

Studies on the inhibition of the "cefuroximase" from *Prot. vulgaris* and the cephalosporinase of *Morganella morganii* by Sawai and Tsukamoto (36) have been reported. The cephalosporinase of *M. morganii* was inhibited in a fashion similar to that reported for the *Ent. cloacae* P99 enzyme (8), in that high concentrations were required to achieve reasonable rates of inactivation. These workers, however, did not detect the recovery of enzyme activity and concluded that the inhibition was irreversible while the P99 β-lactamase slowly recovers activity after the removal of excess inhibitor. The *Prot. vulgaris* enzyme, which, unlike typical cephalosporinases, hydrolyzes amoxicillin and cefuroxime, displayed inhibition kinetics very similar to those seen with TEM-2, with the data suggesting the presence of both transiently stable and irreversible complexes. The K_i of clavulanic acid was reported as 0.35 μM, which is of an order similar to that reported for *Bacteroides* beta-lactamases as well as the sensitive TEM-type enzymes.

Durkin and Viswantha (37) have proposed a complex mechanism for the inhibition of *B. cereus* I beta-lactamase and have invoked conformational changes to explain their results. It is possible, however, that mechanisms similar to those proposed for TEM-2 could apply to this enzyme, but the role of conformational changes during interaction of beta-lactamases with both substrates and inhibitors cannot be ignored.

C. Comparison of Clavulanic Acid with Other Beta-Lactamase Inhibitors

Since the discovery of clavulanic acid a number of inhibitors have been reported which progressively inhibit various beta-lactamases by similar mechanisms. Sulbactam (38)–penicillanic acid sulfone, CP-45,899–is one such compound at present under investigation. It has a spectrum of beta-lactamase inhibitory activity close to that of clavulanic acid but also does incorporate some moderate activity against the class I beta-lactamases (Table 2). Greenwood and Eley (39) have demonstrated that sulbactam synergized the activity of ampicillin against strains of *Enterobacter* and *Serratia* which produced this type of beta-lactamase. Sulbactam in general is less active than clavulanate as a beta-lactamase inhibitor, particularly against chromosomal *Klebsiella* enzymes and plasmid-mediated beta-lactamases (Table 2). With TEM-2 beta-lactamase, for instance, although the K_i value for sulbactam is similar to that of clavulanate, the rate of inactivation is very slow and a large turnover of the compound also occurs. This deficiency is compounded in vivo by poorer penetration into *E. coli* (see Table 8) and the antibacterial activity of sulbactam-penicillin formulations against *E. coli* and *Klebsiella* producing TEM-type enzymes is relatively poor (39,40). The compound, however, is reported to be more stable than clavulanate in both aqueous solution and body fluids (38), although the clinical importance of this is not clear.

The 6β-halopenicillanic acids are further examples of beta-lactamase inhibitors (Table 2), with spectra and potency similar to those of clavulanic acid when tested against cell-free enzyme preparations. Like sulbactam, however, they do have some activity against class I beta-lactamases, yet this is not evident in antibacterial synergy tests (41). A new inhibitor, 6-acetylmethylene penicillanic acid (Ro 151903), has been described recently (42). It has similar activity to sulbactam against the class I beta-lactamases and was reported to be significantly more active than clavulanic acid against plasmid-mediated beta-lactamases, as well as class IV and staphylococcal beta-lactamases when preincubated

Table 2 Beta-Lactamase Inhibitory Activity of Sulbactam, 6-β-Halopenicillanic Acids, and 6-Acetylmethylene Penicillanic Acid in Comparison to Clavulanic Acid

	I_{50} (μg/ml)[a] with (+) and without (-) preincubation									
	Sulbactam		6-β-Bromo-penicillanic acid		6-β-Iodo-penicillanic acid		6-Acetyl-methylene penicillanic acid		Clavulanic acid	
Beta-lactamase	+	-	+	-	+	-	+	-	+	-
Enterobacter cloacae P99	5.8	>50	1.5	>50	5.5	>50	10	>50	110.0	>4000
Pseudomonas aeruginosa A	–	–	–	–	–	–	9	>50	>400	>400
Proteus mirabilis C889	–	–	–	–	–	–	0.007	15.0	0.015	10.0
Klebsiella E70	5.5	20	0.07	12.5	0.014	12.0	0.015	5.2	0.007	0.63
TEM-1	1.4	2.0	0.15	8.0	0.06	5.5	0.005	2.5	0.06	0.7
Staphylococcus aureus (Russell)	1.6	>50	1.5	50	0.7	>50	0.15	>50	0.03	75.0

[a]Concentration required to give 50% protection of a 250-μg/ml nitrocefin substrate after a 5-min reaction time (5).
Source: C. Reading, unpublished results.

Table 3 Hydrolysis of Amoxicillin by Various Types of Beta-Lactamase and Their Susceptibility to Inhibition by Clavulanic Acid

Type of beta-lactamase	Example	Rate of amoxicillin hydrolysis (penicillin G = 100)	Inhibition by low concentration of clavulanic acid
Chromosomal cephalosporinase	*Enterobacter cloacae* P99	5	-
	Pseudomonas aeruginosa A	10	-
	Escherichia coli JT410	2	-
	Bacteroides fragilis	>100	+
Chromosomal penicillinase	*Proteus mirabilis* C889	142	+
Chromosomal broad-spectrum beta-lactamase	*Klebsiella pneumoniae* E70	127	+
	Branhamells catarrhalis 1908	120	+
Plasmid-mediated beta-lactamase	TEM-1 and TEM-2	86	+
	SHV-1	126	+
	OXA type, e.g., OXA-2	162	+
	PSE type, e.g., PSE-4 (Dalgleish)	92	+
Gram-positive penicillinase	*Staphylococcus aureus* (Russell)	168	+

Source: Data from Ref. 60.

with cell-free enzyme preparations. This activity, however, is less marked in the presence of substrate (Table 2). The in vivo and in vitro antibacterial results for this compound, in combination with beta-lactam antibiotics (43), appear disappointing if one compares them with the reported (42) inhibitory activity of the compound against cell-free beta-lactamases.

At present, Augmentin is the only marketed product based on the concept of beta-lactamase inhibition. Sulbactam in its oral prodrug form, sultamicillin, is under investigation. This comprises sulbactam linked by a covalent ester bond

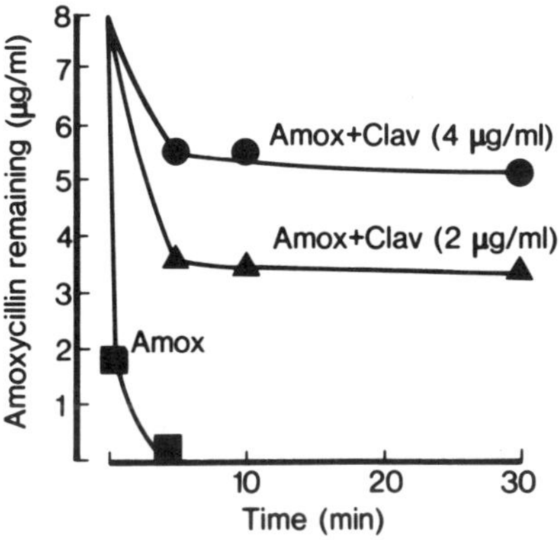

Figure 7 Effect of staphylococcal beta-lactamase on amoxicillin alone and in the presence of clavulanic acid. *Staphylococcus aureus* Russell was grown in the presence of 1 μg/ml methicillin to induce beta-lactamase. The enzyme concentration in the reaction was equivalent to that released by ultrasonication of approximately 2 x 10^8 cells/ml. (Data from Ref. 44.)

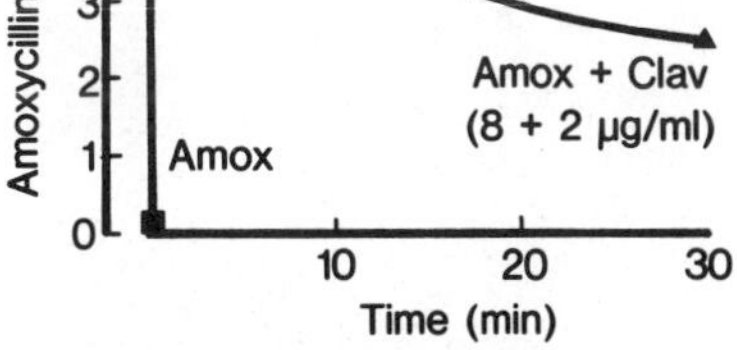

Figure 8 Effect of TEM-1 beta-lactamase on amoxicillin alone and in the presence of clavulanic acid. The TEM-1 beta-lactamase preparation was a cell-free extract of *E. coli* JT4. The enzyme concentration in the reaction was equivalent to that released by ultrasonication of approximately 2 x 10^8 cells/ml. (Data from Ref. 44.)

Table 4 Effect of Clavulanic Acid on the Stability of Amoxicillin to Cell-Free Preparations of Plasmid-Mediated Beta-Lactamases

Strain of *E. coli* producing beta-lactamase	Beta-lactamase type	Enzyme concentration in reaction mixture (units)[a]	Percent amoxicillin (8 μg/ml) remaining after		Percent amoxicillin remaining after 30 min: amoxicillin + clavulanic acid (μg/ml)		
			1 min	30 min	8 + 4	16 + 4	8 + 2
JT-4 (R+)	TEM-1	0.5	<2.5	<2.5	54	53	28
K12 (RP1)	TEM-2	0.33	<2.5	<2.5	48	43	23
K12 J53/2 (pR1010)	SHV-1	2.5	<2.5	<2.5	79	75	62
K12 (RGN 238)	OXA-1[b]	1.6	7	<2.5	44	72	43
K12 (R1818)	OXA-2	0.8	66	<2.5	68	70	45
K12 (R57b)	OXA-3	1.6	71	<2.5	56	57	38
K12 E5/2 (RPL11)	PSE-1	1.25	<2.5	<2.5	48	54	24
K12 E5/2 (R151)	PSE-2	0.3	80	<2.5	79	76	69
K12 E5/2 (Rms149)	PSE-3	2.5	70	<2.5	85	90	85
K12 E5/2 (pMG19)	PSE-4	1.25	<2.5	<2.5	48	52	28

[a]One unit represents the enzyme concentration obtained in solution after ultrasonication of approximately 2 x 10^8 cells/ml and the removal of cell debris.
[b]Enzyme and clavulanic acid preincubated (2 min) before addition of amoxicillin.
Source: Data from Ref. 44.

Table 5 Effect of Clavulanic Acid on the Stability of Amoxicillin to Cell-Free Preparations of Chromosomal Beta-Lactamases and Staphylococcal Beta-Lactamase

Source of beta-lactamase	Enzyme concentration in reaction mixture (units)[a]	Percent amoxicillin (8 μg/ml) remaining after		Percent amoxicillin remaining after 30 min: amoxicillin + clavulanic acid (μg/ml)		
		1 min	30 min	8 + 4	16 + 4	8 + 2
Prot. mirabilis C889	2	<2.5	<2.5	44	40	11
K. pneumoniae ATCC 29665	5	<2.5	<2.5	67	64	49
K. pneumoniae E70	5	19	<2.5	85	85	82
E. coli JT410	0.15	100	96	96	97	96
Ent. cloacae P99	0.01	100	100	97	97	96
Staph. aureus (Russell)	1	8	<2.5	64	68	42

[a]One unit represents the enzyme concentration obtained after ultrasonication of approximately 2 x 10^8 cells/ml.
Source: Data from Ref. 44.

to ampicillin, which on hydrolysis in the blood releases the separate compounds, yielding high blood levels of both components.

D. Beta-Lactamase Stability of Augmentin

The measurement of beta-lactamase inhibitory activity by determining I_{50} values using a chromogenic substrate such as nitrocefin provides useful preliminary data on the spectrum of inhibitory activity. Such methods are also useful for comparing various inhibitors (5). The way in which a beta-lactam antibiotic reacts with beta-lactamase can, however, have a marked effect on the ability of an inhibitor to protect it from hydrolysis. For this reason the stability of a particular formulation must be considered separately from the overall beta-lactamase inhibitory activity of the synergist. The results in Table 3 show that amoxicillin alone has little stability to the majority of beta-lactamase types being hydrolyzed at rates similar to or even greater than those obtained with benzyl-

Table 6 Characteristics of the Interactions Between Clavulanic Acid and Beta-Lactamases

Beta-lactamases	Clavulanic acid affinity constant, K_i (μM)	Clavulanic acid inhibition value to inhibit 50% enzyme activity, I_{50} (μg/ml)	Protection coefficient[a]
Penicillinases			
TEM-1	0.8	0.08	380.0
TEM-2	0.7	0.06	335.0
PIT-2 (SHV-1)	0.6	0.015	790.0
11-03 } (class IV	0.33	0.01	790.0
GN-422 } *Klebsiella*)	0.39	0.07	505.0
OXA-1	31	0.7	1.8
OXA-2	10.3	0.16	5.0
OXA-3	46.0	0.67	2.5
CARB-1 (PSE-4)	0.95	0.06	155.0
CARB-2 (PSE-1)	0.65	0.07	360.0
CARB-3	1.3	0.07	320.0
Cephalosporinases			
E. coli	190.0	95.0	1.0
Prot. vulgaris	0.35	0.06	255.0

[a]Amount of amoxicillin hydrolyzed in a given time relative to the hydrolysis of amoxicillin in the presence of clavulanic acid (2:1).
Source: Data from Ref. 45.

penicillin. Amoxicillin, however, is relatively stable to one group of beta-lactamases, namely, the chromosomally mediated cephalosporinases. The lack of antibacterial activity of amoxicillin against organisms producing this type of enzyme, such as *Pseudomonas aeruginosa,* cannot, therefore, be attributed solely to beta-lactamase.

The ability of low concentrations of clavulanic acid to inhibit the various beta-lactamase types has already been discussed and is also indicated in Table 3. It can be seen that the inhibitor is effective against all the enzymes which readily hydrolyze amoxicillin. Clavulanic acid lacks significant activity only against the cephalosporinases of types Ia, Ib, and Id, the enzymes to which amoxicillin has some intrinsic stability. It can be seen, therefore, that amoxicillin and clavulanic acid are ideal partners for a synergistic formulation. This compatibility also extends to oral absorption and, as will be seen later, both components show similar pharmacokinetic properties.

Studies on the ability of clavulanate to protect amoxicillin from a range of clinically important beta-lactamases (44) were carried out by following the time course of amoxicillin destruction in the absence and presence of the inhibitor using cell-free beta-lactamase preparations. Low concentrations of antibiotic were used in these studies in order to reproduce conditions closer to those likely to be encountered in vivo. Results for staphylococcal beta-lactamase (Fig. 7) show an initial loss of amoxicillin which was rapidly arrested. The extent of this loss was dependent on the inhibitor concentration. These data were consistent with the time-dependent conversion of the staphylococcal enzymes to an inactive complex. For TEM-1 beta-lactamase (Fig. 8), although clavulanic acid immediately reduces amoxicillin hydrolysis, the time taken to completely stop destruction is somewhat longer and again reflects inactivation rates. Competitive inhibition may be improved by increasing the inhibitor concentration, which results in a decrease in amoxicillin loss during the early part of the reaction. Experiments of the type shown in Figures 7 and 8 were carried out for a range of beta-lactamase types and the results are summarized in Tables 4 and 5. These data illustrate the ability of clavulanic acid to protect amoxicillin from beta-lactamases which readily hydrolyze the antibiotic. Labia and Peduzzi (45) have also considered the stability of amoxicillin in the presence of clavulanic acid and have expressed this in terms of a protection coefficient as shown in Table 6. This value was based on the amount of clavulanate required to inhibit 1 unit of enzyme activity and the known kinetic parameters of the interaction of amoxicillin with the various enzymes. The protection coefficient can be considered as the ratio of the amount of amoxicillin hydrolyzed in a set time (15 min) to the corresponding amount of amoxicillin in Augmentin (4:1) hydrolyzed in the same period. The results show good protection for nearly all the plasmid-mediated enzymes tested, while the OXA types were, as mentioned earlier, less readily inhibited. Amoxicillin in the presence of clavulanic acid was relatively stable to the Ic cephalosporinase of *Prot. vulgaris,* but clavulanate did not affect the stability of amoxicillin to the class I beta-lactamase of *E. coli.*

Extrapolation of biochemical inhibition data to antibacterial tests has generally correlated quite well, in that amoxicillin-resistant strains, producing a beta-lactamase which is inhibited by clavulanic acid, are susceptible to Augmentin (46).

III. FURTHER BIOCHEMICAL ASPECTS

A. Induction of Beta-Lactamase by Clavulanic Acid

Inducible beta-lactamases are common in gram-negative bacteria producing chromosomal cephalosporinases, although these class I enzymes can also be constitutive. The penicillinase produced by staphylococci is another example of a clinically important inducible beta-lactamase. It is well known that the synthesis of inducible enzymes from both gram-positive and gram-negative bacteria is derepressed by beta-lactam antibiotics. The inducing power of a beta-lactam is generally higher if it is stable to hydrolysis by the beta-lactamases produced. Hence methicillin is a highly effective inducer of staphylococcal beta-lactamase while 6-APA is extremely effective in inducing the production of the Sabath and Abraham enzyme of *Ps. aeruginosa.* Substrates such as benzylpenicillin are poor inducers when compared to equimolar concentrations of beta-lactamase-stable beta-lactams.

Clavulanic acid is highly stable to beta-lactamases, and this includes enzymes such as the class I beta-lactamases against which the compound has little inhibitory effect (1). As discussed earlier, the mechanism of action of clavulanic acid with some enzymes does involve the hydrolysis of the inhibitor by normal substratelike interactions; the amount of inhibitor which is degraded, however, is insignificant when taken in the normal context of stability to beta-lactamase. It is not surprising, therefore, that clavulanic acid, as a highly beta-lactamase-stable beta-lactam, has the ability to induce beta-lactamase. Clavulanate induces the production of class I enzymes in *Ent. cloacae* GN 5797 (47) and in a strain of *Proteus rettgeri* (48). It has been suggested (49) that induction of class I beta-lactamases by clavulanic acid is responsible for the lack of susceptibility of some strains of *Enterobacter* to Augmentin. This however, seems unlikely to be the case, as will be discussed later in the section covering the antibacterial activity of Augmentin against these organisms.

Where inducible beta-lactamases are susceptible to inhibition by clavulanic acid, it is of course difficult to measure induction by the inhibitor. For inducible enzymes such as those produced by *Prot. vulgaris* (46) and staphylococci (C. Reading, unpublished results) clavulanic acid appears to have little or no effect on enzyme production, but of course if enzyme synthesis were increased, the beta-lactamase would be immediately inhibited by the inducer. It is difficult, therefore, to comment on the ability of clavulanate to induce enzymes of this type.

B. Interaction of Clavulanic Acid and Amoxicillin with Penicillin-Binding Proteins and Penicillin-Sensitive Enzymes

The broad-spectrum antibacterial activity of amoxicillin is well documented and its high intrinsic activity is reflected in the I_{50} values obtained in conventional penicillin-binding protein (PBP) assays in which [^{14}C] benzylpenicillin is used to reveal residual PBPs after interaction of membrane preparations with the test compound. The results in Table 7 were reported by Curtis et al. (50) for the PBPs of *E. coli* DCO and illustrate the high affinity of amoxicillin for several of the essential PBPs.

Table 7 Interaction of Amoxicillin and Clavulanic Acid with Penicillin-Binding Proteins

Penicillin-binding protein	I_{50} (μg/ml) competition against [^{14}C] benzylpenicillin							Reference
	1A	1B	2	3	4	5	6	
E. coli								
Amoxicillin	0.7	2.2	0.9	4.1	2.5	110	9	50
Clavulanic acid	52[a]		4.1	310	11	21	15	52
	I_{50} (μg/ml) competition against [^{125}I] penicillin X							
	1A	1B	2	3	4	5/6		
E. coli								
Clavulanic acid	21	100	3.2	>100	15	20		53
Prot. mirabilis								
Clavulanic acid	14	>300	>300	–	>300	14		53
Acinetobacter calcoaceticus								
Clavulanic acid	51	–	26.5	19	–	–		53
Staph. aureus								
Clavulanic acid	2.1	–	0.64	0.64	2.1	–		53

[a]For PBP 1A and 1B (unseparated).

Clavulanic acid has a low, relatively uniform level of antibacterial activity against most bacteria but does show greater activity against *Neisseria gonorrhoeae*, staphylococci (51), and *Legionella* spp. (16). Studies on the binding of clavulanic acid to the PBPs of *E. coli* using competition with [^{14}C] benzylpenicillin have been reported by Spratt et al. (52). Masson et al. (53) used [^{125}I] penicillin X in their studies on the binding of clavulanic acid to the PBPs of *E. coli* and a number of other bacteria. Similar results were obtained with both methods (Table 7) and showed little binding to the PBPs of *E. coli.* Clavulanic acid had its highest affinity for PBP-2, while PBP-3 was the least readily inhibited enzyme. Spratt et al. described the morphological effects of clavulanic acid (30 μg/ml) on *E. coli* as yielding slightly elongated, swollen, bulging, and lemon-shaped cells. At 50 μg/ml increased amounts of lysis occurred, with the release of spheroplasts. Simple round cell forms that are obtained with mecillinam were less evident with clavulanic acid, although Spratt and co-workers concluded that disruption of cell shape was due to the inhibition of PBP-2.

The mecillinam-like interaction of clavulanic acid with PBP-2 combined with evidence that clavulanate could synergize the action of beta-lactams even against bacteria not producing beta-lactamase led Greenwood et al. (54) to suggest that clavulanic acid could act in several ways. Clearly its main role is to protect the antibiotic from destruction by beta-lactamase, but it seems quite possible that with certain gram-negative bacteria the mecillinam-like properties of clavulanic acid could make a contribution to the overall synergistic effect (54). Masson et al. (53), on the basis of their studies with clavulanic acid and PBPs, have also suggested this possibility.

Studies (53) on the binding of clavulanic acid to the PBPs of *Prot. mirabilis* and *Acinetobacter calcoaceticus* produced a different pattern to that seen for *E. coli*, but the I_{50} values remained unimpressive (Table 7). In the case of *Staphylococcus aureus* improved I_{50} values were obtained (53). The values are correlated with the greater sensitivity of this organism to the antibacterial effects of clavulanate. With another gram-positive organism, *Bacillus subtilis,* Horikawa and Ogawara (55) have reported that clavulanic acid, like nocardicin, has little affinity for the five main PBPs in contrast to the marked inhibition obtained with ampicillin and methicillin, implying high affinity for these drugs. It is of interest that these workers demonstrated an increase in the binding of [^{14}C]-benzylpenicillin in the presence of clavulanate, although the significance of this observation is not clear.

Studies on the inhibition of penicillin-sensitive enzymes by clavulanic acid have also been reported. Oka et al. (56) have demonstrated that the peptidoglycan transpeptidase of *E. coli* which corresponds to PBP-1b was not readily inhibited but the transpeptidase enzyme from *Bacillus megatherium* appeared to be highly sensitive to inhibition by the compound. Brown and Perkins (57) also showed significant inhibition of peptidoglycan biosynthesis by clavulanic acid in

N. gonorrhoeae which correlates with the relatively good MIC values obtained with this organism. With a strain of *Neisseria* producing TEM-1 beta-lactamase it was shown that clavulanic acid protected benzylpenicillin from degradation, in that peptidoglycan biosynthesis was inhibited by benzylpenicillin-clavulanate, but benzylpenicillin alone had no effect. The clavulanic acid concentration present with benzylpenicillin was too low for clavulanic acid itself to have any direct effect on cell wall biosynthesis.

C. Permeability

Beta-lactam antibiotics inhibit enzymes involved in peptidoglycan biosynthesis, which in gram-negative cells are located on the inner cytoplasmic membrane. The ability of beta-lactams to permeate the outer membrane and reach these target sites is obviously crucial to their success. The weak activity of more hydrophobic beta-lactams such as benzylpenicillin and cloxacillin against gram-negative bacteria is considered to be due to their inability to readily pass through the porins, water-filled channels which cross the outer membrane (58) into the periplasmic space. Hydrophilic beta-lactams such as amoxicillin can, however, diffuse via the porins and achieve inhibitory concentrations in the periplasm. In beta-lactamase-producing strains the periplasmic concentration of antibiotic is markedly reduced by the action of the enzyme (59,60). Reduction in sensitivity to beta-lactams, due to the presence of periplasmic beta-lactamase, is greatly assisted by the relatively slow rates (58) at which some of these antibiotics cross the outer membrane of some gram-negative bacteria, and it is a combination of these two effects which often serves as a mechanism of resistance. In order that an efficient beta-lactamase inhibitor also be a good synergist, it must be able to penetrate the outer membrane and protect the antibiotic from periplasmic beta-lactamase. Studies on the penetration of a variety of inhibitors into *E. coli* have been reported (61). Permeability was assessed by determining I_{50} values with both cell-free and whole-cell beta-lactamase. From the ratio of these values, a permeability index could be derived and a value of 1.0 indicates that the outer membrane did not limit the entry of the inhibitor. The results obtained by this method are shown in Table 8. Of the inhibitors tested, clavulanic acid was the most permeable. Sulbactam and the β-halopenicillanic acids were clearly less effective in inhibiting whole-cell beta-lactamase. The olivanic acids were also very inefficient and the hydrophobic penicillin BRL 1437 (2-isopropoxy-1-napthyl penicillin) was highly impermeable. This compound, despite high activity against cell-free TEM-1, only inhibited the periplasmic enzyme when the external concentration was raised by a factor of 30,000.

The ability of clavulanic acid to penetrate the outer membrane of gram-negative bacteria is an extremely important property and it is thus distinguished from other beta-lactamase inhibitors which often fail when tested as synergists against

Table 8 Penetration of Beta-Lactamase Inhibitors into *E. coli* JT4 (TEM-1)

Inhibitor	I_{50} (μg/ml)[a]		
	Cell-free beta-lactamase	Whole-cell beta-lactamase	Permeability index (ratio of I_{50} values)
Potassium clavulanate 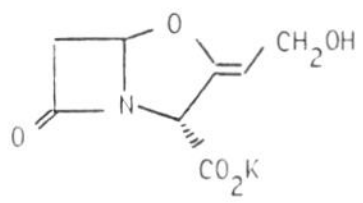	0.056	0.69	12.3
Sulbactam 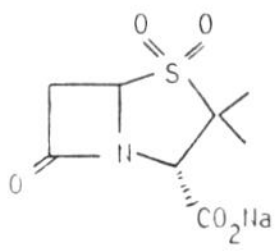	0.3	23.0	77.0
β-Bromopenicillanate 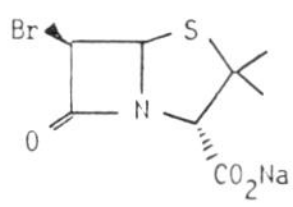	0.45	34	76.0
MM 13902 (olivanic acid) 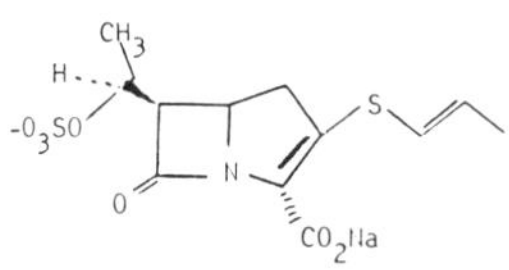	0.015	7.0	467.0
BRL 1437 (penicillin) 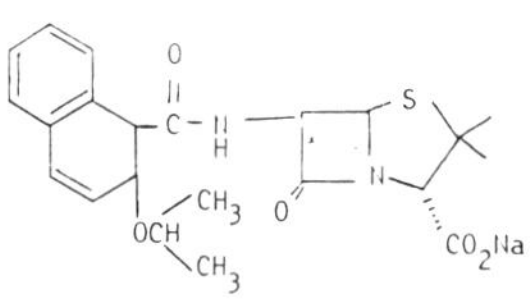	0.0032	110.0	34,375.0

[a]The I_{50} values were determined using cephaloridine as the substrate. For whole-cell beta-lactamase studies the substrate concentration was 1000 μg/ml in the external medium. The periplasmic concentration of cephaloridine under these conditions was calculated and it was this calculated internal concentration which was used in the cell-free beta-lactamase studies. This procedure ensured that the substrate concentration was the same in both whole-cell and cell-free systems. Inhibition of cephaloridine hydrolysis was monitored spectrophotometrically at 290 nm. Substrate and inhibitor were added simultaneously to the enzyme preparations (no preincubation).

Source: Data from Ref. 61.

growing bacterial cells. The combination of clavulanic acid with amoxicillin ensures protection of the antibiotic in the periplasm of a large number of clinical bacteria, thus allowing concentrations of amoxicillin to rise to a level sufficient to inhibit growth and induce lysis.

IV. ASSAY OF AUGMENTIN

As Augmentin is comprised of amoxicillin and clavulanic acid, assay systems must be considered carefully, especially in terms of the effect one component may have on the determination of the other. At present there is no single method which enables the determination of low concentrations of both components in one test. The assay of the individual components will therefore be considered and only methods suitable for the assay of human body fluids will be included in this section. It is recommended (62) that if samples cannot be assayed at the time of collection, they should be stored under the conditions summarized in Table 9.

A. Microbiological Assays

1. Amoxicillin

Agar plate assays using *Sarcina lutea* NCTC 8340 provide a sensitive method for the assay of amoxicillin without interference from clavulanic acid. Inocula are prepared in nutrient broth at 30°C for 48 hr and may be stored for up to 3 months at 4°C. An inoculum of 0.6 ml/100 ml of Antibiotic Medium No. 2 agar (Difco) is used to prepare assay plates. Standards from 0.016 to 1.0 μg/ml are prepared in pooled serum or plasma for the assay of samples in this type of fluid or in Sorensen's 0.1 M citrate buffer, pH 6.5, for other samples. Samples are diluted if necessary in pooled serum or buffer, whichever is appropriate to fall within the concentrations of the standard line. Plates are then incubated at 30°C overnight.

2. Clavulanic Acid

Klebsiella pneumoniae A (NCTC 11228) is grown overnight in tryptone soy broth at 37°C for 18 hr and should be used on the day of preparation. Plates are prepared using nutrient agar (Lab m Ltd.) with a 3% inoculum plus 0.25% addition of a 24-mg/ml solution of benzylpenicillin in sterile water to give a final concentration of 60 μg/ml in the agar. When the plate is incubated, the beta-lactamase produced by the *Klebsiella* destroys the added benzylpenicillin and a normal lawn of growth is produced. When samples of clavulanic acid are applied to the plate, the beta-lactamase is inhibited and the benzylpenicillin exerts its antibacterial effect, producing a zone of inhibition. With this assay the presence of amoxicillin in samples has no effect up to a ratio of 100:1 amoxicillin–

Table 9 Summary of Storage Conditions for Body Fluids Containing Augmentin

Biological fluid	Storage temperature (°C)	Time limit (days)	Comments
Serum	-40 to -70	14	Buffering with CO_2 improved stability at -20 and +4°C
	-20	3	
	+4	2	
Urine	-40 to -70	14	Dilute urine x 10 in pH 6.5 citrate buffer; do not store at -20°C
	+4	5	
Pleural fluid	-40 to -70	14	
	-20	2	
Cerebrospinal fluid	-40 to -70	14	
	-20	2	
Sputum	-40 to -70	14	
	-20	2	
Bile/pus	-40 to -70	14	
	-20	2	

Source: Data from Ref. 62.

clavulanate. Clavulanate standards in serum or buffer are prepared in a fashion similar to that described for amoxicillin to give a range of 0.078-5.0 μg/ml. Samples are diluted if necessary in pooled serum or buffer to fall within this range. Plates are incubated at 37°C overnight.

B. High-Performance Liquid Chromatography Assays

The determination of clavulanic acid in urine using high-performance liquid chromatography (HPLC) has been described by Haginaka et al. (63). A Lichrosorb RP-18 column was eluted with 10 μM tetrabutylammonium bromide in phosphate buffer at pH 7.02 containing methanol (1 part to 10 parts of buffer). This system detected both amoxicillin and clavulanic acid in urine, but a detection limit of 5 μg/ml for the inhibitor meant that this method was not suitable for other body fluids.

An alternative HPLC system has been described by Foulstone and Reading (64) which provides a highly sensitive assay of clavulanic acid. Both compo-

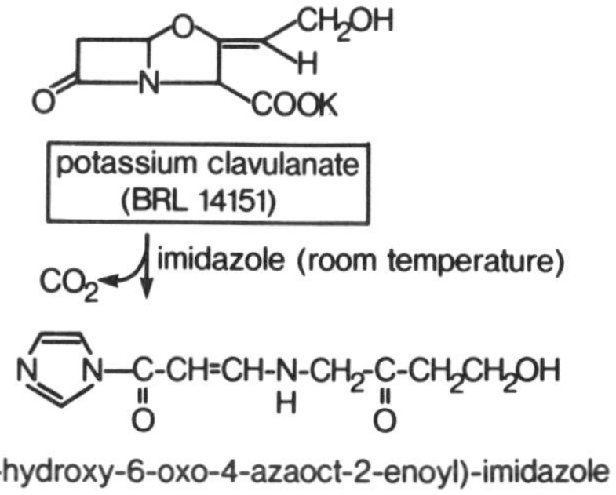

Figure 9 Reaction of imidazole with clavulanic acid. (Data from Ref. 64.)

nents of Augmentin may be determined, but separate assays are performed. Clavulanic acid is reacted with imidazole prior to chromatography to form a derivative (Fig. 9) which absorbs at 311 nm (65). The HPLC determination of this derivative at 311 nm eliminates interference from ultraviolet-absorbing components of serum and urine. Sample (4 parts) is reacted for 10 min at room temperature with reagent (1 part). The reagent is prepared by dissolving 8.25 g of pure imidazole in 24 ml of H_2O plus 2 ml of 5 M HCl, the pH is adjusted to 6.3 with further HCl, and the volume made up to 40 ml with H_2O. Samples of this reaction mixture (25 μl) are chromatographed on a Waters C_{18} μ-Bondapak steel column eluted with 0.1 M phosphate, pH 3.2, containing 4–6% methanol vol./vol.

Serum samples and standards containing amoxicillin and clavulanate may be ultrafiltered before assay using the Amicon MPS-1 system, which provides a simple method of removing protein. This prolongs column life and also reduces interference from serum components (Fig. 10). Serum is diluted with an equal volume of 0.1 M phosphate buffer, pH 7.0, before ultrafiltration in order to prevent a rise in the pH of the filtrate. A portion of the ultrafiltered sample may then be derivatized for clavulanic acid assay or injected directly onto a C_{18} μ-Bondapak column for amoxicillin determination. The eluent for amoxicillin assays is the same as that used for derivatized clavulanic acid but is monitored at 227 nm. Standards of amoxicillin and clavulanate for HPLC are prepared in serum as described earlier for the microbiological assays when assays of serum are to be performed.

For other body fluids, such as urine, where ultrafiltration serves no useful purpose, standards may be prepared in control urine or phosphate buffer. For the assay of amoxicillin in urine, sample blanks may be prepared by treatment with 1 M NaOH (30 min, room temperature) followed by neutralization with 1 M HCl (Fig. 11). This procedure allows the detection of underlying peaks in the

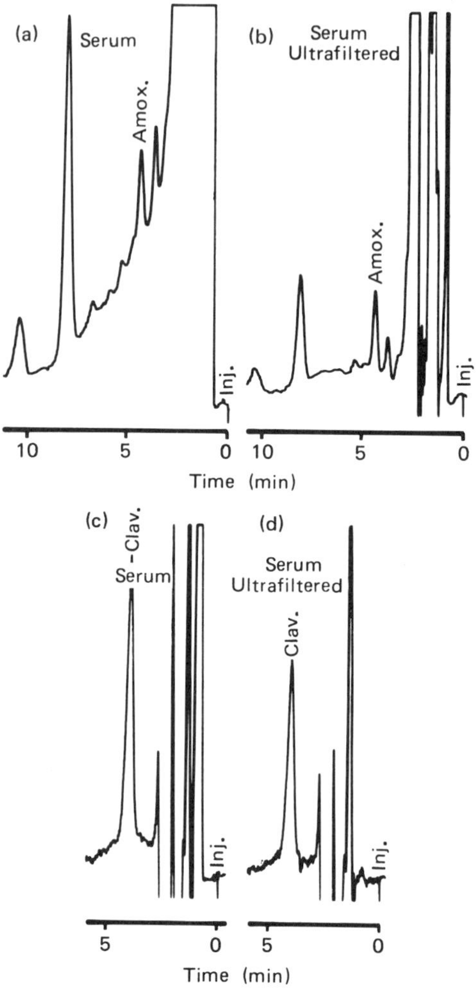

Figure 10 Determination of amoxicillin and clavulanic acid in human serum by HPLC. Samples were chromatographed in 0.1 M potassium phosphate buffer (pH 3.2) + 6% methanol (vol./vol.) and the eluent was monitored at 227 nm and 0.01 AUFS for (a) serum containing 2.5 μg/ml amoxicillin, 25 μl injected [inj] and (b) serum containing 2.5 μg/ml amoxicillin, diluted half into 0.1 M sodium phosphate buffer, pH 7.0, and ultrafiltered, 50 μl injected. For clavulanic acid the eluent was monitored at 311 nm. (c) Serum containing 1.25 μg/ml clavulanic acid was derivatized and 25 μl injected. (d) Serum containing 1.25 μg/ml clavulanic acid, diluted half into phosphate buffer, and ultrafiltered. The ultrafiltrate was derivatized and 50μl injected. (Data from Ref. 64.)

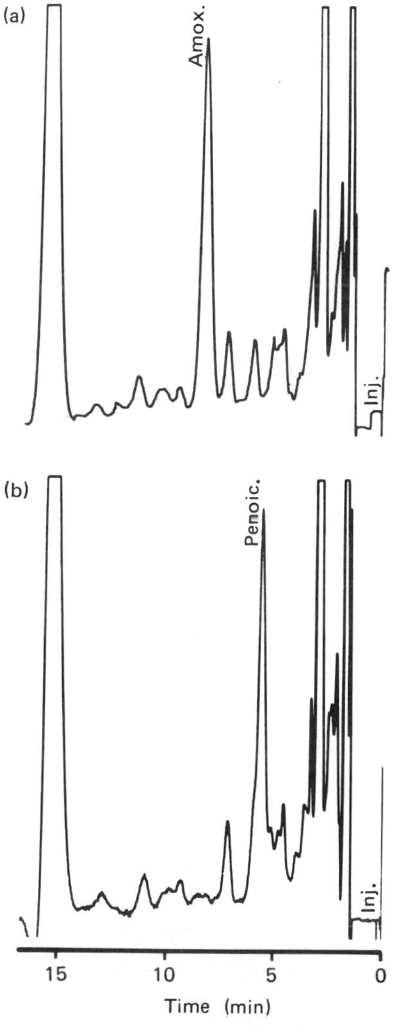

Figure 11 The HPLC determination of amoxicillin (Amox) in urine. Samples were chromatographed in 0.1 M potassium phosphate (pH 3.2) -4% (vol./vol.) methanol. The eluent was monitored at 227 nm and 0.01 AUFS. Amoxicillin (200 μg/ml) in urine was diluted 1/10 into 0.1 M sodium phosphate buffer (pH 7.0). (a) A total of 0.6 ml of diluted urine plus 0.2 ml of buffer (25 μl injected [inj]). (b) A total of 0.6 ml of diluted urine blanked with 0.1 ml of 1 M NaOH (30 min at room temperature) neutralized with 0.1 ml of 1 M HCl (25 μl injected). (Data from Ref. 64.)

amoxicillin position which can affect the accuracy of the method. This particularly applies when measuring low concentrations of amoxicillin in high-osmolality urine.

C. Beta-Lactamase Inhibition Assays

Clavulanic acid may be determined biochemically by relating beta-lactamase inhibitory activity to concentration. Staphylococcal beta-lactamase is the most suitable enzyme for this purpose in that the stoichiometry with clavulanic acid is 1:1, providing a simple linear relationship between concentration and percentage inhibition. A suitably diluted sample is incubated with the enzyme and then residual activity is measured by the addition of a suitable substrate. Automated beta-lactamase inhibition assays (5,32) may be adapted for the assay of clavulanic acid and provide an alternative and highly sensitive method.

D. Stability in Body Fluids

Conditions recommended (62) for the storage of Augmentin samples in body fluids including serum have already been summarized in Table 9. Studies by Haginaka et al. (66,67) on the stability of clavulanic acid in aqueous solution show that the inhibitor is relatively unstable at an alkaline pH. This instability has particular relevance to serum and plasma, which on exposure to air become increasingly alkaline. For this reason stability studies in these media must be carried out under controlled pH conditions if the results are to be related to stability in the body. The pH is conveniently adjusted with CO_2. Under these controlled conditions the half-life of clavulanic acid (50 μg/ml) in human serum is about 17 hr at pH 7.3 and 37°C (62). English et al. have reported a half-life of 12 hr for 100 μg/ml clavulanate in serum (38). If the pH of the serum is not controlled and the sample is exposed to air, then the rate of degradation gradually accelerates as the pH rises. The results in Table 10 show that the half-life of 5 μg/ml clavulanic acid in fresh human serum and plasma, in the absence of pH control, is about 5 hr. It can be seen, however, that when the pH was maintained between 7.0 and 7.3 only a 12-18% loss occurred over the same period. Therefore, the main factor affecting stability in serum or plasma is pH, and under physiological conditions clavulanic acid is relatively stable.

In whole blood, where homeostasis ensures little change in pH, clavulanic acid, as one might expect, has similar stability in both pH-controlled and uncontrolled reactions (Table 10). The half-life in whole blood is about 5 hr at 37°C. Clavulanic acid is therefore less stable in the presence of blood cells than it is in serum or plasma.

Stability in urine is also highly pH dependent. English et al. (38) reported that the half-life of clavulanic acid (100 μg/ml) in urine at pH 4.5 and 37°C was 9.2 hr, while at pH 9.0 this value was reduced to 1.3 hr. An increase in the os-

Table 10 Stability of Clavulanic Acid in Human Blood, Serum, and Plasma

Medium containing clavulanate (5 μg/ml)	Percent clavulanic acid remaining after 5 hr at 37°C: pH controlled at 7.0–7.3[a]	pH uncontrolled
Serum	88	52
Plasma	82	48
Whole blood	50	56

[a]pH adjusted with CO_2.
Source: Data from M. Foulstone, unpublished results.

molality of the urine also decreases the stability of clavulanic acid (M. Kenig, unpublished results), and for this reason urine samples, which are to be stored before assay, should be diluted 10-fold into pH 6.5 citrate buffer.

V. ANTIBACTERIAL ACTIVITY

A. Antibacterial Spectrum

The antibacterial activity of amoxicillin in the presence of clavulanic acid compared with that of amoxicillin and clavulanic acid (2:1) against representative strains of aerobic and anaerobic gram-positive and gram-negative bacteria is illustrated in Tables 11–14. Clavulanic acid alone exhibits a moderate to low level of antibacterial activity against the majority of strains tested (MIC, 8.0–128 μg/ml) (51,68,72); however, against some strains of anaerobic cocci and against *Neisseria* species and *Branhamella catarrhalis,* clavulanic acid is more active (MIC, 0.25–8.0 μg/ml). In general, the activity of amoxicillin against amoxicillin-susceptible strains is not increased by clavulanic acid and the strains are as susceptible to amoxicillin-clavulanic acid as to amoxicillin alone. However, many amoxicillin-resistant bacteria are more susceptible to amoxicillin in the presence of clavulanic acid. These bacteria include strains of *E. coli, K. pneumoniae, Hemophilus influenzae, Br. catarrhalis, N. gonorrhoeae, Staph. aureus, Staphylococcus epidermidis, Bacteroides fragilis,* and other *Bacteroides* species. Amoxicillin-resistant gram-negative bacteria, producing inducible chromosomally mediated class I beta-lactamases (cephalosporinases), however, are not readily inhibited by clavulanic acid and are relatively resistant to amoxicillin-clavulanic acid. Examples of these organisms are *Acinetobacter anitratus, Citrobacter*

Table 11 Antibacterial Spectrum of Amoxicillin, Clavulanic Acid, and Amoxicillin–Clavulanic Acid Against Aerobic Gram-Positive Bacteria

	MIC (μg/ml)		
Organism	Amoxicillin	Amoxicillin + clavulanic acid[a]	Clavulanic acid
Staphylococcus aureus ATCC 25923	0.12	0.12	16
Staphylococcus aureus ATCC 29213[b]	8.0	0.25	16
Staphylococcus aureus NCTC 11561[b]	256	1.0	16
Staphylococcus aureus V532[c]	256	16	512
Staphylococcus epidermidis 810[b]	128	1.0	8.0
Staphylococcus epidermidis 254[c]	256	4.0	64
Staphylococcus saprophyticus 685	0.5	0.25	16
Streptococcus pyogenes 1953	0.01	0.01	8.0
Streptococcus agalactiae 2787	0.06	0.03	32
Streptococcus pneumoniae 1760	0.01	0.01	16
Streptococcus faecalis ATCC 29212	0.5	0.5	512
Listeria monocytogenes 5348	0.25	0.25	32
Nocardia asteroides 406	8.0	8.0	128

[a]Expressed as concentration of amoxicillin (amoxicillin–clavulanic acid, 2:1).
[b]Beta-lactamase producing, methicillin susceptible.
[c]Beta-lactamase producing, methicillin resistant.
Source: Data from Ref. 72.

Table 12 Antibacterial Spectrum of Amoxicillin, Clavulanic Acid, and Amoxicillin–Clavulanic Acid Against Aerobic Gram-Negative Bacilli

	MIC (μg/ml)		
Organism	Amoxicillin	Amoxicillin + clavulanic acid[a]	Clavulanic acid
Escherichia coli ATCC 25922	8.0	4.0	16
Escherichia coli ATCC 35218	>512	4.0	16
Escherichia coli NCTC 11560	>512	8.0	16
Shigella sonnei IP3	8.0	8.0	16
Klebsiella pneumoniae I112	64	2.0	32
Proteus mirabilis 977	1.0	1.0	64
Proteus mirabilis 889	>512	4.0	32
Proteus vulgaris T510	512	2.0	32
Citrobacter koseri 4046	64	2.0	32
Yersinia enterocolitica 10723	32	8.0	32
Enterobacter cloacae T524	512	64	32
Citrobacter freundii T745	128	64	32
Providencia stuartii T90	128	128	64
Providencia rettgeri R110	64	32	64
Morganella morganii R80	64	64	32
Serratia marcescens OG25	64	64	32
Campylobacter jejuni RLH 4864	4.0	4.0	2.0
Pseudomonas aeruginosa ATCC 27853	>512	>512	128
Aeromonas hydrophila U53	256	32	16
Flavobacterium meningosepticum 10580	256	128	16
Acinetobacter anitratus WIG1	>512	32	32

[a]Expressed as concentration of amoxicillin (amoxicillin–clavulanic acid, 2:1).
Source: Data from Ref. 72.

Table 13 Antibacterial Activity of Amoxicillin, Clavulanic Acid, and Amoxicillin–Clavulanic Acid Against *H. influenzae, N. meningitidis, N. gonorrhoeae, Br. catarrhalis,* and *G. vaginalis*

Organism	MIC (μg/ml) Amoxicillin	Amoxicillin + clavulanic acid[a]	Clavulanic acid
Hemophilus influenzae Q1	0.5	0.5	128
Hemophilus influenzae NEMC1[b]	64	0.5	32
Neisseria meningitidis 2062	0.12	0.12	2.0
Neisseria gonorrhoeae L2444	0.5	0.5	2.0
Neisseria gonorrhoeae AX 1729[b]	128	1.0	4.0
Branhamella catarrhalis 1502	0.01	0.01	8.0
Branhamella catarrhalis 2001E[b]	16	0.25	8.0
Gardnerella vaginalis 2297	0.06	0.06	16

[a]Expressed as concentration of amoxicillin (amoxicillin–clavulanic acid, 2:1).
[b]Beta-lactamase producing.
Source: Data from Ref. 72.

freundii, Enterobacter species, *M. morganii, Povidencia* species, *Serratia marcescens,* and *Ps. aeruginosa.*

B. Activity Against Clinical Isolates

1. Gram-Positive Bacteria

In susceptibility studies against amoxicillin-resistant, beta-lactamase-producing clinical isolates of *Staph. aureus* White et al. (68) found 86% of strains to be inhibited by a concentration of 1.25 μg/ml amoxicillin in the presence of 1.25 μg/ml clavulanic acid, and 96% in the presence of 2.5 μg/ml clavulanic acid. Likewise, Verbist (69) reported 90% of 102 isolates inhibited by 2 μg/ml Augmentin (1.35 μg/ml amoxicillin + 0.65 μg/ml clavulanic acid). In a recent study Fuchs et al. (71) found all of 57 amoxicillin-resistant, methicillin-susceptible strains to be inhibited by 8 μg/ml amoxicillin + 4 μg/ml clavulanic acid. Methicillin (oxacillin)-resistant isolates of *Staph. aureus*, producing beta-lactamase, were also more susceptible to amoxicillin–clavulanic acid than to amoxicillin alone. However, these strains were 4- to 16-fold less susceptible (69,71) than the

Table 14 Antibacterial Spectrum of Amoxicillin, Clavulanic Acid, and Amoxicillin–Clavulanic Acid Against Anaerobic Bacteria

Organism	MIC (μg/ml) Amoxicillin	Amoxicillin + clavulanic acid[a]	Clavulanic acid
Peptococcus asaccharolyticus 1011	0.03	0.03	0.25
Peptococcus anaerobius 290.5	0.06	0.03	8.0
Clostridium haemolyticum 9692	0.25	0.12	16
Clostridium difficile 25665	0.5	0.5	128
Clostridium sporogenes 532	0.25	0.12	16
Fusobacterium varium	4.0	4.0	64
Bacteroides fragilis 83	32	0.5	32
Bacteroides melaninogenicus 109	16	0.1	32
Bacteroides thetaiotaomicron 76	32	0.5	32
Bacteroides vulgatus 940	16	0.5	32
Bacteroides uniformis 784.4	32	0.25	16

[a]Expressed as concentration of amoxicillin (amoxicillin–clavulanic acid, 2:1).
Source: Data from Ref. 72.

methicillin-susceptible strains tested as a consequence of the intrinsic resistance of these organisms to beta-lactam antibiotics. The majority (91%) of hospital isolates of *Staph. aureus,* in a recent study reported by Slocombe et al. (72), were beta-lactamase-producing strains resistant to amoxicillin. All were inhibited by 2 μg/ml amoxicillin + 1 μg/ml clavulanic acid, and 63% were susceptible to 1 μg/ml amoxicillin in the presence of 0.5 μg/ml clavulanic acid. Studies on the susceptibility of gram-positive aerobic bacteria isolated from general practice patients and outpatients (73) showed that 95-100% of *Staphylococcus* species, β-hemolytic streptococci, and enterococci were susceptible to amoxicillin-clavulanic acid when tested against a 30-μg disk (20 μg of amoxicillin, 10 μg of clavulanic acid) using a comparative disk-diffusion agar susceptibility test.

2. Gram-Negative Bacteria

Hemophilus influenzae. Strains susceptible to amoxicillin are generally not more susceptible to amoxicillin-clavulanic acid in conventional serial-dilution susceptibility tests, but beta-lactamase-positive strains, resistant to amoxicillin, are rendered susceptible to amoxicillin by the addition of clavulanic acid, as a result of the inhibition of the plasmid-mediated beta-lactamase. In most studies the amoxicillin-resistant isolates were all susceptible to low concentrations of amoxicillin-clavulanic acid, with MIC values ⩽1.0:0.5 μg/ml (68,70,74,75). Strains which were less susceptible to amoxicillin owing to an intrinsic resistance were no more sensitive to amoxicillin-clavulanic acid than to amoxicillin (71, 74).

Neisseria gonorrhoeae. Strains of beta-lactamase-producing *N. gonorrhoeae* are resistant to amoxicillin (MIC, 4-64 μg/ml) but have been shown to be susceptible to low concentrations of amoxicillin in the presence of clavulanic acid (68,76-79), most isolates being inhibited by concentrations of 1 μg/ml amoxicillin or less in the presence of low concentrations of the beta-lactamase inhibitor (⩽0.5 μg/ml). As with isolates of *H. influenzae,* strains of *N. gonorrhoeae*, less susceptible to amoxicillin owing to an intrinsic resistance not related to beta-lactamase, were no more susceptible to amoxicillin-clavulanic acid than to amoxicillin alone.

Branhamella catarrhalis. Branhamella catarrhalis is becoming increasingly recognized as an important pathogen (80) frequently implicated in infections of the lower respiratory tract (81-83) and otitis media (84,85). Many strains of *B. catarrhalis* produce beta-lactamase and are resistant to amoxicillin and ampicillin. However, in the presence of low concentrations of clavulanic acid, beta-lactamase-producing strains were as susceptible to amoxicillin as beta-lactamase-negative strains (68,81,86). In a similar fashion, clavulanic acid has been shown to enhance the antibacterial activity of ampicillin against beta-lactamase-producing isolates of *B. catarrhalis* (83,85).

Enterobacteriaceae

Escherichia coli. The majority of amoxicillin-resistant isolates of *E. coli* producing plasmid-mediated beta-lactamases were susceptible to 12.5 μg/ml Augmentin (amoxicillin-clavulanic acid, 2:1) (51), but only a smaller proportion of isolates were inhibited by 5 μg/ml Augmentin. In a study with 83 isolates, all resistant to amoxicillin, Verbist (69) reported 7% of the *E. coli* to be susceptible to concentrations of 4 μg/ml amoxicillin or less in the presence of 2 μg/ml clavulanic acid, whereas the majority of the strains tested were inhibited by 16 μg/ml amoxicillin in the presence of 8 μg/ml of the inhibitor. Fuchs et al. (71) reported 77% of 30 strains inhibited by ⩽8 μg/ml amoxicillin:4 μg/ml clavulanic acid, and 93% by ⩽32 μg/ml amoxicillin:16 μg/ml clavulanic acid, respectively. Leigh et al. (87) found that none of 32 clinical isolates were inhibited by 15 μg/ml amoxicillin alone, but the same concentration of amoxicillin was inhibitory for 78% of strains in the presence of 7.8 μg/ml clavulanic acid. The susceptibility of amoxicillin-resistant clinical isolates of *E. coli* and other Enterobacteriaceae is illustrated in Table 15 (68), which shows that most strains of *E. coli* tested were more susceptible to amoxicillin-clavulanic acid than to amoxicillin, with 50% of strains inhibited by 12.5 μg/ml amoxicillin + 5.0 μg/ml clavulanic acid, and 72% inhibited by 12.5 μg/ml amoxicillin in the presence of 10 μg/ml clavulanic acid. The minority of strains of *E. coli* isolated, which produce large quantities of chromosomally mediated beta-lactamase (class I cephalosporinase) not effectively inhibited by clavulanic acid, remaining resistant to amoxicillin even in the presence of 10 μg/ml clavulanic acid (51,88).

Klebsiella species. In most in vitro susceptibility studies the strains of *K. pneumoniae* fell into two distinct groups according to their resistance to amoxicillin. In the study reported by White et al. (68) 75% of isolates exhibited a moderate level of resistance to amoxicillin (MIC, 125 μg/ml) and produced a chromosomally mediated class IV beta-lactamase. The remainder of the strains were highly resistant to amoxicillin (MIC >500 μg/ml) and were thought to produce plasmid-mediated beta-lactamase in addition to the chromosomally mediated enzyme. The former group were very susceptible to amoxicillin-clavulanic acid and were inhibited by 5 μg/ml amoxicillin in the presence of 2.5 μg/ml clavulanic acid. The latter group were made resistant to amoxicillin-clavulanic acid but in the presence of higher concentrations of inhibitor, 5.0 or 10 μg/ml clavulanic acid, a significant proportion were sensitive to amoxicillin. Van Landuyt and Lambert (90) found 73% of *K. pneumoniae* isolates to be susceptible to 8 μg/ml Augmentin (5.3 μg/ml amoxicillin + 2.7 μg/ml clavulanic acid). Fuchs et al. (71), using a broth microdilution procedure, found that 97% of 30 *K. pneumoniae* isolates were inhibited by 8 μg/ml or less of amoxicillin in the presence of 4 μg/ml clavulanic acid. Using a disk-diffusion method, Abbas and Francis (89) reported 90% of 3468 clinical isolates of *Klebsiella* species to be susceptible to a 30-μg Augmentin disk. Likewise, Abbas et al. (73), using a similar disk-diffusion method, found 46 urinary isolates (76%) of *K. aerogenes* from hospital inpatients to be sensitive to a 30-μg Augmentin disk.

Proteus species. Beta-lactamase-producing strains of *Prot. mirabilis* were considerably more susceptible to amoxicillin-clavulanic acid than to amoxicillin alone, with most isolates inhibited by 8-16 μg/ml amoxicillin in the presence of 4 or 8 μg/ml clavulanic acid (69-71). *Proteus vulgaris* isolates were particularly susceptible to amoxicillin-clavulanic acid, with 100% of 26 strains (71) inhibited by 8 μg/ml amoxicillin + 4 μg/ml clavulanic acid.

Other Enterobacteriaceae. Numerous investigators (70,76,90-94) have reported that bacteria possessing class I beta-lactamases resistant to inhibition by clavulanic acid, such as *Enterobacter* species, *M. morganii, Providencia* species, *C. freundii,* and *Ser. marcescens,* were not rendered more susceptible to amoxi-

Table 15 Comparative Activities of Amoxicillin Alone and in the Presence of Fixed Concentrations of Clavulanic Acid Against 286 Amoxicillin-Resistant Clinical Isolates

Organism	Number of strains		Inhibitory concentration of amoxicillin (μg/ml)			
			Range	MIC_{50}	MIC_{75}	MIC_{90}
E. coli	68	Amoxicillin	50 ->500	>500	>500	>500
		Amox + CA (2.5)[a]	≤ 1.25- 500	25	50	250
		Amox + CA (5.0)	≤ 1.25- 500	12.5	50	250
		Amox + CA (10.0)	≤ 1.25- 500	12.5	50	125
K. pneumoniae	50	Amoxicillin	25 ->500	125	125	>500
		Amox + CA (2.5)	≤ 1.25->500	2.5	5.0	250
		Amox + CA (5.0)	≤ 1.25->500	2.5	2.5	125
		Amox + CA (10.0)	≤ 1.25- 50	2.5	2.5	5.0
Prot. mirabilis	38	Amoxicillin	≤ 12.5 ->500	125	125	>500
		Amox + CA (2.5)	≤ 1.25- 250	25	50	250
		Amox + CA (5.0)	≤ 1.25- 250	12.5	50	250
		Amox + CA (10.0)	1.25- 250	5.0	12.5	125

Prot. vulgaris	9	Amoxicillin	250 –>500	>500	>500	>500
		Amox + CA (2.5)	≤ 1.25– 50	12.5	12.5	25
		Amox + CA (5.0)	≤ 1.25– 25	5.0	12.5	25
		Amox + CA (10.0)	≤ 1.25– 12.5	5.0	5.0	12.5
Staph. aureus	57	Amoxicillin	5.0 –≤100	50	≤100	≤100
		Amox + CA (1.25)	≤ 0.1 – 5.0	0.5	1.25	2.5
		Amox + CA (2.5)	≤ 0.1 – 2.5	0.5	0.5	1.25
		Amox + CA (5.0)	≤ 0.1 – 1.25	0.25	0.25	0.5
H. influenzae	21	Amoxicillin	2.5 – 25	25	25	25
		Amox + CA (1.25)	0.25– 0.5	0.5	0.5	0.5
		Amox + CA (2.5)	0.25– 0.5	0.25	0.25	0.25
		Amox + CA (5.0)	≤ 0.1 – 0.5	0.25	0.25	0.25
Bact. fragilis	43	Amoxicillin	5.0 –≤100	50	≤100	≤100
		Amox + CA (1.25)	≤ 0.1 – 5.0	1.25	1.25	2.5
		Amox + CA (2.5)	≤ 0.1 – 5.0	0.5	1.25	2.5
		Amox + CA (5.0)	≤ 0.1 – 2.5	0.25	1.25	1.25

[a]Fixed concentration of clavulanic acid (CA) (μg/ml); Amox = amoxicillin.
Source: Data from Ref. 68.

cillin by the addition of the inhibitor. These findings correlate with the poor enzyme inhibitory activity of clavulanic acid observed against Richmond–Sykes class I beta-lactamase (1,95). However, some strains of *Citrobacter diversus* and *Enterobacter agglomerans* were fully susceptible to amoxicillin–clavulanic acid (MIC ⩽8 μg/ml amoxicillin + 4 μg/ml clavulanic acid (71).

Bacteria producing chromosomally mediated cephalosporinases resistant to Augmentin (amoxicillin–clavulanic acid) but susceptible to ampicillin by disk-diffusion testing have been reported (49,96). In a study of 72 strains of bacteria producing inducible cephalosporinase, Griffin and Sutherland (94) showed the organisms to be resistant to both amoxicillin and amoxicillin–clavulanic acid, but that a small proportion of strains (13–18%) were more sensitive to ampicillin than to amoxicillin by agar-dilution and disk-diffusion tests, respectively. These results supported those of Brumfitt et al. (96), who reported that ampicillin was generally more active than amoxicillin against cephalosporinase-producing bacteria and that induction of beta-lactamase by clavulanic acid, as described by Crump and Cansdale (49), was an uncommon occurrence.

3. Miscellaneous Bacteria

Amoxicillin-resistant beta-lactamase-producing strains of the sexually transmitted pathogen *Hemophilus ducreyi,* isolated from patients in Africa, Canada, and the United States, were found to be sensitive to amoxicillin–clavulanic acid (97). The beta-lactamase of *L. pneumophila* is readily inhibited by clavulanic acid (17). Pohlod et al. (98) showed that the mean MIC of amoxicillin for 15 isolates was reduced from 1.95 to 0.61 μg/ml by the addition of concentrations as low as 0.1 μg/ml clavulanic acid. However, the authors also reported that 0.2–0.4 μg/ml clavulanic acid alone inhibited the strains tested. Isolates of *Mycobacterium fortuitum* were shown by Cynamon and Palmer (99) to be more sensitive to amoxicillin in the presence of clavulanic acid than to amoxicillin alone. Acar (18) described 7 of 12 multiresistant isolates of *Noc. asteroides* which were fully susceptible to Augmentin.

4. Anaerobic Bacteria

Bacteroides fragilis, the most frequently isolated pathogen from anaerobic infections, is resistant to amoxicillin as a consequence of inactivation by the beta-lactamases produced by these organisms. These enzymes are readily inhibited by clavulanic acid (11) and, as a result, most isolates tested were susceptible to low concentrations of amoxicillin in the presence of 1.0–2.0 μg/ml clavulanic acid (68,87,100,101). The antibacterial activity of amoxicillin in the presence of clavulanic acid against representative strains of *Bacteroides* species and other anaerobic bacteria is shown in Table 14. Mitsuhashi et al. (101) reported more than 90% of 125 isolates of *Bact. fragilis* were inhibited by 4 μg/ml amoxicillin in the presence of 2 μg/ml clavulanic acid, including strains highly resistant to amoxicillin.

C. Factors Affecting Antibacterial Activity

1. Culture Medium

The activity of amoxicillin in the presence of clavulanic acid is unaffected by the composition or pH of a variety of culture media commonly employed for antibacterial susceptibility testing, such as Mueller-Hinton agar and broth, Isosensitest agar, and diagnostic sensitivity test agar, and the MIC values obtained were similar in media buffered to pH 6.0, 7.4, and 8.0 (51,68).

The antibacterial activity of amoxicillin + clavulanic acid was, however, reduced in tests performed with certain selective media or media supplemented with defined growth additives (102). For example, amoxicillin-clavulanic acid was found to be inactive against beta-lactamase-producing strains of gram-negative enteric bacilli when tested in Endo agar, owing to the inactivation of the beta-lactamase inhibitor by the relatively high concentration of sodium sulfite contained in the medium. Likewise, beta-lactamase-producing strains of *N. gonorrhoeae* were not rendered susceptible to amoxicillin upon addition of clavulanic acid to media supplemented with growth additives (such as Isovitalex, BBL; Vitox, Oxoid; Supplement VX, Difco) recommended for the susceptibility testing of fastidious organisms such as *N. gonorrhoeae* and *H. influenzae.* The antagonistic effect observed was associated with the inactivation of clavulanic acid by the cysteine present in the growth supplements. Thus White and his colleagues (102) urged caution in tests of susceptibility with amoxicillin-clavulanic acid using media containing such additives.

2. Human Serum

Neither amoxicillin (18% bound) nor clavulanic acid (25% bound) is highly bound to human serum proteins, and the antibacterial activity of amoxicillin + clavulanic acid was not reduced when tested in media containing 50% pooled human serum (51,68).

3. Inoculum Size

Amoxicillin alone is generally inactive against large inocula of beta-lactamase-producing strains of *Staph. aureus* and *K. pneumoniae* but may show some activity when tested against a small inoculum of cells. In contrast, the inhibitory activity of amoxicillin-clavulanic acid against these organisms was not greatly affected by large changes in the size of the inoculum tested (68,72).

4. Bactericidal Activity

The results of conventional kill-curve studies to measure bactericidal activity showed that clavulanic acid protected amoxicillin from inactivation by bacterial beta-lactamases, and, as a result, amoxicillin + clavulanic acid exhibited excellent bactericidal activity against bacteria highly resistant to amoxicillin (51,68,88).

For example, Matsuura et al. (88) reported amoxicillin to be bactericidal at concentrations from 3.1 to 10 μg/ml in the presence of 5.0 μg/ml clavulanic acid against beta-lactamase-producing strains of *E. coli, K. pneumoniae, Prot. mirabilis,* and *Prot. vulgaris* not inhibited by high concentrations of amoxicillin (100–800 μg/ml). In a study with an amoxicillin-resistant strain (MIC >500 μg/ml) of *K. pneumoniae,* Comber et al. (51) demonstrated that 5 μg/ml clavulanic acid was effective in protecting amoxicillin from inactivation by beta-lactamase and that amoxicillin–clavulanic acid produced a 99.9% reduction in the initial inoculum within 7 hr. Similar bactericidal effects were observed using conventional test conditions against a beta-lactamase-producing strain of *Staph. aureus,* where a 99.9% reduction was observed after exposing the culture to a concentration of 10 μg/ml amoxicillin in the presence of 2.5 μg/ml clavulanic acid.

In the above studies the organisms were exposed to a static concentration of amoxicillin and inhibitor throughout the course of the test. In the body, however, antibiotic concentrations are subject to fluctuations owing to rates of absorption and excretion, resulting in a relatively short period of exposure of the bacterial cell to the antibiotic, particularly with most beta-lactams. Accordingly, the bactericidal effects produced by amoxicillin, clavulanic acid, and amoxicillin-clavulanic acid have been measured under in vitro conditions in which the concentrations of the antibiotic in the culture medium was constantly adjusted to simulate the concentrations attained in humans following oral or parenteral doses of the amoxicillin–clavulanic acid formulations.

Under conditions which simulated the serum concentrations achieved after oral administration of a single dose of 375 mg of Augmentin (250 mg of amoxicillin + 125 mg of clavulanic acid), Comber et al. (51) showed that the bactericidal activities of amoxicillin-clavulanic acid against beta-lactamase-producing strains of *Staph. aureus* and *K. aerogenes* in the dynamic in vitro model were similar to those obtained following exposure to a constant concentration of 7.5 μg/ml Augmentin, comparable to the peak concentrations attained following oral dosage of 375 mg of Augmentin, and reduced the number of viable cells of both organisms by more than 99.9% over a 24-hr incubation period. Similar bactericidal effects against a beta-lactamase-producing strain of *Staph. aureus* were also produced by concentrations of amoxicillin and clavulanic acid which simulated those measured in serum following a single 625-mg oral dose of Augmentin to human volunteers. In this study (68) the numbers of viable bacteria fell from 3×10^6 to 2×10^2 cells/ml after 8 hr. A second dose, equivalent to a further 625 mg of Augmentin, was given after 8 hr and the numbers of viable cells remained below a detectable level during the following 8-hr period. Against this beta-lactamase-producing strain, amoxicillin in the absence of clavulanic acid was relatively ineffective, such that the bacterial counts of the culture exposed to concentrations simulating a 500-mg dose of amoxicillin alone were similar to those of the antibiotic-free control.

In a similar fashion, it has been shown (A. R. White, unpublished data) that concentrations simulating those achieved following an intravenous bolus dose of 1.2 g of Augmentin (1.0 g of amoxicillin + 200 mg of clavulanic acid) were markedly bactericidal against an amoxicillin-resistant strain of *K. pneumoniae* (MIC >512 μg/ml amoxicillin). For example, when the culture was exposed to amoxicillin + clavulanic acid, the bacterial counts fell rapidly from 8×10^5 to 2×10^2 colony-forming units per milliliter within 3 hr, at which time concentrations of 2.6 μg/ml amoxicillin and 0.6 μg/ml clavulanic acid were measured in the culture medium. In contrast, concentrations of amoxicillin reproducing those measured following a 1-g intravenous bolus dose of amoxicillin to humans were ineffective at reducing the number of viable cells, as were those simulating concentrations of clavulanic acid alone (500-mg intravenous bolus dose). Amoxicillin exhibits rapid bacteriolytic action against amoxicillin-susceptible strains of gram-negative bacilli and in the presence of clavulanic acid has been shown to exhibit marked bacteriolytic effects on the growth of large inocula of amoxicillin-resistant strains of *E. coli* and *K. pneumoniae*, producing plasmid-mediated TEM beta-lactamase (68,72). The morphological changes in the amoxicillin-resistant strain of *E. coli* exposed to amoxicillin–clavulanic acid were the same as those observed with an amoxicillin-susceptible strain, indicating that the amoxicillin had been protected from degradation by the beta-lactamase produced by the bacteria; that is, the formation of spheroplasts associated with subsequent rapid cell lysis, whereas the cells from the culture exposed to amoxicillin alone displayed normal morphology with no evidence of structural damage (68).

D. Activity In Vivo

Studies in laboratory animals have shown that both amoxicillin and clavulanic acid distribute readily throughout body tissues and fluids following oral (103) and parenteral dosing (L. Mizen, unpublished data).

The protection of amoxicillin from inactivation by bacterial beta-lactamases observed in vitro has also been demonstrated in vivo in a number of experimental models of infection, resulting in effective therapy following oral or parenteral administration of amoxicillin with clavulanic acid. The infection models studied include intraperitoneal infections (101,104,106), a mouse pneumonia (104), an experimental pyelonephritis (104,105), localized soft tissue lesions (104), and a neonatal rat meningitis (75), all caused by beta-lactamase-producing organisms. Boon et al. (104) demonstrated that amoxicillin and amoxicillin–clavulanic acid, following oral treatment, were equally effective against an experimental mouse pyelonephritis infection caused by an amoxicillin-suscep-

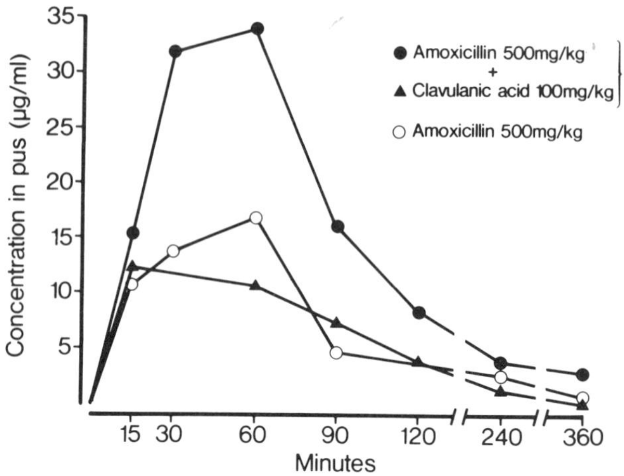

Figure 12 Concentrations of amoxicillin and clavulanic acid in pus following a single subcutaneous dose of amoxicillin or amoxicillin–clavulanic acid to mice infected with *Bact. fragilis* B3. (R. J. Boon, unpublished results.)

tible strain of *E. coli*, but only amoxicillin plus clavulanic acid was effective against a pyelonephritis induced by a beta-lactamase-producing strain. In the study reported by Ritzerfeld (105) the bacterial count in the kidney tissue of rats treated with amoxicillin-clavulanic acid was significantly lower than in the kidneys of rats treated with only amoxicillin.

In experimental localized tissue abscesses (104) caused by the anaerobe *Bact. fragilis*, amoxicillin coadministered orally with clavulanic acid was effective in reducing both the numbers of palpable abscesses and the numbers of viable bacteria in the infected groin tissue, whereas amoxicillin, administered without the inhibitor, was ineffective in reducing either the numbers of abscesses or the numbers of organisms at the site of infection. Boon et al. (104) observed that in a number of tissue fluids the amoxicillin concentrations measured after dosing amoxicillin-clavulanic acid were higher than those found after dosing amoxicillin alone. Similar results have been obtained (R. J. Boon, unpublished data) following subcutaneous dosing of amoxicillin–clavulanic acid. The concentrations of amoxicillin and clavulanic acid measured in pus aspirated from soft tissue abscesses in mice infected with *Bact. fragilis* are shown in Figure 12. In other studies of experimental infections (104) effective therapy with amoxicillin plus clavulanic acid was demonstrated against a pneumonia caused by a strain of *K. pneumoniae* and a staphylococcal thigh lesion in the mouse.

The protection of amoxicillin by clavulanic acid in vivo was also demonstrated in intraperitoneal infections in the mouse by Hunter et al. (106), who showed bacterial counts in the peritoneal cavity to increase rapidly following infection by a beta-lactamase-producing strain of *E. coli* in animals receiving amoxicillin alone. In contrast, in those animals receiving the amoxicillin-clavulanic acid combination, the concentration of amoxicillin in the peritoneal fluid declined less rapidly and there was a rapid fall in the numbers of viable cells. Likewise, Mitsuhashi et al. (101) reported that amoxicillin-clavulanic acid was highly effective against systemic infections in mice caused by beta-lactamase-producing strains of *Staph. aureus, E. coli, K. pneumoniae, Prot. mirabilis,* and *Prot. vulgaris* which were resistant to treatment with amoxicillin alone.

The efficacy of parenteral amoxicillin, alone and in the presence of clavulanic acid, was tested by Yogev et al. (75) in an infant rat model of bacteremia and meningitis caused by ampicillin-resistant strains of *H. influenzae* type b. Of those animals treated with amoxicillin-clavulanic acid, 30 of 33 blood cultures and 29 of 33 cerebrospinal fluid cultures were reported sterile. Neither amoxicillin (27 animals) nor clavulanic acid (20 animals) administered separately was effective in sterilizing the blood or cerebrospinal fluid of the infected animals.

Further evidence of the protection of amoxicillin from degradation by bacterial beta-lactamase in vivo has been demonstrated using infected rat granuloma pouches in which the amoxicillin concentration measured was higher following dosing with amoxicillin plus clavulanic acid than with amoxicillin alone, administered either orally (107) or parenterally (108). Bacterial counts in the pouch exudate were lower after treatment with amoxicillin-clavulanic acid by either route than after treatment with amoxicillin alone.

VI. PHARMACOKINETICS

A. Absorption and Bioavailability

Studies in healthy fasting human subjects have shown that clavulanic acid is well absorbed after oral administration and exhibits pharmacokinetic properties similar to those of amoxicillin (109,110). After single 375-mg doses of Augmentin (250 mg of amoxicillin + 125 mg of clavulanic acid), Ball et al. (111) reported peak serum concentrations of 4.0-4.8 μg/ml amoxicillin and 2.55-3.5 μg/ml clavulanic acid. Administration of a single 625-mg Augmentin dose (500 mg of amoxicillin + 125 mg of clavulanic acid) produced mean peak plasma levels of 6.5 μg/ml amoxicillin and 2.8 μg/ml clavulanic acid (112). After giving healthy human subjects a single film-coated 625-mg Augmentin tablet, Jackson et al. (109) reported peak serum concentrations of 9.73 μg/ml amoxicillin and 3.49 μg/ml clavulanic acid, with a serum elimination half-life of 78 min for amoxicillin and of 59 min for clavulanic acid. As with most oral antibacterial agents, the absorption of clavulanic acid was reported to exhibit considerable interindividual variation (113,114). The absorption characteristics of amoxicillin were not influenced in the presence of clavulanic acid (109,110) and the authors concluded that the absorption of neither component was greatly influenced by food, aluminum hydroxide antacid, or cow's milk (110).

Staniforth et al. (115) compared the effect of probenecid on the bioavailability of amoxicillin and clavulanic acid following an oral dose of 750 mg of Augmentin (500 mg of amoxicillin + 250 mg of clavulanic acid) with that of amoxicillin dosed alone. Probenecid was found to elevate the serum concentration and bioavailability of amoxicillin but had little effect on the bioavailability of clavulanic acid.

Parenteral administration of Augmentin, as a bolus 1.2-g intravenous injection (1.0 g of amoxicillin + 200 mg of clavulanic acid) to healthy subjects produced mean plasma serum concentrations of 105.4 μg/ml amoxicillin and 28.5 μg/ml clavulanic acid, with urinary recoveries of 77.3 and 63.8%, respectively (116). Following an intravenous injection of 575 mg of amoxicillin with 125 mg of clavulanic acid, Lode et al. (117) measured 12.9 μg/ml clavulanic acid at the end of a 15-min infusion and 3.3 μg/ml clavulanic acid after 60 min in the serum of healthy volunteers. The simultaneous infusion, over 2 minutes, of 25 mg of amoxicillin and 5 mg of clavulanic acid to 12 children (mean age 10 years) revealed that the pharmacokinetics of amoxicillin and clavulanic acid were compatible (118). The mean plasma concentrations achieved 15 min after the end of the infusion was 47.4 μg/ml amoxicillin and 11.97 μg/ml clavulanic acid.

B. Metabolism and Excretion

Studies (109,110) have shown that approximately 75% of clavulanic acid is absorbed orally in humans and animals. Metabolism studies in the rat showed that approximately 34% of the dose administered was recovered in the urine, 25% was measured in the feces, 33% found in respired air, and only 1% was detected in the bile. The major metabolites of clavulanic acid in rats and humans have been identified as 1-amino-4-hydroxybutan-2-one (which may dimerize to 2,5-di(2-hydroxyethyl)pyrazine), and carbon dioxide (110).

Urinary excretion of amoxicillin and clavulanic acid over 6 hr after oral administration of 375 mg of Augmentin to normal human subjects, either as a standard or dispersable tablet, amounted to amoxicillin; 69 and 78% amoxicillin, respectively, and 37 and 42% clavulanic acid, respectively (109). Recovery of amoxicillin in the urine following a single oral 625-mg dose of Augmentin was reported to be 56 and 30% clavulanic acid (110). In patients with advanced states of renal insufficiency, Dalet et al. (119) reported that the elimination half-life for amoxicillin increased to approximately 7 hr and that for clavulanic acid to 4.3 hr following a single oral 625-mg dose of Augmentin. Likewise, in a group of patients with severe renal impairment, Boelaert et al. (120) showed that the mean β-elimination half-life for amoxicillin increased 6-fold, whereas that for clavulanic acid increased only 2.6-fold. The authors suggested that the dosage of Augmentin should not be altered in mild renal insufficiency, but that the dosage interval should be increased—to 12-18 hr in cases of moderate insufficiency and to 20-36 hr in severe insufficiency.

C. Distribution

The distribution of clavulanic acid has been measured in a number of body tissues and fluids, including lung tissue, sputum, pleural fluid, bile, peritoneal fluid, and cerebrospinal fluid. Kitzis et al. (121) reported in a study involving 13 patients undergoing pulmonary surgery that amoxicillin and clavulanic acid both penetrate well into pleural fluid after a single oral administration of two 625-mg Augmentin tablets, giving a total dose of 1.0 g of amoxicillin and 250 mg of clavulanic acid. Mean peak serum concentrations of amoxicillin (9.9 ± 1.3 μg/ml) and clavulanic acid (3.8 ± 0.6 μg/ml) were detected 2 hr after dosing, whereas mean peak pleural fluid concentrations of amoxicillin (6.9 ± 0.7 μg/ml) and clavulanic acid (3.1 ± 0.6 μg/ml) were not attained until 4 hr after dosing. In random sputum samples from patients in which concentrations ranging from 0 to 2.0 μg/ml amoxicillin (mean peak, 0.4 μg/ml) were measured, Kosmidis (122) reported clavulanic acid mean peak sputum levels of 0.92 μg/ml 1 hr after a single 750-mg oral Augmentin dose. Graham et al. (123), employing the same dosage, reported median sputum levels of 0.78 μg/ml amoxicillin and less than 0.16 μg/ml clavulanic acid, compared with a median serum level of 8.8 μg/ml amoxicillin and 3.0 μg/ml clavulanic acid.

Munch et al. (124) reported that the penetration of clavulanic acid, like other beta-lactam antibiotics, into the cerebrospinal fluid of patients with noninflamed meninges was relatively poor, with concentrations of less than 0.15 μg/ml detected in 14 of 15 patients given a 250-mg oral dose. Another study reported mean concentrations of 0.34 μg/ml amoxicillin and 0.19 μg/ml clavulanic acid detected in the cerebrospinal of patients measured 4 hr after a single oral dose of 750 mg of Augmentin (125).

Peak amoxicillin concentrations in peritoneal fluid achieved in three patients following oral dosage of two tablets of 625 mg of Augmentin ranged from 0.23 to 20 μg/ml, attained from 1 to 4 hr after dosing (125). Peak concentrations of clavulanic acid in the peritoneal fluid occurred between 2 and 4 hr after administration and ranged from 1.14 to 0.47 μg/ml. The corresponding serum concentrations for clavulanic acid 2-4 hr after administration ranged from 1.8 to 0.41 μg/ml, respectively. Concentrations of amoxicillin in the bile of four patients reached 10.6 μg/ml compared with 12.1 μg/ml in serum 1 hr after oral administration of two 625-mg Augmentin tablets. Peak concentrations of clavulanic acid were 3.3 and 7.7 μg/ml for bile and serum, respectively, achieved approximately 1 hr after administration (125). Kitzis et al. (126) measured the penetration of amoxicillin and clavulanic acid into pus after twice daily oral administrations of 625 mg of Augmentin to patients with infected ischemic leg ulcers. Following oral therapy with 625 mg of Augmentin twice daily for 5 days, the concentrations of amoxicillin and clavulanic acid measured in 10 of 11 patients showed that the extent of penetration of clavulanic acid (49%) was similar to that of amoxicillin (44%) when calculated from the ratio of peak concentrations in pus to serum. For comparison, patients were given oral ampicillin twice daily for 5 days. Bacteria resistant to ampicillin were isolated from the pus of all patients treated with ampicillin (six isolates were penicillinase-producing strains of staphylococci). Ampicillin was undetected in the pus of seven of the nine patients who received oral ampicillin therapy, presumably as a result of inactivation by the bacterial beta-lactamases present at the site of infection.

D. Side Effects

Side effects normally associated with oral dosage of Augmentin are generally characteristic of other oral antibiotic therapy, notably gastrointestinal intolerance which occurs for a short duration and normally resolves with continued therapy. Adverse side effects were reported in 99 of 1460 patients treated and resulted in therapy withdrawal for only about 3% of patients (127). Jackson et al. (110) concluded that in studies conducted with 46 healthy human volunteers there were no major differences in tolerance between Augmentin, cephalexin, and amoxicillin.

VII. CLINICAL THERAPY

A. Urinary Tract Infections

Much of the published clinical experience with Augmentin has been in urinary tract infections, where treatment with 375- or 625-mg oral doses every 8 hr has been shown to be extremely effective in eradicating infections due mainly to amoxicillin-resistant bacteria (127–131). Mashimo (127) showed amoxicillin-clavulanic acid (Augmentin) to be effective in the oral and parenteral treatment of complicated and uncomplicated urinary infections of hospitalized and domiciliary patients caused by amoxicillin-susceptible and amoxicillin-resistant bacteria. Tolkoff-Rubin et al. (129) found that 375 mg, given at intervals of 8 hr, cured 26 of 27 outpatients infected with amoxicillin-resistant bacteria. Likewise, in a randomized double-blind trial involving 21 adult patients with infections of the urinary tract caused by beta-lactamase-producing organisms, Martinelli et al. (130) found that bacteriuria was absent in 85% of patients within 7 days of therapy with 250 mg of amoxicillin + clavulanic acid, whereas only 25% of patients responded to therapy with 250 mg of amoxicillin alone. In patients whose urine was infected with beta-lactamase-producing gram-negative bacteria, Goldstein et al. (131) demonstrated that the urinary concentration of amoxicillin was low after a single 500-mg dose of amoxicillin and large numbers of bacteria were recovered. However, if these patients were given oral Augmentin (500 mg of amoxicillin + 100 mg of clavulanic acid), there was a 10-fold increase in the urinary concentration of amoxicillin and the numbers of infecting organisms were reduced or eliminated.

In a study with 50 patients suffering from pelvic inflammatory disease, Mayer and colleagues (132) showed that Augmentin, 625 mg, administered three times daily for an average of 13.6 days, was fully or partially effective in the therapy of 37 assessable cases.

B. Respiratory Tract Infections

Patients with respiratory tract infections, including chronic bronchitis, acute exacerbations of chronic bronchitis, bronchiectasis, or bronchopneumonia, in general responded favorably to therapy with Augmentin (133-138). In addition, of 24 general practice cases of upper respiratory tract infection treated with 625 mg of Augmentin three times daily (average duration, 7 days), therapy was successful in 22. Of the 26 cases of lower respiratory infection also assessed, all were effectively treated (136). A study conducted by Benard et al. (137) in comparable groups of patients suffering from bronchopulmonary superinfections showed the therapeutic efficacy of Augmentin (two 625-mg tablets given twice daily) to be superior (88%) to that of amoxicillin (two 500-mg doses twice daily) (62%), despite most bacterial isolates being susceptible to amoxicillin. Mehtar (138) also demonstrated the efficacy of oral Augmentin (375 mg, three times daily) in the treatment of 19 of 23 patients with severe respiratory infections caused by beta-lactamase-producing organisms, comprising *Staph. aureus, H. influenzae, Br. catarrhalis,* and mixed anaerobic bacteria, including *Bact. fragilis.* Zaegel et al. (139) reported successful treatment with Augmentin of *Noc. asteroides* pulmonary infections in immunosuppressed patients.

C. Skin, Soft Tissue, and Bone Infections

Leigh et al. (87) reported clinical and bacteriological improvement in 80% of bone infections and 75% of skin infections treated with 250 mg of amoxicillin + 125 mg of clavulanic acid, three times daily for 10 days. Millard and Abbas (140) reported that Augmentin was particularly successful in the therapy of skin and soft tissue infections caused by gram-positive bacteria.

In a larger study involving 107 patients with skin and soft tissue infections, Nakayama (141) reported good to excellent overall clinical efficacy in 81% of patients. In a clinical trial in which Augmentin was administered orally either as single 625-mg doses (31 outpatients) or two 625-mg doses (13 outpatients) twice daily for 6-20 days (mean, 9 days), Garrel et al. (142) reported 36 complete cures, three improvements, and three failures, with two unassessable cases. In a double-blind trial comparing high-dose (625 mg) Augmentin with 500 mg of cefaclor, both administered three times daily to 60 patients with fever or extensive soft tissue infections, Pien (143) reported 68% of 25 patients cured with oral Augmentin and 32% improved, compared with 67% of 30 patients cured and 33% improved after therapy with cefaclor. In another group of patients with major skin infections in the same trial, it was shown that 375 mg of Augmentin given three times daily was effective in eradicating the bacteria in all 13 infections studied, compared with 70% eradication in a similar number of infections after the same daily dosage regimen with 250 mg of cefaclor.

Augmentin has been studied in patients with acute gonorrhoea caused by amoxicillin-resistant *N. gonorrhoeae.* Kumamoto (144) reported the elimination of gonococci, the majority sensitive to amoxicillin, from all 173 male patients treated for 3 days with a daily dose of 1 g of amoxicillin plus 500 mg of clavulanic acid, although a purulent secretion persisted in 3 patients and a serous secretion was evident in 75 patients. Augmentin treatment for 7 days resulted in no purulent secretion in 107 patients, although 14 patients still displayed a persistent serous secretion. Treatment with 1500 mg of Augmentin for 3 days was highly successful in eradicating *N. gonorrhoeae* from 27 of 29 female patients, but a serous secretion persisted in 26 patients. It was thought that the persistent secretion may have been due to a postgonococcal urethritis or residual inflammation of urethral tissue. Lao and Lao (145) were successful in eradicating the infection from 50 male patients with acute gonorrhoea caused by beta-lactamase-producing strains who had failed to respond to previous penicillin treatment. A single oral dose of 3 g of amoxicillin + 125 mg of clavulanic acid successfully treated the infection in 92% of cases, with no adverse side effects. A total of 116 patients with uncomplicated urogenital tract infections caused by beta-lactamase-producing strains of *N. gonorrhoeae* were treated with a single oral dose of Augmentin (amoxicillin, 3 g, with clavulanic acid, 500 mg) and probenecid, 1 g (146). Of the 78 patients who returned for assessment, 73 were successfully treated with Augmentin + probenecid. Nsanze et al. (147) reported effectively treating 65 male patients with chancroid caused by beta-lactamase-producing strains of *H. ducreyi.*

D. Pediatric Infections

Augmentin, dosed either as 156.25 mg in 5 ml of syrup three times daily for a mean period of 6.1 days (age range, 2-5 years) or as 312.5-mg dispersible Augmentin tablets three times daily for mean periods of 7.0-9.8 days, has been successful in treating a variety of infections, including acute tonsillitis, acute and chronic otitis media, acute sinusitis (148,149), and urinary (149,150), gastrointestinal (149), and skin and soft tissue infections (151), with few reported side effects and good clinical tolerance.

E. Parenteral Augmentin

Parenteral 1.2- or 2.2-g Augmentin formulations, comprising 1 g of amoxicillin + 200 mg of clavulanic acid or 2 g of amoxicillin + 200 mg of clavulanic acid, respectively, are currently undergoing clinical investigation to evaluate their efficacy in the treatment of skin and soft tissue, urinary, and respiratory tract infections. Maslak and Heilmann (152) demonstrated that of 40 patients suffering from a variety of systemic infections and receiving parenteral Augmentin therapy (1.2 or 2.2 g) for a mean duration of 7.1 days, 31 were successfully cured. One patient showed improvement and reinfection occurred in two patients after successful initial therapy. Therapy failed in one patient. Of those cases which were assessable at 3 days posttherapy, 94% were cured, 3% showed clinical improvement, and 3% were treatment failures.

In a clinical study (153) involving 54 hospitalized patients with lower respiratory tract infections, many with severe underlying or concomitant diseases, treatment with 2.2 g of Augmentin administered intravenously three times daily was fully effective in 70.4% of cases, with a further 21.8% of cases showing significant clinical improvement. One patient with a lung abscess was reported to have failed therapy.

In a comparative study involving 102 patients, Green-Thompson et al. (154) showed that 1.2 g of Augmentin administered intravenously by bolus injection every 6 hr was significantly more effective against the causative organisms of septic abortion than triple parenteral therapy of ampicillin, kanamycin, and metronidazole.

These preliminary investigations demonstrate that parenteral therapy with Augmentin formulations appears effective and safe in the treatment of a variety of infections caused by gram-positive and gram-negative bacteria.

VIII. CONCLUSIONS

The concept of using a beta-lactamase inhibitor to protect beta-lactamase-labile antibiotics from inactivation became a clinical reality with the discovery of clavulanic acid. The failure of earlier inhibitors to provide effective antibacterial synergy was largely due to their inability to penetrate the outer membrane of gram-negative bacteria and inhibit periplasmic beta-lactamase. On the other hand, clavulanic acid, a small hydrophilic molecule, efficiently inhibits beta-lactamase within the periplasm and has a marked synergistic effect on the antibacterial activity of beta-lactamase-labile antibiotics with which it is combined. This chapter has reviewed the activity and clinical applications of one such formulation of amoxicillin with clavulanic acid (Augmentin).

Clavulanic acid is effective against the majority of beta-lactamases encountered in clinical strains resistant to amoxicillin. Both amoxicillin and clavulanic acid are orally absorbed and show similar pharmacokinetic properties. This enables effective concentrations of both components to be present at the site of infection. The formulation of amoxicillin with clavulanic acid as Augmentin was therefore a logical first step, but a formulation comprising clavulanic acid and ticarcillin (Timentin*) is also undergoing clinical investigation in some countries.

The possibilities of further developments based on either clavulanic acid or other beta-lactamase inhibitors are numerous, and this approach should continue to make significant contributions to antimicrobial chemotherapy in the years ahead.

ACKNOWLEDGMENTS

We would like to acknowledge the helpful discussions and cooperation of our many colleagues. In particular, we wish to thank Janice and Rachael for their patience during the preparation of this chapter. Finally, we are most grateful to the Management of Beecham Pharmaceutical Research Division for their permission to publish this review.

REFERENCES

1. C. Reading and M. Cole. Clavulanic acid, a β-lactamase inhibiting β-lactam from *Streptomyces clavuligerus. Antimicrob. Agents Chemother., 11*:852 (1977).
2. A. G. Brown, D. Butterworth, M. Cole, G. Hanscomb, J. D. Hood, C. Reading, and G. N. Rolinson. Naturally occurring β-lactamase inhibitors with antibacterial activity. *J. Antibiot., 29*:668 (1976).
3. J. D. Hood, S. J. Box, and M. S. Verrall. Olivanic acids, a family of β-lactam antibiotics produced by *Streptomyces* species II. Isolation and characterization of the olivanic acids MM 4550, MM 13902 and MM 17880 from *Streptomyces olivaceus. J. Antibiot., 32*:295 (1979).
4. T. T. Howarth, A. G. Brown, and T. J. King. Clavulanic acid, a novel β-lactam isolated from *Streptomyces clavuligerus*; x-ray crystal structure analysis. *J. Chem. Soc. Chem. Commun.*, 266 (1976).
5. C. Reading and T. Farmer. The biochemical evaluation of β-lactamase inhibitors, in *Antibiotics: Assessment of Antimicrobial Activity and Resistance* (A. D. Russell and L. B. Quesnel, eds.), Academic, London, 1983, p. 141.
6. M. H. Richmond and R. B. Sykes. The β-lactamases of gram-negative bacteria and their possible physiological role. *Adv. Microbiol. Physiol., 9*:31 (1973).

---

*Timentin is a registered trademark of Beecham Group plc.

7. R. Labia, J. Peduzzi, A. Kazmierczak, and A. Phillipon. Inhibition kinetics of 11 penicillinases in relation to the FIC index obtained with clavulanic acid. Paper presented at the 20th Interscience Conference on Antimicrobial Agents and Chemotherapy, New Orleans, American Society for Microbiology, 1980, Abstract 594.
8. C. Reading and T. Farmer. The inhibition of β-lactamases from gram-negative bacteria by clavulanic acid. *Biochem. J., 199*:779 (1981).
9. S. Mitsuhashi and M. Inoue. Mechanisms of resistance to β-lactam antibiotics, in *β-Lactam Antibiotics* (S. Mitsuhashi, ed.), Springer-Verlag, Berlin, 1981, p. 41.
10. K. Hirai, S. Oyobe, M. Inoue, and S. Mitsuhashi. Purification and properties of a new β-lactamase from *Ps. cepacia. Antimicrob. Agents Chemother., 17*:355 (1980).
11. K. Sato, Y. Matsuura, Y. Miyata, M. Inoue, and S. Mitsuhashi. Characterisation of cephalosporinases from *Bacteroides fragilis, Bacteroides thetaiotaomicron* and *Bacteroides vulgatus. J. Antibiot., 36*:76 (1983).
12. J. M. Sherrill and L. R. McCarthy. Comparison of the β-lactamases of *Bacteroides* species. *Curr. Microbiol., 6*:327 (1981).
13. R. Timewell, E. Taylor, and I. Phillips. The β-lactamases of *Bacteroides* species. *J. Antimicrob. Chemother., 7*:137 (1981).
14. I. N. Simpson, C. D. Page, and P. B. Harper. The contribution of β-lactamases to β-lactam resistance in *Bacteroides fragilis. J. Antimicrob. Chemother., 9*:29 (1982).
15. Y. Saino, F. Kobayashi, M. Inoue, and S. Mitsuhashi. Purification and properties of inducible penicillin β-lactamases isolated from *Pseudomonas maltophila. Antimicrob. Agents Chemother., 22*:564 (1982).
16. C. Thornsberry and L. A. Kirven. β-Lactamase of the Legionnaires' bacterium. *Curr. Microbiol., 1*:51 (1978).
17. K. P. Fu and H. C. Neu. Inactivation of β-lactam antibiotics by *Legionella pneumophila. Antimicrob. Agents Chemother., 16*:561 (1979).
18. J. F. Acar. Respiratory tract infection, in *Augmentin: Clavulanate-Potentiated Amoxycillin. Proceedings of the European Symposium* (E. A. P. Croydon and M. F. Michel, eds.), Excerpta Medica, Amsterdam, 1982, p. 314.
19. J. M. Frère, C. Dormans, M. V. Leuzini, and C. Duyckaerts. Interaction of clavulanate with the β-lactamases of *Streptomyces albus* G and *Actinomadura* R39. *Biochem. J., 207*:429 (1982).
20. H. Ogawara and A. Mautoku. Interaction of β-lactamase of *Streptomyces cacaoi* 1. Clavulanic acid and PS-5. *J. Antibiot., 34*:1341 (1981).
21. R. P. Ambler. The structure of β-lactamases. *Philos. Trans. R. Soc. London B, 209*:321 (1980).
22. B. Jaurin and T. Gundström. ampC cephalosporinase of *E. coli* K12 has a different evolutionary origin from that of the β-lactamases of the penicillinase type. *Proc. Nat. Acad. Sci. U.S.A., 78*:4897 (1981).

23. V. Knott-Hunziker, S. G. Waley, B. S. Orlek, and P. G. Sammes. Penicillinase active sites: Labelling of serine 44 in β-lactamase 1 by 6β-bromopenicillanic acid. *FEBS Lett., 99*:59 (1979).
24. S. A. Cohen and R. F. Pratt. Inactivation of *Bacillus cereus* β-lactamase 1 by 6β-bromopenicillanic acid: Mechanism. *Biochemistry, 19*:3996 (1980).
25. S. J. Cartwright and A. F. W. Coulson. Active site of staphylococcal β-lactamase. *Philos. Trans. R. Soc. London B, 289*:370 (1980).
26. J. Fisher, R. L. Charnas, S. M. Bradley, and J. R. Knowles. Inactivation of R-TEM β-lactamase from *Escherichia coli.* Interaction of penam sulfones with enzyme. *Biochemistry, 20*:2726 (1981).
27. V. Knott-Hunziker, S. Petursson, G. S. Jayatilake, S. G. Waley, B. Jaurin, and T. Grundström. Active sites of β-lactamases. The chromosomal β-lactamases of *Pseudomonas aeruginosa* and *Escherichia coli. Biochem. J., 201*: 621 (1982).
28. R. H. Abeles and A. L. Maycock. Suicide enzyme inactivators. *Acc. Chem. Res., 9*:313 (1976).
29. N. Seiler, M. J. Jung, and J. Koch-Weser (eds.). *Enzyme Activated Irreversible Inhibitors,* Elsevier/North-Holland, Amsterdam, 1978.
30. D. G. Brenner and J. R. Knowles. Penicillanic acid sulfone: An unexpected isotope effect in the interaction of 6α- and 6β-monodeuterio and 6,6-dideuterio derivatives with R-TEM β-lactamase from *Escherichia coli. Biochemistry, 20*:3680 (1981).
31. S. J. Cartwright and A. F. W. Coulson. A semi-synthetic penicillinase inactivator. *Nature, 278*:360 (1979).
32. C. Reading and P. Hepburn. The inhibition of staphylococcal β-lactamase by clavulanic acid. *Biochem. J., 179*:67 (1979).
33. J. Fisher, R. L. Charnas, and J. R. Knowles. Kinetic studies on the inactivation of *Escherichia coli* R-TEM β-lactamase by clavulanic acid. *Biochemistry, 17*:2180 (1978).
34. R. L. Charnas, J. Fisher, and J. R. Knowles. Chemical studies on the inactivation of *Escherichia coli* R-TEM β-lactamase by clavulanic acid. *Biochemistry, 17*:2185 (1978).
35. R. L. Charnas and J. R. Knowles. Inactivation of R-TEM β-lactamase from *Escherichia coli* by clavulanic acid and 9-deoxyclavulanic acid. *Biochemistry, 20*:3214 (1981).
36. T. Sawai and K. Tsukamoto. Cefoxitin, N-formimidoyl thienamycin, clavulanic acid and penicillanic acid sulfone as suicide inhibitors for different types of β-lactamases produced by Gram-negative bacteria. *J. Antibiot., 35*: 1594 (1982).
37. J. P. Durkin and T. Viswantha. Clavulanic acid inhibition of β-lactamase 1 from *Bacillus cereus* 569H. *J. Antibiot., 31*:1162 (1978).
38. A. R. English, J. A. Retsema, A. E. Girard, J. E. Lynch, and W. E. Barth. CP-45,899, a β-lactamase inhibitor that extends the antibacterial spectrum of β-lactams: Initial bacteriological characterisation. *Antimicrob. Agents Chemother., 16*:503 (1978).

39. D. Greenwood and A. Eley. *In vitro* evaluation of sulbactam, a penicillanic acid sulphone with β-lactamase inhibitory properties. *J. Antimicrob. Chemother., 10*:117 (1982).
40. A. G. Brown. New naturally-occurring β-lactam antibiotics and related compounds. *J. Antimicrob. Chemother.,* 7:15 (1981).
41. R. Wise, J. M. Andrews, and N. Patel. 6β-Bromo and 6β-iodo penicillanic acid, two novel β-lactamase inhibitors. *J. Antimicrob. Chemother.,* 7:531 (1981).
42. M. Arisawa and R. L. Then. 6-Acetylmethylenepenicillanic acid (Ro 15-1903), a potent β-lactamase inhibitor. *J. Antibiot., 35*:1578 (1982).
43. P. Angehrn and M. Arisawa. 6-Acetylmethylenepenicillanic acid (Ro 15-1903), a potent β-lactamase inhibitor. II. Antibacterial properties. *J. Antibiot., 35*:1584 (1982).
44. C. Reading, T. Farmer, and M. Cole. The β-lactamase stability of amoxycillin with the β-lactamase inhibitor, clavulanic acid. *J. Antimicrob. Chemother., 11*:27 (1983).
45. R. Labia and J. Peduzzi. Augmentin and β-lactamases: Inactivation of β-lactamase by clavulanic acid, in *Augmentin: Clavulanate-Potentiated Amoxycillin. Proceedings of the European Symposium* (E. A. P. Croydon and M. F. Michel, eds.), Excerpta Medica, Amsterdam, 1983, p. 11.
46. P. A. Hunter, K. Coleman, J. Fisher, and D. Taylor. Clavulanic acid, a novel β-lactam with broad spectrum β-lactamase inhibiting properties – Synergistic activity with ampicillin and amoxicillin. *Drugs Exp. Clin. Res., 5*:1 (1979).
47. S. Minami, A. Yotsuji, M. Inoue, and S. Mitsuhashi. Induction of β-lactamase by various β-lactam antibiotics in *Enterobacter cloacae. Antimicrob. Agents Chemother., 18*:382 (1980).
48. A Yotsuji, S. Minami, Y. Araki, M. Inoue, and S. Mitsuhashi. Inducer activity of β-lactam antibiotics for the β-lactamase of *Proteus rettgeri* and *Proteus vulgaris. J. Antibiot., 35*:1590 (1982).
49. J. Crump and S. Cansdale. Enterobacter resistant to amoxycillin/clavulanate. *Lancet, 2*:300 (1982).
50. N. A. C. Curtis, D. Orr, G. W. Ross, and M. G. Boulton. Affinities of penicillins and cephalosporins from the penicillin-binding proteins of *Escherichia coli* K12 and their antibacterial activity. *Antimicrob. Agents Chemother., 16*:533 (1979).
51. K. R. Comber, R. Horton, S. J. Layte, A. R. White, and R. Sutherland. Augmentin antibacterial activity *in vitro* and *in vivo,* in *Augmentin: Clavulanate-Potentiated Amoxycillin. Proceedings of the First Symposium* (G. N. Rolinson and A. Watson, eds.), Excerpta Medica, Amsterdam, 1980, p. 19.
52. B. G. Spratt, V. Jobamputura, and W. Zimmerman. Binding of thienamycin and clavulanic acid to the penicillin-binding proteins of *Escherichia coli* K12. *Antimicrob. Agents Chemother., 12*:406 (1977).
53. J. M. Masson, A. Kazmierczak, and R. Labia. Interactions of clavulanic acid and sulbactam with penicillin-binding proteins. *Drugs Exp. Clin. Res., 9*:513 (1983).

54. D. Greenwood, F. O'Grady, and P. Baker. An *in vitro* evaluation of clavulanic acid, a potent broad-spectrum β-lactamase inhibitor. *J. Antimicrob. Chemother., 5*:539 (1979).
55. S. Horikawa and H. Ogawara. Penicillin binding proteins in *Bacillus subtilis*. The effects of penicillin binding protein and the antibacterial activities of β-lactams. *J. Antibiot., 33*:614 (1980).
56. T. Oka, K. Hashizume, and H. Fujita. Inhibition of peptidoglycan transpeptidase by β-lactam antibiotics: Structure–activity relationships. *J. Antibiot., 33*:1357 (1980).
57. C. A. Brown and H. R. Perkins. *In vitro* synthesis of peptidoglycan by β-lactam-sensitive and resistant strains of *Neisseria gonorrhoeae*: Effects of β-lactam and other antibiotics. *Antimicrob. Agents Chemother., 16*:28 (1979).
58. H. Nikaido. Nonspecific transport through outer membranes, in *Bacterial Outer Membranes: Biogenesis and Function* (M. Inoue, ed.), Wiley, New York, 1979, p. 361.
59. W. Zimmerman and A. Rosselet. Function of the outer membrane of *Escherichia coli* as a permeability barrier to β-lactam antibiotics. *Antimicrob. Agents Chemother., 12*:368 (1977).
60. C. Reading. The biochemistry and mode of action of Augmentin, in *Augmentin: Clavulanate-Potentiated Amoxicillin. Proceedings of an International Symposium* (D. A. Leigh and O. P. W. Robinson, eds.), Excerpta Medica, Amsterdam, 1982, p. 5.
61. C. Reading and T. Farmer. Inhibition of intracellular β-lactamase in *Escherichia coli* by clavulanic acid and other β-lactamase inhibitors. Paper presented at the 23rd Interscience Conference on Antimicrobial Chemotherapy, Las Vegas, American Society for Microbiology, 1983, Abstract 37.
62. Beecham Pharmaceuticals. Clinical pharmacology of Augmentin, in *Augmentin: Clavulanate-Potentiated Amoxicillin. Proceedings of the European Symposium* (E. A. P. Croydon and M. F. Michel, eds.), Excerpta Medica, Amsterdam, 1982, p. 123.
63. J. Haginaka, T. Nakagawa, Y. Nishino, and T. Uno. High performance liquid chromatographic determination of clavulanic acid in human urine. *J. Antibiot., 34*:1189 (1981).
64. M. Foulstone and C. Reading. Assay of amoxycillin and clavulanic acid, the components of Augmentin, in biological fluids with high performance liquid chromatography. *Antimicrob. Agents Chemother., 22*:753 (1982).
65. A. E. Bird, J. M. Bellis, and B. C. Gasson. Spectrophotometric assay of clavulanic acid by reaction with imidazole. *Analyst, 107*:1241 (1982).
66. J. Haginaka, T. Nakagawa, and T. Uno. Stability of clavulanic acid in aqueous solutions. *Chem. Pharm. Bull., 29*:3334 (1981).
67. J. Haginaka, H. Yasuda, T. Uno, and T. Nakagawa. Degradation of clavulanic acid in aqueous solution. *Chem. Pharm. Bull., 31*:1812 (1983).
68. A. R. White, R. J. Boon, P. J. Masters, and R. Sutherland. Antibacterial activity of amoxycillin/clavulanic acid (augmentin) *in vitro*, in *Augmentin: Clavulanate-Potentiated Amoxycillin. Proceedings of the European Symposium* (E. A. P. Croydon and M. F. Michel, eds.), Excerpta Medica, Amsterdam, 1982, p. 21.

69. L. Verbist. Antimicrobial activity of Augmentin *in vitro,* in *Augmentin: Clavulanate-Potentiated Amoxycillin. Proceedings of the European Symposium* (E. A. P. Croydon and M. F. Michel, eds.), Excerpta Medica, Amsterdam, 1982, p. 42.
70. H. W. van Landuyt, M. Pyckavet, and A. M. Lambert. Microbiological testing of the action of Augmentin. *J. Antimicrob. Chemother., 7*:65 (1981).
71. P. C. Fuchs, A. L. Barry, C. Thornsberry, T. L. Gavan, and R. N. Jones. Augmentin: *In vitro* evaluation by broth microdilution and disk diffusion susceptibility testing, regression analysis, tentative interpretative criteria and quality limits. *Antimicrob. Agents Chemother., 24*:32 (1983).
72. B. Slocombe, A. S. Beale, R. J. Boon, K. E. Griffin, P. J. Masters, R. Sutherland, and A. R. White. The antibacterial activity *in vitro* and *in vivo* of amoxicillin in the presence of clavulanic acid, in *Progress and perspectives on beta-lactamase inhibition: A review of Augmentin (amoxicillin plus potassium clavulanate), Postgrad. Med. Custom Communications,* 1984, p. 29.
73. A. M. A. Abbas, B. Chattopadhyay, C. Dulake, T. M. Jones, J. M. Read, M. A. S. Talukder, T. F. Elias Jones, A. H. Quoraish, and R. Sutherland. A multicentre antibiotic sensitivity survey of general practice and hospital isolates, in *Augmentin: Clavulanate-Potentiated Amoxycillin. Proceedings of the First Symposium* (G. N. Rolinson and A. Watson, eds.), Excerpta Medica, Amsterdam, 1980, p. 173.
74. B. Van Klingeren and M. Dessens-Kroon. The influence of clavulanic acid on the susceptibility to amoxycillin of β-lactamase-producing strains of *H. influenzae* using different inoculum sizes. *J. Antimicrob. Chemother., 5*: 322 (1979).
75. R. Yogev, C. Melick, and W. J. Kabat. *In vitro* and *in vivo* synergism between amoxicillin and clavulanic acid against ampicillin-resistant *Haemophilus influenzae* type b. *Antimicrob. Agents Chemother., 19*:993 (1981).
76. P. A. Hunter, K. Coleman, J. Fisher, and D. Taylor. *In vitro* synergistic activities of clavulanic acid with ampicillin, amoxycillin and ticarcillin. *J. Antimicrob. Chemother., 6*:455 (1980).
77. J. M. Miller, C. N. Baker, and C. Thornsberry. Inhibition of β-lactamase in *Neisseria gonorrhoeae* by sodium clavulanate. *Antimicrob. Agents Chemother., 14*:794 (1978).
78. P. Piot, E. van Dyck, J. Colaert, J. P. Ursi, E. Brosmans, and A. Meheus. Antibiotic susceptibility of *Neisseria gonorrhoeae* strains from Europe and Africa. *Antimicrob. Agents Chemother., 15*:535 (1979).
79. B. van Klingeren and L. J. van Winjgaarden. Inhibition of β-lactamase in penicillinase-producing gonococci by clavulanic acid. *J. Antimicrob. Chemother., 8*:79 (1981).
80. C. V. Doern, M. J. Miller, and R. E. Winn. *Branhamella (Neisseria) catarrhalis* systemic disease in humans. *Arch. Intern. Med., 12*:1690 (1981).
81. G. Ninane, J. Joly, M. Kraytman, and P. Piot. Bronchopulmonary infection due to β-lactamase-producing *Branhamella catarrhalis* treated with amoxycillin/clavulanic acid. *Lancet, 1*:257 (1978).

82. D. T. McLeod, F. Ahmad, J. T. Power, M. A. Calder, and A. Seaton. Bronchopulmonary infection due to *Branhamella catarrhalis*. *Br. Med. J., 287*: 1446 (1983).
83. C. V. Doern, K. G. Siebers, L. M. Hallick, and S. A. Morse. Antibiotic susceptibility of beta-lactamase-producing strains of *Branhamella (Neisseria) catarrhalis*. *Antimicrob. Agents Chemother., 17*:24 (1980).
84. L. Wie-Sing, T. Fordham, and J. Alban. Otitis media caused by beta-lactamase-producing *Branhamella (Neisseria) catarrhalis*. *J. Clin. Microbiol., 13*: 222 (1981).
85. P. A. Shurin, C. D. Marchant, C. H. Kim, G. F. van Hare, C. E. Johnson, M. A. Tutihasi, and L. J. Knapp. Emergence of beta-lactamase-producing strains of *Branhamella catarrhalis* as important pathogens of acute otitis media. *Pediatr. Infect. Dis., 2*:34 (1983).
86. E. E. Stobberingh, B. I. Davies, and C. P. van Boven. *Branhamella catarrhalis*: Antibiotic sensitivities and β-lactamases. *J. Antimicrob. Chemother., 13*:55 (1984).
87. D. A. Leigh, J. M. Marriner, M. Freeth, K. Bradnock, and D. Nisbet. Antibacterial activity of Augmentin and treatment of tissue infections, in *Augmentin: Clavulanate-Potentiated Amoxycillin. Proceedings of the First Symposium* (G. N. Rolinson and A. Watson, eds.), Excerpta Medica, Amsterdam, 1980, p. 222.
88. M. Matsuura, H. Nakazawa, T. Hashimoto, and S. Mitsuhashi. Combined antibacterial activity of amoxycillin with clavulanic acid against ampicillin-resistant strains. *Antimicrob. Agents Chemother., 17*:908 (1980).
89. A. M. A. Abbas and R. A. Francis. Antimicrobial activity of Augmentin against amoxycillin-resistant clinical isolates, in *Augmentin: Clavulanate-Potentiated Amoxycillin. Proceedings of the First Symposium* (G. N. Rolinson and A. Watson, eds.), Excerpta Medica, Amsterdam, 1980, p. 67.
90. H. W. van Landuyt and A. M. Lambert. Comparative activity of BRL 25000 with amoxicillin against resistant clinical isolates, in *Current Chemotherapy and Infectious Disease* (J. D. Nelson and C. Grassi, eds.), American Society for Microbiology, Washington, D.C., 1980, p. 334.
91. D. S. Reeves, M. J. Bywater, and H. A. Holt. Antibacterial synergism between beta-lactam antibiotics. Results using clavulanic acid (BRL 14151) with amoxycillin, carbenicillin or cephaloridine. *Infection, 6*:9 (1978).
92. G. Peters, G. Pulverer, and M. Neugebauer. *In vitro* activity of clavulanic acid and amoxicillin combined against amoxicillin-resistant bacteria. *Infection, 8*:104 (1980).
93. A. Thabaut, J. L. Durosoir, and P. Salion. Activité in vitro de l'association acide clavulanique–amoxicilline sur 335 souches d'enterobactéries et de la *Staphylococcus aureus* résistants à l'amoxicilline. *Med. Mal. Infect., 11*: 588 (1981).
94. K. E. Griffin and R. Sutherland. Comparative activities of amoxycillin, ampicillin and amoxycillin/clavulanic acid against Enterobacteriaceae producing Class-I cephalosporinases, in *Proceedings of the 13th International*

Congress of Chemotherapy, Vol. 97 (K. H. Spitzy and K. Karrer, eds.), Egerman Druckerie, Vienna, 1983, p. 1.
95. H. C. Neu and K. P. Fu. Clavulanic acid, a novel inhibitor of β-lactamases. *Antimicrob. Agents Chemother., 14*:650 (1978).
96. W. Brumfitt, J. M. T. Hamilton-Miller, S. Dixson, R. A. Gargan, and A. Gooding. *Enterobacter* resistant to amoxycillin/clavulanate. *Lancet, 2*: 768 (1982).
97. Y. C. Girouard, I. W. Maclean, A. R. Ronald, and W. L. Albritton. Synergistic antibacterial activity of clavulanic acid and amoxicillin against β-lactamase-producing strains of *Haemophilus ducreyi. Antimicrob. Agents Chemother., 20*:144 (1981).
98. D. J. Pohlod, L. D. Saravolatz, E. L. Quinn, and M. M. Somerville. Effect of clavulanic acid on minimal inhibitory concentrations of 16 antimicrobial agents tested against *Legionella pneumophila. Antimicrob. Agents Chemother., 18*:353 (1980).
99. M. H. Cynamon and G. S. Palmer. *In vitro* susceptibility of *Mycobacterium fortuitum* to amoxicillin or cephalothin in combination with clavulanic acid. *Antimicrob. Agents Chemother., 23*:935 (1983).
100. I. D. Farrell and G. R. Brookes. The laboratory efficacy of amoxycillin and clavulanic acid combinations, in *Augmentin: Clavulanate-Potentiated Amoxicillin. Proceedings of the First Symposium* (G. N. Rolinson and A. Watson, eds.), Excerpta Medica, Amsterdam, 1980, p. 54.
101. S. Mitsuhashi, H. Nakazawa, M. Inoue, M. Matsuura, and T. Hashimoto. Antibacterial activity of amoxycillin with clavulanic acid against amoxycillin-resistant strains of clinical isolates, in *Augmentin: Clavulanate-Potentiated Amoxicillin. Proceedings of an International Symposium* (D. A. Leigh and O. P. W. Robinson, eds.), Excerpta Medica, Amsterdam, 1982, p. 22.
102. A. R. White, R. J. Boon, and R. Sutherland. Effect of culture media and supplements on the activity of amoxycillin/clavulanic acid, in *Proceedings of the 13th International Congress of Chemotherapy,* Vol. 55 (D. H. Spitzy and K. Karrer, eds.), Egerman Druckerie, Vienna, 1983, p. 16.
103. L. Mizen, K. Bhandari, J. Sayer, and E. Catherall. Pharmacokinetics and distribution of Augmentin (amoxycillin/clavulanic acid) in laboratory animals. *Drugs Exp. Clin. Res., 7*:263 (1981).
104. R. J. Boon, A. S. Beale, K. R. Comber, C. V. Pierce, and R. Sutherland. Distribution of amoxicillin and clavulanic acid in infected animals and efficacy against experimental infections. *Antimicrob. Agents Chemother., 22*:369 (1982).
105. W. Ritzerfeld. Die Beeinflussung der experimentellen Harnwegsinfektion durch die Kombination Amoxicillin-Clavulansaure. *Urol. Ausg. B, 22*:26 (1982).
106. P. A. Hunter, C. Reading, and D. A. Witting. *In vitro* and *in vivo* properties of BRL 14151, a novel beta-lactam with beta-lactamase inhibitory properties, in *Current Chemotherapy* (W. Siegenthaler and R. Luthy, eds.), American Society for Microbiology, Washington, D.C., 1978, p. 478.

107. L. Mizen, E. Catherall, J. D. Sayer, and R. Sutherland. Distribution of Augmentin in laboratory animals, in *Augmentin: Clavulanate-Potentiated Amoxycillin. Proceedings of the First Symposium* (G. N. Rolinson and A. Watson, eds.), Excerpta Medica, Amsterdam, 1980, p. 112.
108. E. J. Catherall and L. W. Mizen. Pharmacokinetics and activity of parenteral Augmentin (amoxycillin/clavulanic acid) in the rat granuloma pouch infection model, in *Proceedings of the 13th International Congress of Chemotherapy,* Vol. 55 (K. H. Spitzy and K. Karrer, eds.), Egerman Druckerie, Vienna, 1983, p. 31.
109. D. Jackson, D. L. Cooper, T. L. Hardy, P. F. Langley, D. H. Staniforth, and J. A. Sutton. Pharmacokinetic, toxicological and metabolic studies with Augmentin, in *Augmentin: Clavulanate-Potentiated Amoxycillin. Proceedings of the First Symposium* (G. N. Rolinson and A. Watson, eds.), Excerpta Medica, Amsterdam, 1980, p. 87.
110. D. Jackson, D. L. Cooper, R. Horton, P. F. Langley, D. H. Staniforth, and J. A. Sutton. Absorption, pharmacokinetic and metabolic studies with Augmentin, in *Augmentin: Clavulanate-Potentiated Amoxicillin. Proceedings of the European Symposium* (E. A. P. Croydon and M. F. Michel, e eds.), Excerpta Medica, Amsterdam, 1982, p. 83.
111. A. P. Ball, A. M. Geddes, P. G. Davey, I. D. Farrell, and G. R. Brookes. Clavulanic acid and amoxycillin; a clinical, bacteriological and pharmacological study. *Lancet, 1*:620 (1980).
112. G. Hoffken, G. Witkowske, H. Lode, and P. Koeppe. Comparative pharmacokinetics of amoxycillin, clavulanic acid and their combination, in *Augmentin: Clavulanate-Potentiated Amoxycillin. Proceedings of the European Symposium* (E. A. P. Croydon and M. F. Michel, eds.), Excerpta Medica, Amsterdam, 1982, p. 102.
113. R. Munch, R. Luthy, J. Blaser, and W. Siegenthaler. Clavulanic acid: Human pharmacokinetics and penetration into cerebrospinal fluid, in *Current Chemotherapy and Infectious Disease* (J. D. Nelson and C. Grassi, eds.), American Society for Microbiology, Washington, D.C., 1980, p. 345.
114. D. Hoffler and A. Dahloff. Pharmacokinetics of clavulanic acid in patients with normal and impaired renal function, in *Current Chemotherapy and Infectious Disease* (J. D. Nelson and C. Grassi, eds.), American Society for Microbiology, Washington, D.C., 1980, p. 322.
115. D. H. Staniforth, D. Jackson, H. L. Clarke, and R. Horton. Amoxycillin/clavulanic acid: The effects of probenecid. *J. Antimicrob. Chemother., 12*:273 (1983).
116. E. A. P. Croydon, D. Jackson, and D. H. Staniforth. Pharmacokinetics of parenteral Augmentin. Paper presented at the 12th International Congress of Chemotherapy, Florence, July 1981, Abstract 475.
117. H. Lode, G. Hoffken, W. Schmidt, and P. Koeppe. Pharmacokinetic studies of oral and parenteral clavulanic acid, amoxycillin and their combinations (Augmentin), in *Proceedings of the 13th International Congress of Chemotherapy,* Vol. 22 (K. H. Spitzy and K. Karrer, eds.), Egerman Druckerie, Vienna, 1983, p. 17.

118. U. B. Schaad, P. A. Casey, and D. L. Cooper. Single-dose pharmacokinetics of intravenous clavulanic acid with amoxicillin in pediatric patients. *Antimicrob. Agents Chemother., 23*:252 (1983).
119. F. Dalet, E. Cabrera, T. Donate, and G. Del Rio. Pharmacokinetics of the association amoxycillin and clavulanic acid in renal insufficiency and during haemodialysis, in *Augmentin: Clavulanate-Potentiated Amoxycillin. Proceedings of the European Symposium* (E. A. P. Croydon and M. F. Michel, eds.), Excerpta Medica, Amsterdam, 1982, p. 109.
120. J. Boelaert, D. Vogelaers, R. Daneels, M. Schurgers, E. A. Guest, A. M. Lambert, and H. W. van Landuyt. The pharmacokinetics of oral Augmentin in renal impairment, in *Proceedings of the 13th International Congress of Chemotherapy,* Vol. 22 (K. H. Spitzy and K. Karrer, eds.), Egerman Druckerie, Vienna, 1983, p. 33.
121. M. D. Kitzis, M. B. Kitzis, C. Yvelin, J. F. Acar, and B. Andreassian. The penetration of Augmentin into the pleural fluid, in *Augmentin: Clavulanate-Potentiated Amoxycillin. Proceedings of the European Symposium* (E. A. P. Croydon and M. F. Michel, eds.), Excerpta Medica, Amsterdam, 1982, p. 261.
122. J. D. Kosmidis. Pharmacokinetic and clinical experiences with clavulanic acid in association with amoxycillin and ticarcillin, in *Proceedings of the 13th International Congress of Chemotherapy,* Vol. 22 (K. H. Spitzy and K. Karrer, eds.), Egerman Druckerie, Vienna, 1983, p. 50.
123. V. A. L. Graham, J. A. Lowes, E. J. Shaw, and R. J. Davies. An assessment of the value of Augmentin in the management of respiratory tract infections, in *Augmentin: Clavulanate-Potentiated Amoxycillin. Proceedings of an International Symposium* (D. A. Leigh and O. P. W. Robinson, eds.), Excerpta Medica, Amsterdam, 1982, p. 138.
124. R. Munch, R. Luthy, J. Blaser, and W. Siegenthaler. Human pharmacokinetics and CSF penetration of clavulanic acid. *J. Antimicrob. Chemother., 8*:29 (1981).
125. E. A. P. Croydon and A. J. Swaisland. Tissue penetration of amoxycillin and clavulanic acid following oral Augmentin, in *Proceedings of the 13th International Congress of Chemotherapy,* Vol. 22 (K. H. Spitzy and K. Kerrer, eds.), Egerman Druckerie, Vienna, 1983, p. 26.
126. M. D. Kitzis, N. Y. Juillet, J. N. Feissinger, E. Housset, and J. F. Acar. The penetration of Augmentin into ischemic ulcers of the leg, in *Augmentin: Clavulanate-Potentiated Amoxycillin. Proceedings of the European Symposium* (E. A. P. Croydon and M. F. Michel, eds.), Excerpta Medica, Amsterdam, 1983, p. 227.
127. K. Mashimo. The results of clinical studies with BRL 25000 (Augmentin) in Japan, in *Augmentin: Clavulanate-Potentiated Amoxycillin. Proceedings of an International Symposium* (D. A. Leigh and O. P. W. Robinson, eds.), Excerpta Medica, Amsterdam, 1983, p. 227.
128. R. N. Brogden, A. Carmine, R. C. Heel, P. A. Morley, T. M. Spreight, and G. S. Avery. Amoxycillin/clavulanic acid: A review of its antibacterial activity, pharmacokinetics and therapeutic use. *Drugs, 22*:337 (1981).

129. N. E. Tolkoff-Rubin, D. Weber, M. Kelley, R. Wilkinson, and R. H. Rubin. The use of a fixed drug combination of amoxycillin and clavulanic acid (Augmentin) in the treatment of urinary tract infection. A preliminary report, in *Augmentin: Clavulanate-Potentiated Amoxycillin. Proceedings of an International Symposium* (D. A. Leigh and O. P. W. Robinson, eds.), Excerpta Medica, Amsterdam, 1982, p. 57.
130. R. Martinelli, A. A. da Silva Lopes, M. M. M. G. de Oliveira, and H. Rocha. Amoxicillin-clavulanic acid in treatment of urinary tract infection due to gram-negative bacteria resistant to penicillin. *Antimicrob. Agents Chemother., 20*:800 (1981).
131. F. R. Goldstein, M. D. Kitzis, and J. F. Acar. The protective role of clavulanic acid in urinary tract infections, in *Augmentin: Clavulanate-Potentiated Amoxycillin. Proceedings of the European Symposium* (E. A. P. Croydon and M. F. Michel, eds.), Excerpta Medica, Amsterdam, 1983, p. 178.
132. H. O. Mayer, H. Jeschek, and A. Kowatsch. Augmentin in the treatment of urinary tract infection in pregnant women and pelvic inflammatory disease, in *Augmentin: Clavulanate-Potentiated Amoxycillin. Proceedings of the European Symposium* (E. A. P. Croydon and M. F. Michel, eds.), Excerpta Medica, Amsterdam, 1983, p. 207.
133. P. J. Elliott, D. S. Reeves, H. A. Holt, S. T. Chapman, and M. J. Bywater. Evaluation of Augmentin in respiratory tract infections, in *Augmentin: Clavulanate-Potentiated Amoxycillin. Proceedings of the First Symposium on Augmentin* (G. N. Rolinson and A. Watson, eds.), Excerpta Medica, Amsterdam, 1980, p. 269.
134. K. Takebe. The evaluation of Augmentin treatment in respiratory tract infections, in *Augmentin: Clavulanate-Potentiated Amoxycillin. Proceedings of an International Symposium* (D. A. Leigh and O. P. W. Robinson, eds.), Excerpta Medica, Amsterdam, 1982, p. 125.
135. K. Aigner, H. W. Mittermayer, and R. Schindl. Experience with Augmentin in the treatment of chronic bronchitis and bronchopneumonia, in *Augmentin: Clavulanate-Potentiated Amoxycillin. Proceedings of the European Symposium* (E. A. P. Croydon and M. F. Michel, eds.), Excerpta Medica, Amsterdam, 1983, p. 267.
136. G. Kynast. The use of Augmentin in general practice, in *Augmentin: Clavulanate-Potentiated Amoxycillin. Proceedings of the European Symposium* (E. A. P. Croydon and M. F. Michel, eds.), Excerpta Medica, Amsterdam, 1983, p. 278.
137. Y. Benard, J. Lemenager, and C. Morel. A comparative study of amoxycillin and Augmentin in the treatment of bronchopulmonary infection, in *Augmentin: Clavulanate-Potentiated Amoxycillin. Proceedings of the European Symposium* (E. A. P. Croydon and M. F. Michel, eds.), Excerpta Medica, Amsterdam, 1983, p. 282.
138. S. Mehtar. Respiratory tract infections caused by β-lactamase-producing organisms treated with Augmentin. *Scott. Med. J., 27*:24 (1982).

139. R. Zaegel, Y. Gandover, F. W. Goldstein, G. Deloux, and J. Blamontier. New drug combination successfully used for nocardiosis. *Presse Med., 12*:643 (1983).
140. L. G. Millard and A. M. A. Abbas. The treatment of skin and soft tissue infections with Augmentin, in *Augmentin: Clavulanate-Potentiated Amoxycillin. Proceedings of the First Symposium* (G. N. Rolinson and A. Watson, eds.), Excerpta Medica, Amsterdam, 1980, p. 231.
141. I. Nakayama. BRL 25000 – Augmentin: Clinical experience in the treatment of surgical and dermatological infections, in *Augmentin: Clavulanate-Potentiated Amoxycillin. Proceedings of the International Symposium* (D. A. Leigh and O. P. W. Robinson, eds.), Excerpta Medica, Amsterdam, 1982, p. 165.
142. J. P. Garrel, J. M. Sonneck, A. Thabaut, and J. B. Leaute. Augmentin in the treatment of skin infections, in *Augmentin: Clavulanate-Potentiated Amoxycillin. Proceedings of the European Symposium* (E. A. P. Croydon and M. F. Michel, eds.), Excerpta Medica, Amsterdam, 1983, p. 234.
143. F. D. Pien. Double-blind comparative study of two dosage regimens of cefaclor and amoxicillin-clavulanic acid in the outpatient treatment of soft tissue infections. *Antimicrob. Agents Chemother., 24*:856 (1983).
144. Y. Kumamoto. Basic and clinical studies on BRL 25000 – Augmentin treatment of gonorrhoeal infections, in *Augmentin: Clavulanate-Potentiated Amoxycillin. Proceedings of an International Symposium* (D. A. Leigh and O. P. W. Robinson, eds.), Excerpta Medica, Amsterdam, 1982, p. 204.
145. L. M. Lao and M. L. M. Lao. A combination of amoxycillin and clavulanic acid in the treatment of acute male penicillin-resistant gonorrhoea in the Philippines, in *Augmentin: Clavulanate-Potentiated Amoxycillin. Proceedings of an International Symposium* (D. A. Leigh and O. P. W. Robinson, eds.), Excerpta Medica, Amsterdam, 1982, p. 222.
146. G. A. J. de Koning, D. Tio, J. F. Coster, R. A. Coutinho, and M. C. Ansink-Schipper. The combination of clavulanic acid and amoxycillin (Augmentin) in the treatment of patients infected with penicillinase-producing gonococci. *J. Antimicrob. Chemother., 8*:81 (1981).
147. H. Nsanze, P. Karasira, P. Kabuleeta, L. J. D'Costa, M. Fast, F. Plummer, I. Maclean, W. Albritton, and A. R. Ronald. Therapy of genital ulcer disease: A comparison of amoxycillin alone and amoxycillin combined with clavulanic acid, in *Augmentin: Clavulanate-Potentiated Amoxycillin. Proceedings of an International Symposium* (D. A. Leigh and O. P. W. Robinson, eds.), Excerpta Medica, Amsterdam, 1982, p. 195.
148. R. Wielemans and J. P. Gline. Clinical experience with oral Augmentin in the treatment of ear, nose and throat infections in children, in *Augmentin: Clavulanate-Potentiated Amoxycillin. Proceedings of the European Symposium* (E. A. P. Croydon and M. F. Michel, eds.), Excerpta Medica, Amsterdam, 1982, p. 341.
149. H. Debray and A. Galland. Experience with Augmentin in the treatment of infections in children, in *Augmentin: Clavulanate-Potentiated Amoxycil-*

lin. Proceedings of the European Symposium (E. A. P. Croydon and M. F. Michel, eds.), Excerpta Medica, Amsterdam, 1982, p. 347.

150. M. Fink and W. Swoboda. A trial of orally administered Augmentin in the treatment of urinary tract infection and lower respiratory tract infection in a children's hospital, in *Augmentin: Clavulanate-Potentiated Amoxycillin. Proceedings of the European Symposium* (E. A. P. Croydon and M. F. Michel, eds.), Excerpta Medica, Amsterdam, 1982, p. 325.
151. G. R. Fleisher, C. M. Wilmott, and J. M. Campos. Amoxicillin combined with clavulanic acid for the treatment of soft tissue infections in children. *Antimicrob. Agents Chemother., 24*:679 (1983).
152. A. Maslak and H. D. Heilmann. Clinical and bacteriological evaluation of a parenteral formulation of Augmentin (amoxicillin plus clavulanic acid), in *Proceedings of the 13th International Congress of Chemotherapy,* Vol. 55 (K. H. Spitzy and K. Karrer, eds.), Egerman Druckerie, Vienna, 1983, p. 104.
153. F. W. Hulla, G. Kapetanakis, and D. Keratzopoulos. Therapeutic efficacy of intravenous Augmentin in severely ill patients with lower respiratory tract infections, in *Proceedings of the 13th International Congress of Chemotherapy*, Vol. 55 (K. H. Spitzy and K. Karrer, eds.), Egerman Druckerie, Vienna, 1983, p. 88.
154. R. W. Green-Thompson, A. Bhamjee, Y. Coovadia, V. Naidoo, M. Kemp, and N. A. Kritzinger. A comparative study of the efficacy of Augmentin and a triple therapy of ampicillin, kanamycin and metronidazole in the treatment of septic abortion, in *Proceedings of the 13th International Congress of Chemotherapy,* Vol. 79 (K. H. Spitzy and K. Karrer, eds.), Egerman Druckerie, Vienna, 1983, p. 17.

16

Aztreonam (SQ 26,776) and Other Monobactams

EDWARD A. SWABB,* CHRISTOPHER M. CIMARUSTI,†
SHARON A. HENRY, and RICHARD B. SYKES
The Squibb Institute for Medical Research, Princeton, New Jersey

I. INTRODUCTION

Monobactams represent the latest development in the field of beta-lactam antibiotics, an area that has created excitement and interest for over 40 years (Fig. 1). The term *monobactam* was coined to describe a novel group of *mono*cyclic *bac*terially produced beta-*lactam* antibiotics. These naturally occurring compounds have led to the identification of many completely synthetic monobactams. Aztreonam (SQ 26,776, formerly azthreonam) is the first monobactam to enter extensive clinical trials and is the focus of this chapter.

Aztreonam has potent, specific activity against aerobic gram-negative bacteria, but no significant activity against gram-positive or anaerobic organisms. Unlike many other beta-lactam antibiotics, aztreonam is highly stable toward chromosomally and plasmid-mediated beta-lactamases produced by gram-negative bacteria and, in addition, does not induce beta-lactamase production. The antibacterial spectrum of aztreonam serves to preserve the normal bowel flora and reduce the risk of intestinal colonization by pathogenic organisms, pseudomembranous colitis, and disturbances of the blood clotting system. Unlike cephalosporins, aztreonam lacks noteworthy cross-reactivity with penicillin and therefore may have little, if any, potential for inducing immediate hypersensitivity reactions in patients with histories of allergy to beta-lactam antibiotics. Clinically, aztreonam has been used successfully in the therapy of a wide variety of bacterial infections due to susceptible organisms while offering a better therapeutic ratio than aminoglycosides.

**Current affiliation*: Gastrointestinal Research, G. D. Searle, Chicago, Illinois
†*Current affiliation*: Department of Chemical Development, Squibb Chemical Division, Princeton, New Jersey

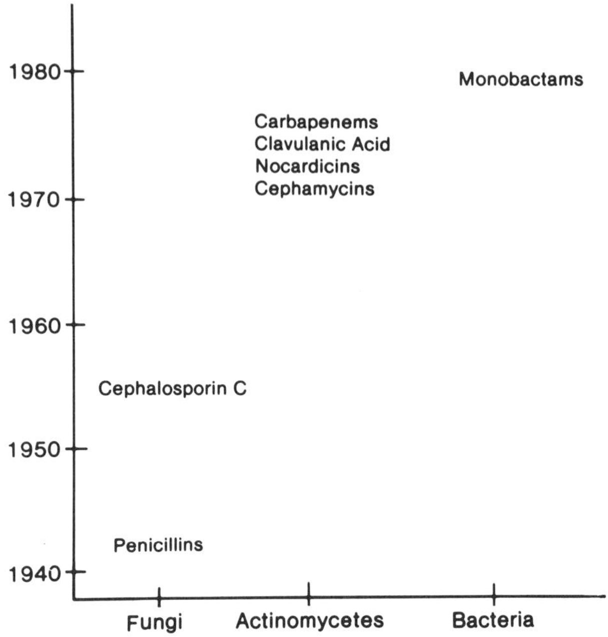

Figure 1 Discovery of naturally occurring beta-lactam antibiotics.

This chapter describes the discovery of monobactams and the synthetic origin of aztreonam, followed by results of extensive microbiological studies. Reported clinical pharmacology studies and therapeutic trials of aztreonam demonstrate its potential application in the therapy of bacterial infections.

II. ORIGIN OF AZTREONAM

A. Discovery of Monobactams

Monobactams were not a discovery of chance, as were the penicillins and cephalosporins, but the products of carefully designed schemes developed to search out novel beta-lactam nuclei. In Japan Kitano and his colleagues (1) mutated strains of *Escherichia coli* to hypersensitivity for beta-lactam antibiotics and used these strains to screen for the occurrence of novel, naturally occurring beta-lactams. The use of such screening mutants led to the discovery of sulfazecin and isosulfazecin, monocyclic beta-lactam antibiotics produced by *Pseudomonas* species (2).

At the Squibb Institute for Medical Research, novel screening procedures were also designed to search specifically for naturally occurring beta-lactam-containing molecules. One such screening procedure involved the use of a strain of *Bacillus licheniformis,* which was highly sensitive to and specific for beta-lactam antibiotics. Over the past 5 years we have isolated and characterized 14 naturally occurring monobactams from gram-negative bacteria (3). Monobactam-producing strains include *Gluconobacter* sp., *Acetobacter* sp., *Pseudomonas* sp. (4), strains of *Chromobacterium violaceum* (5), *Agrobacterium radiobacter* (6) and *Flexibacter* sp. (7,8). Although the majority of these naturally occurring molecules show a high degree of stability to beta-lactamases, none exhibit good antibacterial activity. Thus, although no clinically useful antibiotics were identified by these highly sophisticated screening systems, the knowledge gained from the structures isolated to date may prove even more rewarding.

Discovery of the monobactams led to the synthesis of the novel beta-lactam nucleus 3-aminomonobactamic acid (3-AMA) (9). This nucleus has provided the basis for a whole new generation of beta-lactam antibiotics, of which aztreonam is the first to be developed clinically.

B. Synthesis of Aztreonam

Aztreonam (1) is a totally synthetic analog of the naturally occurring monobactams, a family of monocyclic beta-lactams characterized by the 2-oxoazetidine-1-sulfonic acid moiety (A). This moiety, which distinguishes monobactams from all other families of beta-lactam antibiotics (whether bicyclic or monocyclic), is responsible for many of the unique physical, chemical, and biological properties displayed by aztreonam.

Unlike the naturally occurring monobactams, aztreonam possesses a methyl substituent at the 4-position of the beta-lactam ring. This grouping not only provides the compound a high degree of stability to the plasmid-mediated beta-lactamases of gram-negative bacteria but also increases the intrinsic activity of the compound in comparison with the nonmethylated derivative (10). The aminothiazole oxime side chain provides aztreonam with a high degree of intrinsic activity against aerobic gram-negative bacteria, and the terminal acid contributes significantly to the potent antipseudomonal activity.

The simplest naturally occurring monobactam, SQ 26,180 (2), was the progenitor of aztreonam. Undesirable properties of SQ 26,180 included limited chemical stability and poor antibacterial activity; in addition, it was produced in only limited quantities by fermentation (11). Greatly improved chemical stability attended the replacement of the 3-methoxyl group of SQ 26,180 by a hydrogen atom. The non-methoxylated analog of SQ 26,180, SQ 26,396 (3), is much more stable under physiological conditions. Exchange of the simple methyl side chain of SQ 26,396 for the more complex aminothiazole oxime side chain of SQ 81,402 (4) resulted in a compound with increased intrinsic activity against a broad range of gram-negative bacteria, including *Pseudomonas aeruginosa* (Table 1). This compound, however, proved to be relatively unstable to

Table 1 Antibacterial Activity of SQ 26,396 and SQ 81,402

		Minimal inhibitory concentration (μg/ml) Agar dilution 10^4 CFU[a]	
Organism	SC number	SQ 26,396	SQ 81,402
Staphylococcus aureus	1,276	50	>100
Staphylococcus aureus	2,399	50	>100
Staphylococcus aureus	2,400	50	>100
Staphylococcus aureus	10,165	100	>100
Streptococcus faecalis	9,011	>100	>100
Streptococcus agalactiae	9,287	50	50
Micrococcus luteus	2,495	>100	50
Escherichia coli	8,294	>100	0.4
Escherichia coli	10,857	>100	0.4
Escherichia coli	10,896	>100	0.4
Escherichia coli	10,909	>100	<0.05
Klebsiella aerogenes	10,440	>100	0.4
Klebsiella pneumoniae	9,527	>100	<0.05
Proteus mirabilis	3,855	>100	<0.05
Proteus rettgeri	8,479	>100	<0.05
Proteus vulgaris	9,416	>100	<0.05
Salmonella typhosa	1,195	>100	<0.05
Shigella sonnei	8,449	>100	0.4
Enterobacter cloacae	8,236	>100	0.4
Enterobacter aerogenes	10,078	>100	0.8
Citrobacter freundii	9,518	>100	0.8
Serratia marcescens	9,783	100	0.8
Pseudomonas aeruginosa	9,545	>100	0.4
Pseudomonas aeruginosa	8,329	>100	3.1
Actinobacter calcoaceticus	8,333	>100	100

[a]CFU = colony-forming units.

beta-lactamases, including the plasmid-mediated TEM enzymes (12). This effect was due to replacement of the 3α-methoxyl group in order to increase chemical stability. Like their penicillin and cephalosporin counterparts, 3α-methoxylated monobactams are much more stable to beta-lactamases than the 3-unsubstituted parent molecules (13).

The properties of increased chemical stability, high intrinsic activity, and excellent beta-lactamase stability could be combined in a single molecule, however. Introduction of a 4α-methyl group onto the monobactam nucleus of SQ 81,402 (4) gave SQ 26,726 (5). The corresponding zwitterionic free acid of (5) is aztreonam (1).

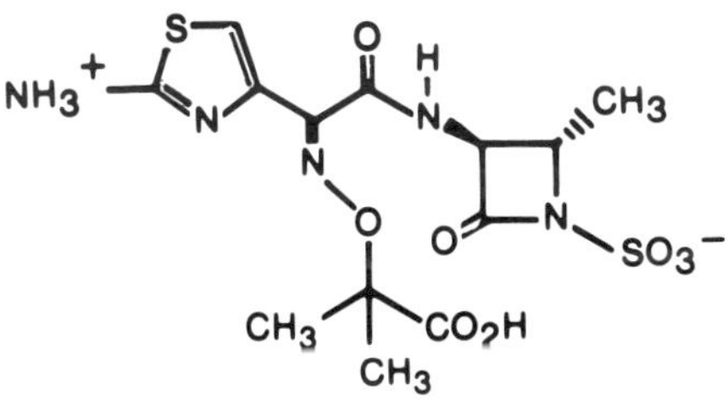

(1) AZTREONAM

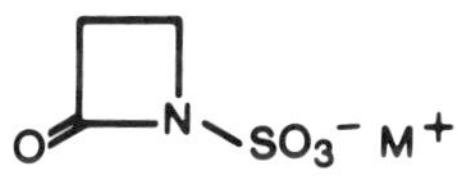

A

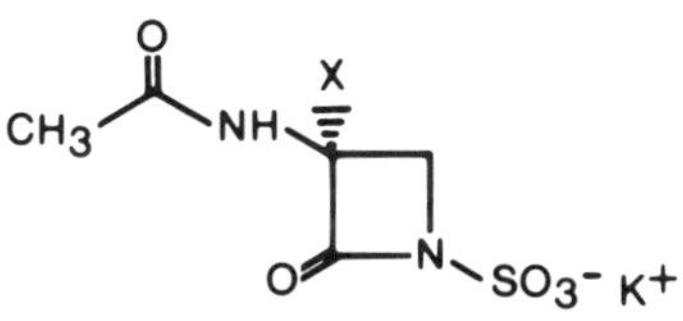

		X
(2)	SQ 26,180	CH_3O
(3)	SQ 26,396	H

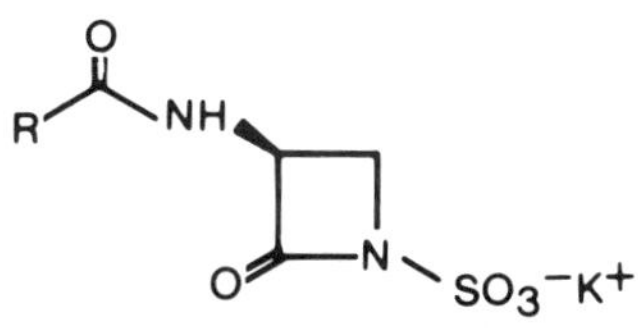

		R
(3)	SQ 26,396	CH_3
(4)	SQ 81,402	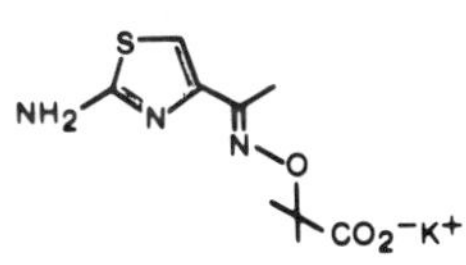

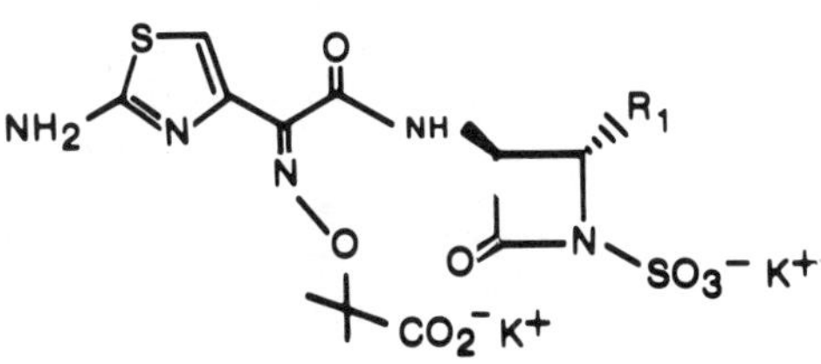

		R_1
(4)	SQ 81,402	H
(5)	SQ 26,726	CH_3

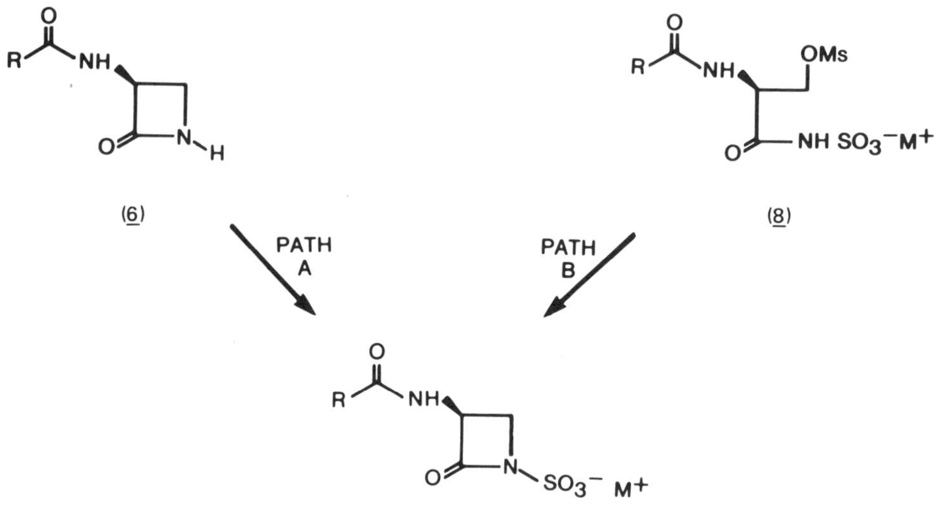

(6) (8) (7)

Two general procedures have been discovered for the synthesis of monobactams. The first (path A) involves sulfonation of an unsubstituted monocyclic beta-lactam (6) to give the corresponding monobactam (7). The second, which we believe mimics their biosynthesis, creates the characteristic 2-oxoazetidine-1-sulfonic acid moiety of monobactams directly from acyclic precursors such as (8). This latter method (path B) is particularly suited to large-scale synthesis and has been chosen for the production of aztreonam.

III. MICROBIOLOGY

A. Mode of Action

Aztreonam, like all members of the beta-lactam family, interferes with the biosynthesis of bacterial cell walls. In aerobic gram-negative bacteria, aztreonam causes filamentation at its lowest effective concentration, a morphological effect identical to that observed with the majority of cephalosporins (14). The penicillin-binding protein (PBP) profile indicates a very high affinity for PBP-3 (complete binding at 0.1 μg/ml) for a wide range of aerobic gram-negative bacteria (15) (Table 2). As would be expected from its relative inactivity against gram-positive bacteria and anaerobes, aztreonam interacts poorly with essential PBPs from these organisms (16). Accordingly, aztreonam has poor activity against *Streptomyces* R61 DD-carboxypeptidase (50% inhibition at >100 μg/ml) and

E. coli peptidoglycan transpeptidase (50% inhibition at 100 μg/ml) (15). Aztreonam, although novel in structure, has a mode of action similar to that of the cephalosporins, specifically affecting septation in susceptible aerobic gram-negative bacteria. As a consequence of this interaction, cell growth is inhibited and death ensues. As for other beta-lactam antibiotics, the bactericidal concentration of aztreonam is either the same or twice the inhibitory concentration (16).

B. Interaction with Beta-Lactam-Hydrolyzing Enzymes

1. Beta-Lactamases

On the basis of their interaction with aztreonam, beta-lactamases from gram-negative bacteria can be divided into three main groups. The first group, representing the broad-spectrum plasmid-mediated enzymes, has little or no observable hydrolytic activity against aztreonam and ceftazidime but notable activity against cephaloridine, cefotaxime, and cefoperazone (Table 3). Aztreonam shows an exceptionally poor affinity for these enzymes (high K_m) and a low rate of hydrolysis (low V_{max}) (12). The second group of enzymes, whose sole representative is the broad-spectrum, chromosomally mediated beta-lactamase produced by certain strains of *Klebsiella,* is one of the few enzymes which have been shown to hydrolyze aztreonam significantly (Table 4). Although aztreonam shows a poor affinity for this enzyme (K_m around 800 μM), the relative V_{max} is half that observed with cephaloridine; consequently, hydrolysis of aztreonam is readily observed and is comparable to that of cefotaxime and cefoperazone but greater than that of ceftazidime (12).

The third and most diverse group of enzymes is represented by the chromosomally mediated cephalosporinases. These are the class I enzymes referred to by Richmond and Sykes (17) and are products of the great majority of gram-negative bacteria. Aztreonam is highly stable to this group of enzymes and has stability equal to or superior to other third-generation cephalosporins (Table 4). With this diverse group of beta-lactamases, the behavior of aztreonam varies from that of a beta-lactamase inhibitor to a poor enzyme substrate. The cephalosporinases produced by strains of *Enterobacter* are strongly inhibited by aztreonam, which has been reported to act as a tight-binding competitive substrate (12) and as a beta-lactamase inactivator for these enzymes. Labia and his colleagues (18) have reported on a time-dependent inactivation of cephalosporinases by aztreonam; covalent enzyme–inhibitor complexes at molar ratios of 1:1 (12) are formed in this reaction. However, with time (over a period of hours) this covalent complex breaks down to give free reactive beta-lactamase. Chromatographic studies have shown that the released product of the covalent complex is the simple beta-lactam hydrolysis product of aztreonam, referred to as SQ 26,992 (9).

Table 2 Binding of Aztreonam and Cephalothin to Penicillin-Binding Proteins (PBPs) of Different Bacteria

		Concentration (μg/ml) for complete Inhibition of Benzylpenicillin Binding		
Organism	Compound	PBP-1	PBP-1a	PBP-1b
Escherichia coli SC 8294	Aztreonam		10	⩾100
	Cephalothin		0.5	100
Proteus mirabilis SC 3855	Aztreonam		2.0	100
	Cephalothin		0.1	10
Proteus vulgaris SC 9416	Aztreonam		10	⩾100
	Cephalothin		0.5	10
Enterobacter cloacae SC 8236	Aztreonam		10	>100
	Cephalothin		0.1	100
Klebsiella pneumoniae SC 9527	Aztreonam		ND	>100
	Cephalothin		ND	30
Pseudomonas aeruginosa SC 9545	Aztreonam		ND	100
	Cephalothin		ND	10
Staphylococcus aureus SC 2399	Aztreonam	>100		
	Cephalothin	0.5		
Bacteroides fragilis SC 11,085	Aztreonam	>100		
	Cephalothin	>100		

[a]MIC = minimal inhibitory concentration.
[b]ND = not detected.
Source: Data from Ref. 15.

The tenacity with which aztreonam and some of the third-generation cephalosporins bind to the *Enterobacter* beta-lactamases has been implicated as an antibiotic resistance mechanism. Trapping of nonhydrolyzable beta-lactams by *Enterobacter* beta-lactamase has been referred to by Then and Angehrn (19) and by Sanders and Sanders (20) as a sponge effect. Extensive studies in a series of *Enterobacter* strains by Sykes et al. (21) have been unable to confirm these observations. Working with multiply-resistant strains of *Enterobacter*, these workers have shown that resistance appears to be a function of cell impermea-

Concentration (μg/ml) for complete inhibition of benzylpenicillin Binding						
PBP-1c	PBP-2	PBP-3	PBP-4	PBP-5	PBP-5/6	MIC[a] (μg/ml)
	>100	0.1	100		100	0.1
	100	2.0	100		>100	1.6
	>100	0.1	100		>100	<0.05
	100	2.0	10		>100	0.8
	ND[b]	0.1	ND		>100	<0.5
	ND	2.0	ND		>100	12.5
	>100	0.1	>100		0.1	0.1
	>100	0.5	100		>100	>100
	>100	0.1	>100		>100	0.1
	100	0.5	30		>100	<0.05
30	>100	0.1	>100		>100	0.2
0.5	>100	2.0	30		>100	>100
	≥100	>100	>100			>100
	0.5	0.5	100			0.1
	100	ND	>100	>100		>100
	>100	ND	>100	>100		>100

bility to the drug and that there is little contact between the periplasmically located beta-lactamase and the potential inhibitor.

Chromosomal beta-lactamases produced by rare strains of *Pseudomonas maltophila*, *Bacteroides fragilis* (22,23), and a strain of *Proteus vulgaris* (24) have been shown to hydrolyze aztreonam.

A further unique aspect of aztreonam in its interaction with beta-lactamases involves the property of inducible enzymes. Class 1 enzyme-producing strains, such as *Enterobacter*, *Serratia*, *Providencia*, *Proteus*, and *Pseudomonas*, charac-

Table 3 Stability of Aztreonam and Comparison Compounds to Plasmid-Mediated Beta-Lactamases Isolated from Gram-Negative Bacteria

	Relative efficacy of hydrolysis by beta-lactamase type							
Compound	TEM-1	TEM-2	OXA-2	SHV-1	PSE-1	PSE-2	PSE-3	PSE-4
Cephaloridine	100	100	100	100	100	100	100	100
Aztreonam	0.04	0.03	1.0	0.1	0.02	5.5	0.8	0.01
Ceftazidime	<0.01	<0.01	<0.5	0.04	0.02	<3.0	0.4	<0.01
Cefotaxime	0.1	0.07	6.0	0.14	0.03	40	0.3	0.03
Cefoperazone	70	60	250	150	260	1900	6	280

Source: Data from Ref. 12, with permission from the American Society for Microbiology, Washington, D.C.

Table 4 Stability of Aztreonam and Comparison Compounds to Chromosomally Mediated Beta-Lactamases Isolated from Gram-Negative Bacteria

	Relative efficiency of hydrolysis by beta-lactamase type						
Compound	*Klebsiella* K1	*Proteus* P1	*Serratia* S1	*Enterobacter* P99	*Enterobacter* E1	*Providencia* PD1	*Bacteroides* B1
Cephaloridine	100	100	100	100	100	100	100
Aztreonam	10	<1.0	<0.2	<0.01	<0.01	0.03	1.1
Ceftazidime	0.01	<0.1	<0.2	0.2	0.04	1.3	4.0
Cefotaxime	5.0	0.6	5.0	5.0	0.02	3.0	30
Cefoperazone	30	>1	30	7.0	5.0	5.0	40

Source: Data from Ref. 12, with permission.

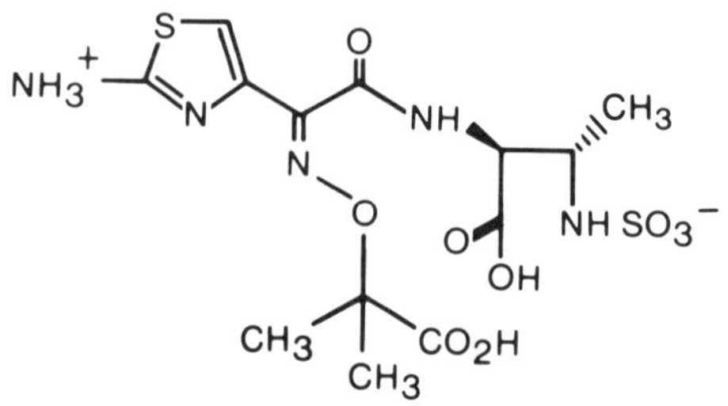

(9) SQ 26,992

teristically produce beta-lactamases which are inducible in the presence of beta-lactam antibiotics (25). Aztreonam is an exception to this rule, because the monobactam fails to induce beta-lactamase activity, unlike cefoxitin, cefoperazone, cefotaxime, and ceftazidime (26). In addition, beta-lactamase activity following incubation with aztreonam is often less than that observed in cultures not exposed to aztreonam, owing to enzyme inhibition (Table 5).

2. Renal Dipeptidase

The renal dipeptidase isolated from swine kidney, although highly potent at hydrolyzing both penems and carbapenem antibiotics, shows no hydrolytic activity against aztreonam (27).

C. Antibacterial Activity

The antibacterial spectrum of aztreonam is unique among beta-lactam antibiotics. Unlike the great majority of beta-lactam compounds, aztreonam generally exhibits little or no activity against gram-positive organisms, such as staphylococci and streptococci, and anaerobic bacteria. In contrast, however, aztreonam is a potent inhibitor of aerobic gram-negative bacteria. It is now well recognized that members of the Enterobacteriaceae and *Ps. aeruginosa* are common causes of nosocomial infections. The activity of aztreonam is directed specifically against these problem organisms. The following results summarize data obtained from studies around the world. Against the Enterobacteriaceae, the great majority of strains are inhibited at less than 1 μg/ml. Particularly sensitive are members of the *Proteus-Providencia* group, *E. coli, Serratia marcescens,* and *Klebsiella pneumoniae* (16,28,29). Similarly, the drug has proved highly active against ampicillin-sensitive and ampicillin-resistant strains of *Hemophilus influenzae* and *Neisseria gonorrhoeae,* with the majority of these strains inhibited at less than 0.1 μg/ml. For 60 strains of *Pseudomonas,* the MIC_{50} value is around 4 μg/ml and the MIC_{90} around 12 μg/ml (Table 6). A second, unpublished survey found an MIC_{90} value of 32 μg/ml for *Ps. aeruginosa* (data on file, The Squibb Institute for Medical Research).

Table 5 Interaction of Aztreonam and Cephalosporins with Organisms Known to Produce Inducible Beta-Lactamases

Organism	No inducer	Relative level of beta-lactamase activity after induction by 10 μg/ml of				
		Cefoxitin	Cefoperazone	Cefotaxime	Ceftazidime	Aztreonam
Proteus SC 10,986	1.0	251	1.1	34.0	13.0	<0.1
Providencia SC 10,188	1.0	5.7	2.0	3.4	1.7	1.1
Enterobacter SC 12,535	1.0	1.3	0.7	0.9	0.6	<0.1
Enterobacter SC 9965	1.0	203	3.8	338	156	1.3
Serratia SC 12,505	1.0	3.1	0.7	1.1	2.2	<0.2
Citrobacter SC 10,204	1.0	20.0	0.3	<0.1	0.9	<0.5

Source: Data from Ref. 26, with permission from the College of Physicians of Philadelphia.

Table 6 Antibacterial Activity of Aztreonam

Organism (number of strains)	MIC_{90} (μg/ml), inoculum 5 x 10^5 CFU
Staphylococcus aureus (20)	>100
Streptococcus pyogenes (20)	12.5
Streptococcus faecalis (20)	>100
Bacteroides fragilis (10)	>100
Escherichia coli (80)	0.2
Klebsiella pneumoniae (70)	0.3
Enterobacter cloacae (30)	12.5
Serratia marcescens (120)	1.6
Proteus mirabilis (25)	<0.1
Indole-positive *Proteus* (50)	<0.1
Providencia stuartii (15)	<0.1
Citrobacter freundii (50)	0.7
Pseudomonas aeruginosa (60)	12.0
Hemophilus influenzae (50)	0.2
Neisseria gonorrhoeae (20)	0.2

Source: Data from Ref. 16, with permission.

Aztreonam is particularly active against multiresistant beta-lactamase-producing gram-negative organisms that are being encountered more frequently and are gaining increased clinical importance. Generally resistant to first- and second-generation cephalosporins and the majority of penicillins, these organisms elaborate a diverse array of beta-lactamases targeted at destroying beta-lactam antibiotics. As already discussed, aztreonam is particularly stable to the plasmid-mediated beta-lactamases including the insidious TEM beta-lactamases produced by a wide range of gram-negative bacteria. The plasmid-mediated genes responsible for enzyme production pass freely among the Enterobacteriaceae, pseudomonads, and now *H. influenzae* and *N. gonorrhoea.* Other beta-lactamases capable of the same promiscuous behavior are the OXA, SHV, and PSE enzymes. Aztreonam shows a high degree of stability to all these beta-lactamases and consequently is highly active against the producing strains.

A further indication of the stability of aztreonam to the action of beta-lactamases is its lack of inoculum effects. Little or no inoculum effect is observed with beta-lactamase-producing strains of *E. coli, Proteus* sp., *Providencia* sp., *Ser. marcescens* and *Ps. aeruginosa* (Table 7). A group of bacteria infrequently isolated in the hospital environment are the nonfermenting gram-negative rods. Among this diverse group of organisms, the pseudomonads and *Acinetobacter* sp. are dominant. Approximately half of these organisms have MIC values for aztreonam of 8 μg/ml or less, but resistant species are evident (31,32) (Table 8). The antimicrobial properties of aztreonam are not affected by pH, media composition, or serum (30,33).

D. Antibiotic Combinations

The directed spectrum of aztreonam will lead in many situations to the use of the drug in combination with other antibiotics. For empiric therapy in seriously ill patients, where broad-spectrum coverage is needed, it is envisaged that the drug will be used in combination with anti-gram-positive compounds or anti-anaerobe compounds. In addition, the use of combination therapy for gram-negative infections is medically acceptable in immunocompromised patients. These clinical situations have prompted the assessment of aztreonam in combination with other antibiotics in the laboratory.

In combination with nafcillin, cloxacillin, erythromycin, or vancomycin, aztreonam produced no deleterious effects on the activity in vitro of these compounds against gram-positive organisms. Likewise, the activity of aztreonam against gram-negative bacteria was unaffected in the presence of these agents (34). On the other hand, aztreonam-aminoglycoside combinations show very positive interactions. In combination with either gentamicin, tobramycin, or amikacin, aztreonam has been reported to exhibit a high incidence of synergistic activity against strains of *Ps. aeruginosa* (35,36) (Table 9). Hindler et al. (38) reported on the synergistic combination of aztreonam and amikacin against amikacin-resistant strains of *Ps. aeruginosa* and *Ps. maltophila.* Stutman et al. (37) have reported synergistic activity with aztreonam and tobramycin against pediatric isolates of *Ps. aeruginosa.*

E. Animal Experimentation

1. Pharmacokinetics

In experimental animals aztreonam shows excellent pharmacokinetic properties, with approximately 40-50% being excreted unchanged in the urine and about 15% appearing in the bile (39,40). Subcutaneously, aztreonam produces high and prolonged serum levels in mice and rats (Figs. 2 and 3). At the 50-mg/kg dose, peak serum levels are in excess of 100 μg/ml at 15 min and are still above 10 μg/ml at 2 hr. Oral administration to mice results in detectable serum levels, but of an order markedly lower than those seen after parenteral administration, because absorption from the gastrointestinal tract is less than 10%. Intramuscular administration to squirrel monkeys gave a serum pharmacokinetic pattern

Table 7 Effect of Inoculum Size on the Activity of Aztreonam and Comparison Compounds Against Strains of *P. aeruginosa* Producing R-Plasmid-Mediated Beta-Lactamases

Beta-lactamase	MIC (μg/ml) at inoculum size (CFU)								
	Aztreonam			Cefotaxime			Ceftazidime		
	10^2	10^4	10^6	10^2	10^4	10^6	10^2	10^4	10^6
TEM-1	1.6	3.1	3.1	3.1	6.3	12.5	3.1	3.1	3.1
TEM-2	1.6	3.1	6.3	6.3	12.5	25	0.4	0.8	0.8
OXA-2	1.6	3.1	6.3	6.3	12.5	25	1.6	3.1	12.5
OXA-3	1.6	3.1	6.3	12.5	12.5	25	3.1	6.3	12.5
SHV-1	1.6	3.1	6.3	6.3	6.3	6.3	0.4	0.8	1.6
PSE-1	0.8	1.6	6.3	3.1	6.3	25	0.8	0.8	1.6
PSE-2	0.8	1.6	6.3	3.1	6.3	25	0.4	0.4	0.8
PSE-3	0.8	1.6	6.3	3.1	6.3	25	0.4	0.8	1.6
PSE-4	0.8	1.6	6.3	3.1	6.3	50	0.4	0.8	1.6

Source: Data from Ref. 16, with permission.

similar to that observed in rodents (Fig. 4). In the three species urinary recovery averaged 40-50% in the first 6 hr, while in mice and rats biliary excretion accounted for about 15% of the administered dose. Tissue levels of aztreonam at 30 and 60 min following subcutaneous administration are shown in Table 10. High levels of aztreonam were found in the kidney and liver, reflecting the excretion of the antibiotic by these routes. In all tissues samples detectable levels of aztreonam were found at 60 min, indicating good penetration. Aztreonam levels in rats were comparable to those for cefotaxime, somewhat lower than those for cefuroxime, but markedly higher than those for gentamicin (Table 10).

Barza and McCue (41) have studied the pharmacokinetics of aztreonam in rabbit eyes after intramuscular, subconjunctival, and intravitreal injections. All methods of administration resulted in potentially therapeutic aztreonam levels in various occular sites.

2. Experimental Infections

In standard mouse protection tests, aztreonam has proved highly efficacious. In general, the efficacy of aztreonam is similar or superior to that observed with the third-generation cephalosporins (Table 11). The efficacy of aztreonam has also been studied in more complex situations, using animal models of human

MIC (μg/ml) at inoculum size (CFU)					
Cefoperazone			Cefsulodin		
10^2	10^4	10^6	10^2	10^4	10^6
6.3	50	>100	25	50	>100
12.5	50	>100	25	50	>100
12.5	12.5	50	1.6	3.1	6.3
12.5	12.5	25	3.1	3.1	6.3
12.5	12.5	>100	0.8	0.8	3.1
12.5	25	50	12.5	12.5	50
12.5	12.5	>100	0.8	3.1	12.5
6.3	6.3	25	6.3	6.3	25
12.5	25	100	6.3	12.5	25

infectious diseases. Examples of such models include ascending urinary tract infection in mice caused by *E. coli*, pneumonia due to *Ps. aeruginosa* and *Ser. marcescens* in rats, *H. influenzae* meningitis in neonatal rats and rabbits, wound infection in mice caused by *Ser. marcescens* and *Proteus rettgeri*, and *Enterobacter* endocarditis in rabbits.

In a model of *H. influenzae* meningitis in infant rats, aztreonam penetrated well into cerebrospinal fluid and showed efficacy against the ampicillin-resistant strain equal to that seen with third-generation cephalosporins (39,42) (Table 12). In a similar model in rabbits, Scheld et al. (43) showed that aztreonam was more efficacious than comparison compounds against infections produced with beta-lactamase-producing and non-beta-lactamase-producing strains of *H. influenzae* and *E. coli*. In the therapy of an *E. coli* experimental cerebritis in rats, aztreonam reduced the number of organisms in rat brain as rapidly as gentamicin (43). In a mouse wound infection caused by beta-lactamase-producing strains of *Prot. rettgeri* and *Ser. marcescens*, aztreonam showed superior efficacy to cefotaxime and piperacillin and was equal to gentamicin (39) (Table 13). Kobasa and Kaye (44) have evaluated the efficacy of aztreonam alone and in combination with gentamicin in an *Enterobacter aerogenes* endocarditis model in rabbits. Although aztreonam was effective in reducing titers in vege-

Table 8 Activity of Aztreonam Against Infrequently Isolated Gram-Negative Bacteria

Organism	MIC (μg/ml)[a]		
	50%	90%	Range
Pseudomonas cepacia	1	2	1 - 16
Pseudomonas diminuta	⩾128	⩾128	⩾128
Pseudomonas maltophilia	⩾128	⩾128	⩾128
Pseudomonas putida	32	64	8 - 64
Pseudomonas stutzeri	2	32	0.5->64
Pseudomonas acidovorans	4	8	2 - 8
Pseudomonas fluorescens	8	64	8 - 64
Acinetobacter anitratus	8	32	4 - 32
Acinetobacter lwoffi	4	64	2 - 64
Acinetobacter biohaemolyticus	8	>64	1 ->64
Acinetobacter bioalcaligenes	4	16	2 - 16
Alcaligenes species	32	64	4 - 64

[a]Here 50% and 90% denote MIC inhibiting 50 and 90% of strains, respectively.
Source: Data from Refs. 32 and 33, with permission from the American Society for Microbiology, Washington, D.C., and S. Karger AG, Basel, respectively.

Table 9 Interaction of Aztreonam with Aminoglycosides Against Gram-Negative Bacteria

Organism group	Number of strains synergistically inhibited[a] (number/total tested)		
	Aztreonam-gentamicin	Aztreonam-tobramycin	Aztreonam-amikacin
Ps. aeruginosa	19/27	24/27	22/27
Acinetobacter	6/25	7/25	8/25
Gentamicin-resistant[b]	12/23	16/23	16/23

[a]Synergy defined as fractional inhibitory concentration index ⩽0.5.
[b]Includes *E. coli* (2), *Serratia* (8), *Klebsiella* (4), *Enterobacter* (3), *Providencia* (4), *Morganella* (1), and *Pseudomonas* (1).
Source: Data from Ref. 34, with permission.

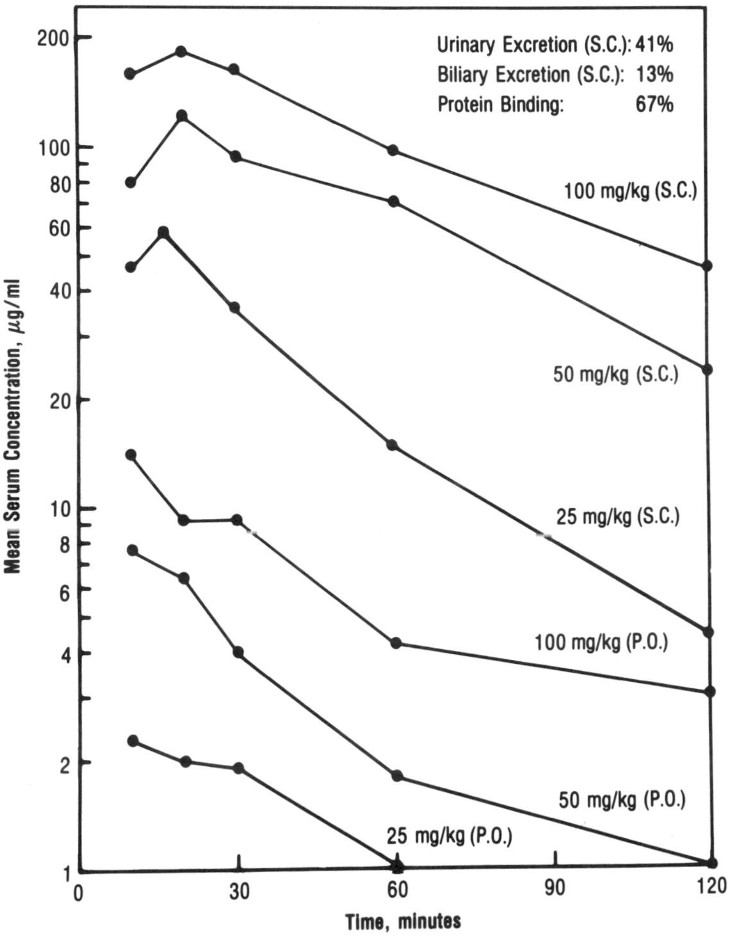

Figure 2 Serum levels of aztreonam in mice after subcutaneous and oral administration. Adapted from Bonner et al. (39,40). Used with permission of Academic Press, New York, and the American Society for Microbiology, Washington, D.C.

tations in rabbits, in combination with gentamicin the effectiveness of aztreonam was significantly enhanced (Table 14).

Antibiotic combinations have also been used to treat experimental mixed infections in mice (45). In a *Staphylococcus aureus/Ser. marcescens* infection, both organisms responded equally well to aztreonam plus clindamycin or aztreonam plus nafcillin where the individual drugs were ineffective. In a *Pseudomonas* infection synergistic activity was observed between aztreonam and gentamicin.

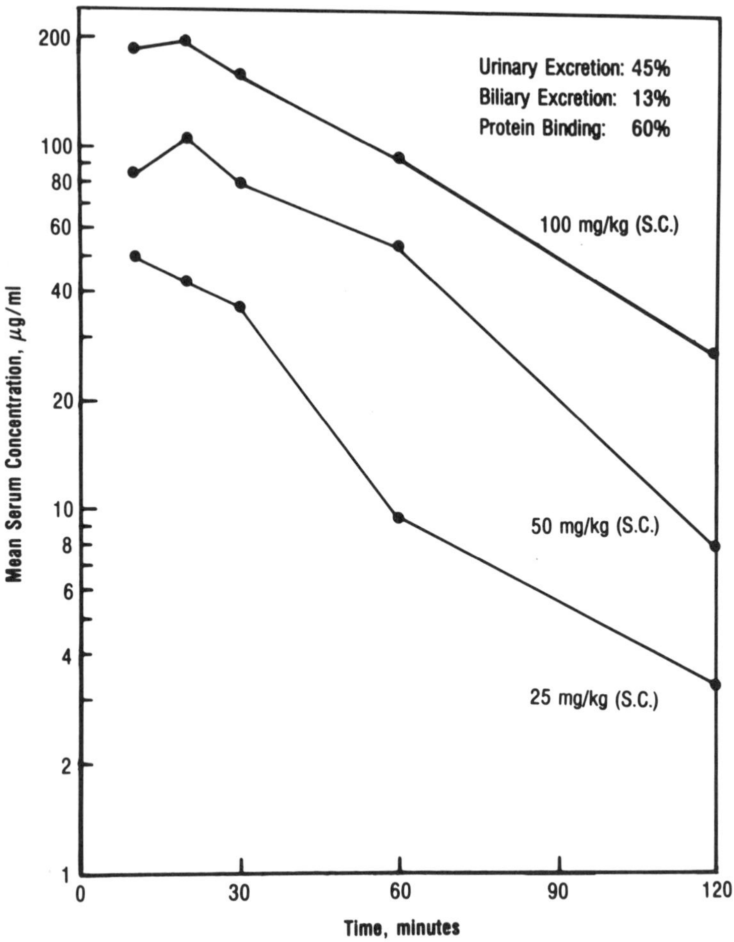

Figure 3 Serum levels of aztreonam in the rat after subcutaneous administration. Adapted from Bonner et al. (39,40). Used with permission of Academic Press, New York, and the American Society for Microbiology, Washington, D.C.

Hospital-acquired infections are frequently observed when patients become immunocompromised. To determine the potential utility of aztreonam in such cases, immunocompromised mice with systemic infections caused by *E. coli*, *Ser. marcescens*, and *Ps. aeruginosa* were treated. In these severe infections aztreonam proved to be highly effective (46). In a model *K. pneumoniae* septicemia in neutropenic rats, aztreonam was shown to be superior to cefazolin and gentamicin (47).

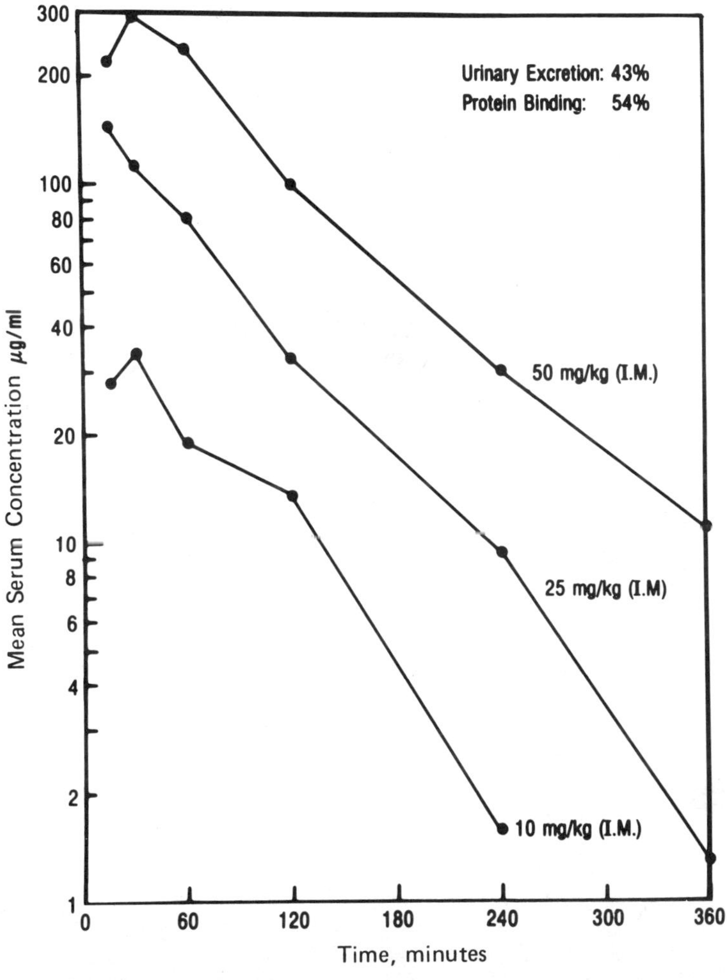

Figure 4 Serum levels of aztreonam in squirrel monkeys after intramuscular administration. Adapted from Bonner et al. (39,40). Used with permission of Academic Press, New York, and the American Society for Microbiology, Washington, D.C.

3. Effect on Fecal Flora

A normal healthy body rarely succumbs to bacterial infections. One of the major protecting mechanisms is the immune response. Additional protection is provided by the normal bacterial flora of the skin and mucosal surfaces of the

Table 10 Tissue and Organ Distribution of Aztreonam in Female Rats

Test drug[a]	Dose (mg/kg)	Time after dosing (min)	Organ/tissue concentration (μg/g)[b]							Serum concentration (μg/ml)[b]
			Genital tract	Heart	Kidney	Liver	Lung	Muscle	Spleen	
Aztreonam	50	30	22.3	8.5	46.9	71.0	16.0	4.0	4.5	60.0
		60	9.3	4.8	24.8	52.7	8.3	2.9	2.4	31.0
Cefotaxime	50	30	24.0	5.2	20.0	5.6	10.0	2.8	2.9	65.5
		60	7.1	1.8	10.4	2.7	5.5	1.4	2.5	27.8
Cefuroxime	50	30	50.4	17.6	78.4	122.4	28.0	8.8	12.8	95.0
		60	36.0	ND[c]	97.6	50.4	14.4	ND	ND	43.0
Gentamicin	50	30	2.2	2.0	10.8	<0.4	1.3	<0.4	0.6	36.0
		60	3.3	1.4	8.4	<0.4	0.8	<0.4	0.6	38.0

[a]Administered subcutaneously.
[b]Determined by microbiological assay.
[c]ND = not detected.
Source: Data from Ref. 40.

Table 11 Efficacy of Aztreonam in Systemic Murine Infections

Pathogen	Aztreonam MIC[a] (μg/ml)	Aztreonam ED_{50}[b] (mg/kg)	Cefotaxime MIC (μg/ml)	Cefotaxime ED_{50} (mg/kg)	Ceftazidime MIC (μg/ml)	Ceftazidime ED_{50} (mg/kg)	Cefoperazone MIC (μg/ml)	Cefoperazone ED_{50} (mg/kg)
E. coli SC 8294	0.4	0.4	0.1	0.2	0.4	<0.1	0.8	0.2
Shigella sonnei SC 8449	0.2	0.3	<0.1	0.08	0.2	0.2	0.4	0.5
S. chottmulleri SC 3850	<0.1	0.2	<0.1	0.2	0.1	0.2	<0.1	0.7
K. pneumoniae SC 12216	0.1	0.4	<0.1	0.2	0.4	0.3	3.1	7.9
C. freundii SC 10204	0.1	0.9	0.1	3.1	0.4	0.5	0.2	1.0
Ent. cloacae SC 9965	0.1	3.7	0.1	24.4	0.2	3.6	0.4	5.9
Prot. rettgeri SC 8217	<0.1	0.6	<0.1	0.3	<0.1	0.7	1.6	65.2
Prov. stuartii SC 12375	<0.1	0.4	1.6	7.0	3.1	18.8	12.5	>100
H. influenzae SC 10556	<0.1	0.4	<0.1	<0.1	<0.1	0.1	50	0.1
Ser. marcescens SC 9782	0.2	0.5	1.6	0.6	0.2	0.7	1.6	28.5
Ps. aeruginosa SC 8392	3.1	24.7	12.5	48.0	1.6	37.0	3.1	>200

[a]Determined at an inoculum of 10^5 CFU.
[b]ED = effective dose.
Source: From Ref. 16, with permission.

Table 12 Therapy of Ampicillin-Resistant *H. influenzae* SC 10556 Meningitis in Infant Rats

Test compound[a]	MIC[b] (μg/ml)	CD_{50}[c] (mg/kg per day)
Aztreonam	<0.1	5
Ampicillin	>100	171
Piperacillin	>100	>50
Cefoperazone	50	3
Cefotaxime	<0.1	3
Ceftazidime	<0.1	8
Ceftizoxime	<0.1	4
Moxalactam	<0.1	8
Chloramphenicol	0.6	>200

[a]Administered subcutaneously, twice daily, for 2 days.
[b]Minimum inhibitory concentration: agar dilution procedure, inoculum = 5 x 10^5 CFU.
[c]Median curative dose.
Source: Data from Ref. 42, with permission.

Table 13 Efficacy of Aztreonam in Mouse Wound Infections

Pathogen	Test compound[a]	MIC (μg/ml)	ED_{50}[b] (mg/kg)
Prot. rettgeri SC 8217	Aztreonam	<0.05	7.7
	Cefotaxime	0.1	>200
	Piperacillin	1.6	>200
Ser. marcescens SC 9782	Aztreonam	0.1	19.0
	Cefotaxime	0.2	186.0
	Gentamicin	0.8	4.0

[a]Compound administered subcutaneously 1 and 5 hr postinfection; wounds cultured 18 hr postinfection.
[b]Based on 3 $\log_{10}$ reduction in CFUs from untreated controls.
Source: Data from Ref. 39, with permission from Academic Press, New York.

Table 14 Effect of Aztreonam Alone and in Combination with Gentamicin in Reducing Titers of *Ent. aerogenes* Aortic Vegetations in Rabbits

Duration of therapy (days)	Mean ± SD $\log_{10}$ CFU per gram of vegetation (number sterile/total)					
	Aztreonam	Aztreonam + gentamicin	Cefoperazone	Cefoperazone + gentamicin	Gentamicin	Controls (untreated)
5	7.1 ± 1.2 (0/9)	3.8 ± 1.7 (3/8)	8.4 ± 1.2 (0/10)	4.4 ± 2.8 (3/12)	5.9 ± 2.6 (1/11)	9.2 ± 0.7 (0/12)
10	6.2 ± 3.0 (1/7)	2 ± 0 (6/6)	6.3 ± 2.1 (1/7)	2 ± 0 (4/4)	4.8 ± 1.3 (0/7)	9.5 ± 0.3 (0/3)

Source: Data from Ref. 44, with permission.

body. These organisms exist in a symbiotic relationship with their host. The large intestine contains billions of bacteria which, in addition to protecting the gut from colonization and invasion by potential pathogenic microorganisms, are responsible for producing essential body nutrients. An undisturbed gut flora represents a normal defense capacity. If these protecting enzymes are disturbed or destroyed, the gut becomes vulnerable to invasion by potential pathogens. Interference with the normal gut flora by the use of broad-spectrum antibiotics results in a decreased defense capacity and opens the way to intestinal colonization by pathogenic organisms.

To maintain colonization resistance, therapy directed specifically against the invading pathogen is preferred (46). The general use of broad-spectrum antibiotics has resulted in increased gastrointestinal complications caused by disturbances of intestinal microflora. The most serious manifestation is seen in pseudomembranous colitis, which has been associated with the multiplication of *Clostridium difficile* and other *Clostridium* species in the large intestine depleted of its normal anaerobic bacterial flora (47). Cytotoxins produced by *Cl. difficile* are responsible for the lesions of this disease. An animal model for antibiotic-induced colitis has been developed (48) in which antibiotics causing pseudomembranous colitis in humans also cause *Cl. difficile* toxin-mediated hemorrhagic cectitis in hamsters (49). When broad-spectrum antibiotics such as cefoperazone are given parenterally to hamsters, a dramatic increase in the normal intestinal anaerobic flora is evident by 24 hr (50) (Fig. 5). This allows for an invasion and proliferation of nonindigenous organisms, such as *Cl. difficile.* Within 4 days of cefoperazone administration, all the hamsters so treated died from hemorrhagic cectitis, and *Cl. difficile* and its toxins could be demonstrated in the ceci of these animals.

In contrast, when hamsters were treated with aztreonam, either parenterally or orally, the animals remained alive and healthy. Neither *Cl. difficile* nor its toxins could be demonstrated in the ceci of the treated animals. In these experiments aztreonam allowed the anaerobic microflora to remain unchanged, thus protecting the colonization resistance mechanisms. While aztreonam does eliminate the intestinal coliforms (Fig. 5), this does not adversely affect the hamsters. On the contrary, in hospital situations it has been found beneficial to selectively eliminate aerobic gram-negative bacteria from the intestinal microflora of immunocompromised patients, because serious systemic infections due to these organisms frequently arise from the gastrointestinal tract (51).

4. Immunology

Penicillin and cephalosporin antibiotics have proven to be immunologically cross-reactive to various degrees, owing to similar nuclear structures, despite marked differences in side-chain configuration (52-54). This cross-reactivity of available penicillins has hampered clinical administration of these antibiotics.

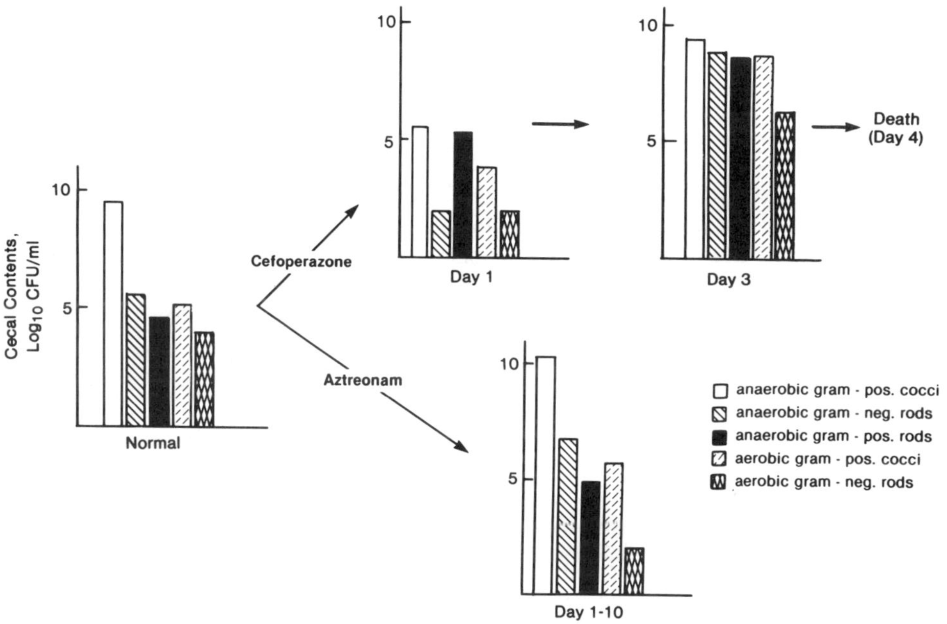

Figure 5 Comparative effects of cefoperazone and aztreonam on hamster intestinal microflora. Adapted from Fernandes et al. (50). Used with permission of the Laux Company, Inc., Ayer, MA.

The monocyclic beta-lactam nucleus of aztreonam is markedly different from the bicyclic nuclei of available beta-lactam compounds; therefore studies were undertaken by Adkinson et al. (55) to assess the immunological cross-reactivity among aztreonam, benzylpenicillin, and cephalothin.

Rabbits were immunized with protein conjugates of benzylpenicillin, cephalothin (CEPH), and aztreonam (AZ). The resulting anti-benzylpenicilloyl (BPO) and anti-CEPH rabbit IgG antibodies showed negligible cross-reactivity with aztreonam conjugated to human serum albumin (AZ-HSA); similarly, rabbit anti-AZ IgG showed negligible cross-reactivity with BPO-HSA and CEPH-HSA. Unlike benzylpenicillin and cephalothin, unconjugated aztreonam was as effective as aztreonam conjugated to ϵ-aminocaproic acid (Az-EACA) in inhibiting binding of homologous antibody. Immunoglobulin G anti-AZ was found to be entirely side-chain specific in studies with various analogs of aztreonam.

In a separate study the inhibition of binding of human IgE anti-penicilloyl to BPO-HSA was investigated in the presence of AZ-EACA, BPO-formyllysine, and CEPH-EACA. Whereas CEPH-EACA displayed 3% cross-reactivity with BPO-lysine, AZ-EACA showed little or no cross-reactivity (<<0.9%). The findings suggest that at least those penicillin-allergic patients with major determinant (penicilloyl) allergy may receive treatment with aztreonam with little likelihood of cross-allergenicity (55).

IV. CLINICAL PHARMACOLOGY

The safety, absorption, distribution, metabolism, and elimination of aztreonam has been investigated in healthy volunteers. The disposition of aztreonam has also been studied in volunteers with impaired excretory function and patients with infections under treatment with aztreonam. The pharmacodynamics of aztreonam have been described by measuring bactericidal activity in body fluids after drug administration. The effect of aztreonam on fecal flora and the immunology of aztreonam have also been investigated.

A. Healthy Subjects

The pharmacokinetics of aztreonam in animals was extrapolated (based on empiric correlations of serum clearance and volume of distribution with body weight) to humans in order to plan the first clinical pharmacology study of aztreonam, administered as a single 0.125- to 4-g intravenous dose to healthy volunteers (56). Aztreonam was first administered to humans in April 1981.

Aztreonam is measurable in human serum and urine by microbiological and high-pressure liquid chromatography (HPLC) methods, which give similar results, indicating the lack of microbiologically active metabolites (57).

The serum and urinary concentrations of aztreonam administered as a single 0.5-g intravenous (3-min infusion), intramuscular (gluteus maximus), or oral (solution) dose are given in Table 15 (58–60). The highest serum levels are achieved after intravenous dosing; however, the serum levels 1 hr after equal intravenous and intramuscular doses are similar. A 0.5-g dose given parenterally achieves potentially therapeutic urinary levels for 12–24 hr after dosing. Aztreonam is eliminated primarily unchanged in the urine. The oral bioavailability of aztreonam is less than 1%.

Serum and urinary concentrations after 1-g doses (intravenous and intramuscular) and after a 2-g dose (intravenous) are given in Table 16 (58,60). As before, doses given intravenously were infused over 3 min and doses given intramuscularly were administered into the gluteus maximus. Urinary levels of aztreonam were very high, consistent with the function of the kidney as the primary excretory organ for this monobactam.

The serum levels of aztreonam after 0.5-, 1-, and 2-g intravenous 3-min infusions and after 0.5- and 1-g intramuscular injections are compared with the in vitro MIC_{90} values (16) for various gram-negative bacteria in Figure 6. All doses achieve potentially therapeutic levels for most Enterobacteriaceae, as well as

Table 15 Serum and Urinary Concentrations (μg/ml, mean ± SEM) of Aztreonam After a 0.5-g Parenteral or Oral Dose in Healthy Volunteers

Time postdose	Route of administration		
	Intravenous (N=6)	Intramuscular (N=6)	Peroral solution (N=15)
Serum			
5 min	50 ± 3	4.8 ± 1.0	–
1 hr	23 ± 1	22 ± 2	0.11 ± 0.02
4 hr	6.7 ± 0.2	8.9 ± 0.5	0.11 ± 0.02
6 hr	2.9 ± 0.2	3.8 ± 0.3	0.08 ± 0.02
8 hr	1.3 ± 0.1	1.7 ± 0.2	<0.04
12 hr	0.26 ± 0.04	0.30 ± 0.05	<0.04
AUC[a] (μg hr/ml)	94 ± 2	84 ± 3	0.45 ± 0.08
Urine			
0-2 hr	1400 ± 200	520 ± 190	2.9 ± 0.7
4-6 hr	330 ± 57	420 ± 87	6.6 ± 1.4
8-12 hr	50 ± 8	27 ± 8	1.4 ± 0.2
16-24 hr	1.9 ± 0.4	1.3 ± 0.3	0.31 ± 0.05
Percent recovery	69 ± 2	62 ± 4	0.7 ± 0.1

[a]AUC = area under the curve.
Source: Data from Refs. 58-60, with permission.

Hemophilus and *Neisseria*, for 8-12 hr. A 2-g intravenous dose achieves mean serum concentrations of aztreonam exceeding the MIC_{90} of *Ps. aeruginosa* and *Enterobacter cloacae* for about 4-6 hr.

Two studies of aztreonam administered as 0.5-, 1-, and 2-g 30-min intravenous infusions to healthy volunteers have confirmed the linearity and predictability of aztreonam kinetics and the previously mentioned implications regarding therapeutical potential (61,62). Comparative studies in healthy volunteers have shown that aztreonam has a pharmacokinetic profile similar to that of moxalactam (63) and cefoperazone (64).

Aztreonam has been administered to four groups of nine healthy volunteers according to various multiple-dose regimens: 0.5 and 1 g intravenously every 8 hr for 7 days, and 0.5 and 1 g intramuscularly (gluteus maximus) every 8 hr for 7 days (65). The pharmacokinetic profiles of aztreonam after the first and last doses were very similar (Fig. 7) and corresponded to those seen after single 0.5-

Table 16 Serum and Urinary Concentrations (μg/ml, mean ± SEM) of Aztreonam After a 1- or 2-g Parenteral Dose in Healthy Volunteers

Time postdose	1-g dose Intravenous (N=6)	1-g dose Intramuscular (N=6)	2-g dose (N=6)
Serum			
5 min	125 ± 4	8.6 ± 2.3	242 ± 20
1 hr	49 ± 2	46 ± 3	91 ± 6
4 hr	13.2 ± 0.3	18.4 ± 0.6	26 ± 2
6 hr	6.0 ± 0.3	8.2 ± 0.4	13 ± 1
8 hr	2.7 ± 0.1	3.5 ± 0.2	6.0 ± 0.6
12 hr	0.51 ± 0.02	0.65 ± 0.09	1.2 ± 0.1
AUC[a] (μg hr/ml)	191 ± 5	180 ± 4	379 ± 23
Urine			
0-2 hr	3000 ± 1200	1200 ± 320	6500 ± 1100
4-6 hr	720 ± 190	640 ± 200	1800 ± 520
8-12 hr	70 ± 10	140 ± 28	180 ± 58
16-24 hr	2.8 ± 0.5	5.0 ± 2.7	9.8 ± 3.1
Percent recovery	74 ± 3	69 ± 3	65 ± 3

[a]AUC = area under the curve.
Source: Data from Refs. 58 and 60, with permission.

and 1-g doses (Tables 15 and 16). Though serum levels of aztreonam were essentially constant, indicating no apparent accumulation of the antibiotic.

A study of the metabolism of aztreonam in healthy subjects given single 0.5-g intravenous and intramuscular doses of ^{14}C-labeled drug showed that aztreonam is excreted primarily unchanged in the urine, although the unchanged antibiotic can also be found in small amounts in the feces (66). The most prominent metabolite is SQ 26,992, the microbiologically inactive compound resulting from the hydrolytic opening of the beta-lactam ring. This compound is analogous to the penicilloate metabolite of penicillins.

Table 17 reviews the pharmacokinetic parameters for aztreonam (60). The 101% bioavailability (F), time to peak serum concentration of 1.0 hr, and half-life for absorption of 0.4 hr indicate that absorption of aztreonam from an intramuscular injection site is rapid and complete. The α-phase half-life of 0.2 hr indicates that distribution of aztreonam is rapid. Aztreonam is 56% bound to

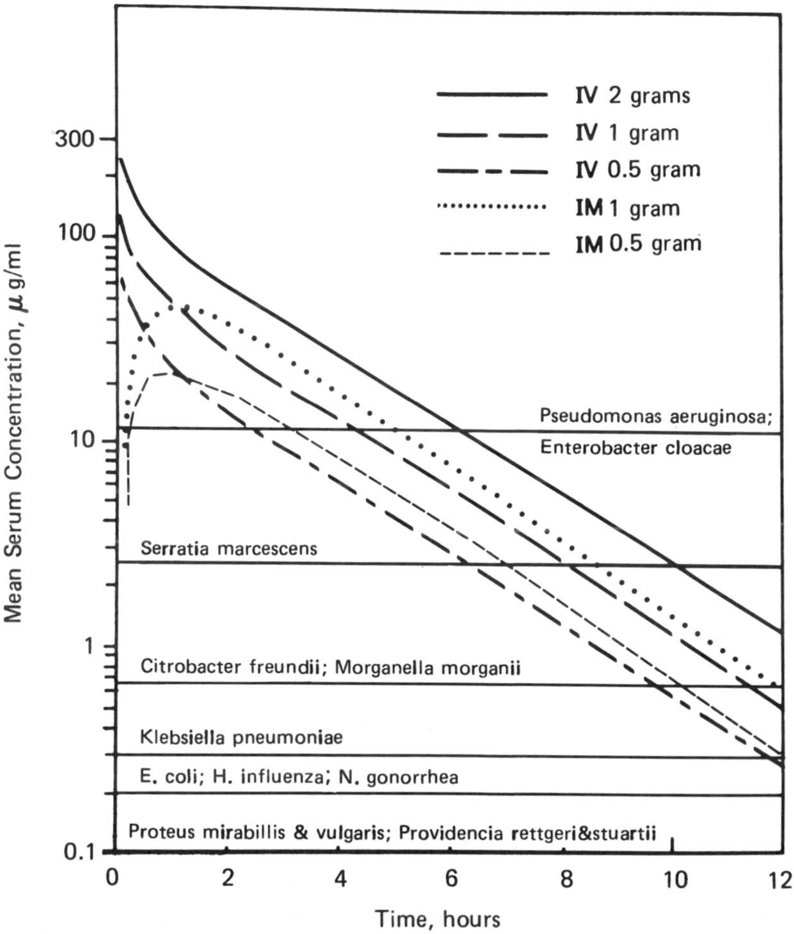

Figure 6 Comparison of pharmacokinetic profile of aztreonam in serum of healthy subjects with antibacterial activity of aztreonam in vitro. Adapted from Swabb et al. (57,58) and Sykes et al. (16). Used with permission of Academic Press, New York, and the American Society for Microbiology, Washington, D.C.

serum protein and has a steady-state volume of distribution (V_{SS}) of 0.18 liters/kg. The percent excretion of aztreonam, SQ 26,992, and unknown metabolites is listed in Table 17 and indicates that two-thirds of a dose of aztreonam is eliminated unchanged in urine, while 6.9% of a dose is excreted as SQ 26,992 by the kidneys. Approximately 1% of a dose is excreted unchanged in the feces, indicating probable biliary secretion of aztreonam. The serum clearance of aztreonam is

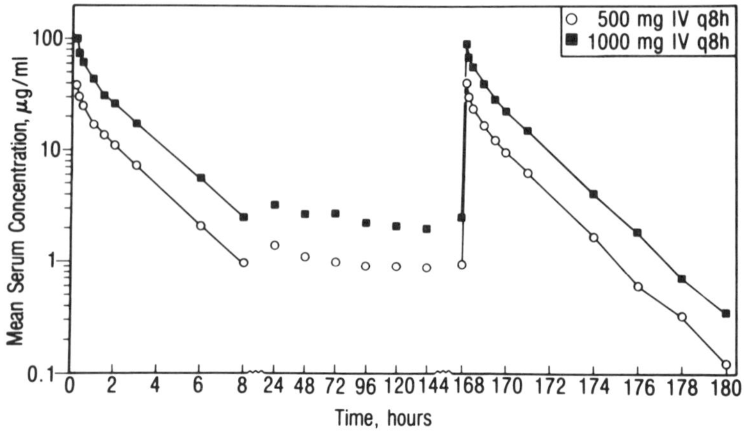

Figure 7 Multiple-dose pharmacokinetics of aztreonam in healthy subjects. Adapted from Swabb et al. (65). Used with permission of the American Society for Microbiology, Washington, D.C.

about 1.5 ml/min per kilogram and the half-life for elimination ($t_{1/2\beta}$) is 1.7 hr. Analysis of renal excretion rates indicates that SQ 26,992 has an apparent elimination half-life over 10 times that of aztreonam. The penicilloate metabolites of penicillins are also reported to be eliminated more slowly than the parent compound (67,68).

The renal handling of aztreonam has been described by studying the renal excretion of aztreonam and inulin under steady-state conditions. Loading doses followed by continuous intravenous infusions of both agents were administered in the presence and absence of probenecid treatment (69). Serum clearance of unbound aztreonam was due to (a) renal tubular secretion (two-fifths of serum clearance), (b) glomerular filtration (two-fifths), and (c) nonrenal mechanisms (one-fifth). Probenecid reduces renal tubular secretion of aztreonam by about 50% without altering aztreonam clearance by glomerular filtration and nonrenal routes. Probenecid tends to slightly increase the steady-state serum concentration and elimination half-life of aztreonam, but not to a significant extent (Fig. 8).

The safety of aztreonam administered to healthy volunteers has recently been reviewed and is summarized in Table 18 (60). The most common clinical finding was mild transient taste sensation during the intravenous infusion in about 6% of subjects. All clinical findings were mild and reversible. Transiently elevated serum transaminases in 4.6% of subjects was the most common laboratory finding. The laboratory abnormalities were reversible and not associated with

Table 17 Summary of the Pharmacokinetics of Aztreonam in Healthy Volunteers

	Parameter	Mean ± SD
Absorption	Extent	
	F(i.m.) (%)	101 ± 6
	F(p.o.) (%)	0.6 ± 0.3
	Rate	
	t peak (i.m.) (hr)	1.0 ± 0.3
	t peak (p.o.) (hr)	2.1 ± 1.5
	$t_{1/2a}$ (i.m.) (hr)	0.4 ± 0.2
Distribution (i.v.)	Extent	
	V_1 (liter/kg)	0.10 ± 0.02
	V_{SS} (liter/kg)	0.18 ± 0.04
	Percent bound in serum	56 ± 2
	Rate	
	$t_{1/2\alpha}$ (hr)	0.2 ± 0.1
	k_{12} (hr^{-1})	1.5 ± 0.4
	k_{21} (hr^{-1})	1.8 ± 0.3
Elimination (i.v.)	Extent	
	Percent excreted urine: unchanged	65.9 ± 3.0
	Percent excreted urine: SQ 26,992	6.9 ± 1.0
	Percent excreted urine: unknowns	3.2 ± 4.4
	Percent excreted feces: unchanged	1.4 ± 0.1
	Percent excreted feces: SQ 26,992	3.4 ± 0.2
	Percent excreted feces: unknowns	7.5 ± 0.2
	Serum clearance (ml/min per kg)	1.5 ± 0.3
	Rate	
	$t_{1/2\beta}$ (hr)	1.7 ± 0.1
	k_{10} (hr^{-1})	0.9 ± 0.1

Source: Data from Ref. 60.

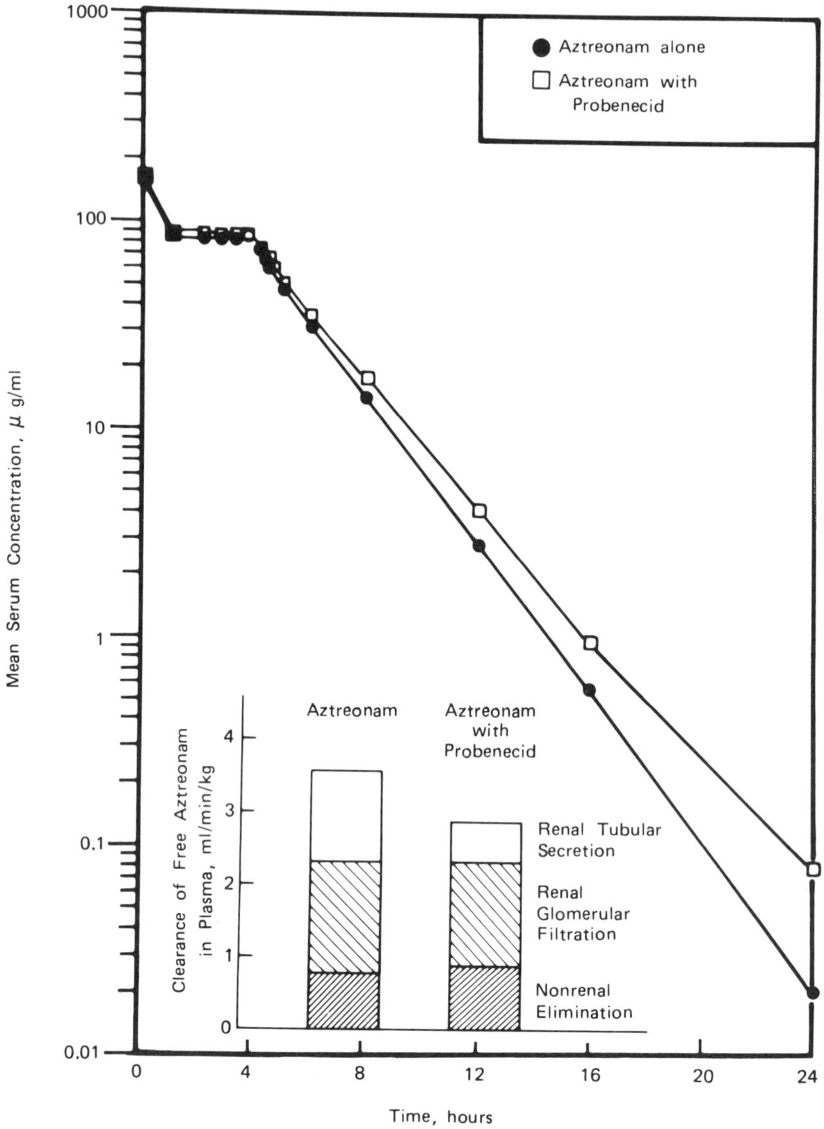

Figure 8 Influence of probenecid on the disposition of aztreonam in healthy subjects. Aztreonam was administered as an intravenous loading dose of 1.2 g over 2 min followed by a continuous infusion of 0.5 g/hr for 4 hr with and without oral probenecid (1 g b.i.d. for 2 days before aztreonam infusion and during the day of infusion). Adapted from Swabb et al. (69). Used with permission of the C.V. Mosby Company, St. Louis, MO.

Table 18 Summary of Safety Data from Clinical Pharmacology Studies of Aztreonam

Side effect	Percent (number/total subjects)
Mild taste sensation during intravenous infusion	6.0 (7/117)
Mild fatigue	2.6 (4/153)
Mild pruritic, erythematous rash	1.3 (2/153)
Sneezing and nasal congestion	0.6 (1/153)
Loose stools within 0.5-1.5 hr of dosing	0.6 (1/153)
Fever (100.4°F), headache, and malaise	0.6 (1/153)
Elevated SGOT and/or SGPT two to three times the ULN[a]	4.6 (7/153)
Elevated LDH	2.0 (3/153)
Elevated GGTP	1.3 (2/153)
Elevated alkaline phosphatase	1.3 (2/153)
Relative eosinophilia	0.6 (1/153)

[a]ULN = upper limit of normal range.
Source: Data from Ref. 60 (based upon 153 subjects).

apparent symptoms or physical findings of organ injury. Similar transient elevations of serum transaminase values are seen with penicillins and cephalosporins.

The urinary excretion of N-acetyl-β-glucosaminidase, alanine aminopeptidase, and β_2-microglobulin, as well as serum creatinine and urinary creatinine clearance, during a 7-day multiple-dose study (0.5 or 1 g every 8 hr) showed no renal dysfunction associated with aztreonam (65). There were no abnormalities of hemostasis, as judged by multiple determinations of prothrombin time and partial thromboplastin time and multiple injection site evaluations (65).

B. Patients with Renal or Hepatic Insufficiency

The pharmacokinetics of 1-g intravenous doses of aztreonam in 18 patients with various degrees of chronic renal insufficiency and 6 subjects with normal renal function are summarized in Table 19 and Figure 9 (70). The serum clearance of aztreonam was linearly related to urinary creatinine clearance, as described by the regression equation in Table 19. In the presence of severe renal insufficiency the mean serum clearance of aztreonam is about one-fourth normal and the

Table 19 Effect of Renal Insufficiency on the Pharmacokinetics of Aztreonam

Parameter[a]	Category of creatinine clearance (ml/min) >80 (N=6)	30–80 (N=6)	10–29 (N=6)	<10 (N=6)
Mean creatinine clearance (ml/min per 70 kg)	106	42	19	4
V_{SS} (liters/kg)	0.22	0.17	0.18	0.19
$t_{1/2}\beta$ (hr)	2.0	3.4	4.8	6.0
Serum aztreonam clearance (ml/min)	107	46	34	29
Percent excreted in urine unchanged	58	40	21	1.4
Percent free in serum	42	51	57	64

[a]Aztreonam clearance = 0.80 creatinine clearance + 26.6, r = 0.97.
Source: Data from Ref. 70, with permission.

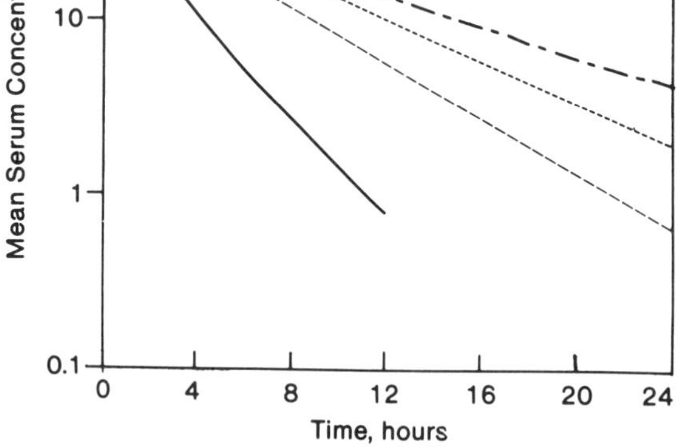

Figure 9 Influence of renal insufficiency on the pharmacokinetic profile of aztreonam in serum after a 1-g intravenous dose. Adapted from Mihindu et al. (70). Used with permission of the American Society for Microbiology, Washington, D.C.

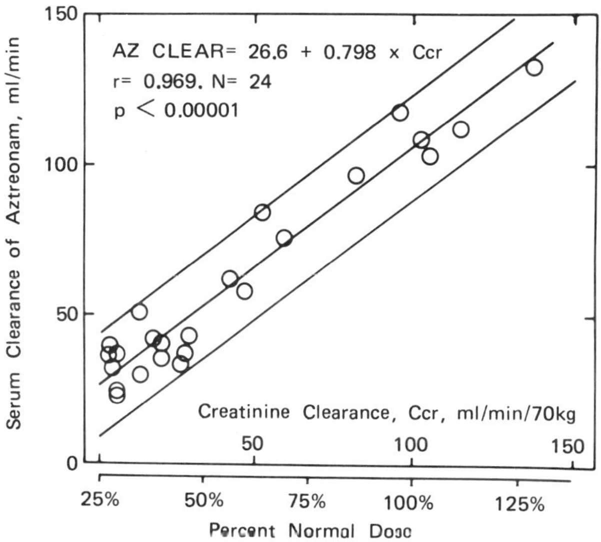

Figure 10 Relationship between serum clearance of aztreonam and creatinine clearance, with recommended dosage adjustment. Adapted from Mihindu et al. (70). Used with permission of the American Society for Microbiology, Washington, D.C.

mean elimination half-life is about three times normal. A nomogram has been proposed to guide dosage adjustment (Fig. 10). Similar results have been obtained by other investigators (71). Serum protein binding of aztreonam declines slightly with increasing renal insufficiency, as has been reported for other drugs in the presence of uremia.

Aztreonam is cleared by both hemodialysis and chronic ambulatory peritoneal dialysis (71-73). A standard 4-hr hemodialysis treatment will remove about half of a 1-g dose administered just prior to dialysis. In a group of six patients supported by hemodialysis the serum half-life for aztreonam was 7.9 hr between dialysis sessions and 2.7 hr during hemodialysis. In contrast, chronic ambulatory peritoneal dialysis (6-hr dwell time) removed about 10% of a 1-g intravenous dose in 48 hr. Clearance of aztreonam by either method of dialysis was approximately 30% that of urea. The systemic bioavailability of intraperitoneally administered aztreonam was approximately 60-70%.

The half-life of aztreonam in patients with biliary cirrhosis and alcoholic cirrhosis was 2.2 and 3.2 hr, respectively, compared to 1.9 hr in concurrently studied healthy subjects (74). Alcoholic cirrhotics also had a 24% drop in serum clearance and a 50% decrease in nonrenal clearance compared to healthy volunteers.

C. Infected Patients

In patients undergoing treatment with intravenous aztreonam for lower respiratory tract or urinary tract infections (75), there was a notable increase in the elimination of aztreonam from the first or second day to the last day of therapy. This could be explained by concurrent improvement in renal function, typically related to reversal of dehydration or resolution of pyelonephritis. Serum protein binding of aztreonam averaged 30% in patients and about 50% in fresh serum from healthy volunteers, probably owing to undefined factors relating to infection or uremia. Another study of patients with urinary tract infections and renal insufficiency found that serum levels of SQ 26,992 increased by 4- to 11-fold during therapy in patients with creatinine clearances of less than 25 ml/min (76).

D. Penetration into Body Fluids and Tissues

Aztreonam was secreted into bile (77) and reached a mean peak concentration of 43 μg/ml 2.4 hr after administration of a 1-g intravenous dose in postcholecystectomy patients with a T-tube in place for partial collection of bile output. In contrast, patients with complete biliary obstruction due to carcinoma of the pancreas or ampulla had an average maximum biliary concentration of aztreonam of 14 μg/ml 1.0 hr after drug administration. Only 0.2% of the 1-g dose was recovered in 12-hr quantitative bile collections from the latter patients. Of the 14 patients in this study, only 1 had quantitatively detectable SQ 26,992 in the bile.

In contrast to the results given above, approximately 12% of a 0.5-g parenteral dose of ^{14}C-labeled aztreonam was recovered in the feces of healthy subjects (66), suggesting that biliary obstruction inhibits aztreonam secretion in the bile.

After a 1-g, 2-min intravenous infusion of aztreonam in nine healthy subjects, the maximum mean saliva level was 0.2 μg/ml at 0.5 hr (data on file, The Squibb Institute for Medical Research).

In patients with normal meninges receiving a 2-g intravenous dose of aztreonam, the mean cerebrospinal fluid (CSF) concentrations were 0.5 and 1 μg/ml at 1 and 4 hr, respectively (78). In contrast, mean levels were 2 and 3.2 μg/ml at 1 and 4 hr, respectively, in the presence of meningitis, indicating that meningeal inflammation produced approximately three to four times higher CSF levels of aztreonam than those reached in the absence of inflammation. Maximum CSF levels were found at 2-4 hr after dosing. These results were confirmed in a separate study of single 2-g intravenous doses in patients with meningitis (79). The pharmacokinetics of aztreonam indicated that a 2-g, every 6- or 8-hourly intravenous dosage regimen would be potentially therapeutic for members of the Enterobacteriaceae commonly responsible for gram-negative baciliary meningitis.

Intravenously administered aztreonam entered artificially produced blister fluid in six healthy subjects and reached a maximum concentration of 20 μg/ml 1 hr after dosing, after which blister fluid levels were comparable to serum drug levels and declined in parallel (80).

In a study of 15 patients receiving aztreonam therapy for intra-abdominal infections, aztreonam penetrated into peritoneal fluid, achieving a peritoneal fluid to serum concentration ratio of 0.95:1.0 (81); the ratio of the peritoneal fluid concentration to the infecting organism MIC was typically in excess of 10:1 for gram-negative isolates.

Aztreonam levels of 2.1 to 12.5 μg/ml have been reported in the aqueous humor of patients who received multiple 1- or 2-g parenteral doses (82). In four patients undergoing nephrectomies a single 2-g intravenous dose of aztreonam achieved concentrations in the renal cortex, medulla, and papilla of 4.6-70, 31-61, and 34-103 μg/ml, respectively (83).

E. Special Studies

Aztreonam was administered as 1-g doses infused intravenously over 30 min every 8 hr for 6-9 days to patients receiving cancer chemotherapy and residing in sterile isolation rooms in order to investigate the effects of the antibiotic on oral and fecal flora and the pharmacokinetics of the drug (84). Although there was no evident effect on the numbers of oral aerobic bacteria and fungi, there was a dramatic decline in fecal counts of aerobic gram-negative bacilli, without notable alterations in the other aerobic or anaerobic bacteria or fungi. Aerobic gram-negative rods were initially present in the feces of eight of nine patients and were completely eradicated at the end of therapy in five of eight (62.5%) patients.

Similar results were found when aztreonam was administered in multiple oral doses (20, 100, and 500 mg every 8 hr for 5 days) to healthy volunteers. There was a dramatic decrease in aerobic gram-negative bacteria, without noteworthy changes in anaerobes or fungi (85). These results suggest that aztreonam has a potential application in the oral prophylaxis of infection in immunocompromised patients, because the drug can selectively decontaminate the intestinal tract without impairing the colonization resistance function of anaerobes in the gut.

In studies of 36 healthy subjects receiving multiple parenteral doses of aztreonam (65), the incidence of a detectable aztreonam antibody response was 0 out of 36 for IgE and 1 out of 36 for IgG, suggesting that aztreonam is only weakly immunogenic in humans not previously exposed to the drug (55). The IgG antibody to aztreonam was not cross-reactive with penicillin in vitro. To assess the potential for aztreonam to cross-react with IgE antibodies directed against penicillin derivatives, 41 penicillin-skin-test-positive and 40 control subjects were skin tested with aztreonam, SQ 26,992, and SQ 26,992 conjugated to polylysine (86). No evidence was found for immunological cross-reactivity between aztreonam and penicillin. As discussed previously, studies in vitro have shown a lack of immunological cross-reactivity of aztreonam with benzylpenicillin and cephalothin, as might be expected for a beta-lactam compound having a radically different (monocyclic, as opposed to bicyclic) chemical structure (55).

Early results from an investigation of the pharmacokinetics of aztreonam (single 30-mg/kg intravenous dose) in pediatric patients indicate that, as expected, clearance of the monobactam is slower in newborns, particularly in patients under 1 week of age and 2.5 kg body weight (87).

V. THERAPEUTIC USES

Reported therapeutic trials of aztreonam can be divided into studies having a single treatment group and comparative studies involving randomization of an aztreonam treatment regimen and an alternate antimicrobial regimen. Some of the larger early studies in these categories are summarized in this section and Table 20. Many other studies are in progress and will be the subjects of future publications.

A. Studies Having a Single Treatment Group

The earliest and largest reported study in this category was performed by Scully and Neu (88) in 74 critically ill patients. The majority of patients received intravenous infusions of 1 g of aztreonam over 30 min every 8 hr. Some patients having pulmonary infections due to *Pseudomonas* received 1.5 or 2 g every 8 hr. The duration of therapy ranged from 5 to 47 days (mean, 14 days). Patients who were considered to be possibly infected with gram-positive aerobes or anaerobic organisms were given either oxacillin or vancomycin, or clindamycin or metronidazole. The 77 treated infections consisted of bacteremia (12 patients), respiratory infection (23 patients), soft tissue infection (5 patients), osteomyelitis-septic arthritis (9 patients), intra-abdominal infection (4 patients), and urinary tract infections (24 patients). Causative organisms included *Ps. aeruginosa* (47), *Klebsiella* (8), *Enterobacter* (6), *E. coli* (12), *P. alcaligenes* (1), *H. influenzae* (2), *Serratia* (7), *Proteus mirabilis* (2), *Providencia stuartii* (1), and *Citrobacter freundii* (1). The overall clinical cure and bacteriological eradication rates were 88 and 57%, respectively.

Aztreonam displayed a good safety profile, and no major adverse effects were noted: 1 patient had a rash, 3 had eosinophila, and 15 had minor increases in SGOT and SGPT. Aztreonam was judged to be a safe alternative to aminoglycosides and an antibiotic useful for providing more directed therapy of hospital-acquired infections.

Table 20 Design of Reported Therapeutic Trials of Aztreonam

Aztreonam dosing	Single-treatment[a] indication	Randomized treatments: Indication	Comparison drug[b]	Additional drug common to both treatments
Single dose	–	Acute uncomplicated gonorrhea	Spectinomycin (93, 94)[c]	–
Multiple dose	UTI[d] (88–90, 92)	UTI	Cefamandole (95)	–
	LRTI[e] (88–92)		Gentamicin (96)	–
	Intra-abdominal (88, 89, 91)		Tobramycin (97)	–
	Bone and joint (88, 90–92)	LRTI	Tobramycin (98, 99)	Clindamycin
	Skin and skin structure (88, 90–92)			
	Septicemia (88, 89, 91, 92)	Gynecological	Gentamicin (100)	Clindamycin or metronidazole
	Gynecological (90)			

[a]Additional antibiotics were often administered for coverage of gram-positive organisms.
[b]Randomized in a ratio (aztreonam:comparison drug) of 1:1, except for UTI and LRTI, where a 2:1 ratio was used.
[c]References in parentheses.
[d]UTI = urinary tract infection.
[e]LRTI = lower respiratory tract infection.

A second study of aztreonam therapy in 24 high-risk patients was conducted by Garcia-Rodriguez et al. (89), who used a treatment regimen of 1 g intravenously every 6 hr. Five patients with polymicrobial infections received, in addition, metronidazole, gentamicin, or amikacin. Infections consisted of pneumonia, sepsis, peritonitis, or urinary tract infection and were due to a variety of susceptible organisms [*E. coli* (13), *Klebsiella* (5), *Ser. marcescens* (6), and *Prot. mirabilis* (3)]. Overall clinical cure and microbiological eradication rates were both 79%. Superinfections due to *Candida albicans* were noted in three patients, two of whom were receiving multiple antibiotics.

Greenberg et al. (90) treated 35 patients with aerobic gram-negative infections. Patients appearing septic or with an infection due to a *Pseudomonas* species received intravenous aztreonam at a dose of 2 g every 6 hr. Other infections were usually treated intravenously or intramuscularly with 1-2 g every 8-12 hours. Duration of therapy ranged from 5 to 42 days. Antibiotics for gram-positive aerobic or anaerobic organisms included penicillin, oxacillin, vancomycin, and clindamycin and were administered to 13 patients. Infections consisted of pyelonephritis (25 patients), pneumonia (5 patients), soft tissue infection (2 patients), osteomyelitis (2 patients), and postoperative endometritis (1 patient). Bacterial isolates included *E. coli* (11), *Prot. mirabilis* (8), *Klebsiella* species (7), *Enterobacter* species (4), *Pseudomonas fluorescens* (4), *Citrobacter* species (3), *Ps. aeruginosa* (2), and *Prov. stuartii* (1). Overall clinical cure and bacterial eradication rates were 89%. Minor reactions included phlebitis (4 patients), rash (1 patient), pruritis (1 patient), and mild transient elevations in liver function tests (11 patients). Superinfections due to enterococci (1 patient) and *Staph. aureus* (1 patient) were noted.

Mokhbat et al. (91) treated 27 patients with infections (urinary tract, bacteremia, intra-abdominal, soft tissue, osteomyelitis, pneumonia) due to a variety of gram-negative organisms—*E. Coli* (14), *Ps. aeruginosa* (10), and others. Other antibiotics, (e.g., benzylpenicillin, nafcillin, clindamycin, metronidazole, and vancomycin) were added to treat gram-positive or gram-negative anaerobic organisms. The overall clinical cure and microbiological eradication rates were 65 and 73%, respectively. Adverse effects consisted of elevations in hepatic enzymes (seven patients), diarrhea (four patients), bleeding disorders (two patients), and local irritation (one patient). Superinfections were noted at the original infection site in seven patients. In two patients *Ps. aeruginosa* strains isolated during therapy were resistant when compared to baseline organisms; this apparent increased resistance was not confirmed by serotyping. One of the patients was a clinical failure. Of the 27 patients, 5 had histories of allergic reactions to penicillins or cephalosporins but tolerated aztreonam without any manifestation of hypersensitivity.

Giamarellou et al. (92) administered aztreonam to 23 patients according to an intramuscular, 1-g every 8 hr dosage regimen, and to 10 patients as an intravenous, 2-g every 8 hr treatment regimen. The infections consisted of upper urinary tract infections (23 patients), exacerbation of chronic osteomyelitis (3 patients), bronchopneumonia (3 patients), soft tissue infection (3 patients), and septicemia (1 patient). The following microorganisms were isolated from cultures: *E. coli* (12), *Prot. mirabilis* (5), *Ent. cloacae* (4), *Ent. aerogenes* (1), *C. freundii* (3), and *Ps. aeruginosa* (8). The MICs for *Enterobactericeae* were less than 0.5 μg/ml and those for *Ps. aeruginosa* were 2-16 μg/ml. Overall clinical cure and microbiological eradication rates were 88 and 90%, respectively. Side effects consisted of pain at the intramuscular injection site (seven patients), elevated serum transaminases (three patients), prolonged prothrombin time (one patient), and allergic purpura (one patient). It was noted that none of the patients had diarrhea, and it was speculated that this was due to the lack of influence of aztreonam on colonization resistance of the gut.

B. Studies Using Randomization of Treatments

Studies in this category consisted of single-dose treatment of acute gonorrhea and multiple-dose therapy of urinary tract, lower respiratory tract, and gynecological infections.

1. Gonorrhea

Mogabgab et al. (93) treated 263 patients with known or suspected acute uncomplicated gonorrhea with 1 g of aztreonam or 2 g of spectinomycin using intramuscular injections. No penicillinase-producing *N. gonorrhoeae* were encountered. In 184 evaluable patients, microbiological eradication was achieved in 23 of 25 (92%) males with urethral infections and in 68 of 68 (100%) females with urethral, endocervical, or anal canal infections. For spectinomycin the corresponding rates were 24 of 24 (100%) and 65 of 67 (97%), respectively. Adverse effects consisted of mild pain or discomfort at the injection site in 30% of the aztreonam recipients and 40% of the spectinomycin group. Three patients with histories of penicillin allergy received aztreonam without reaction.

Miller et al. (94) treated 112 men with gonococcal urethritis, of whom 93 were evaluable: 51 received aztreonam and 42 received spectinomycin. Both drugs were 100% effective in the therapy of urethritis produced by both penicillin-sensitive and penicillin-resistant strains of *N. gonorrhoeae*. There were no reported side effects in either group.

2. Urinary Tract Infection

Randomized clinical trials have compared the efficacy and safety of aztreonam with cefamandole, gentamicin, and tobramycin in the therapy of urinary tract infections.

Childs et al. (95) entered 111 patients into a study in which treatment with aztreonam (1 g intravenously every 8 hr in the first 32 patients, then 1 g every

12 hr in following patients) or cefamandole (1 g intravenously every 8 hr) was randomized in a 2:1 ratio. Most patients had cystitis or pyelonephritis; the mean duration of therapy was 7 days in all treatment groups. Complicating factors, such as neurogenic bladder, renal calculi, prostatic obstruction, surgery, or instrumentation existed in 64-72% of patients in the three treatment groups. Causative organisms generally consisted of *E. coli, Klebsiella,* and *Prot. mirabilis.* Overall clinical response was judged satisfactory in 21 of 21 (100%), 49 of 50 (98%), and 28 of 32 (88%) evaluable patients receiving aztreonam three times daily, aztreonam twice daily, and cefamandole, respectively; the corresponding microbiological eradication rates were 57, 64, and 34%, respectively. The differences in clinical response and bacteriological eradication rates (aztreonam versus cefamandole) were clinically significant. The most common reinfecting or superinfecting organisms were enterococci in the aztreonam groups (11 patients) and *Ps. aeruginosa* in the cefamandole group (10 patients). Whereas reinfection or superinfection with enterococci was frequently asymptomatic and, if necessary, treatable on an outpatient basis, the superinfections and reinfections with *Pseudomonas* in cefamandole-treated patients were usually symptomatic and required additional hospitalization for parenteral antibiotic therapy. Adverse reactions consisted of stomatitis and glossitis in one aztreonam patient and mild reversible elevations in serum transaminases in approximately 10% of aztreonam- and cefamandole-treated patients.

Sattler et al. (96) randomized treatment with aztreonam or gentamicin in a 2:1 ratio to 59 patients with urinary tract infections. Patients normally received 1 g of aztreonam or 1 mg/kg gentamicin every 8 hr intravenously or intramuscularly, while patients with presumed bacteremia received 2 g and 1.7 mg/kg, respectively. The mean duration of therapy was 6.7 and 6.2 days in the aztreonam and gentamicin groups, respectively. Infecting organisms consisted primarily of *E. coli, Ps. aeruginosa, Klebsiella,* and *Proteus.* A favorable microbiological response was achieved in 35 of 35 (100%) patients treated with aztreonam and in 13 of 16 (81%) treated with gentamicin, while favorable clinical responses were found in all patients in both treatment groups. In both groups relapse, reinfection, and failure were associated with an anatomical or physiological abnormality of the urinary tract. Group D streptococcal colonization was evident in 11 aztreonam-treated and 1 gentamicin-treated patient but typically did not require specific therapy. Adverse reactions in the aztreonam-treated group consisted of bad taste after each infusion (one patient), *Candida* vaginitis (one patient), and asymptomatic liver test abnormalities (seven patients). In patients treated with gentamicin adverse reactions consisted of liver test abnormalities (two patients) and elevations in serum creatinine (four patients).

In a similar study of 45 male patients with urinary tract infections (97), aztreonam (1 g every 8 hr) and tobramycin (1 mg/kg every 8 hr) were administered intramuscularly for 7-10 days. The rate of eradication of infecting organisms (primarily *E. coli, Citrobacter, Klebsiella, Proteus,* and *Pseudomonas*) was 65% in the aztreonam group and 73% in the tobramycin group. Persistence and superinfection in the aztreonam group were due to *Streptococcus faecalis*. There were no adverse reactions noted, except for mild pain at the intramuscular injection site.

3. Lower Respiratory Tract Infection

Two studies compared the efficacy of aztreonam and tobramycin in lower respiratory tract infections due to gram-negative pathogens. Radriguez and Ramirez-Ronda (98) enrolled 40 patients who received, in a randomized 2:1 fashion, either aztreonam (1-2 g every 8 hr) or tobramycin (80-100 mg every 8 hr) for 6-27 days. All patients also received clindamycin (2.4 g/day). Infecting organisms that were isolated in the aztreonam group consisted of *K. pneumoniae* (5), *E. coli* (5), *Ps. aeruginosa* (4), *Enterobacter* (2), and three others, while organisms in the tobramycin group consisted of *E. coli* (4), *K. pneumoniae* (2), and two others. Overall clinical cure and bacterial eradication rates were 92 and 100%, respectively, in aztreonam-treated patients, and 86 and 100%, respectively, in tobramycin-treated patients. Adverse reactions in the aztreonam group consisted of thrombocytosis (five patients), elevated alkaline phosphatase (one patient), elevated serum transaminases (two patients), and eosinophilia (two patients). The tobramycin group had the following adverse reactions: rash (one patient), reversible changes in renal function (one patient), thrombocytosis (three patients), eosinophilia (one patient), and elevated serum transaminase (one patient).

Nolen et al. (99) studied 34 patients using aztreonam (1-2 g every 8 hr) and tobramycin (5 mg/kg per day) intravenously and randomized in a 2:1 ratio. Clindamycin (600 mg every 8 hr intravenously) was also administered for coverage against possible gram-positive and anaerobic organisms. Treatment lasted 5-14 days. Causative organisms isolated from the aztreonam group consisted of *Ps. aeruginosa* (9), *E. coli* (3), *Prot. mirabilis* (3), and 11 others, while the tobramycin group had *Ps. aeruginosa* (6), *Prot. mirabilis* (2), and 3 others. Microbiological eradication rates were 81 and 9% in the aztreonam and tobramycin groups, respectively. It was noted that the response to tobramycin was lower than expected; however, the number of patients in this group was limited, and many of these patients had been previously treated with aminoglycosides. Adverse reactions consisted of rash (one patient), and mild diarrhea (one patient) in the aztreonam group and hearing loss (one patient), transient increase in serum creatinine (one patient), and transient abnormal liver function tests (one patient) in the tobramycin group.

4. Gynecological Infection

Gibbs and Blanco (100) treated 45 patients with endometritis after cesarean section with either aztreonam (2 g every 8 hr) or gentamicin (1.5 mg/kg every

8 hr) intravenously, according to a 1:1 randomization scheme. All patients also received clindamycin (600 mg every 6 hr) intravenously. Infecting organisms consisted of a variety of gram-positive and gram-negative aerobic and anaerobic bacteria. The overall cure rate was 95% in both treatment groups. Adverse reactions consisted of diarrhea in one patient in each group.

VI. CONCLUSION

The discovery of monobactams is a clear demarcation point in beta-lactam chronology. The bacterial origin of the monobactams and their uniquely activated monocyclic structure set them apart from all of their beta-lactam predecessors. Freed from the constraints imposed by a second fused ring, rapid progress has been made in the synthesis and evaluation of new monocyclic beta-lactams. Aztreonam is the first monobactam to undergo extensive clinical trials.

Aztreonam is a novel, completely synthetic, monocyclic beta-lactam antibiotic with a spectrum of activity that is specifically for the treatment of patients with infections due to aerobic gram-negative bacteria. Studies of aztreonam in vitro have shown potent activity against aerobic gram-negative bacteria, including many drug-resistant and beta-lactamase-producing strains. Most genera of Enterobacteriaceae, as well as most strains of *H. influenzae* and *N. gonorrhoeae,* are inhibited by aztreonam concentrations below 1 μg/ml, while *Ps. aeruginosa* is typically inhibited by concentrations of 12 μg/ml or lower. In addition, microbiological studies have demonstrated synergism when aztreonam is combined with an aminoglycoside for the eradication of certain strains of *Pseudomonas.* Aztreonam fails to induce bacterial production of beta-lactamases.

Aztreonam lacks notable activity against gram-positive bacteria and anaerobes and therefore has less potential for harming normal bacterial flora (a problem associated with the use of broad-spectrum antibiotics). This monobactam also lacks significant immunological cross-reactivity with penicillin in vitro and therefore has less potential for evoking hypersensitivity reactions in individuals who are allergic to other beta-lactams. Aztreonam offers potent therapy targeted against aerobic gram-negative bacteria without the risk of ototoxicity and nephrotoxicity associated with aminoglycosides.

In clinical pharmacology studies in healthy volunteers and patients aztreonam has shown a favorable pharmacokinetic profile. Serum and urine levels after 0.5-, 1-, and 2-g doses are potentially therapeutic for gram-negative organisms that are susceptible to aztreonam. Aztreonam is widely distributed in the body, and concentrations exceeding the MIC values of important gram-negative pathogens are attained in these compartments in which infections are most common. Aztreonam is primarily eliminated unchanged in the urine, although it also undergoes biliary secretion and biotransformation to a minor extent. Elimination of aztreonam can be significantly impaired in the presence of renal insufficiency. Aztreonam can be cleared by hemodialysis and, to a minor extent, by peritoneal dialysis. As has been demonstrated in animal models, parenterally and orally administered aztreonam will selectively reduce the population of aerobic gram-negative bacteria in the gut without notably altering the numbers of anaerobic organisms, thereby providing colonization resistance. Finally, volunteers with penicillin allergy have not demonstrated IgE-mediated cross-allergenicity with aztreonam based upon skin-test studies. Results of the early clinical pharmacology studies, along with knowledge of the microbiological properties of aztreonam, provided the scientific basis for the treatment regimens used in subsequent therapeutic trials.

Early clinical trials of parenterally administered aztreonam have shown the drug to be effective in the therapy of septicemia and infections of the urinary tract, lower respiratory tract, skin and skin structures, peritoneum and adjacent structures, bone and joint tissues, and female pelvic tissues, when these infections are due to susceptible organisms (most genera of the Enterobactericeae, as well as *Ps. aeruginosa*, *Neisseria gonorrhoeae*, and *Hemophilus influenzae*). Microbiological cure rates were in the range of 90%, and superinfection was infrequently encountered. Apparent increased resistance was reported in only two patients but was not confirmed by serotyping. Adverse effects have been minimal. Except for patients with acute, uncomplicated gonorrhea, for whom single 1-g doses are adequate, adults require doses ranging from 0.5 to 2 g, administered intravenously or intramuscularly every 6-12 hr. For empiric therapy when the casusative organisms have not yet been identified or for mixed infections aztreonam may be administered concurrently with appropriate antibiotics active against gram-positive and anaerobic organisms.

Aztreonam has a pattern of side effects qualitatively similar to those reported for other beta-lactam antibiotics, for example, eosinophila, rash, transiently elevated liver function test values, and mild gastrointestinal disorders. Very few patients have experienced side effects prompting discontinuation of therapy. There has been little pain or discomfort at the injection site. Based on early clinical trial reports, aztreonam appears to have a low incidence of diarrhea and therefore a low potential for impairing colonization resistance. In addition, in 134 patients receiving aztreonam and having histories of allergies to beta-lactams, only 1 (0.7%) had a possible IgE-mediated hypersensitivity reaction to aztreonam.

Aztreonam appears to be potentially very useful as a replacement for many broad-spectrum agents when more directed therapy is necessary, or for aminoglycosides in many situations where antibacterial activity against *Enterobacteriaceae* and *Pseudomonas* is needed.

REFERENCES

1. K. Kitano, K. Kintaka, S. Suzuki, K. Katamoto, K. Nara, and Y. Nakao. Screening of microorganisms capable of producing β-lactam antibiotics. *J. Ferment. Technol., 53*:327–338 (1975).
2. A. Imada, K. Kitano, K. Kintaka, M. Muroi, and M. Asai. Sulfazecin and isosulfazecin, novel β-lactam antibiotics of bacterial origin. *Nature, 289*:590–591 (1981).
3. R. B. Sykes, W. L. Parker, and J. S. Wells. β-Lactam antibiotics produced by bacteria, in *Trends in Antibiotic Research, Genetics, Biosyntheses, Actions and New Substances* (H. Umezawa, A. L. Demain, T. Hata, and C. R. Hutchinson, eds.), Japan Antibiotics Research Association, Tokyo, 1982, pp. 115–124.
4. W. C. Liu, W. L. Parker, J. S. Wells, P. A. Principe, W. H. Trejo, D. P. Bonner, and R. B. Sykes. EM5210 (SQ 26,445), a novel monobactam, in *Current Chemotherapy and Immunotherapy Proceedings of the 12th International Congress of Chemotherapy* (P. Periti and G. G. Grassi, eds.), American Society for Microbiology, Washington, D.C., 1982, pp. 328–329.
5. J. S. Wells, W. H. Trejo, P. A. Principe, K. Bush, N. H. Georgopapadakou, D. P. Bonner, and R. B. Sykes. SQ 26,180, a novel monobactam. I. Taxonomy, fermentation and biological properties. *J. Antibiot., 35*:184–188 (1982).
6. J. S. Wells, W. H. Trejo, P. A. Principe, K. Bush, N. H. Georgopapadakou, and R. B. Sykes. EM5400, a family of monobactam antibiotics produced by *Agrobacterium radiobacter*. I. Taxonomy, fermentation and biological properties. *J. Antibiot., 35*:295–299 (1982).
7. P. D. Singh, J. H. Johnson, P. C. Ward, J. S. Wells, W. H. Trejo, and R. B. Sykes. SQ 28,332, a new monobactam produced by a *Flexibacter* sp. Taxonomy, fermentation, structure determination and biological properties. *J. Antibiot., 34*:1245–1251 (1983).
8. R. Cooper, K. Bush, P. A. Principe, W. H. Trejo, J. S. Wells, and R. B. Sykes. Two new monobactam antibiotics produced by a *Flexibacter* sp. I. Taxonomy, fermentation, isolation and biological properties. *J. Antibiot., 34*:1252–1257 (1983).
9. R. B. Sykes, C. M. Cimarusti, D. P. Bonner, K. Bush, D. M. Floyd, N. H. Georgopapadakou, W. H. Koster, W. C. Liu, W. L. Parker, P. A. Principe, M. L. Rathnum, W. A. Slusarchyk, W. H. Trejo, and J. S. Wells. Monocyclic β-lactam antibiotics produced by bacteria. *Nature, 291*:489–491 (1981).
10. W. H. Koster, C. M. Cimarusti, and R. B. Sykes. Monobactams, in *Chemistry and Biology of β-Lactam Antibiotics,* Vol. 3 (R. B. Morin and M. Gorman, eds.), Academic, New York, 1982, pp. 339–375.
11. W. L. Parker, W. H. Koster, C. M. Cimarusti, D. M. Floyd, W. C. Liu, and M. L. Rathnum. SQ 26,180, a novel monobactam. II. Isolation, structure determination and synthesis. *J. Antibiot., 35*:189–195 (1982).

12. K. Bush, J. S. Freudenberger, and R. B. Sykes. Interaction of aztreonam and related monobactams with β-lactamases from gram negative bacteria. *Antimicrob. Agents Chemother., 22*:414–420 (1982).
13. R. B. Sykes, D. P. Bonner, K. Bush, N. H. Georgopapadakou, and J. S. Wells. Monobactams – Monocyclic β-lactam antibiotics produced by bacteria. *J. Antimicrob. Chemother. Suppl. E, 8*:1–16 (1981).
14. A. D. Russell. *In vitro* studies on SQ 26,776, a new monobactam antibiotic. *J. Antimicrob. Chemother. Suppl. E, 8*:81–88 (1981).
15. N. H. Georgopapadakou, S. A. Smith, and R. B. Sykes. Mode of action of aztreonam. *Antimicrob. Agents Chemother., 21*:950–956 (1982).
16. R. B. Sykes, D. P. Bonner, K. Bush, and N. H. Georgopapadakou. Aztreonam (SQ 26,776), a synthetic monobactam specifically active against aerobic gram negative bacteria. *Antimicrob. Agents Chemother., 21*:85–92 (1982).
17. M. H. Richmond and R. B. Sykes. The β-lactamases of gram-negative bacteria and their possible physiological role, in *Advances in Microbial Physiology,* Vol. 9 (A. H. Rose and D. W. Tempest, eds.), Academic, New York, 1973, pp. 31–88.
18. R. Labia, A. Morand, and A. Kazmierczak. Kinetic studies on the interactions of aztreonam with beta-lactamases, in *Program and Abstracts of the Twenty-Third Conference on Antimicrobial Agents and Chemotherapy,* American Society for Microbiology, Washington, D.C., 1983, p. 142.
19. R. L. Then and P. Angehrn. Trapping of nonhydrolysable cephalosporins by cephalosporinases in *Enterobacter cloacae* and *Pseudomonas aeruginosa* as a possible resistance mechanism. *Antimicrob. Agents Chemother., 21*: 711–717 (1982).
20. C. C. Sanders and W. E. Sanders. Emergence of resistance during therapy with the newer β-lactam antibiotics: Role of inducible β-lactamases and implications for the future. *Rev. Infect. Dis., 5*:639–648 (1983).
21. R. B. Sykes, D. P. Bonner, K. Bush, N. H. Georgopapadakou, and S. K. Tanaka. Interaction of aztreonam, ceftazidime, moxalactam and thienamycin with β-lactamase producing strains of *Enterobacter* sp., in *Program and Abstracts of the Twenty-Third Interscience Conference on Antimicrobial Agents and Chemotherapy,* American Society for Microbiology, Washington, D.C., 1983, p. 162.
22. A. Percival, E. Thomas, C. A. Hart, and P. Karayiannis. *In vitro* activity of monobactam SQ 26,776 against gram negative bacteria. *J. Antimicrob. Chemother. Suppl. E, 8*:49–55 (1981).
23. I. Phillips, A. King, K. Shannon, and C. Warren. SQ 26,776: *In vitro* antibacterial activity and susceptibility to β-lactamases. *J. Antimicrob. Chemother. Suppl. E, 8*:103–110 (1981).
24. J. Siegel, P. Ryan, D. April, and J. Christenson. Unusual β-lactamase stability of Ro 17-2301 (AMA-1080), a new monocyclic β-lactam, in *Program and Abstracts of the Twenty-Third Interscience Conference on Antimicrobial Agents and Chemotherapy,* American Society for Microbiology, Washington, D.C., 1983, p. 189.

25. R. B. Sykes and M. Matthew. The β-lactamases of gram negative bacteria and their role in resistance to β-lactam antibiotics. *J. Antimicrob. Chemother., 2*:115-157 (1976).
26. K. Bush and R. B. Sykes. Interaction of new β-lactams with β-lactamases and β-lactamase-producing gram negative rods, in *New β-Lactam Antibiotics: A Review from Chemistry to Clinical Efficacy of the New Cephalosporins*, Vol. 1 (H. Neu, ed.), College of Physicians of Philadelphia, Philadelphia, 1982, pp. 47-63.
27. H. Mikami, M. Ogashiwa, Y. Saino, M. Inoue, and S. Mitsuhashi. Comparative stability of newly introduced β-lactam antibiotics to renal dipeptidase. *Antimicrob. Agents Chemother., 22*:693-695 (1982).
28. R. B. Sykes and I. Phillips (eds.). Aztreonam, a synthetic monobactam. *J. Antimicrob. Chemother. Suppl. E, 8* (1981).
29. A. G. Paradelis, J. Tselentis, L. Crassaris, and C. Triantaphyllidis. *In vitro* activity of aztreonam (SQ 26,776), a new monobactam antibiotic. *Drugs Exp. Clin. Res., 9*:325-329 (1983).
30. H. Neu and P. Labthavikul. Antibacterial activity of a monocyclic β-lactam SQ 26,776. *J. Antimicrob. Chemother. Suppl. E, 8*:111-122 (1981).
31. R. Wise, J. M. Andrews, and J. Hancox. SQ 26,776, a novel β-lactam: An *in vitro* comparison with other antimicrobial agents. *J. Antimicrob. Chemother. Suppl. E, 8*:39-47 (1981).
32. D. A. Standberg, J. H. Jorgensen, and D. J. Drutz. Activities of aztreonam and new cephalosporins against infrequently isolated gram negative bacilli. *Antimicrob. Agents Chemother., 24*:282-286 (1983).
33. P. C. Appelbaum, J. Tamin, G. A. Pankuch, and R. C. Aber. Susceptibility of 324 nonfermentative gram negative rods to 6 cephalosporins and aztreonam. *Chemotherapy, 29*:337-344 (1983).
34. S. K. Tanaka, D. P. Bonner, and R. B. Sykes. *In vitro* activity of aztreonam in combination with aminoglycosides and other β-lactams against gram positive and gram negative bacteria, in *13th International Congress of Chemotherapy Proceedings* (K. H. Spitzy and K. Karrer, eds.), Egerman, Vienna, 1983, pp. 27/1-27/5.
35. S. K. Tanaka, R. A. Schwind, B. F. Minassian, L. Lalama, D. P. Bonner, and R. B. Sykes. Synergistic activity of aztreonam-aminoglycoside combinations against antibiotic resistant and susceptible aerobic gram negative bacilli, in *Program and Abstracts of the Twenty-Third Interscience Conference on Antimicrobial Agents and Chemotherapy*, American Society for Microbiology, Washington, D.C., 1983, p. 85.
36. S. J. Rehm, C. S. Hall, A. Alanis, A. J. Weinstein, and T. L. Gavan. *In vitro* effects of combinations of aztreonam with tobramycin, piperacillin and moxalactam against *Pseudomonas aeruginosa* and *Serratia marcescens*, in *Program and Abstracts of the Twenty-Third Interscience Conference on Antimicrobial Agents and Chemotherapy*, American Society for Microbiology, Washington, D.C., 1983, p. 84.
37. H. R. Stutman, R. K. Scribner, D. F. Welch, and M. I. Marks. Aztreonam: *In vitro* antimicrobial activity alone, and in combination against pediatric

pathogens, in *Program and Abstracts of the Twenty-Third Interscience Conference on Antimicrobial Agents and Chemotherapy,* American Society for Microbiology, Washington, D.C., 1983, p. 84.

38. J. A. Hindler, W. L. Hewitt, I. Ioka, R. L. Muench, and L. S. Young. *In vitro* activity of aztreonam in combination with amikacin and moxalactam, in *Program and Abstracts of the Twenty-Second Interscience Conference on Antimicrobial Agents and Chemotherapy,* American Society for Microbiology, Washington, D.C., 1982, p. 88.
39. D. P. Bonner, R. R. Whitney, C. O. Baughn, B. H. Miller, S. J. Olsen, and R. B. Sykes. *In vivo* properties of SQ 26,776, *J. Antimicrob. Chemother. Suppl. E., 8*:123-130 (1981).
40. D. P. Bonner, C. O. Baughn, S. J. Olsen, R. R. Whitney, B. H. Miller, and R. B. Sykes. SQ 26,776: Pharmacokinetics in experimental animals, in *Program and Abstracts of the Twenty-First Interscience Conference on Antimicrobial Agents and Chemotherapy,* American Society for Microbiology, Washington, D.C., 1981, Abstract 883.
41. M. Barza and M. McCue. Pharmacokinetics of aztreonam in rabbit eyes. *Antimicrob. Agents Chemother., 24*:468-473 (1983).
42. R. R. Whitncy, D. P. Bonnor, S. J. Olsen, B. H. Miller, and R. B. Sykes. Treatment of experimental *Haemophilus influenzae* meningitis with SQ 26,776, in *Program and Abstracts of the Twenty-First Interscience Conference on Antimicrobial Agents and Chemotherapy,* American Society for Microbiology, Washington, D.C., 1981, Abstract 888.
43. W. M. Scheld, J. P. Brodeur, J. C. Gratz, P. Foresman, and G. Rodeheaver. Evaluation of aztreonam in experimental bacterial meningitis and cerebritis. *Antimicrob. Agents Chemother., 24*:682-688 (1983).
44. W. Kobasa and D. Kaye. Aztreonam, cefoperazone, and gentamicin in the treatment of experimental *Enterobacter aerogenes* endocarditis in rabbits. *Antimicrob. Agents Chemother., 24*:321-324 (1983).
45. D. P. Bonner, P. B. Fernandes, and R. B. Sykes. Aztreonam in combination with other antibiotics as therapy for single and mixed bacterial infections in mice, in *13th International Congress of Chemotherapy Proceedings* (K. H. Spitzy and K. Karrer, eds.), Egerman, Vienna, 1983, Paper PS 4.1/3.14.
46. D. van der Waaij and W. Hofstra. Effect of aztreonam on the colonization resistance of the digestive tract, consequences for selective decontamination, in *Program and Abstracts of the Twenty-Second Interscience Congress on Antimicrobial Agents and Chemotherapy,* American Society for Microbiology, Washington, D.C., 1982, p. 89.
47. E. Magliulo, G. Piantieri, D. Tosre, and M. Crucianni. Activity of gentamicin, cefazolin and aztreonam in *Klebsiella pneumoniae* septicemia in neutropenic rats. *Chemotherapia, 2*:203-206 (1983).
48. R. H. Lusk, R. Fekety, and J. Silva. Clindamycin induced colitis in hamsters. *J. Infect. Dis., 137*:464-475 (1978).
49. J. R. Ebright, R. Fekety, J. Silva, and K. H. Wilson. Evaluation of eight cephalosporins in a hamster colitis model. *Antimicrob. Agents Chemother., 19*:980-986 (1981).

50. P. B. Fernandes, D. P. Bonner, and R. B. Sykes. Aztreonam: A new concept in β-lactam antibiotics. *Comprehens. Ther., 9*:21-26 (1983).
51. D. T. Sleyfer, N. H. Mulder, and H. G. DeVries-Hospers. Infection prevention in granulocytopenic patients by selective decontamination of the digestive tract. *Eur. J. Cancer, 16*:859-869 (1980).
52. F. R. Batchelor, J. M. Dewdney, R. D. Weston, and A. W. Wheeler. The immunogenicity of cephalosporin derivatives and their cross-reaction with penicillin. *Immunology, 10*:21-33 (1966).
53. M. W. Brandriss, J. W. Smith, and H. G. Steinman. Common antigenic determinants of penicillin G, cephalothin and 6-aminopenicillanic acid in rabbits. *J. Immunol., 94*:696-704 (1965).
54. B. B. Levine. Antigenicity and cross-reactivity of penicillins and cephalosporins. *J. Infect. Dis., 128*:S364-S366 (1973).
55. N. F. Adkinson, Jr., E. A. Swabb, and A. A. Sugerman. Immunology of the monobactam aztreonam. *Antimicrob. Agents Chemother., 25*:93-97 (1984).
56. E. A. Swabb and D. P. Bonner. Prediction of aztreonam pharmacokinetics in humans based on data from animals. *J. Pharmacokinet. Biopharm., 11*: 215-223 (1983).
57. E. A. Swabb, M. A. Leitz, F. G. Pilkiewicz, and A. A. Sugerman. Pharmacokinetics of the monobactam SQ 26,776 after single intravenous doses in healthy subjects. *J. Antimicrob. Chemother. Suppl. E, 8*:131-140 (1981).
58. E. A. Swabb, A. A. Sugerman, T. B. Platt, F. G. Pilkiewicz, and M. Frantz. Single-dose pharmacokinetics of the monobactam aztreonam (SQ 26,776) in healthy subjects. *Antimicrob. Agents Chemother., 21*:944-949 (1982).
59. E. A. Swabb, A. A. Sugerman, and M. Stern. Oral bioavailability of the monobactam aztreonam (SQ 26,776) in healthy subjects. *Antimicrob. Agents Chemother., 23*:548-550 (1983).
60. E. A. Swabb. Human pharmacology of aztreonam, in *13th International Congress of Chemotherapy Proceedings* (K. H. Spitzy and K. Karrer, eds.), Egerman, Vienna, 1983, pp. 15/23-15/29.
61. B. E. Scully, E. A. Swabb, and H. C. Neu. Pharmacology of aztreonam after intravenous infusion. *Antimicrob. Agents Chemother., 24*:18-22 (1983).
62. M. Nakashima, T. Uematsu, and M. Takashima. Pharmacokinetics and safety of aztreonam in Japanese healthy volunteers, in *13th International Congress of Chemotherapy Proceedings* (K. H. Spitzy and K. Karrer, eds.), Vienna, 1983.
63. R. Luthy, B. Joos, U. Borschberg, R. Putzi, and R. Wehrli. Comparative pharmacokinetics and bactericidal activity of aztreonam and moxalactam, in *13th International Congress of Chemotherapy Proceedings* (K. H. Spitzy and K. Karrer, eds.), Egerman, Vienna, 1983, pp. 27/13-27/17.
64. Y. van Laethem, J. Klastersky, D. Daneau, and A. van Houcke. Serum bactericidal activity and killing activity of aztreonam, cefoperazone, amikacin, aztreonam plus amikacin, and aztreonam plus cefoperazone against *Escherichia coli, Klebsiella pneumoniae, Serratia marcescens,* and *Pseudo-*

monas aeruginosa, in *Program and Abstracts of the Twenty-Third Interscience Conference on Antimicrobial Agents and Chemotherapy,* American Society for Microbiology, Washington, D.C., 1983, Abstract 369.

65. E. A. Swabb, A. A. Sugerman, and D. N. McKinstry. Multiple-dose pharmacokinetics of the monobactam azthreonam (SQ 26,776) in healthy subjects. *Antimicrob. Agents Chemother., 23*:125-132 (1983).
66. E. A. Swabb, S. M. Singhvi, M. A. Leitz, M. Frantz, and A. A. Sugerman. Metabolism and pharmacokinetics of aztreonam in healthy subjects. *Antimicrob. Agents Chemother., 24*:394-400 (1983).
67. M. Cole, M. D. Kenig, and V. A. Hewitt. Metabolism of penicillins to penicilloic acids and 6-aminopenicillanic acid in man and its significance in assessing penicillin absorption. *Antimicrob. Agents Chemother., 3*:463-468 (1973).
68. J. Birner. Determination of phenoxymethyl penicilloic acid and phenoxyethyl penicilloic acid in urine in the presence of the parent penicillins. *J. Pharm. Sci., 59*:757-760 (1970).
69. E. A. Swabb, A. A. Sugerman, M. Frantz, T. B. Platt, and M. Stern. Renal handling of the monobactam azthreonam in healthy subjects. *Clin. Pharmacol. Therap., 33*:609-614 (1983).
70. J. C. L. Mihindu, W. M. Scheld, N. D. Bolton, D. A. Spyker, E. A. Swabb, and W. K. Bolton. Pharmacokinetics of aztreonam in patients with various degrees of renal dysfunction. *Antimicrob. Agents Chemother., 24*:252-261 (1983).
71. A. Leroy, J. P. Fillastre, G. Humbert, and J. P. Morin. Pharmacokinetics of aztreonam (SQ 26,776) in subjects with normal and impaired renal function, in *Program and Abstracts of the Twenty-Third Interscience Conference on Antimicrobial Agents and Chemotherapy,* American Society for Microbiology, Washington, D.C., 1983, Abstract 405.
72. J. Gerig, N. D. Bolton, W. M. Scheld, E. A. Swabb, and W. K. Bolton. Pharmacokinetics of aztreonam in patients on chronic hemodialysis, in *13th International Congress of Chemotherapy Proceedings* (K. H. Spitzy and K. Karrer, eds.), Vienna, 1983: Part No. 94.
73. N. D. Bolton, J. Gerig, W. M. Scheld, E. A. Swabb, and W. K. Bolton. Pharmacokinetics of aztreonam in patients on chronic ambulatory peritoneal dialysis, in *13th International Congress of Chemotherapy Proceedings* (K. H. Spitzy and K. Karrer, eds.), Vienna, 1983: Part No. 94.
74. C. M. LacLeod, E. A. Bartley, J. A. Payne, and R. G. Devlin. Aztreonam handling in cirrhosis, in *13th International Congress of Chemotherapy Proceedings* (K. H. Spitzy and K. Karrer, eds.), Vienna, 1983, PS 4.1/3-16.
75. D. M. Janicke, R. F. Cafarell, S. W. Parker, M. A. Apicella, and W. J. Jusko. Pharmacokinetics of aztreonam in infected patients, in *13th International Congress of Chemotherapy Proceedings* (K. H. Spitzy and K. Karrer, eds.), Vienna, 1983, pp. 27/23-27/26.
76. F. R. Sattler, M. Schramm, and E. A. Swabb. Pharmacokinetics and safety of aztreonam and SQ 26,992 in renal failure, in *Program and Abstracts of the Twenty-Third Interscience Conference on Antimicrobial Agents and*

Chemotherapy, American Society for Microbiology, Washington, D.C., 1983, Abstract 408.

77. O. V. Martinez, J. U. Levi, and R. G. Devlin. Excretion of aztreonam in patients with biliary tract disease, in *Program and Abstracts of the Twenty-Third Interscience Conference on Antimicrobial Agents and Chemotherapy,* American Society for Microbiology, Washington, D.C., 1983, Abstract 412.
78. R. J. Duma, S. M. Smith, A. J. Berry, J. W. Baggert, E. A. Swabb, and T. B. Platt. Study of the pharmacology of aztreonam in human cerebrospinal fluid, in *13th International Congress of Chemotherapy Proceedings* (K. H. Spitzy and K. Karrer, eds.), Vienna, 1983, pp. 27/18-27/22.
79. R. Greenman, S. Arcey, G. Dickinson, J. Mokhbat, L. Sabbath, and L. Friedhoff. Penetration of aztreonam (SQ 26,776) into human cerebrospinal fluid in the presence of meningeal inflammation, in *Program and Abstracts of the Twenty-Third Interscience Conference on Antimicrobial Agents and Chemotherapy,* American Society for Microbiology, Washington, D.C., 1983, Abstract 410.
80. R. Wise, A. Dyas, A. Hegarty, and J. M. Andrews. Pharmacokinetics and tissue penetration of azthreonam. *Antimicrob. Agents Chemother., 22*: 969–971 (1982).
81. J. J. Schentag, P. B. Wels, G. W. Simons, E. A. Swabb, A. Vigano, D. P. Reitberg, I. L. Smith, D. J. Swanson, R. J. Lascola, P. Walczak, and T. Ryan. Abdominal fluid penetration of aztreonam versus tobramycin in patients with abdominal sepsis, in *13th International Congress of Chemotherapy Proceedings* (K. H. Spitzy and K. Karrer, eds.). Egerman, Vienna, 1983, pp. 27/27–27/28.
82. H. Giamarellou, G. Petrikkos, G. Koratzanis, E. Panopoulou, N. Galanakis, and G. K. Daikos. Pharmacokinetic studies with aztreonam, in *13th International Congress of Chemotherapy Proceedings* (K. H. Spitzy and K. Karrer, eds.), Egerman, Vienna, 1983.
83. A. J. Watson, R. L. Stout, D. K. Sood, and A. Whelton. The tissue stability and intrarenal distribution of aztreonam in health and disease, in *13th International Congress of Chemotherapy Proceedings* (K. H. Spitzy and K. Karrer, eds.), Egerman, Vienna, 1983.
84. G. P. Bodey, L. Jadeja, E. A. Swabb, R. Bolivar, and V. Fainstein. Pharmacokinetic studies of aztreonam, in *Program and Abstracts of the Twenty-Third Interscience Conference on Antimicrobial Agents and Chemotherapy,* American Society for Microbiology, Washington, D.C., 1983, Abstract 411.
85. D. van der Waaij, H. G. de Vries-Hospers, and G. W. Welling. Selective decontamination of the digestive tract with aztreonam; a study in ten human volunteers, in *13th International Congress of Chemotherapy Proceedings* (K. H. Spitzy and K. Karrer, eds.), Egerman, Vienna, 1983, pp. 15/–15/22.
86. A. Saxon, A. Hassner, E. A. Swabb, B. Wheeler, N. F. Adkinson, Jr. Lack of cross reactivity between the monobactam, aztreonam, and penicillin in penicillin-allergic subjects. *J. Infect. Dis., 149*:16–22 (1983).
87. H. R. Stutman, E. A. Swabb, T. B. Platt, and M. I. Marks. Pharmacokinetics and safety of aztreonam in pediatric patients, in *Program and Abstracts*

of the Twenty-Third Interscience Conference on Antimicrobial Agents and Chemotherapy, American Society for Microbiology, Washington, D.C., 1983, Abstract 408.
88. B. Scully and H. C. Neu. Aztreonam therapy of critically ill patients, in *13th International Congress of Chemotherapy Proceedings* (K. H. Spitzy and K. Karrer, eds.), Vienna, 1983, pp. 15/37–15/42.
89. J. A. Garcia-Rodriguez, M. Capurro, and J. Prieto. The use of aztreonam in high risk patients in the intensive care unit, in *13th International Congress of Chemotherapy Proceedings* (K. H. Spitzy and K. Karrer, eds.), Vienna, 1983, pp. 27/48–27/52.
90. R. N. Greenberg, P. Reilly, K. Luppen, and R. McMillian. Aztreonam treatment in gram-negative infections, in *13th International Congress of Chemotherapy Proceedings* (K. H. Spitzy and K. Karrer, eds.), Egerman, Vienna, 1983.
91. J. E. Mokhbat, M. M. Munyan, T. L. Pruett, and L. D. Sabath. Clinical evaluation of aztreonam in the treatment of serious gram-negative infections, in *13th International Congress of Chemotherapy Proceedings* (K. H. Spitzy and K. Karrer, eds.), Vienna, 1983.
92. H. Giamarellou, N. Galanakis, G. Koratzanis, K. Kanellakopoulou, M. El-Messidi, H. Kouroumalis, and G. K. Daikos. Aztreonam therapy in "difficult to treat" infections, in *13th International Congress of Chemotherapy Proceedings* (K. H. Spitzy and K. Karrer, eds.), Egerman, Vienna, 1983, pp. 27/53–27/56.
93. W. J. Mogabgab, B. Lutz, R. Thurm, T. Newman, and R. Beville. A comparison of aztreonam and spectinomycin for the treatment of gonorrhea, in *13th International Congress of Chemotherapy Proceedings* (K. H. Spitzy and K. Karrer, eds.), Egerman, Vienna, 1983.
94. L. K. Miller, P. L. Sanchez, S. W. Berg, S. B. J. Kerbs, and W. O. Harrison. Effectiveness of aztreonam, a new monobactam antibiotic, against penicillin-resistant gonococci. *J. Infect. Dis., 148*:612 (1983).
95. S. J. Childs, W. G. Wells, and S. Mirelman. Treatment of urinary tract infections with aztreonam: Comparison with cefamandole, in *13th International Congress of Chemotherapy Proceedings* (K. H. Spitzy and K. Karrer, eds.), Vienna, 1983.
96. F. R. Sattler, J. E. Moyer, M. Schramm, J. O. Lombard, and P. C. Applebaum. Aztreonam compared to gentamicin for therapy of serious and nosocomial urinary tract infections, in *13th International Congress of Chemotherapy Proceedings* (K. H. Spitzy and K. Karrer, eds.), Egerman, Vienna, 1983, pp. 27/57–27/60.
97. P. C. Frimodt-Moller and P. O. Madsen. A comparative study of aztreonam and tobramycin in treatment of complicated urinary tract infections, in *13th International Congress of Chemotherapy Proceedings* (K. H. Spitzy and K. Karrer, eds.), Egerman, Vienna, 1983, pp. 27/38–27/41.
98. J. Rodriguez and C. H. Ramirez-Ronda. Aztreonam vs. tobramycin: Report of a continuing randomized study in gram-negative lower respiratory tract

infections: The first 40 patients, in *13th International Congress of Chemotherapy Proceedings* (K. H. Spitzy and K. Karrer, eds.), Egerman, Vienna, 1983, pp. 15/31–15/36.

99. T. M. Nolen, H. L. Phillips, H. J. Hall, D. Smith, and M. Jackson. A comparison of aztreonam and tobramycin in the treatment of gram negative lower respiratory infections, in *13th International Congress of Chemotherapy Proceedings* (K. H. Spitzy and K. Karrer, eds.), Egerman, Vienna, 1983, pp. 27/33–27/37.

100. R. S. Gibbs and J. D. Blanco. A comparison of aztreonam plus clindamycin with gentamicin plus clindamycin in the treatment of endometritis after cesarean section, in *13th International Congress of Chemotherapy Proceedings* (K. H. Spitzy and K. Karrer, eds.), Egerman, Vienna, 1983, pp. 27/42–27/44.

Index

B

T